Sex and Gender

Current Clinical Concepts and Practices

edited by
Frederick L. Peterson, Jr., PsyD
Jill W. Bley, PhD

Professional Resource Press
Sarasota, FL

Published by Professional Resource Press
(An Imprint of Professional Resource Exchange, Inc.)
Post Office Box 3197
Sarasota, FL 34230-3197
www.prpress.com

Printed in the United States of America

Cover image by iStock/Getty Images.

Library of Congress Control Number: 2022940428
Paperback: ISBN: 978-1-56887-227-8
Electronic: ISBN: 978-1-56887-234-6

To Christina Colleen Muenchau-Peterson (1977 - 2021).
Thank you for the time and love we had with you.
We are better people for these gifts.
-Frederick Leo
-Frederick Dane
-Frederick Alexander

To my grandchildren
Carli, Dominic, Kara, Nina, and Reece
and all young people who might benefit from reading this book.
-Jill W. Bley

About the Editors

Frederick L. Peterson, Jr., PsyD, is a clinical psychologist and sexual health specialist who was the last Clinical Fellow trained at the famous Masters and Johnson Institute (which served as the historical basis for the SHOWTIME series, *Masters of Sex*). He worked extensively as a change agent within the Department of Veterans Affairs (as Director of Medical Education and the Director of a Psychology Internship) and as clinical faculty for the Psychology Residency with the 88th Medical Operations Readiness Squadron at Wright-Patterson Air Force Base Medical Center. He holds academic appointments at the Department of Specialty Medicine, Heritage College of Osteopathic Medicine, Ohio University as well as Wright State University's School of Medicine (Department of Psychiatry). He has co-authored or co-edited four books on sexual health topics, including the 2020 college textbook, *The Gender Revolution & New Sexual Health* (Cognella Academic Press). He has served as Behavioral Health Consultant for integrated medicine at the Samuel U. Rodgers Health Center and Kansas City University. He is currently a Behavioral Health Psychologist at Community Health Centers of Greater Dayton and conducts a private practice in Southwest Ohio which includes court evaluations. He promotes and researches programs for risk-reduction for at-risk mothers and family-centered perinatal interventions. Finally, he is an enthusiast for bee keeping, civil liberties, and democracy in Yellow Springs, Ohio. He can be contacted at Docpete2022@gmail.com or through his website: Docpeterson.com.

Jill W. Bley, PhD, is a clinical psychologist in private practice. She received her doctorate from the University of Cincinnati in 1980. She was affiliated with the University of Cincinnati as an adjunct associate professor of psychology from 1982 until 1994. During that time she taught sex therapy to graduate students in psychology. She was a founder of Women Helping Women/Rape Crisis Center in Cincinnati in 1972. Dr. Bley became certified as a sex therapist in 1982 and a sex therapy supervisor in 1988 by the American Association of Sex Educators, Counselors and Therapists (AASECT). She authored a column entitled "Speaking of Sex" which was published in the Cincinnati Downtowner newspaper from 1989 until 2002. She is a co-editor and author of *Innovations in Clinical Practice: Focus on Sexual Health* (2007) and co-author of *The Gender Revolution & New Sexual Health* (2020). She received the Distinguished Alumnae Award presented by the University of Cincinnati Alumni Association for Friends of Women's Studies. She can be reached at drjillbley@cinci.rr.com.

About the Contributors

Bran Allen is currently a Research Assistant who, in the past, has played many roles within the mental health field. They had yet to finish their undergraduate degree when they first started working on the research for the chapter on whether men use pornography as a maladaptive coping behavior. Bran has been accepted to the doctoral (PsyD) Clinical Psychology program at Nova Southeastern University and will start in the Fall of 2023. Email: brandi.allen3000@gmail.com.

Lorenzo E. Aranda, PsyD, earned his doctorate in Clinical Psychology from The Chicago School of Professional Psychology-Irvine in 2021. He also obtained a masters in Mental Health Counseling from the University of Phoenix in 2014. Licensed in the state of Virginia, he currently serves as an active duty Air Force Licensed Clinical Psychologist providing evidence-based mental health care to service members and veterans. He is a member of the American Psychological Association, the Society for Military Psychology, and the Society of Air Force Psychologists. His areas of interest include complex trauma, personality disorders, psychological assessment, Schema Therapy, and Art Therapy. He is currently in the process of pursuing a Post-Master's Art Therapy Certificate and Board Certification in Clinical Psychology. Email: lorenzoaranda@hotmail.com.

Meghan M. Bailey, MSW, is a Clinical Social Worker for the United States Air Force. She completed her Master's Degree from the University of Louisville in 2019 with a specialization in Mental Health and completed her Social Work Residency at Wright Patterson AFB in 2020. Email: Meghan.m.bailey3.mil@mail.mil.

Pamela Broderick, MD, has served 17 years in the United States Air Force as a Forensic Psychiatrist. Dr. Broderick was commissioned into the Air Force following graduation from the United States Air Force Academy, then continued her education at the University of Oklahoma College of Medicine. She completed her residency in Psychiatry at Wright Patterson Air Force Base and her Forensic Psychiatry Fellowship at the University of Cincinnati. Dr. Broderick is currently the David Grant Medical Center Mental Health Medical Director at Travis Air Force Base, California. Email: pamela.j.broderick2.mil@health.mil.

Dalton Bourke, MD, completed medical school at Creighton University, adult psychiatry residency at Wright State, and will finish child psychiatry fellowship as chief fellow at Boston Children's Hospital in 2023. He is an active duty Captain in the United States Air Force and will be working with service members and their families as an Air Force psychiatrist once his training is complete. He is passionate about medical education and helping guide the next generation of psychiatrists. Email: daltonbourke@creighton.edu.

Ronald Skip Carter, MA, MS, LPC, is a Sexual Health Educator and a licensed Mental Health Therapist who specializes in sexual health issues, relationships, and alternative relationships. Skip has researched CNM relationships for numerous years, is researching how CNM impacts the positive psychological aspects of one's primary relationship for his doctoral dissertation, and counsels numerous couples participating in the CNM lifestyle. Skip has a Bachelor's degree in Health & Physical Education, Master's degree in Human Sexuality Education, and Master's degree in Clinical Mental Health Counseling. Skip is currently earning a PhD in General Psychology. He has taught Human Sexuality for Sinclair Community College and the University of Dayton. Ronald can be reached at skip.carter68@gmail.com.

Belinda J. Chaffins, PsyD, is a licensed clinical psychologist specializing in sexual health, women's issues, and treatment of the LGBTQ+ population. She earned her doctoral degree from Wright State University School of Professional Psychology in Dayton, Ohio, and was the first in her family to graduate from college. A strong interest in sexual health led Dr. Chaffins to pursue training and certification through the American Association of Sexuality Educators, Counselors and Therapists (AASECT). Her psychology training and employment background include behavioral health in primary care, college counseling and community care centers, crisis, cognitive and disability evaluation, and private practice. She has over 19 years experience as a psychologist with 13 years of service at the Department of Veterans Affairs. Dr. Chaffins identifies as a cisgender woman as well as an ally and advocate for the LGBTQ+ population. Dr. Chaffins has a passion in helping clients learn accurate information about sexual health due to the culture of shame, myths, and silence that is still prevalent in America. Hence, she is experienced in providing presentations to client groups and training to psychology and psychiatry residents. Email: belinda@chaffins.net.

Emily Chriswell, PsyM, is a 4th year Clinical Psychology doctoral student at Wright State University, School of Professional Psychology. Her interests are in clinical sexuality and sex research as well as treatment of anxiety and trauma. Email: Chriswell.2@wright.edu.

Jennifer Cohen, PhD, was born and raised in China by her mother Jing An Li for the first 16 years of her life. She came to the U.S. and was adopted by her stepfather Benjamin S. Cohen. She earned her doctorate degree in Clinical Psychology from Alliant International University in Los Angeles. Her research and clinical experiences focused on immigration and culture, adolescents' sexuality, posttraumatic growth, various types of health and presurgical evaluations, as well as behavioral threat assessment and management. She worked for the Veteran's Health Administration in multiple states for many years before transitioning to her current role as a Social Scientist with the Department of Homeland Security. Email: jennifer_91106@yahoo.com.

Sarah Dalton, PhD, LPC, NCC, is a private practice therapist and Counselor Educator in Pittsburgh, Pennsylvania. She is certified by the American Association of Sexuality Educators, Counselors and Therapists (AASECT) as a sex therapist. Dr. Dalton also holds certifications as a Licensed Professional Counselor in Pennsylvania and a Nationally Certified Counselor. In addition to private practice, Dr. Dalton is a Counselor Educator in a CACREP-accredited master and doctoral program. She frequently presents on topics related to sexual health, the LGBTQ+ communities, and patient well-being to various community education and counseling groups. Email: sarah.dalton.phd@gmail.com.

Mischa Dansby, APRN, is an Advanced Practice Registered Nurse specializing in Women's Health and Mental Health. For 27 years she served in the United States Air Force integrating the best evidence from research, clinical expertise, and patient preference into the highest quality care. Mischa is committed to supporting women on their personal journey towards optimal wellness and healing. Email: mischadansby@gmail.com.

Ronald DeLong, PhD, PCC, CCCJS, completes evaluations and treatment of general psychological clients, as well as sexual and forensic offenders throughout the State of Ohio. His services to agencies and courts consist of sexual and criminal offender evaluations, risk assessments, evaluations for predator status, forensic evaluations, and individual and group treatment strategies. He also has consulted for the Internet Crimes Against Children Task Force (ICAC), particularly dealing with sex offender strategies, internet sex offenders, and child pornography. He is a Clinically Certified Criminal Justice Specialist, Certified Sex Offender Treatment Specialist, and Fellow with the Association for the Treatment of Sexual Abusers (ATSA). Dr. DeLong has more than 30 years of experience working with general psychological issues, sexual offenders, and other forensic populations. He has also completed advanced training with the Academy Group, Inc., (former FBI profilers and crime scene evaluators) regarding crime scene analysis and some profiling of sexually violent/deviant offenders. He is owner of the private practice Ronald L. DeLong, Ph.D. & Associates, LLC focusing on the evaluation and treatment of general populations, sexual offenders, and forensic clientele. Dr. DeLong is currently an adjunct professor at the University of Dayton, and previously at Ohio Northern University for 8 years and 2 years with Indiana Institute of Technology. He also has published articles regarding internet sex offenders. Email: drrondelong@gmail.com.

Jon Dembski, BA, earned his Bachelors in Psychology from Wright State University. Besides contributing as a co-author, he served as the first production assistant of this book project. He can be reached at jvdembski@gmail.com.

R. Brian Denton, PsyD, PhD, is a licensed psychologist in the state of Ohio. He is an Assistant Professor and Clinical Faculty at University Hospitals Department of Urology in Cleveland, OH. He is the former Co-Founder and Co-Director of the Ohio Center for Relationship & Sexual Health and the Sexuality Training Institute. Dr. Denton specializes in sexuality, sex therapy, and integrating mindfulness-based treatment approaches (specifically Acceptance and Commitment Therapy [ACT]) to a variety of mental health difficulties including sexual health and treatment. He has specialized in the treatment of trauma-based difficulties, mood disorders, and anxiety disorders. He further specializes in working with individuals who are experiencing difficulties in their sexual lives, including but not limited to sexual anxiety and functioning difficulties, problematic sexual behavior, sexual and gender identity, polyamory and consensual non-monogamy, and kink exploration and fetish behavior. Dr. Denton has published on mindfulness-based treatment approaches as the lead author of the chapter "Clinical Uses of Mindfulness" in *Innovations in Clinical Practice: Focus on Sexual Health*, and as third author of the book *Mindfulness in Clinical Practice*, a primer of mindfulness-based treatment approaches. He is an experienced and sought-after presenter on a wide range of topical areas, and in particular for training around mindfulness, ACT, inclusion/diversity, and sexuality. Dr. Denton may be contacted at rdenton@dentonpsychotherapy.com.

Danielle M. F. Dockery, is a Licensed Clinical Social Worker in the Air Force stationed at Eglin AFB. She is currently the Mental Health Officer in Charge and has experience in holding the Family Advocacy Officer and Social Work Residency Director position. She completed her Master's Degree from the University of West Florida in May 2015. Email: danielle.foley2002@gmail.com.

Nicole Feno, MS, is a therapist at Las Vegas Therapy. She received her Bachelor of Arts in Psychology and Master's from the Couple and Family Therapy Program from the University of Nevada, Las Vegas. Email: nicolefenomft@gmail.com.

Zane Ferguson, MEd, BCBA, COBA, is a Board Certified Ohio Behavior Analyst, Trained Sex Educator, Clinical Supervisor, and Social Groups Lead at an Applied Behavior Analysis clinic out of Centerville, Ohio. Zane received his Bachelor of Science in Psychology from Wright State University and his Master of Education from University of Cincinnati. Mr. Ferguson is currently working toward becoming a certified sex educator and obtaining a PhD in Behavioral Psychology. Email: zferguson2016@gmail.com.

Kimberly Fuller, PhD, LISW-S, CST, is an Assistant Professor in the School of Social Work at Cleveland State University. She researches the relationship experiences of LGBTQ+ adults and gaps in sex education for LGBTQ+ youth. She is the owner of Cleveland Sex & Intimacy Counseling located in Cleveland, Ohio. Email: kimberly.a.fuller@gmail.com.

Teja Fuller is a doctoral level student who is currently enrolled in a Health Psychology program at Kansas City University. Teja is originally from Alexander City, AL but currently calls Jacksonville, FL home. She and her co-author created the Sexual Health Word Cue Paradigm (pp. 585-588) as a means of capturing unconscious thoughts about sex and addressing any perceptions associated with those unsolicited thoughts. Email: teja.fuller@kansascity.edu.

Kayla Gallagher is a clinical psychology doctoral student at Kansas City University. She is currently in her third year of training and just received her Master's within the program. In 2020 she received a BS in Psychology with a minor in child advocacy from Oklahoma City University. Since 2021, Kayla has worked as a Registered Behavior Technician (RBT) providing applied behavioral analysis for children and adolescents on the autism spectrum. Her current areas of interest include providing diagnostic assessment and therapy to children and adolescents with developmental disabilities. Email: kayla.gallagher@kansascity.edu.

Ashley N. Grinonneau-Denton, PhD, CST, CSTS, is a Professional Clinical Counselor and a Marriage and Family Therapist, both with Supervisor designation, as well as being an AAMFT supervisor. She is a board-certified sex therapist (CST) and supervising sex therapist (CSTS) through the American Association of Sexuality Educators, Counselors and Therapists (AASECT). She is Co-Founder and Co-Director of the Ohio Center for Relationship & Sexual Health and the Sexuality Training Institute in University Heights, Ohio. Dr. Grinonneau-Denton specializes in working with individuals, relationship partners and couples, and sex therapy approaches. She treats a wide variety of sexual health concerns such as sexual dysfunction, paraphilias, sexual abuse and trauma, sexual fetishism, sexually compulsive behaviors across the lifespan, pelvic pain, infertility, sexual health in postpartum, infidelity, non-monogamy, kink, and gender identity exploration. Dr. Grinonneau-Denton has taught and presented workshops in the field of sexuality at the national level, and has served as an academic consultant and instructor. Dr. Grinonneau-Denton may be contacted at Dr.Ashley@ocrsh.org.

Capt. Keith Happawana, PhD, is an active duty Air Force staff psychologist at Joint Base Elmendorf-Richardson, Alaska. He is currently the Officer-In-Charge for the partial hospitalization program, manages an outpatient clinic caseload, and also maintains an active private practice. Other duties include leading after-hours emergency and hospital consultation services for high-risk patients and functioning as a base consultant for transgender care. Research interests include advancing data analysis techniques and the implementation of psychological and neuropsychological assessment in multidisciplinary settings, especially for military environments. Email: KeithHappawana@icloud.com.

Sallie N. Henderson is currently a Clinical Social Work Resident at Wright-Patterson AFB, Ohio. Having recently completed her Master's Degree in Social Work (LMSW), Sallie is in the process of completing the required postgraduate clinical hours necessary to obtain full licensure, title of Licensed Clinical Social Worker (LCSW). Email: sallie.henderson82@yahoo.com.

Eva M. Hernandez-Cuevas, MA, is a doctoral candidate for the clinical psychology program at Kansas City University (KCU). Eva is also a University of Puerto Rico at Rio Piedras (UPRRP) alumni, in which she obtained her BA in general psychology. Currently, Eva is a volunteer at Jennifer Fugate, PhD's ABLE (Affect Behavior Learning and Embodiment) Lab, focusing on embodied cognition. Eva has provided bilingual therapy and assessment services as a practicum student at Samuel U. Rodgers Health Center, a community health center in Kansas City and at Osawatomie State Hospital, an inpatient psychiatric hospital treating severe mental health and competency restoration. At KCU, Eva is president of the Latinx Student Association and aims to increase access to mental health services and decrease mental health stigma in underserved populations. Eva is currently working on her dissertation, which will research the use of embodied cognition in neurorehabilitation for neurological disorders. For more information on Eva's work, feel free to read her work on Research Gate (https://www.researchgate.net/profile/Eva-Hernandez-Cuevas) or LinkedIn (https://www.linkedin.com/in/eva-m-hernandez-cuevas-m-a-29857b141/). Email: eva.hernandez-cuevas@kansascity.edu.

Katherine M. Hertlein, PhD, is a Professor in the Couple and Family Therapy Program in the Department of Psychiatry and Behavioral Health at the University of Nevada, Las Vegas. She received her doctorate in marriage and family therapy from Virginia Tech. Dr. Hertlein may be contacted at katherine.hertlein@unlv.edu.

Jonathan Reid Hester, MD, is currently a staff psychiatrist on faculty at Wright State University. He practices clinical psychiatry in an outpatient mental health clinic as well as providing consultation/liaison services in emergency and inpatient medical settings. Additionally, he provides formal didactic instruction for the psychiatry residency at Wright State University Boonshoft School of Medicine. Dr. Hester maintains formal academic interests in consultation/liaison psychiatry, treatment of substance use disorders, and intellectual disability psychiatry. Email: Jonathan.Hester@wright.edu.

Carol M. Jaxson-Jager, EdD, LPC, CST, CCTP, CSOTP, is a Licensed Professional Counselor in the States of Ohio and Michigan, is a Certified Sex Therapist, has Certified Clinical Trauma Competency, is a Certified Sex Offender Treatment Professional, and has maintained a mental health treatment practice since returning to the United States from employment with the Department of Defense in Berlin, Germany at the US Army Base, Misawa, Japan AFB, and Lakenheath AFB in England. Her employment as a speech and hearing and language therapist, in a suburban Ohio school system, led her to the counseling profession. Dr. Jaxson-Jager, in addition to regular counseling duties working for the Department of Defense, has managed and conducted programs in Personal Growth and Development (sex education), Bullying, the school-wide national testing program involving faculty and administration protocols, and the Mentor program which allowed her to work closely with active duty military members and families. Dr. Jaxson-Jager's counseling practice, in Centerville, Ohio schedules patients who have distressing issues that interfere with their everyday functioning, at home, school, or in the workplace. Email: drcarol.jaxsonjager@gmail.com.

Racheal L. Johnson, DO, is a board certified adult psychiatrist. She completed her Psychiatric residency at Wright State University in Dayton, Ohio after graduating medical school from Lake Erie College of Osteopathic Medicine. She is the Mental Health Medical Director for the 81st Operational Medical Readiness Squadron at Keesler AFB, part of the clinical faculty for the Interservice Physician Assistant Program, and contributes to the education of Nurse Practitioners and Physician Assistants. She holds the appointment as Clinical Assistant Professor for Wright State University Psychiatric Residency where she is a psychotherapy educator. She enjoys reading, mindfulness, and yoga. Email: racheal.johnson81@gmail.com.

Stacy Leet, MSW, is a Licensed Clinical Social Worker serving active duty in the US Air Force. Stacy Completed her MSW degree at the University of Southern Maine and joined the Air Force in June of 2020. She completed a year-long intensive social work residency program at Wright Patterson AFB. Email: sa.leet29@gmail.com.

Gabriele Mamone is a doctoral level student who is currently enrolled in a Health Psychology program at Kansas City University. She is a native of Orlando, Florida. She and her co-author created the Sexual Health Word Cue Paradigm (pp. 585-588) as a means of capturing unconscious thoughts about sex and addressing any perceptions associated with those unsolicited thoughts. Email: gabriele.mamone@kansascity.edu.

Christopher Marett, MD, MPH, is an Associate Professor, Director of the Forensic Psychiatry Division, and Director of the Forensic Psychiatry Fellowship training program in the University of Cincinnati Department of Psychiatry. He earned a Bachelor of Science from the University of Notre Dame, a Doctor of Medicine and a Master of Public Health from the Ohio State University, and he completed general adult residency and forensic psychiatry fellowship training at the University of Cincinnati. Dr. Marett practices clinical psychiatry in the University of Cincinnati psychiatric emergency services and in consultation to correctional and public health clinics. He also conducts civil and criminal independent forensic psychiatric evaluations. Dr. Marett maintains academic interests in risk assessment, violent extremism, forensic psychiatry issues related to addiction and victimization, and psychiatric malpractice issues. He is the 2019 recipient of the Howard H. Sokolov Forensic Leadership Award which recognizes excellence in the Ohio forensic mental health system. Email: marettcr@ucmail.uc.edu.

David Miller is currently a Social Worker who works extensively with active-duty military members within the Department of Defense. Having completed his Master's Degree in Social Work from The University of Southern California, David is in the process of finalizing his clinical licensure within the state of Ohio, while also completing the Air Force Social Work Residency Program. Email: davidmiller311@gmail.com.

Timothy Pagano, PhD, serves as an active-duty officer and psychologist in the United States Air Force. Dr. Pagano received his Doctorate in Counseling Psychology from the University of North Dakota. Dr. Pagano has presented at local, state, national, and international conferences. His publications in national journals focused on military children and families and mental health practitioner training. Clinically, Dr. Pagano's work focuses on behavioral and cognitive therapies, posttraumatic stress, administration of a clinic's Alcohol and Drug Abuse Prevention and Treatment program, and the management of an intensive outpatient program. Email: pagano.tim@gmail.com.

Heidi Pence, BA, is currently working at a local hospital in Dayton, Ohio as an Obstetrician Technician where she helps with the deliveries of expectant mothers. Heidi graduated from Wright State University in 2020 with her Bachelor of Arts in Psychology. She was a member of the Wright State Chapter of PSI CHI, The International Honor Society in Psychology, and the Psychology Club. Heidi is currently working to further her education by going back to school for her Master's in Social Work so that she can continue with a career and focus in Family Centered Perinatal Education. When Heidi is not busy with working or going to school, she enjoys traveling, reading, and spending time with her husband and daughter. Email: hpence9215@gmail.com.

Molly Peters is currently working in specialized education and is pursuing a Master's degree at Wright State University. Molly has a strong interest in research on human sexuality, especially as it relates to trauma. Email: mollyr306@gmail.com.

Jouhaina Razzouk, PsyD, has lived and studied in West Africa, the Middle East, and the United States. She is the owner of her private practice Haven Psychotherapy as well as the clinical director at MedOptions, a behavioral health company. Dr. Razzouk's research and clinical experiences include multicultural therapy, gender issues, relationships, trauma, and geriatrics. She earned her doctorate degree in clinical psychology from Wright State University in 2004. E-mail: j_razzouk@yahoo.com.

Ruth A. Roa-Navarrete, PsyD, MS, received her Doctorate in Clinical Psychology from Nova Southeastern University. After some years of practice as a clinical psychologist, she completed a Postdoctoral Fellowship in Clinical Psychopharmacology at Alliant International University, San Francisco and Eglin Air Force Base, Florida. She currently works as one of a few uniformed pre-scribing psychologists in the Department of Defense, in addition to her role as Clinic Chief at Kunsan Mental Health Clinic in the Republic of Korea. She has previously functioned as Clinical Psychology Internship Training Director at Wright Patterson Air Force Base, Ohio, and Staff Psychologist, Chief of Mental Health Services, Director of Alcohol and Substance Abuse Services, and Mental Health Department Head at different clinics throughout the Air Force in deployed locations. Dr. Roa-Navarrete has also been a faculty member at Wright-Patterson's internship training program, adjunct faculty to Alliant's Masters in Psychopharmacology program, faculty of the Social Work Residency program at Eglin Air Force Base, and psychiatry, psychiatric nurse practitioner, physician assistant, and medical students' preceptor. Her interests include psychopharmacology, ethnic/cultural issues in psychological practice, military issues, and the assessment and treatment of chronic and severe mental illness. Email: ruth.a.roanavarrete.mil@mail.mil.

Richard Rothenberg, PsyD, is a clinical psychologist and a member of the Association for the Treatment and Prevention of Sexual Abuse (ATSA). He completed his doctorate in clinical psychology at Xavier University. Dr. Rothenberg is currently serving as a clinical faculty member at the University of Cincinnati in their College of Medicine, and primarily functions as a therapist in the outpatient department. He has experience treating children, adolescents, and adults who have been the victims of sexual abuse and individuals with a variety of different sexual behavioral problems. He also conducts risk assessments for both adolescents and adults with sexual behavior problems who are involved with the criminal justice system. He spends his free time running and playing golf. Email: rothenrd@ucmail.uc.edu.

Elizabeth Sarnoski, MD, graduated from the Virginia Commonwealth University Medical College of Virginia in 2007 and completed a general psychiatry residence at the University of Texas Health Science Center at San Antonio in June 2011. She completed a Forensic Psychiatry Fellowship at the University of Cincinnati College of Medicine in 2021. She has served as Associate Professor of Psychiatry at the Boonshoft School of Medicine at Wright State University. Email: sarnoskieg@gmail.com.

Patricia Schiml, PhD, is a Senior Lecturer and Research Professor at Wright State University in Dayton, Ohio. She received her Doctorate from the University of California at Davis in 1996 and completed an NIH-funded post-doctoral fellowship at the University of Virginia in 1999. Her current research interests focus on the impact of social relationships on physiology and behavior. Email: patricia.schiml@wright.edu.

Emma B. Schmidt, PhD, has a doctorate in Clinical Sexology, is a Professional Clinical Counselor, Supervisor, and Certified Sex Therapist through the American Association for Sex Educators, Counselors and Therapists (AASECT) as well as the American Board for Christian Sex Therapists (ABCST). She is the owner of Emma Schmidt and Associates, a therapy group practice (located in Ohio, Indiana, and Kentucky) that focuses on sex and relationship therapy. Dr. Schmidt received her Bachelor of Arts in Biblical Studies and Psychology as well as a Master of Arts in Counseling from Cincinnati Christian University. She received her doctorate from Modern Sex Therapy Institutes. Dr. Schmidt's research has focused on EMDR as a modality for General Pelvic Pain and Penetration Disorder. Email: Emma@Emma-Schmidt.com.

Kylie Sheaffer is a freelance lifestyle and consumer writer and editor based in Brooklyn, New York. Her writing has been showcased in numerous blogs and websites and has been featured with Rewire. She also edits sensual erotica and other works for independent authors. This is her debut in writing about human sexuality. Kylie is an avid learner and passionate humanitarian with a hope of encouraging widespread and accessible sex education for all. She is a graduate of the University of South Carolina. Email: ky.shea11@gmail.com.

Regina D. Shillinglaw, PhD, is a faculty member and the Associate Training Director in the Doctoral Psychology Internship Program at Wright Patterson Air Force Base. She is board certified in Behavioral and Cognitive Psychology. Special areas of interest include suicide and PTSD treatment. She completed her doctorate in Clinical Community Psychology from the University of South Carolina in 1998 after completing an Air Force internship at Wright Patterson Air Force Base Medical Center. She then served as an Active Duty Air Force psychologist from 1998 until 2001 serving as the Chief of Psychological Services at Robins Air Force Base. After working in private practice for several years treating adults with depression, anxiety, and trauma-related problems, she returned to working with the military population in 2008 at Wright Patterson Air Force Base. She can be reached at: drreginashillinglaw@yahoo.com.

John Skicki earned his doctorate in clinical psychology in 2021 after completing the Psychology Residency at the Medical Center of the Wright-Patterson U.S. Air Force Base in Fairborn, Ohio. He is currently an active duty Captain and Clinical Psychologist providing evidence-based mental health care to service members and veterans at the Cannon Air Force Base in Clovis, New Mexico. He can be reached at john.f.skicki2.mil@health.mil.

Judith Skillings, PsyD, is a clinical psychologist with a specialty in psychological evaluations. Although she is currently retired from full time work, she keeps herself busy writing and facilitating workshops aimed at raising awareness about various types of privilege and managing our privileges more responsibly. Email: judithskillings@yahoo.com.

Tori E. Stevens, PhD, LPCS, CST, is a psychologist and the co-owner/co-founder of the Oklahoma Sex & Relationship Institute. She specializes in working with non-monogamous clients in her practice and she provides training to other mental health clinicians regarding this population. Additionally, Dr. Stevens is an adjunct professor in the areas of counseling and sexuality, relationship and family therapy, conceptualization and diagnosis, and ethics. Email: toristevens412018@outlook.com.

Tonie Taft, APRN, MSN, FNP-C, PMHNP-BC, works as a Psychiatric Mental Health Nurse Practitioner (PMHNP) in the Emergency Department at UC Health University Hospital and is employed as an Instructor in the Psychiatry Department at The University of Colorado Denver Anschutz Medical Campus. Tonie received a Bachelor of Arts in Psychology from Bates College, a Bachelor of Science in Nursing at SUNY Binghamton University, a Masters of Arts in International Relations and Religion at Boston University, a Master of Science in Nursing with a specialty as a Family Nurse Practitioner (FNP) at The University of Virginia, and a postgraduate certificate as a PMHNP at The University of Cincinnati. She is a Veteran of the United States Navy Nurse Corps and a Returned Peace Corps Volunteer in Honduras. Tonie has lived and worked in Latin America, East Asia, and the United States and is dedicated to promoting the health and well-being of vulnerable individuals and communities in a variety of clinical settings. Email: tonietaft@gmail.com.

W. Spencer Vicente, MSW, received his Master's from the University of Southern California with a concentration in youth, children and families, and military social work. Captain Vicente is currently an Active Duty Clinical Social Worker in the United States Air Force and is currently stationed in Texas, where he oversees the base's Alcohol and Drug Abuse Prevention and Treatment program and Family Advocacy Program. Captain Vicente is a licensed independent social worker and recently received his Board Certified Diplomate status from the American Board of Clinical Social Work. Email: wsvicente7@gmail.com.

William "Bill" Wall, LICSW, BCD, is an AF retired Lt. Col. who has a 40-year professional career which spans 30 years of service in the Army and Air Force. He has provided a broad range of clinical services to military, first responders, Veterans, family members, organizations, and communities. He was deployed in 2004-2005 as a combat stress team commander for Operation Iraqi Freedom and learned first-hand the dynamics of combat stress and its relation to PTSD. During his Air Force career, he served in the Command Surgeon's office as the chief of behavioral health for Air Force Materiel Command at Wright-Patterson Air Force Base. Following his AF retirement, he was selected by the Dayton VA Medical Center as the program manager for the Freedom Center, the Dayton VA's OEF and OIF Post Deployment Clinic from 2007 to 2017, serving over 9,000 Veterans and their families. During this period, he was member of state level Ohio Cares/ISFAC committee serving the Ohio National Guard. From 2018 to 2020, he was employed as a senior clinical social worker at the Wright Patterson Medical Center, working in the outpatient mental health clinic and providing clinical supervision, medical board, and separation assessments. Currently in the community, he is in a private practice, with The Center for Life Stress and Psychotherapy, LLC and serves as an active mental health team member for the Southwest Ohio Critical Incident Stress Team. In 2019, he was selected for the Lifetime Achievement Award in Clinical Social Work by the State of Ohio's National Association of Social Workers. He continues to enjoy teaching as an Adjunct Instructor since 2016, at Wright State University, in the College of Health, Education, and Human Services. Email: williamandmary77@gmail.com.

Gerald R. Weeks, PhD, ABPP, is Professor Emeritus at the University of Nevada–Las Vegas. He has published 30 books in the areas of individual, couple, sex, and family therapy. Dr. Weeks is best known for his work in sex therapy having published nine books specifically on this topic. He is the founder of the Intersystem Approach to sex and couple therapy. Email: gerald.weeks@unlv.edu.

Julie Lynn Williams, PsyD, ABPP - I am: White, Upper SES, Dwarf, Hard of Hearing, Queer, cisgender woman, professor, psychologist, and a closet optimist who loves puppies. I do: work as a Professor of Psychology at WSU School of Professional Psychology and am Board Certified Rehabilitation Psychologist. I teach about the struggle for inclusion, equity, and justice as the source of marginalization and suffering in oppressed communities. I strive to speak my truths, own my privilege, and locate myself at the source of suffering. Finally, I encourage my students to find their personal/professional agency to become change agents. I hope for solidarity across and within groups and a space to celebrate the mind/body in all its forms. As a presenter and teacher who identifies as hard of hearing, Dwarf, cisgender woman, and queer, I believe the dialogue is a critical strategy to remove the social distance and promote collective healing and ultimately liberation. Email: julie.williams@wright.edu.

Sarah E. Wright, PsyD, CST/S, is a first-generation college student who earned her Doctorate in Clinical Psychology from the School of Professional Psychology at Wright State University in Dayton, Ohio, and is an AASECT-Certified Sex Therapist and Supervisor. She has worked clinically with issues of sexual health since 2005 in settings ranging from the Veterans Administration to various college counseling centers, and has engaged in extensive supervision training both domestically and internationally. Since 2007, Dr. Wright has worked full time in the counseling center at the University of South Carolina in Columbia. She maintains a small private practice and provides general supervision and sex therapy-focused supervision for those wanting to pursue certification. Dr. Wright is a highly accomplished and sought-after speaker and trainer to a range of professional and general audiences, providing workshops and interactive trainings on clinical sexual health, multicultural issues, LGBTQIAA2+ topics, the impact of stress and trauma on the brain, and more. Dr. Sarah has two published book chapters: "Live Supervision of Sex Therapy" which appears in *The Art of Sex Therapy Supervision* (edited by James C. Wadley and Richard Siegel) and "A Cultural Transformation Approach in the Group Treatment of Addiction" which appears in *Innovations in Clinical Practice: Focus on Group, Couples, and Family Therapy* (edited by Leon VandeCreek and Jeffery B. Allen). Her first book was published in 2020, entitled *Redefining Trauma: Understanding and Coping with a Cortisoaked Brain*. Dr. Wright can be reached through her website: www.DrSarahEWright.com.

Preface

The completion of any book project is challenging enough. Doing so during a pandemic which claimed over one million American lives was extraordinarily unbelievable. Certainly, the editors, contributors, and publisher whose work is contained within this text did not anticipate such challenges. However, adjustments were made as to contributions added and lost. While having very few topics of sexual health not included in this final production, this text represents a very comprehensive review of clinical sexuality. *Sex and Gender: Current Clinical Concepts and Practices* is just as the title describes.

The goal of this text is to assist all mental health professionals to gain the "3 C's": confidence, comfort, and competence in responding to a client's questions about sexual health. Hence, some of the "basics" are addressed in Section I to build some fundamental understanding and move forward toward the stated goal of the book, including the "why" it is important to even be concerned with the sexual health of our clients. A key emphasis of the contributors is to *supply clinically applicable information that is immediately employable in daily practice.* Hence, "how-to topics" such as how to conduct a sexual health assessment and utilize sexual health measurements are part of Section I. Also included are excellent coverage of the effects of aging and the effects on sexual expression from commonly used medications. Finally, the professional ethics of practicing sex therapy are detailed.

Section II contains chapters with exciting next-level thinking regarding sexual health, most of which you will not find from any other authors or sources. Fundamental concepts of sexuality are reexamined for expanded understanding of how to help clients use new models and learning tools toward the goals of increased enhanced satisfaction and self-acceptance. These new models explore the meaning of sexual identity, expression, and the neurochemistry of the "sexual brain." The concept and practice of mindfulness is applied to sexuality in innovative ways. Finally, the amazing model of the Sexual Tipping Point is tweaked a bit and applied in new ways for treating sexual compulsivity.

Section III addresses how to evaluate and treat the most common sexual concerns that present in most general mental health practices. Both men and women present with complaints about low sexual interest as well as sexual trauma (women more than men). Sexual health concerns more specific to women are covered in chapters related to arousal and orgasm as well as sexual pain issues. Sexual health concerns more specific to men are covered in chapters related to erection and ejaculatory problems.

Section IV addresses how to conduct therapy concerning sexual issues for clients within specific populations, such as LGBTQA, polyamorous, consensually non-monogamous, and individuals with varied abilities. Included in this section are chapters that address the needs of clients at different stages of life, including pregnant women, postpartum mothers, and individuals who identify as "seniors." Of special note is a chapter on the general considerations that all mental health professionals should attend to related to cultural sensitivity and competency.

Section V addresses the most damaging effects of sexual expression and topics which often create the most trepidation among mental health therapists – sexual compulsivity, pornography use, and sexual offending. These chapters assist mental health professionals to manage these presenting concerns, and to know when to refer clients to specialists, especially when legal issues are involved. Speaking of such, an excellent guide to consulting with the court system guides practitioners when they do have clients involved in the legal system. In the final chapter, an amazing point-of view story describes the intersectionality of a sex offender's identity and his search for personal redemption as he faces his mortality.

The concluding section (Section VI) is full of helpful therapist guides and patient handouts related to sexual health. Therapist guides include a sexual health history questionnaire and public domain instruments for evaluating erection function, women's sexual function, and satisfaction levels with multiple dimensions of sexuality. Therapist guides also include a word association measure for sexually related terms and a sample treatment plan for an older couple. The patient handouts include exercises on how to increase sensual pleasure, Kegel exercises, how to prevent relapse of unwanted sexual behaviors, mobile apps to augment psychotherapy, how to practice self-affirmations to enhance sexual health, and contemporary sexual myths.

The editors hope you enjoy both the broad scope of sexual health topics as well as the in-depth discussion (with specific examples) of how to assist your clients concerning the many challenges to intimacy that couples face. You are also encouraged to take advantage of the American Psychological Association sponsor-approved home study continuing education program that provides significant continuing education hours/credits.

Frederick L. Peterson, Jr.
Jill W. Bley

Table of Contents

SECTION III: SEXUAL DYSFUNCTIONS AND DISORDERS

SECTION IV: SEX THERAPY WITH SPECIAL POPULATIONS

SECTION V:
SEXUAL COMPULSIVITY AND SEX OFFENDING

SECTION VI:
THERAPIST GUIDES AND PATIENT HANDOUTS

Therapist Guides

Section I

Introduction to the Science and Art of Sex Therapy

1

Making Sexual Health a Part of Your Mental Health Practice

Jill W. Bley and Frederick L. Peterson, Jr.

"We as a nation must address the significant public health challenges regarding the sexual health of our citizens" (U. S. Surgeon General, 2001, p. i). In his call to action, U. S. Surgeon General Dr. Satcher was referring not only to the urgent need for health care professionals to respond to the AIDS epidemic, and other sexually transmitted diseases, but to the problems faced by teens as they attempt to cope with their sexuality, dissemination of accurate information about sexual health issues, intervention strategies, and a method of evaluating the effectiveness of those strategies. The report encouraged health care professionals to make programs available that promote awareness and prevention of sexual abuse and coercion. It also emphasized the fact that the health interests of adults and children can be hurt within relationships with sexual health problems. Therefore, when a mental health professional is entrusted with the task of helping couples and families, ignoring their sexual health may mean that those couples and families will not be able to achieve an optimal level of healthy functioning.

That call to action was published 21 years ago. Sadly, the call was largely ignored by the mental health community. The sexual health of our citizens continues to present a challenge. That call went out due to the evidence seen in studies which showed that there were an alarming number of people suffering from some type of sexual dysfunction. Bartlik and Goldberg (2000) found that "a significant proportion of women in all age groups are affected by female sexual arousal disorder" (p. 86). They estimated that one in five premenopausal women and two in five postmenopausal women suffer from this disorder. There has been no significant change in the prevalence of these disorders (Khajehei et al., 2015; McCabe et al., 2016). In fact, one study states, "Sexual problems are common in women of all ages. Despite their frequency and impact, female sexual dysfunctions are often unrecognized and untreated in clinical settings" (Parish et al., 2019, p. 842). Women who come to therapy with this problem are usually baffled about what might be causing it. Similarly, therapists untrained in sex therapy are sometimes baffled, not only about what might be the cause of the problem but what to do about it.

The National Health and Social Life Survey (a representative sample of men ages 18 to 59), which was conducted by Lauman et al. (1994), found that 10.4% of men reported being unable to achieve or maintain erection during the past year (complete erection dysfunction). Feldman et al. (1994) reported, in The Massachusetts Male Aging Study (a community-based survey of men between the ages of 40 and 70 years), that 52% of respondents had some degree of erectile difficulty. Again, the McCabe et al. (2016) study found that the incidence of sexual dysfunctions in males remains high. That study did, however, point out that there has been more research focused on male sexual dysfunctions than female sexual dysfunctions. It also indicated that erection disorders (ED) in men are being widely treated medically since the advent of and easy access to medications that treat the lack of blood flow to the penis, which is the cause of some ED problems.

Mental health professionals are trained to treat both the mind (psychological, emotional) and body (somatic) manifestations of mental health issues. However, very few have been trained to assess, much less treat, the sexual problems that may affect their clients' minds and bodies. The mental health professional who is not trained to deal with the sexual problems with which their clients may be struggling might, in some cases, be in danger of doing harm to them. There are so many sexual myths and so much sexual misinformation in our culture. Untrained mental health professionals are not immune to believing and endorsing those myths and misinformation and passing them on to their clients.

The Department of Labor Bureau of Labor Statistics (2021) reported data from 2016-2017 that there are over 577,000 licensed mental health professionals in the United States. Therefore, it is surprising that only about 2,200 mental health providers are trained and certified to provide sexuality therapy to their clients.

AMERICA'S SEXUAL HERITAGE AND THE PROBLEM OF SEXUAL MYTHS

A working definition of sexual health was published by the World Health Organization as follows:

> *. . . a state of physical, emotional, mental and social well-being in relation to sexuality; It is not merely the absence of disease, dysfunction or infirmity. Sexual health requires a positive and respectful approach to sexuality and sexual relationships, as well as the possibility of having pleasurable and safe sexual experiences, free of coercion, discrimination and violence. For sexual health to be attained and maintained, the sexual rights of all persons must be respected, protected and fulfilled.* (WHO, 2006)

Hence, sexual misinformation and myths interfere with the intellectual understanding of sexuality, which in turn can affect perceptions of self and others (emotional and social aspects) as well as increase the risk for disease transmission and even sexual violence (physical aspects).

Sexual myths plague most of our sexual lives. The Kinsey Institute of Indiana University surveyed nearly 2,000 American adults to document how sexually illiterate we are as a nation. Of the eighteen questions of basic sexual literacy, 55% of the sample failed to produce ten correct answers (earning an "F") and another 27% supplied 10 to 11 correct answers, earning a "D" (Reinisch & Beasley, 1990). Less than one in five people sampled passed the sexual literacy test with a "C" or better. This study and others (Lewis & Bor, 1994; Muller & Lief, 1976) demonstrate the great prevalence of sexual misinformation in our culture and why the former Surgeon General felt compelled to implore health care professionals of all disciplines to aid Americans in achieving sexual health (Satcher, 2001).

It is easy to understand how sexual myths get perpetuated, as an estimated three of every five people in the Kinsey sample reported that they got their sexual information from either friends (42%) or a partner (17%) (Reinisch & Beasley, 1990). Mental health professionals are not immune from sexual myths. Most of them grew up in homes where sex was a taboo topic, just like the vast majority of Americans. Therapists are encouraged to rid themselves of sexual myths and become more sexually literate in order to assist clients to correct sexual misinformation, which may adversely affect their self-esteem and sexual relationships as well as complicate treatment.

Related to the problem of sexual myths, American culture has been described as sex-negative and sexophrenic (Peterson, 1999). "Sexophrenia" is an informal (nondiagnostic) term that describes a state of dissonance resulting from conflict between feeling pleasure from sexual activity and the negative messages learned about the same behavior. Sex-negative messages may be so potent within a person's thinking that they generate significant anxiety and guilt, which then prevents the person from either engaging in the activity or blocks enjoyment of the activity. Throughout American history, negative stereotypes about any sexual behavior other than heterosexual intercourse have been described as unnatural, sinful, selfish, immoral, unhealthy, or a sign of insanity and disease. In short, the perpetuation of sexual myths serves as an obstacle to an individual achieving sexual health.

A common sexual myth is that people have to be young and beautiful to be attractive to others, and sexually happy. Many people reach a certain age and stop being sexually active, not because they don't have sexual feelings and thoughts but because they think they are not supposed to be sexual at their age. This particular sexual myth is derived from the primary directive of most world religions, to "go forth, be fruitful, and multiply." This clearly is a direct prescription for procreational sex. Over the millennia, most (far from all) societies have upheld the primary directive by creating traditions and incentives that support procreational sex while instituting significant social sanctions against all other forms of sexual expression. This historical process was accomplished in part by making all sexual variations (other than penile vaginal intercourse) either a crime or a medical condition, especially homosexuality, anal sex, and masturbation.

The sexual heritage of traditional American majority culture is based upon the Anglo-puritan values of people who were so sex-negative they used to cover the legs of furniture with cloth skirts for propriety's sake. During the 18th and 19th century, a doctrine of health came to be accepted within the American scientific-medical community, which perceived good health as the result of good food, good exercise, good rest (with plenty of fresh air), and good sex (defined as sexual abstinence with occasional practice for procreation). Restraint even from marital procreational sex was advised as a caution from excessive seminal loss and general overexcitement of the nervous system (Money, 1985).

Because every variety of non-procreational sex was not socially sanctioned, each variety was considered deviant and quite literately believed to lead to disease and disability, including insanity and death. Perhaps the most fascinating example of the medicalization of sexuality in our American heritage is masturbation, also known at various times in this country as self-abuse, self-vice, self-pollution, and the disease of onanism (mistakenly referring to the Old Testament character Onan). During most of American history, masturbation was considered a disease requiring medical treatment. Medical experts of the time believed masturbating would develop into a condition known as "sexual neuroanesthenia" and result in a host of dreaded symptoms, ranging from acne and isolating oneself for long periods in the bathroom to general weakness, blindness, or insanity (Masters et al., 1995; Robinson, 1934). Countless youth were needlessly tormented by such antimasturbation home remedies as tying hands to the bedposts at bedtime, "medical treatments" such as circumcision (for both girls and boys), and castration. Masturbation and seminal loss were so vilified that even involuntary nocturnal ejaculations (wet dreams) were medicalized as the disease of spermatorrhea (Robinson, 1934).

Did you know graham crackers and corn flakes were invented as "antimasturbation foods" to prevent the ill effects of the disease of masturbation? Famous health advocates such as Reverend Sylvester Graham and Dr. John Harvey Kellogg popularized the 19th century doctrine of good health (which excluded sex except for procreation). Rev. Graham was so closely associated with this doctrine of good health that some food products today still bear his name (Graham flour and crackers). Dr. Kellogg and his wife Ella originally invented baked flakes of corn as an antimasturbation food served to the patients of the Battle Creek Sanitarium (Money, 1985). The story of Dr. Kellogg was popularized in the movie *The Road to Wellville* (Abraham, 1994).

Through the first half of the 20th century, masturbation was still referred to as "self-abuse" in medical dictionaries (Gould, 1949; Robinson, 1934). The sexual revolution of the 1960s has helped to change the way we think about this activity. Masturbation is often referred to now as "self-pleasuring" and considered a healthy part of sexual expression. Modern concerns about masturbation are limited to teaching children discretion about the "where and when" of masturbation ("yes, it is normal son, but not at the dinner table"), parental overreaction and punitive responses ("You will go to hell for that!"), guilt resulting from the behavior ("this feels too good not to be bad"), and excessive masturbation that falls into the range of compulsive sexual behavior ("I can't seem to stop doing this even when I want to stop").

The sexual myth about masturbation has been addressed but is only one of a multitude of sexual myths that are far beyond the scope of this chapter. This myth was selected as an example of the devastating effects misinformation can have on the lives of everyday people. Sexual myths abound regarding children and adolescents, seniors, people living with disabilities, gay and lesbians, bisexual and transgendered individuals, and racial/ethnic groups, as well as pregnancy, contraception, abortion, and sexual performance (to name a few).

Sexual literacy is needed by mental health therapists to effectively respond to client needs for accurate sexual information and they are referred to other sources for further reading (Peterson, 1999; Reinisch & Beasley, 1990). Alternatively, readers may reference the patient handout "A Health Care Professional's Guide to Contemporary Sexual Myths" on pages 607-612 or *50 Great Myths of Human Sexuality* by Martha Kempner (2015). Healthcare professionals, especially mental health professionals, are encouraged to use this handout for the sexual health education of their clients.

THE ORIGINS OF SEX THERAPY

In the United States, the development of sex therapy over the last 40 years as an interdisciplinary profession has been built on a confluence of five significant historical influences: (a) The invention of the "talking cure" by Sigmund Freud and others, and the psychoanalytic movement within American psychiatry (Bankhart 1996); (b) the reaction against psychoanalysis and the development of behaviorism within American psychology (O'Donohue & Kitchener, 1999); (c) the application of empirical methods to the study of sexuality and establishment of a sexual science in America, beginning with the pioneers Robert Dickinson (Hartman & Fithian, 1997), Alfred Kinsey (Kinsey et al., 1948, 1953), and William Masters and Virginia Johnson (1966). The empirical methods in sexology led, ultimately, to the advent of oral contraceptives and oral sexual stimulants; (d) the sexual revolution of the 1960s that began the relaxation of the social conventions of previous decades, the questioning of the sexual repression of American women, the allowance of access to sexual literacy, and the creation of a consumer demand for sexual health services; and (e) the social conservatism of American academia that prevented established professions, such as medicine or psychology, from overcoming the effects of the taboos surrounding the teaching of sexuality (other than the traditional teaching in medical schools related to making sure the "plumbing" works, fertility issues, and birthing).

There are likely to be nearly as many perspectives on the history of sex therapy as there are different sexological practitioners and researchers. We believe there are many ways to conceive and outline this history, depending on which set of lenses you use to look back over the 20th century. To gain another perspective, other than our own, we consulted Dennis Sugrue, a past president of the American Association of Sex Educators, Counselors and Therapists (AASECT).

Confluent with the first three key historical influences the authors believe contributed to the advent of sex therapy as an interdisciplinary field, Dr. Sugrue summarizes the sex therapy field as developing over four distinct periods: orthodoxy predating sex therapy, the commercialization of sex therapy, the professionalization of sex therapy, and the postmodern period of sex therapy.

American psychiatry and the psychodynamic model was the gold standard of medical care in the first half of the century. All deviations from expectations of "normal sexuality" were viewed as pathology requiring psychoanalysis. Early behavioralists, such as Joseph Wolpe and Arnold Lazarus, countered this orthodoxy by quietly treating sexual dysfunctions and publishing results as sort of an "underground movement" toward sex therapy. The commercialization of sex therapy occurred with the enormous contributions of Masters and Johnson, who conducted pioneer sex research, applied their research results (as well as incorporated many of the behavioral strategies published by others), packaged it all into a "new sex therapy," and legitimized this treatment with the mantle of a medical context. This was the start of sex therapy proper.

The professionalization of sex therapy occurred over time with mental health professionals (Helen Singer Kaplan, Harold Lief, Joseph LoPiccolo, David Barlow, and others), unable to replicate the results of Masters and Johnson, synthesizing new approaches from their own research and clinical work to effectively resolve the sexual problems their patients presented. Related to the professionalization movement, new professional associations were developed to promote sexual literacy (SIECUS; Sexual Information and Education Council of the U.S.), the continuation of sound sex research (SSSS; Society for the Scientific Study of Sex), and the professional credentialing of sex therapy services (AASECT). The postmodern age of sex therapy which we are currently practicing has brought many changes to the field, including but not limited to more sophisticated and integrative approaches to treatment (cognitive-behavioral, pharmacologic, systemic), the medicalization of sex therapy with the Viagra revolution, the reconceptualization and emphasis on female sexuality, and the broadening of sex therapy to be responsive to cultural and technological shifts such as compulsive sexual behaviors, the cybersex phenomena, and transgenderism (D. Segrue, personal communication, December, 2005).

When we (Bley and Peterson) published our first book in 2007, we saw the field of sex therapy as having evolved through four overlapping stages of development, or "generations." Now, in 2022, we think that we should consider a Fifth Generation or stages of development in the field of sex therapy. A brief review of the development of the field will show that the First Generation of sex therapists began with Masters and Johnson's (1966) initial launching from the sexual science base (1966) into the clinical application of their work (1974). The Second Generation sex therapists, branching out from the medical model, took the basic behavioral exercises of Masters and Johnson and added their own unique variations. Helen Singer Kaplan laid the groundwork for the emergence of the Third Generation of sex therapists when she published *The New Sex Therapy* (1974) and introduced the concept of "desire" as the first phase of sexual response, calling her model the Tri-phasic nature of sexual response, which, she suggested, necessitated the combination of psychotherapy with the Masters and Johnson exercises. Therapists of this generation advocate a "systems" or "integrated" approach. The Fourth Generation of sex therapists must work within a post-Viagra context. Therefore, modern sex therapy reflects a dynamic tension between the medicalization of sexuality and the sexual health paradigm.

The Fifth Generation has embraced a new paradigm related to how we view gender issues as they relate to healthy sexuality. In our book *The Gender Revolution & New Sexual Health: Celebrating Unlimited Diversity of the Human Sexuality Hypercube* (2020), we endeavor to expand our understanding of sexual identity and sexual expression in a time when the LGBTQTA community is becoming increasingly visible and vocal. Mental Health professionals are beginning to understand that gender is not a binary, male-female, dimension. It is so much more than that.

THE FIRST GENERATION

Dr. Alfred Kinsey's groundbreaking "Kinsey reports" (Kinsey et al., 1948, 1953) brought about numerous changes in how Americans perceive sex, including greater understanding of the incredible diversity in sexual behaviors, most of which are now considered within a typical "normal" range of sexual activity (e.g., masturbation and homosexuality). Many of the contributions Kinsey made to sexual science and his effect on shifting sexual norms are reflected in the Fox film release of *Kinsey* (Mutrux, 2004).

While Alfred Kinsey opened the door to America's bedrooms, it was William Masters and Virginia Johnson who brought us to an understanding of what happens under the covers. Between 1954 and 1966, Masters and Johnson observed and measured over 10,000 orgasms under laboratory conditions (Masters et al., 1995). The publication of their 1966 volume marked the beginning of all contemporary sex therapy (Lieblum & Rosen, 2000). Their research led them to develop behavioral techniques that they labeled "Sensate Focus Exercises" (Masters & Johnson, 1974). Sensate focus exercises progress from nongenital pleasuring (Sensate Focus I) to intercourse pleasuring (Sensate Focus III) (see the patient handout on pp. 589-593 for a description of these exercises). David Schnarch has called this linear, "stage," or "phase" theory and practice of sex therapy the "first generation" approach (1991).

THE SECOND GENERATION

The basic Sensate Focus exercises provided the foundation for innovative techniques that were developed by a few sex therapists during the 1970s to help men and women who could not become aroused (lubrication in women and erection in men) and/or control their orgasm (inhibited or premature orgasm). Women and men learned to explore their bodies, relax, and overcome their fears, the antisex societal conditioning and performance anxieties that inhibited their sexual response.

We see this as the second generation of sex therapists because these clinicians took the behavioral techniques of Masters and Johnson and added a cognitive therapy approach that allowed the therapist to explore the cognitions of the patients that may have contributed to the sexual problem. They recognized that sexual problems were not all related to performance anxiety that would easily respond to sensate focus exercises alone. They worked to help patients understand how their culture, lack of accurate information about sex, religion, family attitudes, and values and morals impacted their sexual functioning. As mentioned previously, Sugrue refers to this development as the professionalization of sex therapy.

In 1976, Julia Heiman and Joseph LoPiccolo published their book, *Becoming Orgasmic: A Sexual and Personal Growth Program for Women.* The focus was on helping individual women achieve orgasm by self-pleasuring as well as with a partner. The program provided information that increased their sexual pleasure by expanding sexual literacy and practicing specific exercises designed to help women gradually and systematically achieve orgasm with or without a partner.

In 1978, Bernie Zilbergeld's book *Male Sexuality* described the myths and misinformation that have contributed to the creation of many sexual problems for men. He also used the basic Sensate Focus techniques to describe exercises that men can do, individually, to help them learn to focus their attention on pleasure instead of performance. He guided men in learning how to achieve erections and to prolong the pleasures of arousal so that they could overcome the embarrassments created by premature ejaculation. He included advice on how to transfer these new experiences to a sexual encounter with a partner. In 1992 he published a revised edition, *The New Male Sexuality*, which included information about all of the newest techniques for enhancing male sexuality, such as the use of new medications which cause vasodilation and enhance erections for men.

In 1980, Lonnie Barbach published an important book that outlined her approach to helping women achieve orgasm using a group sex therapy modality. She designed a 10-week group therapy program that provided a step-by-step model for therapists to follow that incorporated individual therapy and group therapy techniques in a group therapy approach. During the first few weeks of the group, the therapist focuses on each woman's individual issues. The therapist uses this information to design a treatment plan for each woman in the group. As the group progresses and each woman begins to do her own individualized homeplays (exercises), the dynamics inherent in group therapy begin to enhance the therapeutic interventions made by the therapist.

THE THIRD GENERATION

Masters and Johnson's conceptualization of the sexual response cycle was that sexual response progressed in phases that they called excitement, plateau, orgasm, and resolution. Helen Singer Kaplan's 1974 book pointed out that, although the plateau phase and the resolution phase may be useful to medical sexologists, they were of no practical use to sex therapists. The major thrust of her message was that sexual response is really "Triphasic" and that Masters and Johnson had failed to address the issue of sexual desire, probably because desire could not be measured in the laboratory. By highlighting the issue of desire phase disorders, Kaplan paved the way for the next generation of sex therapists. She forced them to recognize that sexual response in humans is much more than "stages" or "phases" of physical reactions to sexual stimuli. Understanding the many facets of sexual desire caused researchers, practitioners, and theorists to broaden their scope to take into consideration the context of the entire person including their body, mind, spirit, and relationship.

Research on arousal disorders in males and females indicates that problems with lubrication in females and erection in males are problems that are widespread and cause much distress in those who experience these disorders. However, low sexual desire is the most common presenting complaint of clients seen in sex therapy clinics (Pridal & LoPiccolo, 2000) and probably in private sex therapy practices. Sexual desire disorders are also the most difficult to understand and treat.

Desire phase dysfunctions are resistant to the standard Sensate Focus exercises because people who have no motivation to have sex have little to no motivation to do these exercises because the underlying causes of their avoidance of sex had not been explored. Therefore, the etiology was not understood and so could not be treated. The treatment, according to Kaplan, must be a combination of psychodynamic, sexual, marital, and behavioral therapies.

Kaplan was perhaps the first, but not the only, clinician to recognize that the basic Sensate Focus exercises did not provide the therapist with enough tools to be as effective as possible. LoPiccolo and Friedman (1988) proposed a "broad-spectrum" treatment which would incorporate cognitive, behavioral, and systemic treatment approaches. Pridal and LoPiccolo (2000) maintain that "therapy with low desire clients can be quite successful if the treatment addresses cognitive, affective, behavioral, and systemic elements" (p. 57). Insight and understanding comprise part of their treatment as well.

In 1991, David Schnarch published *Constructing the Sexual Crucible: An Integration of Sexual and Marital Therapy*. His work represented a milestone contribution to the understanding and treatment of sexual problems. Schnarch demonstrated the need for clinicians to make a radical change in their treatment approach by shifting their emphases from sensate-based behavioral-only treatment, analyzing resistances, individual pathology, and/or relational dysfunctions to developing a nonpathological model that focuses on the natural unfolding of human differences. He stressed the need for the development of a multisystem approach to sexual therapy that allows for differentiation as it manifests in sex and intimacy in committed relationships (Schnarch, 1991). Gerald Weeks (a contributor to this volume) also espouses the use of an integrated model of marital and sex therapy (Weeks, 2005).

These important developments in the understanding of the treatment of sexual problems within the context of a committed relationship make it clear that practitioners must increase and expand their knowledge, training, and expertise if they hope to alleviate the distresses endured by couples who experience sexual/relationship issues. They need to become expert in the theory and practice of treating every aspect of sexuality including sexual addiction, sexual abuse, and intimacy disorders, due to the profound impact of these issues on the sexuality of the individual and the sexual relationship of a couple.

THE FOURTH GENERATION

During the 1990s and 2000s, there has been a focus on medicalizing sex therapy. The Fourth Generation of sex therapists are practicing in a post-Viagra world where they must inform themselves, as never before, about the pros and cons of the use of medications to resolve sexual problems. Pharmacological interventions for a patient's sexual concerns has a long history going back to antiquity from the Ayurvedic medical texts in India (rock salt) and early philosophers in Greece (satyrion). In America, Robinson (1934) discussed using the bromides of strontium and sodium, small dosages of atropine, as well as "administrations of thyroid extract and adrenal substance" to treat the pseudodisease of masturbation (pp. 48-49). In the United States, as early as 1890, Robert Dickinson, M.D. began to collect sex histories from his patients. He published extensively on the sexual problems of women (Hartman & Fithian, 1997).

William Masters, also a physician, along with Virginia Johnson, studied the anatomy and physiology of human sexual response and published those results in 1966. Masters and Johnson's research led them to the conclusion that many sexual dysfunctions were psychogenic and should be treated with behavioral-type therapy (1974) which took the emphasis of treatment away from the medical model for approximately 30 years.

In the 1980s, a number of medical treatments became available for erection dysfunctions (ED). One, injections of vasodilators, such as papaverine, was touted as a new "cure" for impotence, because it allowed full tumescence independent of sexual desire (Broderick, 1998; Montague, 1998). Americans had to wait until 1995, however, for the first prescription drug for impotence, prostaglandin E1, which was prescribed as the self-injected medication Caverject (American Association of Clinical Endocrinologists [AACE], 1998). A year and many sore penises later, an intraurethral suppository form of alprostadil (another vasodilator) was approved and released under the commercial name of MUSE (Process of Care Panel of the University of Medicine and dentistry, New Jersey, 1998). The hormones testosterone and estrogen and yohimbine, which is a tree bark extract, have also been used as "sexual medicine." The surgical implantation of penile prostheses was also a fairly common medical answer to erectile dysfunctions. Those treatments, however, were isolated to the practice of urology.

When sildenafil citrate (Viagra) hit the market, medical practitioners were able to prescribe, for the first time in history, an oral medication that actually worked to "cure" many men with erectile dysfunction. The incredible impact of Viagra on American culture as a whole, and sex therapy specifically, is related to three key differences between Viagra and previous sexual medications. First, Viagra was made as an effective and easily-taken oral medication perfect for a "take-a-pill-to-fix-it" American culture. Second, the release of Viagra was accompanied by an effective and unparalleled marketing campaign that recruited the likes of presidential candidates sharing their impotence with the world. Finally, and most importantly, there was a historical shift that occurred with consumers moving away from urology and psychiatry specialists and going to primary care, family medicine, and general internists, who are now the primary professionals prescribing Viagra (Peterson, 2000).

Sex therapists began to worry that there would be a "medicalization" of all erectile problems and possibly of all sexual problems which would then cause most people with sexual issues to look for a pill that would fix them and would set the course for primary care physicians to be the only professionals involved in the evaluation and treatment of erection disorders. While recognizing that this has happened to some extent, it is important to acknowledge how beneficial these drugs have been to many men and to their relationships.

Since the advent of these drugs, drug companies have invested huge amounts of time and money in trying to develop medications that will cure/treat Female Sexual Dysfunction (FSD). Raymond Moynihan, a journalist, published an article in 2003 in which he reported on meetings between clinicians, researchers, and drug company representatives "to discuss the future direction of clinical trials" of medications intended to treat FSD. He stated that this was happening even though there is "widespread lack of agreement about the definition" of FSD. He wrote that Dr. Sandra Leiblum, Dr. John Bancroft, Dr. Leonore Tiefer, and Dr. Raymond Rosen, all leading sex therapists and researchers, have expressed concerns about the "medicalization" of sexuality. Dr. Tiefer was quoted as saying that pharmacological research may oversimplify sexual difficulties because it "promotes genital function as the centrepiece of sexuality and ignores everything else" (Moynihan, 2003, p. 46).

Some sex therapists have postulated that the major emphasis of the first-generation models of "phases" and "stages" had been too focused on what is known about male sexual response, and often overlooked much evidence that suggested that female sexual response may be very different (Stayton et al., 2005; Whipple, 2002). Belinda Chaffins has written an excellent chapter for this book titled "Female Sexual Arousal and Orgasm: Pleasures and Problems" (Chapter 13, see pp. 215-233) in which she discusses the importance of alternative models that may help therapists better understand these differences. Basson's (2003) Non-Linear Model postulates that responsive desire, which is the type of desire reported by most women, is probably more important than spontaneous desire because intimacy is the important component of responsive desire. The new emphasis on a team approach (comprised of sex therapist, medical doctor, and/or physical therapist) to the treatment of female genital pain disorders (as described in Chapter 14) is further evidence of the changes that are moving practitioners toward this Fourth Generation approach to sex therapy.

This historic shift necessitates that several demands be placed on modern mental health professionals as well as, and to a greater degree, sex therapists. First, mental health professionals need to be informed of product information related to the sexual psychopharmacology that is available to clients as well as the "clinical pathways" that have been developed to recommend sequential steps to assessment and treatment of some sexual concerns, such as erection dysfunction (Department of Veterans Affairs, 1999; Process of Care Panel of the University of Medicine and Dentistry, New Jersey, 1998).

Second, because of the direct marketing (as opposed to the traditional marketing to providers) and the availability of information about sexual medicines on the internet, mental health professionals and sex therapists find themselves working with consumers who are familiar with the product information of sexual medicines. These clients may be getting sexual medicine through medical providers or through the internet, bypassing their primary care and specialty providers. Often, clients are presenting for therapy after, not before, trying one or more of the sexual medicines, such as oral medications or hormonal treatments.

Third, mental health and sex therapy practitioners have a greater need to work with colleagues with prescription privileges, which involves professional relations with physicians, physician assistants, or nurse practitioners. Gone are the days that mental health therapists can work "in a bubble" with little interaction with the client's medical care providers. The need for therapists to work collaboratively with medical care providers is not a one-way street, however. Mental health professionals who develop sex therapy competence will find that many of the medical care providers need them as well. They need someone to whom to refer patients who present with sexual concerns, which the medical professional often does not know how to treat effectively. Very few medical care providers have training in sexual health issues beyond the basics they learned in medical school and what they learn from drug company representatives. Therefore, most medical professionals are eager to provide a referral for their patients with sexual concerns to a competent mental health provider with expertise in this area.

It is imperative that fourth-generation sex therapists ensure they work together to provide men and women, who come to them with sexual concerns, with the best information about what is available to help them. This could be Sensate Focus exercises, couples therapy, individual therapy, pharmacological therapy, understanding the cultural/historical/religious context of the problem, or some combination of these.

Raymond Rosen (2000) describes a new process-of-care algorithm for the evaluation and treatment of ED, whereby psychological and sex therapy treatments are strongly emphasized either in conjunction with or as an alternative to medical therapies. This new process could be applied to the treatment of all sexual dysfunctions and usher in the fourth generation of sex therapists, who, by necessity, must be well educated, trained, and knowledgeable about all aspects of sexuality, including mind, body, spirit, culture, religion, relationship, and pharmacology.

THE FIFTH GENERATION

In 1979, endocrinologist and sexologist Harry Benjamin advocated for professionals to learn how to treat transsexual clients. He published the original *Standards of Care* (SOC) manual in order to set guidelines for their treatment. His work evolved into the World Professional Association for Transgender Health (WPATH). WPATH states "Thus, transsexual, transgender, and gender nonconforming individuals are not inherently disordered" (2012, p. 6). There is a long history of clinicians and researchers attempting to study what were originally called sexual "deviations and perversions." In 1886, Richard von Kraft-Ebing published *Psychopathia Sexualis* in which he documented and classified those sexual "pathologies." What he wrote back then is difficult for our modern 21st century eyes to read, but back in the Victorian Era it was extremely "progressive." Another important early pioneer, Magnus Hirschfeld, was beaten and left for dead after he produced the first gay rights film *Different from the Others* in 1919 and advocated for transgender people (Wolff, 1986). Karl Ulrichs, a German lawyer advocated for gay rights and provided the first theoretical study of homosexuality in the 1860s and has been dubbed "the grandfather of the gay liberation" (Bullough, 1994).

In 1948, Alfred Kinsey published *Sexual Behavior of the Human Male* and shocked the nation when his study showed that in young unmarried men, 27.3% reported having had a homosexual experience. Among men aged 36 to 40, the reported incidence was 38.7%. Kinsey's research brought national attention to the reality of how many American men admit that they are homosexual or bisexual or have had at least one homosexual experience. All of these early clinicians and researchers have laid the groundwork for the Fifth Generation of sex therapists. The mental health providers who have been in charge of defining pathology and developing the "Bible" that we call the *Diagnostic and Statistical Manual of Mental Disorders* (*DSM*) have been forced to rethink how they classify gender issues. *DSM I* classified homosexuality as a paraphilia. *DSM II* called it a "sexual orientation disturbance." *DSM III* stated that only "Ego Dystonic" (those people who were very upset about being homosexual) homosexuals should be diagnosed, and then *DSM-III-R* dropped any reference to homosexuality as a disorder.

The United States has made major changes in terms of how sexual diversity is treated at governmental and legal levels. We have moved over the last 50 years from not allowing homosexuals and transsexual people to serve in the military, to "Don't Ask, Don't Tell," to allowing sexually diverse individuals to serve their country openly. We have moved from making homosexuality illegal behavior, to recognizing same-sex civil unions, to a Supreme Court ruling that has made same-sex marriages legal marriages with all of the rights bestowed on opposite sex marriages.

All over America, people are learning to ask what pronoun(s) they wish to be referred to as. Many include their preferred pronouns on the signature line of their emails or on their business cards.

Mental health professionals who have helped to lay the groundwork for this Fifth Generation must continue that work by helping to educate other health providers about the "unlimited diversity of the human sexuality hypercube" (Peterson et al., 2020).

What is the human sexuality hypercube? It is a more complex way to think about sexual identity and expression. It takes into account the fact that humans can and do make transitions across their lifespans in terms of their sexual identity, sex orientation, and sexual orientation. To name just one complexity about human sexuality, there are over five biological and three psychosocial variables to comprehensively classify sex status (Peterson et al., 2020).

These changes in how we understand sex, gender, and sex roles necessitate changes in how we educate our population, especially all providers of health services. We can then ensure that all people, no matter how they define who they are, receive quality health care no matter where they go to receive treatment. Therefore, it is crucial that those providing mental health services are on the front line of advocating for and practicing truly informed, well-educated counseling and therapy to these diverse populations.

HOW AND WHERE TO GET SEX THERAPIST/COUNSELOR TRAINING*

There are three paths to practicing as a sex therapist. First, get a graduate degree in human sexuality that has a clinical emphasis (e.g., clinical sexology). Second, develop a specialty in a particular area of sex therapy, such as "sex addictions." Finally, work on certification through the American Association of Sex Educators, Counselors and Therapists (AASECT).

Regarding the first option of getting an academic degree, here are some options:

- University of Michigan Sexual Health Certificate Program in Sex Therapy. This is offered part in-person and part online.
- Modern Sex Therapy Institute, Advanced Mental Health Training Institute, West Palm Beach, Florida. This is a blended program of online and in-person, or all online.
- Widmer University Center for Human Sexuality Studies, Chester, PA. This program is advertised as one of the only doctoral programs in human sexuality studies at a fully accredited university in the United States.
- Sexual Health Alliance. This program is an online program that can be accessed at www.sexualhealthalliance.com
- According to the website for The Society for the Scientific Study of Sexuality (SSSS; www.sexscience.org), 44 universities offer sex therapy training in their graduate programs but only the programs mentioned above grant academic degrees in human sexuality.

Deciding to treat sexual problems only within special populations, such as men with erection dysfunction, is a second option. It is possible for a psychotherapist who has not been trained as a sex therapist to successfully treat some individuals who present with a particular sexual concern. However, as the foregoing information in this chapter suggests, it is never advisable to try to treat any sexual problem with no training in the area whatsoever.

The third option, pursuing AASECT certification while continuing one's clinical practice, is recommended. Since this choice requires multiple steps, one should start by going to www.aasect.org/certification.cfm. The requirements for certification as a sex counselor are less stringent than those

*Portions of this section were adapted from F. Peterson and J. Bley (2005), "The Development of a Sexual Health Component To Your Mental Health Practice," in L. VandeCreek (Ed.) *Innovations in Clinical Practice: Focus on Health and Wellness,* © 2005, Professional Resource Press. Adapted with permission.

required for certification as a sex therapist. Requirements for sex counselor and sex therapist certification are summarized here, and details are listed on the AASECT site:

1. One must possess state certification or a license to practice in a related field, such as, psychology, social work, medicine, and so forth, and be a member of AASECT.
2. There is a requirement for sexuality education of 90 clock hours for a sex counselor and 90 clock hours for a sex therapist. For sex therapist certification, 75 hours can be eLearning. One can also earn Continuing Education Units by reading books on the topic, such as this one.
3. At least 60 hours of clinical training in one's field must be in sex counseling. There are seven core areas of training listed for certification at the sex therapist level.
4. A minimum of 10 clock hours of Attitudes/Values Training.
5. A minimum of 100 hours of supervised sex counseling for sex counselor certification and 300 hours of supervised sex therapy; 50 of those hours must be with an AASECT Certified Supervisor of Sex Therapy for sex therapy certification.

There are options for a combination of one-to-one and group supervision.

If you have a minimum of 10 years of post-degree clinical experience in sex therapy, you will need only 25 hours of supervision and an endorsement of clinical skill history by an AASECT Certified Sex Therapist. Table 1 below gives a summary of all of the information provided on the AASECT website for both sex therapists and sex counselors. For more complete information about both of these certifications, consult the AASECT website.

Table 1: American Association of Sex Educators, Counselors and Therapists Summary and Comparison of Certification Requirements

	Sex Counselor	Sex Therapist
Membership	Yes	Yes
Code of Ethics	Yes	Yes
Academic & Professional Experience	BA + 2 years (minimum)	MA + 2 yrs or Doc. + 1 year
General Eligibility	Clinical license not required	State license required
Human Sexuality Education	90 clock hours	90 clock hours
Sex Counseling or Sex Therapy Training	60 clock hours (30 general / 30 sex)	60 clock hours (30 general / 30 sex)
Sexual Attitudes & Values Training Experience	10 clock hours	10 clock hours
Clinical Training or Professional Experience	100 hours of supervised sex counseling	300 hours of supervised sex therapy
Application Process	$300 and documentation	$2000 and documentation

Although this third pathway for adding a sex therapy component to your practice is time consuming, it is the best because you will be able to feel very confident that you are well trained and have had the opportunity to use the expertise of a supervisor who will have had many years of experience in the field.

DISCUSSION

Psychiatrists and psychologists are generally perceived today as having expertise in human behavior and behavior change through psychopharmacology and psychotherapy, respectively. However, neither professional organization has divisions or programs within their organizations designed to help its members overcome their own feelings of discomfort in dealing with client concerns about sexuality or developing clinical skills to resolve these concerns. The same can be said for the national associations for counselors and social workers. The challenge to all mental health disciplines is to expand efforts and resources devoted to promoting sexual health and developing skills in clinical sexology.

This volume, as well as other excellent references on sexual health (most notably Leiblum & Rosen, 2000; Levine et al., 2003; and Peterson et al., 2020), is designed to assist mental health therapists of all disciplines to overcome obstacles, expand knowledge base, increase skills, and incorporate sexual health into their clinical practice.

REFERENCES

Abraham, M. (Executive Producer), & Parker, A. (Director). (1994). *The road to Wellville* [Film]. Columbia/Tristar Studios.

American Association of Clinical Endocrinologists (AACE). (1998). AACE clinical practice guidelines for the evaluation and treatment of male sexual dysfunction. *Endocrine Practice, 4*(4), 220-235.

American Association of Sex Educators, Counselors and Therapists. (2003). *Standards for certification.* Retrieved June 30, 2004 from http://www.aasect.org.

Bankhart, C. P. (1996). *Talking cures: A history of western and eastern psychotherapies.* Wadsworth.

Barbach, L. G. (1975*). For yourself: The fulfillment of female sexuality.* Doubleday.

Barbach, L. G. (1980). *Women discover orgasm: A therapist's guide to a new treatment approach.* Free Press.

Bartlik, B., & Goldberg, J. (2000). Female sexual arousal disorder. In S. Leiblum & R. Rosen (Eds.), *Principles and practice of sex therapy* (3rd ed., pp. 85-117). Guilford Press.

Basson, R. (2003). Women's difficulties with low sexual desire and sexual avoidance. In S. B. Levine, C. B. Risen, & S. E. Althof (Eds.), *Handbook of clinical sexuality for mental health professionals* (pp. 111-130). Brunner/Rutledge.

Broderich, G. (1998). Impotence and penile vascular testing: Who are these men and how do they evaluate the etiology and severity of their complaints? *Journal of Sex Education and Therapy, 23*(3), 197-206.

Bullough, V. (1994). *Science in the bedroom: A history of sex research.* Basic Books.

Bureau of Labor Statistics, U.S. Department of Labor. (2021). Occupational employment statistics. http://www.bls.gov/oes/

Department of Veterans Affairs. (1999). *The primary care management of erectile dysfunction* (published by the Pharmacy Benefits Management Strategic Healthcare Group and the Medical Advisory Panel, Publication No. 99-0014). U.S. Government Printing Office.

Feldman, H. E., Goldstein, I, Hatzichristov, D., Krane, R., & McKinlay, R. (1994). Impotence and its medical and psycho-social correlates: Results of the Massachusetts male aging study. *Journal of Urology, 151,* 54-61.

Gould, G. (1949). *Gould's pocket pronouncing medical dictionary of the principal words used in medicine and the collateral sciences* (11th ed.). P. Blakiston's Son & Co.

Hartman W., & Fithian, M. (1997). Sexual dysfunctions, counseling, and therapies: A brief history of American sexual therapy. In R. T. Francoeur (Ed.), *The international encyclopedia of sexuality* (Vol. I-III). Retrieved October 28, 2005, from http://www2.rz.hu-berlin.de/sexology/GESUND/ARCHIV/IES/USA15.HTM

Heiman, J., & LoPiccolo, J. (1976). *Becoming orgasmic: A sexual and personal growth program for women.* Prentice Hall.
Kaplan, H. S. (1974). *The new sex therapy*. Brunner/Mazel.
Kaplan, H. S. (1995). *The sexual desire disorders: Dysfunctional regulations of sexual motivation.* Brunner/Mazel.
Kempner, M. (2015). *50 great myths of human sexuality.* Wiley-Blackwell.
Khajehei, M., Doherty, M., & Tilley, P. J. (2015). An update on sexual function and dysfunction in women. *Archives of Women's Mental Health 18*(3), 423-433. https://doi: 10.1007/s00737-015-0535-y.
Kinsey, A., Pomeroy, W., & Martin, C. (1948). *Sexual behavior in the human male*. W. B. Saunders.
Kinsey, A., Pomeroy, W., Martin, C., & Gebhard, P. (1953). *Sexual behavior in the human female*. W. B. Saunders.
Krafft-Ebing, R. von (1900). *Psychopathia sexualis: With especial reference to antipathic sexual instinct.* [Only authorized English translation of the 10th German edition.] Keener.
Lauman, E., Gagnon, J., Michael, R., & Michaels, S. (1994). *The social organization of sexuality: Sexuality practices in the United States*. University of Chicago Press.
Leiblum, S. R., & Rosen, R. C. (Eds.). (2000). *Principles and practice of sex therapy* (3rd ed.). Guilford Press.
Levine, S. B., Risen, C. B., & Althof, S. E. (2003). *Handbook of clinical sexuality for mental health professionals*. Brunner-Routledge.
Lewis, S., & Bor, R. (1994). Nurses knowledge of and attitudes towards sexuality and the relationship of these with nursing practice. *Journal of Nursing, 20*(2), 251-259.
LoPiccolo, J., & Friedman, J. M. (1988). Broad-spectrum treatment of low sexual desire: Integration of cognitive, behavioral, and systemic therapy. In S. R. Leiblum & R. C. Rosen (Eds.), *Sexual desire disorders* (pp. 107-144). Guilford Press.
Masters, W. H., & Johnson, V. E. (1966). *Human sexual response*. Little, Brown.
Masters, W. H., & Johnson, V. E. (1974). *Human sexual inadequacy.* Little, Brown.
Masters, W. H., Johnson, V. E., & Kolodny, R. C. (1995). *Human sexuality* (5th ed.). HarperCollins College Publishers, Inc.
McCabe, M. P., Sharlip, I. D., Lewis, R., Atalla, E., Balon, R., Fisher, A. D., Laumann, E., Lee, S. W., & Segraves, R. T. (2016). Incidence and prevalence of sexual dysfunction in women and men: A consensus statement from the Fourth International Consultation on Sexual Medicine 2015. *The Journal of Sexual Medicine, 13*(2), 144-152. https://doi.org/10.1016/j.jsxm.2015.12.034
Money, J. (1985). *The destroying angel.* Prometheus Books.
Montague, D. (1998). Erectile dysfunction: The rational utilization of diagnostic testing. *Journal of Sex Education and Therapy, 23*(3), 194-196.
Moynihan, R. (2003). The making of a disease: Female sexual dysfunction. *British Medical Journal, 326,* 45-47. Retrieved October 26, 2005, from http://bmj.bmjjournals.com/cgi/content/full/326/7379/45.
Muller, W. R., & Lief, H. I. (1976). Masturbatory attitudes, knowledge, and experience: Data from the Sex Knowledge & Attitude Test (SKAT). *Archives of Sexual Behavior, 5*(5), 447-467.
Mutrux, G. (Producer), & Condon, B. (Director). (2004). *Kinsey* [Film]. Fox Studios.
O'Donohue, W., & Kitchener, R. (1999). *Handbook of behaviorism*. Academia Press.
Parish, S. J., Hahn, S. R., Goldstein, S. W., Giraldi, A., Kingsberg, S. A., Larkin, L., Minkin, J., Brown, V., Christiansen, K., Hartzell-Cushanick, R., Kelly-Jones, A., Rullo, J., Sadpvsky, R., & Faubion, S. S. (2019). The international society for the study of women's sexual health process of care for the identification of sexual concerns and problems in women. *Clinical Practice Guidelines, 94*(5), 842-856. https://doi.org/10.1016/j.mayocp.2019.01.009
Peterson, F. L., Jr. (1999, March 11). Sexual myths. *Impact Weekly,* pp. 10-13.
Peterson, F. L., Jr. (2000). The assessment and treatment of erection dysfunction. In L. VandeCreek & T. Jackson (Eds.), *Innovations in clinical practice: A source book* (Vol. 18, pp. 57-71). Professional Resource Press.
Peterson, F., & Bley, J. (2005). The development of a sexual health component to your mental health practice. In L. VandeCreek and J. B. Allen (Eds.), *Innovations in clinical practice: Focus on health and wellness* (pp. 159-168). Professional Resource Press.
Peterson, F., Bley J., & Frabotta, R. (2020). *The gender revolution & new sexual health: Celebrating unlimited diversity of the human sexuality hypercube.* Cognella Academic Publishing.
Pridal, C., & LoPiccolo, J. (2000). Multi-element treatment of desire disorders: Integration of cognitive, behavioral and systemic therapy. In S. Leiblum & R. Rosen (Eds.), *Principles and practice of sex therapy* (3rd ed., pp. 57-81). Guilford Press.
Process of Care Panel of the University of Medicine and Dentistry, New Jersey. (1998). *The process of care model for the evaluation and treatment of erection dysfunction.* [Unpublished manuscript used for continuing education, UMDNJ-Center for Continuing Education], Princeton, New Jersey.

Reinisch, J., & Beasley, R. (1990). What you must know to be sexually literated. *The Kinsey Institute new report on sex.* St. Martin's Press.

Robinson, W. J. (1934). *Sexual impotence* (19th ed.). Eugenics Publishing Company.

Rosen, R. (2000). Medical and Psychological Interventions for Erectile Dysfunction: Toward a combined treatment approach. In S. Leiblum & R. Rosen (Eds.), *Principles and practice of sex therapy* (3rd ed., pp. 276-304). Guilford Press.

Satcher, D. (2001). *The Surgeon General's call to action to promote sexual health and responsible sexual behavior.* Office of the Surgeon General (US). https://www.ncbi.nlm.nih.gov/books/NBK44216/

Schnarch, D. M. (1991). *Constructing the sexual crucible: An integration of sexual and marital therapy.* W.W. Norton & Company.

Society for the Scientific Study of Sexology. (2003). *Educational opportunities in human sexuality: A sourcebook.* Retrieved June 30, 2004 from www.sexscience.org.

Stayton, W., Angelo, M., & Kaye, S. (2005, May). Erotic stimulus pathways: The new sexual response cycle [presentation]. Annual conference of the American Association of Sex Educators, Counselors and Therapists, Portland, OR, United States.

U.S. Surgeon General. (2001). *The surgeon general's call to action to promote sexual health and responsible sexual behavior* (Office of the Surgeon General, Rockville, MD). U.S. Government Printing Office. https://www.ncbi.nlm.nih.gov/books/NBK44216/

Weeks, G. R. (2005). The emergence of a new paradigm in sex therapy: Integration. *Sexual and relationship therapy, 20*(1), 89-103.

Whipple, B. (2002). Women's sexual pleasure and satisfaction: A new view of female sexual function. *The Female Patient, 27,* 39-44.

Wolff, C. (1986). *Magnus Hirschfeld: A portrait of a pioneer in sexology.* Quartet Books.

World Health Organization. (2006). *Sexual and reproductive health. Human reproduction programme, research for impact.* www.who.int/reproductivehealth

World Professional Association for Transgender Health (WPATH). (2012). *Standards of care for the health of transsexual, transgender, and gender-nonconforming people* (7th ed). https://www.wpath.org/publications/soc

Zilbergeld, B. (1978). *Male sexuality*. Little, Brown.

Zilbergeld, B. (1992). *The new male sexuality* (rev. ed.). Bantam, .

2

How to Do a Great Sexual Health Assessment

R. Brian Denton and Ashley N. Grinonneau-Denton

While recorded human history has shown many examples of our societal struggles to integrate sexuality in a healthy manner, the 19th and 20th centuries have provided a great deal of change in regard to a sexual revolution and a focus on defining and working towards a greater understanding of sexual health and sexual functioning. In 2006 the World Health Organization revised their definition of Sexual Health as:

> … a state of physical, emotional, mental and social well-being in relation to sexuality; it is not merely the absence of disease, dysfunction or infirmity. Sexual health requires a positive and respectful approach to sexuality and sexual relationships, as well as the possibility of having pleasurable and safe sexual experiences, free of coercion, discrimination and violence. For sexual health to be attained and maintained, the sexual rights of all persons must be respected, protected and fulfilled. (WHO, 2006a) (https://www.who.int/health-topics/sexual-health#tab=tab_2)

Mental Health providers have a unique place in furthering this mission of integrating sexual health in the holistic treatment of clients. However, comprehensive training on human sexuality is not often a part of clinical training, and providers are often less comfortable addressing sexuality both in their initial intake interview process and throughout treatment (Cupit, 2010; Grinonneau-Denton, 2019). Mental health clinicians work with human psychological experience and behavior. In the clinical realm, they work to promote discussion and interventions that target a wide range of those experiences and behaviors from cognition, emotion, physiology, and many more topics that relate to psychological well-being. Sexuality is an innate aspect of human experience, therefore, the absence of training around sexual health for mental health clinicians is a serious oversight. This lack of training leads to negligence in asking about sexual functioning early in the therapy process. Clinicians may default to a stance of "If sexuality is a concern for clients, I wait for them to bring it up." The authors of this chapter hold that neglecting to ask these important questions in the initial clinical interview can give the implicit message that sexuality is not a welcome topic in the setting. This neglect may leave gaps in understanding the full picture of the client's functioning. Furthermore, this gives the message that sexuality should only be discussed if there is a problem. In contrast, by opening the conversation about sex and sexuality early in the therapy process, the mental health clinician normalizes sex as a natural human experience and this can help promote healthy messages around sex and sexuality. It also gives the client permission to feel at ease bringing up sexual issues in the therapy environment.

This of course may not be an easy ask! The fact is, many mental health clinicians grow up in the same environments that our clients do, where discussion about sexuality was absent, confusing, or downright negative. Talking about sex can bring up feelings of discomfort within the clinician, and therefore, can be a default stance to not ask. The goal of this chapter is to help mental health clinicians develop a framework and comfort in doing a good sexual health interview. This chapter will outline process considerations of completing a sexual health assessment, as well as some of the conceptual considerations for what to include in a comprehensive sexual health assessment. One important note the authors would like to make is that while the proposed information about how to conduct what may seem to be a singular activity, they assert that a good sexual health assessment (like any mental health assessment) is an ongoing process and may continue to build on itself as the therapy process continues. Furthermore, information obtained in the sexual health assessment can be referred to throughout therapy, making it a living document, updating it as necessary during the treatment process.

THE PROCESS OF CONDUCTING A SEXUAL HEALTH ASSESSMENT

Why is a Sexual Health Assessment Important?

Sexuality is an innate part of the human experience, yet many individuals do not voluntarily discuss their sexual health or bring up difficulties they are experiencing early on in treatment. This can be due to their own upbringing, societal messages around sexuality, and/or their fear of creating an embarrassing or awkward conversation with their provider. Practitioners are occasionally initially presented with specific questions about some aspect of sexual health, including topics such as safe sexual practice, sexual side effects of medication, changes in functioning, sexual identity, and so forth. Conducting a sexual history interview in these specific situations is clearly indicated. However, even when a client does not specifically identify sexuality as a reason for seeking treatment, conducting a sexual history interview is an overt statement by the practitioner that says, "Sexuality is important, and discussion about sexuality as a part of your treatment is welcome and invited." Many clinicians have been heard saying they will wait for their clients to bring up sexuality before "going there." Upon investigation, many are fearful that by bringing up the topic it will be "off-putting to the client" or may seem "too intrusive." Our experience has demonstrated that on many occasions, when presented in a confident and open manner, clients respond well and report feeling relieved that they can discuss those intimate parts of their life. In many instances when a client is coming in for a reason that is not directly related to sexuality, having them take the sexual health assessment may not be directly relevant to the situation at hand, but it makes clear the openness to discuss direct or indirect effects of their issues on sexuality. Hesitation in preemptively addressing sexuality has as much to do with the practitioner's discomfort as it does the client's. Practitioner comfort in addressing sexuality may be a key factor in addressing difficulties (Cupit, 2010; Grinonneau-Denton, 2019).

The authors' opinion is that conducting a health assessment can be done for every client that walks through your door. Some of the main reasons for this has to do with the previously asserted statement that sexuality is an innate human quality. Everyone has their own thoughts, feelings, or experiences related to sex, their sexual identity, and their gender identity, among other things related to sexuality. These experiences are integral to how they view themselves as individuals, within relationships, and within the greater context of society and the world.

Often, these experiences and social messages cause individuals to keep their sexual concerns under close guard. They may present to therapy talking about their feelings of anxiety and/or depression as a generality, for fear of bringing up their real concerns about their sexuality. While these concerns may show up on their own, giving the client permission to discuss sexuality early in the treatment process allows them to discuss these topics more quickly. Feelings of embarrassment about what is considered by many to be a "private topic" that is only discussed in the confines of their relationship (and often not even there!) can be a large barrier to discussing those concerns in treatment. The truth is that this barrier often exists for clinicians as well! Although many clinicians may not outwardly express discomfort, for most there has never been formal education and practice in discussing sexuality with clients in a clinical setting. The lack of education in various aspects of sexual health may lead to a lack of confidence in conducting a sexual health assessment. The clinician's comfort in asking questions pertaining to a client's sexual health is mitigated by their willingness and personal comfort around sexual discussion. Some authors (Grinonneau-Denton, 2019; Risen, 2007) note that practitioners have barriers to asking in-depth questions and may fall under the following (nonexhaustive) categories:

1. Not wanting to be perceived as prying into "irrelevant topics" if a client does not overtly present with sexual concerns.
2. Being personally uncomfortable with the subject of sexuality and sexual behavior.
3. Not feeling confident in their ability to respond to what is disclosed ("I won't know what to say").
4. Not wanting to accidentally offend or respond unfavorably to what is disclosed.
5. Fear of misperception about why questions about sexuality are being asked, which may lead to the client's belief that the therapist has a sexual interest in the client, and subsequently initiating an ethical investigation.
6. Discomfort in using sexual language and terminology, such as penis, vulva, vagina, and so forth.

One clear distinction to be made is that this assessment is not a disease-centric line of questioning meant specifically for diagnosis. The purpose is to understand the sexual lives and experiences of the client and develop an assessment of their sexual health. This shift in focus emphasizes a sex-positive approach and an introspection of the client's sexual life helping them work toward a healthy relationship with their sexuality. For many, this is a far cry from the models they received in sex education programs that focused solely on basic anatomy, function, pregnancy, and disease-prevention. From the onset of the initial sexual health assessment, we are modeling for our clients that there is a perspective that embraces sexuality as a vital component to overall physical, psychological, mental, and behavioral health. We want to know what is going right in their sexual lives as much as we want to screen for what is not going as well or creating difficulties. Questions that are created with this in mind will emphasize their relational and sexual strengths as well as their difficulties. More than simply a mechanical description of their sexuality and a focus on genital functioning, we want to know about their relational histories that include parental/caregiver models of expressing love and sexuality, early peer and dating relationships, familial and cultural messages they heard in their youth about how sexuality was to be viewed, and early sexual experiences. This detailed account can help us as clinicians understand the complexity of the messages and experiences that creates a person's sexual life, and how these relate to their sexuality in the world and in their relationships with others.

Why then does there seem to be a gap in questioning related to sexuality for many clinicians? Much of this may be attributed to the knowledge gap in training programs (Grinonneau-Denton, 2019) combined with the general attitudes about sexuality in the majority culture that makes discussing sexuality difficult for the clinician. We may hear things like, "I don't want to pry into such personal details," "I wait for the client to bring it up first so that I'm not pushing my own agenda," or more directly "Because I don't want to." We must reflect on the truth that those of us who work in the mental health field are products of the same (or similar) cultural attitudes as our clients, and while there tends to be an openness to emotional experience, there is often still an underlying conservatism about sexuality within the overarching mental health field. Furthermore, cursory discussions about sex can often give the impression of openness, but assessing the more intimate details of sexuality (such as the client's range of sexual expressions) can push the boundaries of the therapist's comfort level. When this occurs, the unspoken (yet palpable) anxiety of the mental health provider occupies a large space in the room and creates a barrier to the work we are all there to do. As stated previously, clinicians likely did not get much help in overcoming this barrier in their education and training. Human Sexuality generally, and Sex Therapy specifically, are often at best elective courses and at worst absent all together. This unfortunate gap in training and the resultant anxiety about addressing the topic in the therapy room can translate to our clients in a way that they feel further marginalized in their sexuality.

Clinicians are often embarrassed to admit how anxious they feel about actually saying out loud basic sexual terms such as "penis," "vagina," "clitoris," "masturbation," and "orgasm." This is often not because the words are unknown, but rather a sudden recognition of how infrequently we vocalize these words. The surge of anxiety and embarrassment can cause a tight feeling and possibly some avoidance. Nevertheless, if we are to fully address the scope of sexuality that our clients experience, it is up to us to go first (i.e., to say the words out loud so that the client can follow suit). To gain some confidence and competence in using sexual language, we must do our own exposure therapy of sorts. Saying the words that we know, asking about terms we do not know, and repeating this process setting to setting (so we become proficient in accessing that language in a natural manner) helps to overcome this hurdle.

Over time, our lexicon of expressive sexual language and commonly used slang terms will grow both technically and formally. Beyond the feeling of awkwardness in using sexual language, there are concerns that therapists have about the perception given to clients through their questioning and discussion. There is often a fear of being perceived as "nosy," "intrusive," and/or "voyeuristic." This fear can increase or decrease depending on a client's ease in sharing sexual information. If the client's difficulty increases, it can lead to more discomfort for the clinician to sit with the topic. If the client seems uncomfortable and/or unable to respond to a simple question, it is natural to want to avoid. However, a little persistence can pay off in many ways and is often the key to helping the client become more comfortable in their own approach to the topic. Consider the following example:

Therapist: We've been talking about the difficulty you and your fiancée are having in balancing the change in living arrangements and work schedule. How does that affect your sex life?

James: What do you mean? I'm not sure that it does (client looks visibly uncomfortable).

Therapist: What I mean is, that the different parts of our relationships do not exist in a vacuum. Day-to-day relationship conflicts can show up in the bedroom and in our sex lives.

James: That makes sense. To be honest, we really haven't been having sex very often. Not like we did when we lived in different places and when my job was less demanding. Most of the time we don't talk about it because it just ends up in a fight.

Therapist: Can you tell me a bit more about what the fight about sex is?

James: She wants me to be more sexual and feels like I don't find her attractive anymore. The truth is, I find her incredibly attractive, but I am just exhausted from a heavy workload and when we fight about things like the dishes it just kills my drive. I feel a bit like I'm less of a man because I'm not as interested as she thinks I should be.

At the start of this excerpt, James appears to feel a bit uncomfortable about the topic. The presenting difficulty is about the communication around household tasks and work/life balance in a new job and living situation. Sex has become a touchy topic in his relational life. He grew up in a home where sexuality was never a part of the conversation. If we took his response of "I'm not sure that it does" at face value, we could assume that either there were no problems or that there was no change in their sexual life. By expounding on the topic just a bit and giving permission to speak about it more, James is able to talk a bit more about the difficulties that have shown up.

When it comes to addressing therapist discomfort, we first need to acknowledge where the discomfort is coming. Perhaps your own upbringing was absent of direct communication and acknowledgment of sexuality. Maybe the client is presenting a topic or language with which you are unfamiliar. These issues can bring up discomfort or anxiety because you may feel your own resistance to the topic, you may have internalized biases regarding the topic, or you simply have little experience with the topic. Our own questions of competence or a feeling of "imposter syndrome" can show up during these occurrences. We may ask ourselves questions like: Am I going to seem knowledgeable about what my client is talking about? What if a patient sees that I am unfamiliar with what they are talking about and feels as though I can't be of any help? You have a choice to make in this instance. If you are unfamiliar with what someone is talking about, you can model curiosity for the person you are working with by asking questions to help illuminate what they are talking about.

Therapist: So, tell me what's been going on and why you are seeking therapy at this time.

Lars: Well, I'm having a bit of difficulty with my manhood.

Therapist: Okay, let's talk about that. I'm not sure specifically what you mean when you say "manhood." What does that mean to you?

Lars: You know Doc, my manhood . . . (client raises eyebrows).

Therapist: I have some ideas about what you might mean when you say that, but I want to make sure that I am hearing you correctly. Are you experiencing some difficulties with feelings of masculinity? Are there some difficulties with getting or keeping your erection? What specifically are you wanting help with?

Lars: Well, specifically I am having trouble keeping it up with my partner. He really wants me to penetrate him, but if I can't keep my erection that's just not going to happen.

In this example, the therapist had some ideas about what the client was wanting to discuss but wanted further clarification. By reflecting on the use of specific language and that "manhood" could imply a couple of different topics, it allowed the client to further express distinct details about what the problem was.

As touched upon briefly, all of us have sets of values and moral standards that we live by. These are constructed by our familial, cultural, religious, and other influential voices, as well as through our own individual experiences. At times, we may have internalized reactions to things that differ from those values. We run the risk of taking a strong judgmental stance or we may pathologize a difference of values or sexual expression. Clients are sensitive to these judgments because they may be coming to a professional to gain validation, to see if their desires or behaviors are "normal," or to see a model for a set of values and standards. Imposing our own value system onto others can induce feelings of shame or can shut down further communication. This is not to say that we cannot share our own beliefs, but we must be cautious in how we share them so we do not suggest that our personal values and beliefs are the "right ones." Consider the following example:

Gina: I am just so lonely. I started dating a new person 2 weeks ago and we had sex for the first time last week. The problem is, I am still occasionally sleeping with my ex-boyfriend and slept with him last night. Now I feel so terrible that I did that and feel like I have cheated on both of them even though there has been no discussion of being exclusive. I feel icky.

Therapist: Gina, this seems to be about self-respect. How can you expect that any new person you date will respect you if you have been so promiscuous and don't have enough self-respect to only give your body to people you are in a committed and loving relationship with?

This response is clearly based on the therapist's own belief system and is wrought with judgment and shame. Gina will most likely refrain from ever communicating about these difficulties and dilemmas in the future should she even return to therapy. Let us look at an alternative response:

Therapist: I can see that you are upset about these recent decisions. Can you tell me a bit about what feels icky to you?

This second response allows Gina to be more invited to express what she thinks and feels about the decisions she made, and may give us some insight into the messaging and values she holds onto or has been judged on in her life. From there, the therapist can begin to explore around what Gina truly wants in her relationships outside of the shame and judgment.

Therapist self-reflection and self-awareness are invaluable tools in any therapeutic setting, and dare we say, crucial in working in the realm of human sexuality. By deliberately and consciously working on yourself as a therapist, you can begin to address your own ambivalence or discomfort when talking about sexual matters and learn to respond with awareness. As with many things, if addressing these topics is a new skill for you, greater comfort comes with continued practice. Give yourself permission to lean into the discomfort and make continued attempts to bring sexuality into your therapeutic space. The implicit messages that never allow sexuality to come up can do more harm than bringing it up and having a stumble or two. Patience, persistence, and a sense of humor will help you get through the processes of gaining experience. Through persistence of holding that space, the initial awkwardness and even the initial pushbacks from clients will model sexuality as a positive and important aspect of your client's life. Acknowledge any of your own hesitancy and keep at it!

When Do You Conduct a Sexual Health Assessment?

There is no one answer to this question, and certainly no absence of opinions. The authors of this chapter run a practice that specifically addresses sexuality concerns. We include a sexual history questionnaire along with their initial intake forms so that the client can fill them out at their leisure and ahead of the first meeting. This gives us the chance to look through them prior to the meeting and sets the tone that sexuality is prioritized and will be a conversation in their treatment. For those clinicians who do not specifically focus on sexuality but are working to have a more sex positive and/or sex inclusive practice, including a sexual history questionnaire in the initial contact may not be the best approach. However, putting it off too long, indefinitely, or waiting until the client brings it up may inadvertently reinforce the idea that it is a taboo subject, and suddenly bringing the topic up further down the line of treatment may increase the discomfort. As discussed earlier, a common mistake is to believe that if the topic is important, the client will bring it up. However, because we believe that sexuality is a topic that is a particularly difficult topic for clients to broach, the therapist must assume responsibility for introducing it as an area of possible relevance. The most natural time to include this is during the phase of treatment which is focused on psychosocial and developmental history. If you do not have a secondary form that includes sexual history, you can integrate asking about sexuality as you explore developmental histories. For example, as one is inquiring about childhood history, significant events, issues, and problems, there can be a natural lead-in to inquiring about sexual matters as they relate to the topic areas. Examples of natural transitional questions could be as follows:

- We've been talking a lot about your romantic relationship(s) today. What is the sexual relationship between you and your partner(s)?
- I have asked you a lot of questions about your childhood and family of origin. How did you learn about sex while growing up, and what kinds of things did you learn about? How was love, affection, and sexuality modeled to you by the adults in your family?
- You have discussed experiencing a great deal of anxiety. How has your anxiety level affected your sex life?

The major advantage of including a sexual health assessment early on is that it gives the client explicit permission to speak of sexual issues at any time and highlights this area of functioning as important and a topic that you, the clinician, are willing to work on. But what if you are already working with a client and this is all new? No problem, it is never too late to bring sexuality into the mix. To aid in reducing any feelings of awkwardness, just simply address the lack of inclusion. By introducing the topic, you are giving recognition that it is a valid part of the dialogue. We do not want to assume that sexuality is not an important area just because the client has not mentioned it. We have countless examples of cases where the individual and/or couple has been in therapy previously and had never discussed sex with their therapist(s) even though it was a major part of the difficulty and/or dissatisfaction in their relationship.

- It came to my realization that, in our direct focus on the difficulties you brought in at the beginning of our work, I've neglected to ask you about your sexual life and the sexual relationship(s) you have with your partner(s). How do you think these difficulties have translated to the bedroom?

Who Needs a Sexual Health Assessment?

With the exception of a very short-term, narrow-in-focus, problem-focused therapy course, our belief is that every single client from preadolescence (and even earlier for some) through later adulthood can benefit from a sexual health assessment and the ability to have sexuality as a valid and approachable topic. For younger children, questions may be more general unless there is a specific sexual concern. However, more specific questions regarding sexual development and discussions about sexual topics can be addressed with the parents of younger children. This allows you as a provider to offer specific suggestions on raising sexually healthy youth. Many clinicians can feel apprehensive about bringing up the topic of sex with preadolescent clients. If this is you, we recommend reflecting on where this apprehension has its origins. Chances are, it causes some dissonance based on your own internalized messages about the appropriateness of the subject.

We also offer the reality that children have an ever-present exposure that implicitly contains sexuality, such as television programming, advertisements, and peer influence. In addition to this, the ability for youth to access sexual imagery and content has grown exponentially. This includes sexual messages, images and video content, and terminology, much of which they may find themselves confused about. Without a safe space to ask questions, they are left to figure it out on their own, or they may ask their peers who, like them, do not have a reference point regarding sexual health.

Realistically speaking, many preadolescent children may have already had sexual experiences, either wanted or unwanted, and may need a nonjudgmental space to help to understand those experiences. As discussed earlier and to further drive home this message, most youth sexual education programs are lacking in a comprehensive approach and focus predominantly on basic anatomy and function, and the prevention of sexually transmitted infections and pregnancy. Because of this, most youth have unanswered questions about contraception, safer sex practices, pregnancy, pleasure-focused sex, and the social-emotional and relational components of sexual health. If the awkwardness of direct questioning is met with some resistance from the youth, approaching the question with a "What are your friends doing?" or "What have friends told you about sex?" type of questioning may be a good initial segue to their experiences.

Another often neglected demographic is adults of advanced age. Therapists often do not or are reluctant to inquire about the sexual feelings and activities of the elderly. This, too, is wrought with internalized biases that are present in the fabric of culture. The emphasis on youth and subjective beauty creates a desexualization of aged adults. It can also bring up feelings of discomfort in thinking about older individuals involved in sexual encounters, and maybe even the countertransference of thinking of one's own parents' sex life, or fears of one's own! This bias may also affect older adults in their own comfort or embarrassment in admitting that they continue to have sexual feelings, fantasies, and/or behavior. If we spend a bit of time thinking about it, it seems silly to assume that there is an age limit to the need for physical affection, closeness, intimacy, and sexual gratification. One of my first clinical experiences in working with an aged population (20 some years ago and early in the career of the first author) taught me a lot about how disempowering those messages can be on people. The following dialogue with a client in her early 70s is a recounting of what was said in the initial assessment.

Therapist: Tell me a bit about your current sex life.
Cora: Oh honey, there is nothing to tell.
Therapist: When was the last time you were engaged in any sexual activity?
Cora: Well, I will have to think about that. My husband died about 8 years ago, but he had prostate cancer well before that which made having sex pretty much impossible for anything to happen. So, that was pretty much the end of that! So, I would say it has been at least 20 years. I don't know why anyone would be interested in hearing about an old lady's sex life.
Therapist: My belief is that sexuality can be an important part of people's lives throughout the lifespan. I imagine that there were a lot of feelings around that part of your life changing so drastically following your husband's cancer.
Cora: There was, but at the time there didn't seem like there was an option so I just pushed those notions away.
Therapist: How do you experience physical closeness in your life now, and do you still have sexual thoughts and desires?
Cora: Well, I do think about it from time to time, but never really considered it an option. Most of my physical closeness is with my grandchildren. That has been the case for a long time.

From this conversation, you can see where Cora felt that she did not have any option for engaging her sexual life following her husband's loss of erectile functioning. Chances are, they were both experiencing some grief over the loss of their sexual life but did not have any model for how to continue to engage that part of their relationship. Furthermore, without the ability to talk about this drastic change that occurred in their 50s, they handled it by avoiding the topic. By opening up this topic in her 70s, space was created to discuss her feelings and was likely the first acknowledgment of having continued sexual thoughts even years later.

The take-home message here is that other than the rare instance, a sexual health assessment should be included for all clients, and to not make any assumptions regarding the potential benefits of doing so no matter how young or how old a client may be.

How Do You Conduct a Great Sexual Health Assessment?

Doing a good Sexual Health Assessment is far beyond simply asking a series of questions and information gathering. To really make the sexual health assessment useful, we want to utilize our questions to help elicit the client's personal experience of sexuality more so than simply a series of answered questions. There are many ways to do this, from presenting specific questions in the form of a sexual timeline or by using open-ended questioning to encourage the individual to use their own language to answer the questions. For example, imagine how differently one could answer the following questions:

At what age did you first have sex?
vs.
Tell me a bit about your first sexual experience.

We want to emphasize that there is no "better question." While open-ended questions can possibly give you more information from the client's own words and experience, they can be a bit overwhelming for some clients who are not used to discussing these topics. For the more inhibited clients, more direct questioning like the first of the examples above may help to get at information. Be patient and allow for some space for the client to answer any inquiry. Additionally, note that you understand that this is not the typical conversation, and offer a patient and calm encouraging attitude.

Another way to really do a great job in conducting your sexual health assessment is to recognize that questions about sexuality do not have to be limited to sex. Expand the topic to the many arenas of life experience that are likely to give both implicit and explicit messages about the topic. Some examples may be as follows:

- Family/religious messages about sex during childhood
- Sexual experiences in childhood (wanted or unwanted)
- Discovery of sexual feelings/masturbation
- Timing and experience of puberty
- Body image
- Awareness of same-gender or other-gender attraction
- Dating history and experience
- First and subsequent partnered sexual experiences
- First and subsequent experiences of romance and love relationships
- Problems with any aspect of sexual functioning
- Contraception and safer sex practices
- Pregnancy/childbirth knowledge and/or history
- Chronic illness
- Gender and sexual identity/expression

Each of these pieces of information help to develop our understanding of the client's sexual story, and how we understand the current difficulties (if any) that are present.

Using the Sexual Health Assessment With Couples

So far, we have discussed the sexual history in the context of working with an individual client. For many presenting difficulties with sexuality, working with partnered systems is the treatment of choice. Additionally, partnered systems may present initially for therapy to focus on problems they are having in their relationship, sexuality related or otherwise. The predominant presentation often leads with interpersonal conflict. Even when the main presenting problem is not centered around a sexual difficulty, understanding how the partners relate to one another in their sexual lives adds further detail to the understanding of how their relationship(s) function. When we extend the sexual health assessment to working with partners, we need to consider a few more components.

The first consideration is the general cultural trend of partners not communicating well regarding their sexual relationship. The same lack of comfort in communication discussed earlier plays out in this partnered scenario, with the added assumption that a good relationship will naturally produce a good sex life. Couples who do not talk about sex will often feel uncomfortable at first, particularly when discussing their sex lives in front of another person.

Furthermore, partners can often have differing views about the quality and satisfaction found in their sexual relationship. It is an often-found phenomenon that out of love and a desire to avoid hurting the feelings of their partner(s), individuals will avoid confronting each other about what they find dissatisfying about the sex they are having. This allows for consideration of the vulnerability of discussing more intimate details about past sexual experiences, and sexual thoughts and fantasies that they may feel unwilling to share with their partner. For the therapist who is working with the partnered system there is a bit of a dance that happens here. The therapist must keep in mind that there needs to be some trust in exploring inner thoughts and fantasy without feeling as though they will be thrust into sharing them when they are not ready (if ever). Additionally, there may be information shared that is crucial to understanding the difficulties in the relationship. Therapists should consider how they might handle a situation where they are told information that may be crucial to a successful outcome of therapy (and if disclosed to the partner, may cause the client to feel exposed and vulnerable).

When conducting a sexual health assessment with a partnered system, the initial introduction of the topic with the partners creates the expectation that the topic of sex will be included for a full understanding of the partnership. Initial topics can be explored while all partners are present to get an overall sense as to what, if any, difficulties are present and to understand the strengths of the partners' sexual relationship. It is highly recommended by the authors that the therapist meets with each partner in an individual assessment session as a routine part of the initial assessment. From experience, the depth of information that is gathered from those individual assessment sessions allows the therapy to get to dynamics that may have taken much longer to get to had they not met individually.

Whether individual or in a partnered system, the inclusion of sexuality as a vital part of your client's story can lead to a richness in the therapy process that cannot be there without it. Furthermore, the skills you develop in working through your own hesitancies and discomfort in having sexual discussions with clients will develop your overall comfort in assessment inquiry.

THE COMPONENTS OF A SEXUAL HEALTH ASSESSMENT

In the first half of this chapter, we discussed the process of overcoming inhibitions, getting the conversation started, and taking a stance of open curiosity and nonjudgment. These process-oriented skills will certainly go a long way in helping clients to discuss their sexual lives. However, these interpersonal skills alone will not fill in the gaps that clients may have in their language, gaps in knowledge, and readiness to talk about details. For this reason, content-specific questions that reflect a comprehensive knowledge of the topic are used to guide the assessment process. One way that we can break down the term "sexuality" is into three components: Sexual Identity, Sexual Function, and Relational Meaning (Risen, 2007).

Sexual Identity

The first component of a sexual health assessment is sexual identity. Sexual identity is more than a single concept, with each underlying feature helping to create the understanding of one's sexual self. Major features of sexual identity include gender, sexual orientation, and sexual expression. Gender identity goes well beyond the biological sex assigned at birth (SAAB). The SAAB may be assigned male at birth (AMAB), assigned female at birth (AFAB), or intersex/different sexual development (DSD). These distinctions are based simply on different biological and physiological characteristics such as chromosomes, hormones, and reproductive organs. While historically there was a general practice to assign sex at birth for individuals with DSD, there have been strides made to not do so, and organizations like the Intersex Society of North America (ISNA) are advocating for change. Gender, on the other hand, is the felt sense of being that relates to aspects of femininity, masculinity, or absence of the binary distinction of those. Our understanding of gender has advanced in recent years, recognizing that gender does not exist solely in the binary. The World Health Organization defines Gender as "the characteristics of women, men, girls and boys that are socially constructed. This includes norms, behaviours and roles associated with being a woman, man, girl or boy, as well as relationships with each other. As a social construct, gender varies from society to society and can change over time" (WHO; 2021, para. 1). While the World Health Organization expands this gender definition, there continues to be an emphasis on the binary of men and women. We recommend that clinicians, who are less familiar with the range of gender, expand their knowledge through additional study. Gender identity interacts with biological sex but is not determined by genetics alone. Gender identity, therefore, refers to a person's deeply felt, internal, and individual experience of gender, which may or may not correspond to the person's physiology or SAAB. Also related to gender identity is gender expression. This too can vary outside of the traditional binary of what is "masculine" and "feminine."

Assessment of gender identity and associated features is important for a comprehensive sexual health assessment. Whether cisgender, transgender, intersex, gender queer, and so forth, there may be feelings associated with their gender identity and the expression of that gender. Assessment about body image, gender role expectancies, gendered relationship history, and social isolation and/or marginalization are all important.

Sexual orientation is another aspect of sexual identity. It includes the subjective sense of attraction as well as sexual behavior with a partner. Orientation points to the experience of sexual feelings and attraction to another person, and represents an enduring pattern of emotional, romantic, and/or sexual attractions. Sexual orientation can be seen as a continuum where individuals may have exclusive attraction to persons of a particular sex/gender or may be more expansive to include a multiplicity of sex/gender persons. While not an exhaustive list, persons may identify their orientation in many ways including heterosexual, homosexual (gay/lesbian), bisexual, pansexual, queer, and more. Sexual orientation should not be conflated to other components of biological sex, gender, social gender roles, and so forth. For example, a transfeminine woman who has sexual attraction and behavior with other women may identify as a lesbian.

Furthermore, sexual orientation is relational in nature in that we understand sexual orientation in context of an individual's relationship to another person. For example, a cisgender male person having sex with another cisgender male person does not alone relate to a specific sexual orientation. In assessing, the therapist/clinician needs to be careful to not equate behavior alone to orientation, but rather to assess the subjective and objective factors of identity in the person.

We can attend to these subjective and objective qualities in our sexual health assessment by asking questions that elicit answer to these two areas. For example, asking questions about the sex/gender of individuals that they have sexual encounters with in the past and currently will gauge the objective behavioral component of sexual behavior expression. Additionally, asking about the sexual fantasies of the individual to include sex/gender of the person or persons in their fantasy can get to some of the subjective experience of attraction. Further questions regarding the subjective feeling of attraction towards individuals of differing sex/gender, or even the absence of felt attraction found in asexuality, can give valuable information about the sexual orientation of your client.

We have discussed the need for awareness around our own internal biases throughout this chapter, and this area is another in which it is important to not make assumptions as to the sexual orientation of the person being interviewed due to our own internal hetero-normative assumptions and bias. Other objective data, such as marital status, gender expression, physical appearance, religious background, or any other characteristics should be understood as independent characteristics that do not point directly towards orientation. For this reason, asking orientation questions that allow for a variety of responses is important. Instead of "Who was your first girlfriend/boyfriend?," consider "Who was your first love interest?" or "Who was your first sexual partner?" Another follow-up question might be "Have you had interest in same (or other) sex/gender experiences?"

At times, your client may appear surprised or even angry and defensive that you have asked a question such as this. Be careful not to dismiss it too quickly. For many individuals, there has been little safety in discussing their interests, and by simply moving away from the topic you are furthering that avoidance. Rather, you can respond in a way that validates that humans have a range of interests, fantasies, and experiences. You also do not want to make assumptions about them without giving them a chance to tell you directly. Our goal here is to encourage clients to speak about all their sexual feelings and behaviors, including those that they may be reluctant to reveal. Consider the following dialogue:

Therapist: Thank you for your openness in telling me about that first sexual experience you had in high school with Laurie. What about same sex/same gender experiences or interest? Have you ever had attraction or sexual experiences with another man?

Joe: What?! Why would you ask me that? What do I look like?

Therapist: I ask because for many people, they may have experiences or fantasies that they keep hidden from others because they have never had a place to discuss those before. It isn't about what you look like, it's about what your personal feelings and experience is. I would hate to make assumptions about you based on the way you look instead of taking the time to really get to know the real you!

Notice here that the therapist responds to Joe in a manner that reflects permission to speak freely about his experiences without having to defend the question or to run away from it. A secondary benefit of this response is to let Joe know that the therapist is going to work to avoid biased assumptions in favor of really knowing who Joe is!

Sexual Functioning

The next component of a sexual health assessment is sexual functioning. This overarching category of sexual functioning involves honing in on specific sexual behavior and anatomical functioning. For those who specialize in working with sexuality, a common presenting problem is a complaint about a partner's difficulty in sexual functioning, especially differences in sexual desire and/or sexual frequency. The various types of presenting problems are beyond the scope of this chapter. For the purposes of this chapter, we want to have you consider the types of questions that you can ask to gain information for making a solid assessment of the functional components of sexuality, and for possible diagnosis.

While many present in our offices to address these difficulties, as we discussed earlier, clients/patients often lack the comfort or language to describe these difficulties in depth. To truly glean the depth of what the client's experience is, we need to ask questions that allow us to understand the functional aspects of desire and arousal, activities of stimulation, ejaculation, orgasm, and more. Because clients are often not used to having direct conversations, our comfort in asking specific detailed questions is important in gathering that information, as well as to put the client at ease by trusting the professionalism of the questioning. For a direct assessment, sexual functioning can be broken down into three separate but related components: desire, arousal, and orgasm.

Sexual desire is a topic that can be discussed in a chapter of its own, with many models to consider in how sexual desire is experienced. Most models have components of internally derived feelings of desire, as well as reference to external elements that influence responsive desire. We consider in our assessment that sexual desire has interactive components of biological urge (often referred to as "sex drive" or "libido"), a cognitive desire to engage in sexual behavior, and an emotional willingness to respond to a sexual experience. Some models of desire focus more on biological drive, and others expand out and recognize that the influence of those other factors weigh heavily on desire.

Dual process models, such as the Sexual Tipping Point (STP) model (Perelman, 2009), identify that desire and sexual response can be influenced by both "Excitation" and "Inhibition" factors of two categories labeled M (Mental) and P (Physical). These mental and physical factors are bridged together by an A (And), to signify an understanding that the mental and physical become progressively more permeable with greater understanding of how thoughts become translated into biological response components. The Mental category include, but are not limited to, factors related to cognition, emotion, social/interpersonal, and culture. The Physical category include, but is not limited to, factors related to anatomy, genetics, endocrinology, drugs, disease, surgery, and environment. The STP model is a valuable aid to client sexual health literacy and is described in-depth in a later chapter.

Another model, proposed by Rosemary Basson (2000), discusses the need for a nonlinear model of sexual desire, particular as related to cisgender female desire. She proposed a circular model of desire that includes more of the receptive qualities of desire and arousal. Within this model, we see the possibility of internal and spontaneous arousal (biological urge) interacting with willingness and emotional satisfaction, external sexual stimuli, and arousability. Like Perelman's STP model, these factors interact to increase or decrease the possibility of desire occurring (Basson, 2000).

As suggested by these models, sexual desire is complex, and we cannot understand how desire functions for an individual (or partnered systems) through a single question. To capture the full picture of how desire is experienced, we must ask several questions that give us data on many of the factors discussed in the illustrated models. We may ask questions such as the following:

1. How often do you feel like having sex?
2. How often would you have sex if you could?
3. Do you initiate sex with your partner(s)?
4. How do you feel when your partner(s) initiates sex?
5. What makes you want to have sex? What are your "turn ons?"
6. What gets in the way of your wanting to have sex? What are your "turn offs?"

Sexual arousal is closely related to desire and refers to the active change in energy that stimulates the body into sexual excitement. Sexual arousal can be in response to physical touch or sensation or could be initiated by internal thoughts and fantasies. In older models, such as the Masters and Johnson linear model of sexual response (Masters & Johnson, 1970), arousal follows desire. However, this is not always the case. Sexual arousal can most certainly happen prior to desire, and for some can be the initial responsive ingredient that leads to desire in the first place. With sexual arousal, there typically comes a physiological change. This may include increases in blood flow in the body and in the genitals, including penile and vulvar tissue. This can lead to (but not always) penile erection or clitoral engorgement, and vaginal lubrication in preparation for possible sexual activity.

Similarly with desire, a single question about sexual arousal is not adequate to understand how individuals experience sexual excitation. Possible questions about arousal might include:

1. How do you know that you are getting aroused?
2. Do you have any difficulty getting or staying aroused?
    a. Are you able to maintain an erection for a time that you are satisfied with?
    b. Do your difficulties with arousal happen in both partnered and solo sex (masturbation)?
    c. Do you have any difficulties with vaginal lubrication?
    d. Do you enjoy stimulation on your clitoris?
3. How does it feel when your body and/or genitals are touched? Do you enjoy it?
4. Does your arousal build up as stimulation continues? If not, what happens for you?
5. What kinds of stimulation are you most aroused by?
6. What kinds of stimulation are you least aroused by?

Orgasmic response is the final area that we will touch on regarding sexual functioning. An orgasm, also known as "sexual climax" or the more informal expression "to cum," refers to the rhythmic contractions of the genital and pelvic musculature and accompanying pleasurable sensations that occur through the building of sexual arousal. Of importance to note is that while orgasm can often include the experience of ejaculation, they are not one and the same. For some individuals they may experience a "dry orgasm," where the pleasurable sensation of orgasm occurs without the expulsion of semen down the urethra. This is particularly true for individuals who have had surgeries (like seen in prostate cancer treatment) that disallow the production of semen into the seminal vesicles.

Difficulties with orgasm is an issue that may bring individuals into treatment. For some, it may be frustrations with how quickly they climax, and for others it may be related to having a delayed or absent climax. It is important to ask detailed questions regarding the individual's experience of heightened arousal and orgasm (or lack thereof) to help determine possibilities of physiological and psychological/cognitive/emotional contributions to the difficulties. Possible questions may be:

1. Have you ever experienced an orgasm? (It is possible that a client may say "I don't know," in which case you may need to explain what an orgasm experience may have been like.)
2. Do you experience orgasm during partnered sex?
3. Do you experience orgasm during solo sex (masturbation)?
4. Do you orgasm more quickly than you would like?
5. Does it take you longer to climax than you would like?

The final important detail regarding assessing sexual functioning is the timeline and associated features of the difficulties. This is particularly true when individuals are reporting difficulties in functioning that may correspond with a diagnosable sexual dysfunction as defined in the *Diagnostic and Statistics Manual of Mental Disorders* (5th ed.; *DSM-5*; American Psychiatric Association, 2013). For some individuals, these difficulties may have been present for a longer period. One example may be as follows:

> Jenny is a cisgender, heterosexual, married woman who has had two male sexual partners in her lifetime and has never experienced an orgasm. She experiences pain during vaginal penetration but has never spoken up about this difficulty because she does not want to offend her partners. She also has a deeply held belief that men will cheat if they do not get enough sex, and it is her responsibility to satisfy her partner sexually. Because of this pain, Jenny has increasingly felt anxious regarding sexual activity, experiences very little arousal leading up to penetrative sex, and her desire to have sex or initiate sex is very low.

As you can see with Jenny, we have components of all the above areas, from sexual identity and role expectancies, as well as desire, arousal, and orgasm difficulties. Contributions to Jenny's experience are a lifelong inability to experience orgasm and the experience of vulvar pain during sexual activity. What we do not know from this vignette are some associated features that may give us clues as to what may be contributing factors. We do not know if Jenny engages in solo touch (masturbation), we do not know what kinds of touch are happening with a partner, history of trauma, medications taken, relational and family histories, and more. By fleshing out some of these details, the sexual health assessment can help to understand the systemic contributions to Jenny's experience of absent climax. For other individuals, the difficulties may be more acute or acquired during the course of their sexual life. This is certainly the case for difficulties like Peyronie's Disease which causes physical injury to the penis, but the difficulties may also be due to a decrease in sexual desire following the start of a medication like an SSRI. When assessing difficulties, the assessor should always screen for contributing physiological factors like illness/disease, medication changes, substance use, and injury.

In addition to screening for a timeline, we must also assess for how difficulties are experienced across situations. For example, some difficulties may happen in any setting, and during both solo-sex (masturbation) and partnered sex. And some may only happen during partnered sex and not during self-stimulation.

When assessing sexual health functioning difficulties, a complete assessment also investigates the learning history of the individual's experiences, the models from their family of origin and psychosocial influencers, and how these impact current functioning. Additionally, for the more acute changes that do not appear to have a physiological etiology, looking to understand the more immediate relational change and/or challenge will help to understand what may be driving the difficulties. Screening for associated mental health difficulties like anxiety, depression, adjustment difficulties, trauma responses, and so forth, may help to understand those contributions as well.

Relational Meaning

The choice to engage our sexuality with another person, whether in the context of a long-term relationship or the fleeting one-night stand, carries some relational value. This could be as simple as "I like having sex, and you are attractive to me." Or it could carry a more emotional valence like "I feel connected to you on an emotional and intellectual level, and I want to express that connection through a physical sexual connection as well." And many more!

It is important to take some time to understand this third component of a sexual health assessment, the motivations and relational meaning that the individual experiences in their sexual expression. This could vary depending on life stage, current partnered system, and other factors. The responses to questioning your client's values, beliefs, and experiences will help to shape their sexual story and your understanding of who they are in their sexual selves. Much of this relational meaning can be derived from a person's family history and the modeling they received from childhood into adulthood. Their current patterns may be a repetition of what they were exposed to in their homes or may be a reactionary deviation from that model to be different from what they experienced in their family of origin. For this reason, having questions regarding their family of origin and how sexuality was modeled is important. Some questions to consider are:

1. How was sexuality discussed in your family home growing up?
2. How did your parents/caregivers express sexuality? Were there open displays of affection?
3. What messages (either implicit or explicit) did you get regarding sexuality from your parents/caregivers?

For some individuals, the relational meaning also carries an element of exploration or desire to engage power differentials with the engagement of pain, control, humiliation, domination, submission, and other variations. It is of great importance to note that the variation of sexual expression is vast, and simply having the presence of these dynamics is not to be equated to pathology. Here is another example of watching one's own internal biases and assumptions. When those dynamics occur in a manner that impedes on another person's right to consent, creates nonconsensual harm to another, or is bound by compulsion and distress, these may fall under the umbrella that the *DSM-5* (American Psychiatric Association, 2013) defines as paraphilias. The term is of Greek origin; "para" means on the side of "philia" or love. Included in these are Voyeuristic Disorder, Exhibitionistic Disorder, Frotteuristic Disorder, Sexual Masochism Disorder, Sexual Sadism Disorder, Pedophilic Disorder, and Fetishistic Disorder. It is extremely important to differentiate kink behavior from disorder, and because these types of dynamics are not as accepted by the general public without judgment and shaming messages, great care in assessing these dynamics should be observed. Possible questions may include:

1. As an adult, have you ever experienced sexual attraction to a minor child? If so, were they prepubescent or postpubescent.
2. Have you ever had the urge to (or have you) exposed yourself to an unwilling participant?
3. Have you ever watched people undress or having sex without their consent?
4. Have you ever engaged in consensual sexual play involving bondage, discipline, dominance, submission, sadism, or masochism (collectively referred to as BDSM)?
5. Have you ever had any sexual arousal and/or engaged in sexual exploration with inanimate objects?

CONCLUSION AND FINAL REMARKS

Whether you are aspiring to focus your clinical practice on working with human sexuality and sexual difficulties or you are working towards becoming a more sex-positive and sex-inclusive professional, including a Sexual Health Assessment is a positive way to understand the full scope of your client's lives, including their sexual functioning. Additionally, the availability to discuss sexuality with your clients can be an extremely rewarding and healing process. The sexual health assessment questionnaires, semi-structured interviews, and other tools offered in this text can further assist you build your comfort and confidence responding to your client's sexual concerns and questions.

We hope that you find the discussion in this chapter gets you thinking about how to include a more comprehensive sexual health assessment in your professional work, and gives you some opportunities to explore your own history. Addressing these concepts, for your own self as a therapist or consultant, will certainly give you pause to challenge your own biases and assumptions and help you develop personal comfort in addressing sexuality with others.

These final few words are offered as an invitation to view this chapter as a starting point for developing competency in conducting a sexual history, and an invitation to keep learning and growing. The information here is certainly not exhaustive. The language used, the investigation of human sexuality, and the sexual variances are ever growing. Harness an attitude of curiosity for yourself and for your clients, and your sexual health assessments will be greatly enhanced.

REFERENCES

American Psychiatric Association. (2013). *Diagnostic and statistical manual of mental disorders* (5th ed.). https://doi.org/10.1176/appi.books.9780890425596

Basson, R. (2000). The female sexual response: A different model. *Journal of Sex and Marital Therapy, 26,* 51-65.

Basson, R., Gilks T. (2018). *Women's sexual dysfunction associated with psychiatric disorders and their treatment.* Women's Health. https://journals.sagepub.com/doi/pdf/10.1177/1745506518762664

Brennan, D. (2021, June 28). *BDSM: What does it mean?* WebMD. https://www.webmd.com/sex/what-is-bdsm-sex

Cupit, R. (2010). *Counselors' comfort levels and willingness to discuss sexual issues with couples they work with* (Doctoral dissertation, University of New Orleans). University of New Orleans Theses and Dissertations (1150). https://scholarworks.uno.edu/td/1150

Grinonneau-Denton, A. (2019). *MFTS' comfort and the extent to which they discuss sexual issues with couples with whom they work* (Doctoral Dissertation, University of Akron). https://etd.ohiolink.edu/

Kaplan, H. S. (1995). *Sexual desire disorders.* Brunner-Routledge.

Masters, W., & Johnson, V. (1970). *Human sexual inadequacy.* Little, Brown.

Perelman, M. A. (2009). The sexual tipping point: A mind/body model for sexual medicine. *The Journal of Sexual Medicine, 6*(3), 629-632. https://doi.org/10.1111/j.1743-6109.2008.01177.x

Risen, C. (2007). How to do a sexual health assessment. In L. VandeCreek, F. Peterson, & J. Bley (Eds.), *Innovations in clinical practice: Focus on sexual health* (pp. 19-33). Professional Resource Press.

World Health Organization. (2006). *Sexual health.* https://www.who.int/health-topics/sexual-health-health#tab=tab_2

World Health Organization. (2021). *Gender.* https://www.who.int/health-topics/gender#tab=tab_1

3

Sexual Health Assessment Tools and Measurements

Frederick L. Peterson, Jr. and Lorenzo E. Aranda

INTRODUCTION

There is an undeniable need for professionals to provide care in the area of sexual health. There is also a relative need for the added skill of the selection and administration of measurements related to sexual health by the professionals that specialize in this area of psychotherapeutic service. Over the last 4 decades there has been an upsurge in designing and rating instruments for assessing various aspects of sexual health, sexual dysfunction, and sexual disorders (Grover & Shouan, 2020).

Most of these measures do not require any sort of formal training, paid workshops, or online video libraries to view. All that is required is the critical thinking that we, as mental health professionals, are trained to employ in the consideration of any material we might use with our clients. However, as it will be stressed throughout this chapter, such measures should only be used as a secondary source of information in making any diagnostic formulation or in the construction of a treatment plan. In routine clinical settings, the standardized rating scales can aid in the detection of symptoms, in serial monitoring, and evaluating the effectiveness of various treatment strategies. At the same time, due to the availability of multiple scales to assess the various aspects of sexuality, clinicians and researchers often face challenges when selecting a scale for use.

Adopting a sexual health framework to enhance traditional interventions could ensure that a greater variety of important factors in sexual behaviors are addressed more comprehensively and efficiently (Higgins et al., 2011). Although there is an abundance of measures available to providers which assess various aspects of sexual health, it can be a daunting and confusing task to sort through which are considered valid, which are accepted within the field of sexual health, and which have no empirical basis for use by professionals. There are those that are open source or public domain, and those that are copyrighted and structured under a pay-for-use system. In this chapter, we will review some of the better known and widely utilized measures of sexual health. We will offer a brief description of each and point to some of the research which credits their design. Finally, we will introduce some informal questionnaires and structured interviews that are very helpful with clients who present to your practice with specific concerns regarding their sexual health.

LITERATURE REVIEW OF PUBLISHED AND VALIDATED MEASURES

The following may have happened to you before. You found an instrument through an online search that seemed ideal because, unlike many of the other instruments reviewed, this one was designed specifically with your population of focus in mind. Then you found out that the information about the instrument's reliability and validity was lacking. It was then that you learned that it is not enough to find a measure that appears to be right for your patient at first glance. You need to know how to choose an appropriate instrument, assess its quality, and use it ethically.

A clinician must sort through the appropriateness for the demographics of the patient, whether it measures the same construct that is desired, the time it takes to administer, and the potential costs associated with access to it. Finally, and most critically, it must be verified that the instrument is both reliable and valid. It must not only produce the same result each time you administer it, but it must also measure what it's supposed to measure. Regardless of the measure used, and the validity established with it, they should only be used to indicate areas of *further inquiry*. It is not good practice to depend on the results of any single measurement as a sole basis for diagnosis.

A key challenge for all research into the development of measures of sexual health is to ensure they are impartial, accurate, and representative of behavioral patterns for the population of the individual you are evaluating. A shortcoming that resides with some of these measures is an issue that has previously been identified as problematic with many psychological measures in general. Specifically, many measures were developed and initially validated among young, literate, predominantly Caucasian participants in North America and Europe (Esho et al., 2019). This presents a significant psychometric challenge. There is a myriad of cultural considerations in the creation and administration of measures of sexual health. These measures are designed to capture perceptions and beliefs regarding sexual life and experiences within the context of autonomy, safety, and satisfaction.

At the same time, self-reported measures may also be unreliable because they are subject to the possibly biased interpretation of the respondent, including reporting and recall bias. This can especially be true for the topic of sexuality, as it remains a charged issue which carries a potential for stigma substantiated by social norms (DiClemente et al., 2011). Since sexual behavior is often thought to be a sensitive and private activity, responding to related questionnaire items is subject to varying degrees of social, cultural, religious, moral, and legal norms and constraints (Fenton et al., 2001).

There are culturally specific values and norms that undeniably play a role in how the respondent perceives questions on this topic. The data may be difficult to gather because the content demands from the respondent a certain degree of vulnerability. These measures depend on the respondents' willingness to report sensitive information and sometimes risk being socially criticized. Some measures may even ask clients to disclose illegal behaviors. To one respondent, the behavior being inquired about may be culturally sanctioned. However, for another respondent, that same behavior may be punishable by death (such as homosexuality) in some parts of the world. Patterns of sexual meaning and satisfaction are shaped by the interaction of individual factors as well as social and cultural environment (Higgins et al., 2011).

Even the way in which the measure is constructed may dilute the potential quality of the resulting data. The difference between using a five-point and four-point Likert scale for the embedded questions might mean that specificity or severity of the construct is lost. Also, the way a construct is defined may not account for culturally sensitive interpretations. For example, Sanders and Reinisch (1999) found that 60% of a sample of college students did not consider oral sex alone to be "having sex."

Interview factors may also influence the endorsement of measure items. Research has shown that people tend to report more sexual information to female interviewers (Anderson & Broffitt, 1998). To avoid interpersonal bias factors, self-completion questionnaires are believed to be valuable as part of an overall assessment. Self-completion questionnaires reduce the need for respondents to disclose sensitive behaviors to the interviewer and may yield more valid results than interviews themselves (Catania et al., 1995).

Another issue in the measurement of sexual health relates to the classic adage "correlation does not equal causation." Determining the dynamics of general behavior is challenging enough, but when we look at the complexities of intimate interpersonal interaction, those challenges increase dramatically. For instance, if a measure identifies a link between engaging in certain sexual behaviors and contracting a sexually transmitted infection (STI), is it the behaviors themselves that are responsible or the absence of safety measures while engaging in those activities that facilitates the transmission of an STI?

Very importantly, there can be difficulty establishing construct validity in creating measures of sexual health. The administrating clinician must be sure that the measure used is assessing exactly what they intended. Is the clinician trying to gather a general understanding of sexual health or a more specific aspect of it, such as individual sexual self-image, sexual literacy, or sexual competency? Sexual competency can be conceived as sexual well-being through individuals' perceptions and beliefs regarding their sexual life and experience within the context of autonomy, safety, and satisfaction (Folch et al., 2018). The different dimensions or composite indicators as a proxy might mean that the measure does not necessarily match the situation.

Another example is the Sexual Health and Well-being Satisfaction (SHAWS; Peterson et al., 2020) scale (a semi-structured interview questionnaire discussed later in this chapter). The measure is designed to be an indicator of overall satisfaction regarding 25 dimensions of one's sexuality. The following are some appropriate questions for the SHAWS, as well as any measure: What construct is exactly being measured and what does the score mean? Does a high score on an item indicate a high level of satisfaction because a person truly has a high level of health related to that item (such as an absence of an STI) or because they are not aware of the STI they have? (Peterson, 2020).

RESOURCES DESCRIBING AND DISTRIBUTING MEASURES OF SEXUAL HEALTH

The following is a list of resources that describe and distribute measures of sexual health to researchers and clinical providers. It is not all-inclusive, and you are encouraged to consider alternative sources as well. Resources reviewed here include (a) the Mental Measurement Yearbook and Tests in Print, (b) the APA Database Suite, and (c) the Health and Psychosocial Instruments (HAPI) database.

Mental Measurement Yearbook and Tests in Print

To find commercially available tests, the Buros Institute's *Test Reviews Online* (www.unl.edu/buros) is a great place to begin. This database contains information on thousands of commercially available psychological measures dating back to the mid-1970s. Searching by keywords in the "scores" category will yield measures that assess for constructs that may not be in the measure's title. From there, test reviews can be purchased for $15 each. You can also consult the volume of Buros's "Mental Measurements Yearbook" that contains the desired review. Buros's "Tests in Print" also allows for a search of measures according to what they measure. The book contains information about every commercially available English-language test currently in print.

APA Database Suite

The American Psychological Association (APA) PsycINFO database is another resource. A centralized database of scholarly research in psychology, in general, it also hosts documents with appended measures. In addition to searching by instrument name, you can also search by area and then check the "tests and measures" information in the abstracts of published articles. Within the PsycINFO suite of databases, PsycTests is an extensive collection of items associated with psychological measures, scales, surveys, and other instruments. This resource also contains instrumentation tools developed for research but not made commercially available. Access to both PsycINFO and PsycTests databases are included in the APA's membership fees. A subscription to other research archive providers, like ProQuest and EBSCO, also allows access.

The Health and Psychosocial Instruments

The Health and Psychosocial Instruments (HaPI) database is created by Behavioral Measurement Database Services and is available at most physical and virtual libraries through the bibliographic database OVID. HaPI describes measures appearing in journals dating back to 1985. In addition to its database, the company has hundreds of measures on file that it can mail to researchers and clinicians for a handling fee of $20 per measure.

COMMERCIALLY AVAILABLE INSTRUMENTS

If you are thinking about using a commercial product, keep in mind that many are either pay-per-use or by subscription. This means that you might have to incur cost each time you administer the measure to a patient, or you might have to pay a monthly fee to have access to the platform that administers and interprets the measure. Costs can range from a few cents for each copy of a questionnaire to several dollars. You may also have to buy a manual or send data to the publisher for scoring, which can potentially increase the costs. Three commercially available instruments are highlighted below: (a) the Abel Assessment for Sexual Interest (AASI), (b) the Multiphasic Sex Inventory (MSI), and (c) the Clarke Sex History Questionnaire for Males – Revised (SHQ-R).

Abel Assessment for Sexual Interest (AASI)

The AASI for Men and Women, now in its third revision, is an empirically validated comprehensive evaluation that measures sexual interests and involvement in abusive or problematic sexual behaviors. Aside from baseline data, it also offers treatment planning guidance and aids in risk assessment. Available in both English and Spanish versions, the AASI is administered via a Windows platform computer. The AASI for Boys and Girls is similar to the adult version but structured to be administered to adolescents and teens ages 12 to 17. The full assessment includes six objective measures and ten self-report measures. The objective measures assess for sexual interest in children, sexual recidivism risk, cognitive distortions, social desirability, sexual victimization, and probability of past child sexual abuse acts. The self-report measures assess for internet child pornography use, child sexual contact, danger to children, admitted sexual behaviors, sexual health concerns, sexual abuse victimization history, sexual behaviors, sexual fantasies, criminal infraction history, arousal to children and adults, and alcohol and drug use. In the AASI, the respondent is shown photos depicting various gender and age categories to determine interest or arousal. This is accompanied by a 600-item questionnaire. Once the respondent completes the assessment, the evaluator sends the resulting data to Abel Screening for processing and a detailed report is then returned within minutes.

The robustness of the assessment is due, in part, to the continued effort of Abel Screening to collect and maintain data to refine the evaluation of those with sexual behavioral problems. Though the AASI has shown to have acceptable test-retest reliability, there is no shortage of criticisms regarding its validity. One repeated criticism is regarding the proprietary nature of its scoring and interpretation platform (similar to other frequently used psychological tests). Since these algorithms are unknown, one can test the "formula" only by inference from the results. However, experts in the field of sex offense risk assessment often recommend the use of objective measures as part of a comprehensive evaluation of sex offenders. They detail many advantages of the AASI over traditional utilization of penile plethysmography (the peter-meter) as a proxy measure for sexual arousal (Abel et al., 2007; Peterson, 2020). These advantages and the inherent traits of the AASI allow the instrument to meet the *Daubert* standards used in court to establish the acceptability as evidence and to achieve wide acceptance among practitioners as well as jurisdictions across the country.

Multiphasic Sex Inventory II (MSI II)

The MSI, now in its second revision, is a comprehensive 300-item true/false self-report instrument designed specifically for assessing sex offenders. Scores on the MSI are often used to assess levels of pedophilic interest (Nichols & Molinder, 1984). The MSI includes 20 scales for evaluating sexually deviant behaviors, cognitions, and attitudes. The MSI scales demonstrate moderate to high levels of internal consistency, and considerable convergence and divergence with other measures (Kalichman et al., 1992). The MSI's most notable limitations are its face validity and potential contamination by response biases.

The MSI is frequently used in the assessment of individuals suspected of having pedophilia, primarily via the Child Molest (CM) scale. The CM scale yields significantly higher scores from child sex offenders than other sex offenders (Dowling et al., 2000). Two additional MSI scales are linked to distorted thinking that enables or justifies sexual offending against children: the Sexual Obsessions (SO) scale and the Cognitive Distortions/Immaturity (CDI) scale. These scales are also sensitive to general sexual deviance, such as having extrafamilial victims, having male victims, and having multiple victims (Freund & Watson, 1991; Seto & Lalumière, 2001).

Given that the MSI also includes an Antisocial Personality Disorder Scale, it can be used in support of arriving at a formal diagnosis for the disorder. However, the measure is based on *DSM-III* criteria which was heavily criticized for its focus on overt behavioral indicators over more covert ones (Houser, 2015). Beginning with the *DSM-IV*, the "Associated Features" section of diagnostic criteria was added to summaries underlying personality traits that may support the diagnosis (American Psychiatric Association, 2000). There is some disagreement on how the results of the MSI should be interpreted when assessing for pedophilia (Mackaronis et al., 2011). Because no existing evidence has conclusively determined whether pedophilia has a categorical or continuous latent structure, it is unclear whether MSI scores should be treated as a continuous measure of severity or whether a cutoff score should be used to categorize individuals as pedophilic.

Clarke Sex History Questionnaire for Males–Revised (SHQ-R)

The SHQ-R is a fully validated and standardized self-report assessment of an individual's sexual history. It has been widely used to assess male offenders, and to evaluate their risk to others and their potential for rehabilitation. It investigates the frequency, desire for, and aversion to a wide range of sexual behaviors, including atypical paraphilic behaviors (Paitich et al., 1977). The original version of the measure (of which the current 2002 one is based) consisted of 24 scales and 255 items (Langevin & Paitich, 2002). The assessment currently consists of 23 scales covered by 508 items in a multiple-choice format, and it explores six areas of male sexuality. There is a scale addressing Childhood and Adolescent Sexual Experiences which includes abuse that might have occurred during those years. There is a Sexual Dysfunction scale which evaluates conditions such as impotence, hypersexuality, and premature (or rapid) ejaculation. There are seven scales that address Adult Age/Gender Sexual Outlets, including the frequency of various sexual activities with adults, children, and adolescents. There are three scales within the area of Fantasy and Pornography that measure sexual fantasies involving women, men, and the use of pornography. Three scales cover Transvestism, Fetishism, and Feminine Gender Identity which evaluate personal experiences regarding transvestism, sexual fetishes, and identification with female gender traits. A total of six scales address Courtship Disorders, which take into consideration conditions such as voyeurism, exhibitionism, obscene telephone calls, frotteurism, and sexual assault. There are also two validity indicators: a "Lie Scale" measuring insincere responding and an "Infrequency Scale" measuring infrequent responding. Scoring and interpretation is done either via the purchased software package with unlimited usage or a pay-per-use format via the developer's website.

PUBLIC DOMAIN INSTRUMENTS AND ASSESSMENT TOOLS (VALIDATED)

Because public domain instruments are readily available, they can be a cost-effective way to assess patients. This is especially true if such measures are used often, such as with the continued monitoring of a patient's presentation or progress over time. However, one hazard of public domain instruments is the fact that patients are also able to gain access to them. Advanced awareness of a measure's questions, and its interpretation instructions, means that a patient could potentially produce intentional results. First, two formally validated instruments will be briefly discussed: (a) the Female Sexual Function Index (FSFI), and (b) the International Index of Erectile Function (IIEF). Next, several public domain self-administered structured interviews will be discussed, which are less formal assessment tools that have not had validity/reliability studies published but have high face validity and practical value working with clients who present with sexual health concerns.

Female Sexual Function Index (FSFI)

The diagnosis of female sexual dysfunction (FSD) is based mainly on a detailed sexual and reproductive history and may be followed by a specific questionnaire to gather a clearer picture of the dynamics of the client's clinical presentation (Barber, 2007). Though there are several instruments used to measure sexual function in women, the FSFI is one of the most widely used measures of female sexual dysfunction. It is a 19-item self-report questionnaire that assesses 6 domains: desire, arousal, lubrication, orgasm, satisfaction, and pain. It is easily understood, brief, and has been replicated in several languages (Rosen et al., 2000). Items are scored on a five-point Likert scale with low scores indicating lower levels of sexual functioning. The measure is provided at the back of this book (see pages 557-562).

Validation studies in women aged 21 to 70 have demonstrated excellent internal consistency and 2- to 4-week test-retest reliability for each subscale (Goldfarb et al., 2013). Discriminant validity was significant for all subscales, as well as the summary score. In the FSFI validation study, an analysis of sensitivity and specificity yielded a cutoff score of 26.55 for the identification of women with sexual dysfunction (Wiegel et al., 2005). It has been validated both in healthy women and women with chronic medical conditions. This instrument was developed to measure sexual function in women who were sexually active over the prior 4 weeks. Since this measure contains questions asking respondents to reflect on their recent experiences with a current sexual partner, it may not be appropriate for those clients who have multiple concurrent sexual partners and those who have not had sexual relations with others recently.

Approximately 10 years after the creation of the original FSFI, attempts were made to offer an abridged version to provide a fast screener of FSD for easy use in outpatient visits, epidemiological studies, and assessment of treatment response (Isidori et al., 2010). This iteration, referred to as the

FSFI-6, takes no more than 3 minutes to complete. A total score of less than 19 indicates the need for further inquiry, including the full-length FSFI and a dedicated interview. The initial study, conducted by Isidori et al. (2010) included 200 women attending outpatient clinics for sexual and reproductive medicine. Reliability, internal consistency, and stability on retest were found to be good, though not as promising as the original version. Although it has not gained the same traction as the original, it serves as a novel tool that can help any clinician (mental health or medical) to detect FSD rapidly and efficiently.

International Index of Erectile Function (IIEF)

The 15-question IIEF is a validated, multidimensional, self-administered questionnaire that is widely accepted by both the regulatory agencies and scientific journals as a valid and reliable measure of sexual functioning in men (Rosen et al., 2002). It consists of 15 items, on a five-point Likert scale, that ask respondents questions about the effects that their erection problems have had on their sex life over the last 4 weeks. The instrument provides accurate and reliable information as a quantitative index of ED severity which may be of value to clinicians in diagnosing the disorder (Rosen et al., 1997). The measure is provided at the back of this book (see pages 553-556).

The IIEF meets psychometric criteria for test reliability and validity, has a high degree of sensitivity and specificity, and correlates well with other measures of treatment outcome. It has demonstrated consistent and robust treatment responsiveness in studies in the U.S., Europe, and Asia, as well as in a wide range of etiological subgroups. A brief screening version of the instrument has also recently been developed. Interesting to note, improvements in IIEF scores were found to be highly correlated with improvements in mood (Rosen et al., 2002).

The measure examines four main domains of male sexual function: erectile function, orgasmic function, sexual desire, and intercourse satisfaction. The IIEF is limited by the superficial assessment of psychosexual background and the very limited assessment of partner relationship, both important factors in the presentation of male sexual dysfunction. However, it cannot capture any physiological components that may account for the patient's erectile difficulties. Interpretation of this questionnaire should, therefore, be viewed as an adjunct to, rather than a substitute for, a thorough sexual history and physical examination. As such, a referral to a medical provider to aid in establishing medical rule-outs (e.g., diabetes) should be paired with psychotherapy for this population of patients.

Patients with low IIEF scores (<14 out of 30) in Domain A (erectile function) may be referred to a medical provider for consideration for a trial course of medication, such as Sildenafil. If medication trials are unsuccessful, this is typically followed by a referral to a specialist (particularly a sex therapist). Patients demonstrating primary orgasmic or ejaculatory dysfunction (Domain B) should also be referred for specialist investigation. Patients with reduced sexual desire (Domain C) require testing of blood levels of androgen and prolactin per best practice clinical guidelines (see Chapter 15 on the assessment and treatment of ED, pp. 255-273). Sex therapy should be strongly considered if low scores are recorded in any domain as there is typically an emotional overlay to any sexual dysfunction regardless of the etiology. This is even true when there is only a moderately lowered score (14 to 25) in Domain A (erectile function).

A disadvantage of this measure is that it provides only a limited assessment of the domains of sexual desire and orgasmic dysfunction. It also does not differentiate between different types of sexual desire disorders (e.g., primary vs. secondary) or to distinguish between premature ejaculation and other types of male orgasmic disorders (Rosen et al., 2002). The instrument appears heterosexist, as it focuses specifically on vaginal intercourse. It will not properly capture the nuances related to issues associated with same-sex activity.

PUBLIC DOMAIN CLINICAL TOOLS (WITHOUT VALIDITY STUDIES)

There are several assessment tools in the public domain for use by anybody, including clinicians seeking helpful tools to better understand nuanced details of their client's sexual development and current sexual status. As previously noted, these public domain tools are less formal and have not had validity/reliability studies published yet have high face validity and practical value working with clients who present with sexual health concerns. While different from the validated instruments discussed thus far, these evaluative tools have high utility as a short-cut means of learning much about the intimate details of a client's sex life and providing information for generating hypotheses relative to diagnosis and treatment. All the evaluation tools discussed in this section have been found "tried and true" in clinical practice and are shared to promote effective clinical assessment of the sexual health concerns of clients. Except the first one below, these tools have been previously published in *Innovations in Clinical Practice: A Focus on Sexual Health* (2007) and *The Gender Revolution and New Sexual Health* (2020). They are all represented in Section VI of this book.

Sexual Health Assessment Questionnaire

Using a questionnaire for data collection on a client's sexual health history is a huge time-saver for the clinician and money-saver for the client. It could easily take 2 hours (or more) of an in-person interview to cover the history reported in the questionnaire. This sexual health assessment questionnaire (see pp. 539-551) can be completed in your office or sent out for the client to complete in the comfort of their own home. It is recommended that the client be screened first before they attempt to complete the questionnaire, so you have a sense that the client has some initial rapport established, that they understand that this is a legitimate part of an overall sexual health evaluation, and that they have the "ego strength" to take on such an extensive inquiry of their sex life without being triggered or offended.

The questions are comprehensive, covering the client's lifespan and uses language appropriate for clients who identify with varied sexual identities. The authors' instructions below give clients not only an explanation for the need of the information disclosed but also informs them that the client's answers (and possibly questions) will be discussed in session:

> *This questionnaire is provided so that we can address sexuality as part of normative human functioning as quickly as possible. Even if you are not coming in with an acute sexual issue, opening the door to conversation on sexuality early helps to create a positive and open space to include it in treatment when relevant . . . There are no "right" or "wrong" answers to these questions, please answer them in a way that is accurate for you. The information gathered here is important for our assessment of the difficulties you are experiencing and for development of our course of treatment. . . . We will review your answers together in our session and ongoing as needed.*

Assessment of Family Support For Healthy Sexual Development

This 25-item self-assessment questionnaire (see pp. 564-568) is a means to gather relevant clinical data about the client's childhood/adolescence, and then review the same with the client to ensure accuracy of responses (and the client understanding the question) or ask more detailed follow-up questions to their response. Alternatively, the questionnaire can be used as a structured interview (especially if the client was not able to complete it in advance of meeting with the clinician). The measure covers all the typical developmental milestones of sexual development, traumatic events (such as assault, unplanned pregnancies, etc.), and the client's emotional experience going through childhood. It is helpful for gauging personal satisfaction (or lack thereof) regarding how they view their *past* sexual experiences. It also provides the clinician insight into which of three general developmental pathways people have walked before they found their way to a therapist's office:

1. An overall sex-positive development as a child/teenager with a minimal number of adverse effects from family influences and sex-induced anxiety during maturation.
2. An overall sex-neutral or sex-ambivalent development as a child/teenager with a moderate number of adverse effects from family influences and sex-induced anxiety during maturation.
3. An overall sex-negative development as a child/teenager with a high number of adverse effects from family influences and sex-induced anxiety during maturation.

This questionnaire is based completely upon client responses from a specialized sex therapy practice. Hence, interpretive statements above should not be considered generalizable to people who do not go to therapy (or even to other clients). Therefore, caution is to be exercised while applying any descriptive language. In other words, this questionnaire is a general indication of how your client did or did not feel supported as a kid learning about sexuality.

Assessment of Sexual Health and Well-being Satisfaction (SHAWS)

As the questionnaire discussed above focuses on the client's level of satisfaction regarding their past experiences, the SHAWS is designed to measure the client's level of satisfaction regarding 25 dimensions of their current sexual self (see pp. 569-574). The 25 items of the SHAWS asks clients to rate their satisfaction across four domains of being a sexual entity:

- **Sexual Self-Satisfaction** (items like sexual health literacy, self-image, self-pleasuring)
- **Relational Sexual Satisfaction** (items like attraction, libido, partnered pleasuring)
- **Medical Sexual Satisfaction** (items like sexual pain, STI, reproductive status)
- **Sexual Identity Satisfaction** (items like sex, sexual, and sex-role orientations)

Areas of sexual health that have the highest and lowest levels of satisfaction are of keen interest and have specific purposes. Areas of highest satisfaction may represent your client's strengths and are important in not only "counter-balancing" other areas of low satisfaction, but possibly assisting in selection of strategies to enhance their sexual satisfaction. Conversely, areas of lowest satisfaction may represent areas of your client's greatest sexual concerns and can serve as a guide in focusing efforts on your client's self-improvement journey, recovery program, and/or therapy strategies. These are the areas deserving particular attention in order to focus on increasing client satisfaction.

Assessment of Your Big Wheel of Health and Well-being

A clinician cannot accurately assess a client's sexual health without understanding the larger context of their overall health and well-being, especially if they have significant chronic illnesses that interfere with sexual function. The "Big Wheel" questionnaire (pp. 575-578) is designed to measure the client's satisfaction with 25 health indicators across eight dimensions of their health. Each of the eight dimensions can be thought of as a "Spoke in the Big Wheel." Clients are asked to state their level of satisfaction about three items across all eight dimensions, which are as follows:

- **Nutrition and Health Literacy** (nutrition, BMI, health literacy)
- **Medical Health** (blood pressure, cholesterol level, any chronic illnesses)
- **Lifestyle Health Factors** (tobacco and alcohol use, exercise/health maintenance)
- **Environmental Health** (reliable shelter, clean water/food supply, no environmental hazards as well as having an environment free of violence and coercion)
- **Mental Health** *(*anxiety, depression, and self-esteem)
- **Relational Health** (emotional connection to others, social support from your friends and family, sense of spiritual connection to the larger world and/or sense of meaning)
- **Work and Financial Health** (work satisfaction, productivity, financial status)
- **Sexual Health** (sexual identity, sexual function, overall sexual health)

How satisfied your clients are about different areas of their general health is only a proxy indicator for actual measures of the health (e.g., blood pressure, cholesterol, etc.). Clients may not know their actual health status and often do not know their testosterone level or that they have hypertension (high blood pressure is referred to as the silent killer). Therefore, they are asked to have physical examinations with their primary care provider (or urologist or other specialist) and understand what their values are on all laboratory results.

Generally, high satisfaction is associated with better-than-average health (assuming they are honest with themselves). They are most likely able to achieve optimal health through their own determination and self-help strategies. However, moderate range of satisfaction with overall health indicates that clients have some areas of strength, that they feel good about many areas of their health. At the same time, they need professional help and are recommended to work with their health team of providers. They are recommended to use self-help strategies but really need to work with professionals to help get where they want to go. Clients with pervasive low satisfaction about many areas of their health means there is a good chance they likely have general dissatisfaction with many areas of life. Their low satisfaction likely indicates that they may be experiencing important health challenges and there is no question that they need professional assistance to help find the way back to the days when they felt good about their health and life.

DISCUSSION

This chapter introduced clinicians to some of the most common assessment instruments employed to evaluate the sexual health concerns of clients. The assessment instruments presented here can be found in several resource databases, are commercially available, or are in the public domain. The assessment instruments described here are far from a comprehensive list of measurements related to sexual health, and their coverage is beyond the scope of this chapter. Those presented here represent some of the most used and familiar to the authors.

In addition, helpful clinical tools in public domain were presented for therapists to use and increase their comfort and competency evaluating sexual health concerns of their clients. As previously noted, the last few clinical tools discussed are less formal and do not have validity/reliability studies published. It was decided to include them in this chapter as they have face validity and high practical value working with clients. It is the hope of the authors, who are full-time clinicians, to collaborate with academic colleagues to eventually conduct such studies. Until then, use these last few evaluative tools as a short-cut means of learning much about the intimate details of a client's sex life (in a shorter time frame) and providing information for generating hypotheses relative to diagnosis and treatment. All the evaluation tools discussed here have been found to have high utility in clinical practice and are highlighted in this chapter to facilitate effective clinical assessment and treatment for the promotion of our client's sexual health.

REFERENCES

Abel, G. G., Wiegel, M., & Osborn, C.A. (2007). Pedophilia and other paraphilia. In L. VandeCreek, F. Peterson, & J. Bley (Eds.), *Innovations in clinical practice: Focus on sexual health* (pp. 157-175). Professional Resource Press.

American Psychiatric Association. (2000). *Diagnostic and statistical manual of mental disorders* (4th ed. text rev.).

Anderson, B., & Broffitt, B. (1998). Is there a reliable and valid self-report measure of sexual behaviour? *Archives of Sexual Behavior, 17*(6), 509-525. https://doi.org/10.1007/BF01542339.

Barber, M. (2007). Outcomes and quality-of-life measures in pelvic floor research, In M. Walters & M. Karram (Eds.), *Urogynecology and reconstructive pelvic surgery* (pp. 499-511). Mosby.

Catania, J., Binson, D., & Van der Straten, A. (1995). Methodological research on sexual behavior in the AIDS era. *Annual Review of Sex Research, 6,* 77-125.

DiClemente, R., Sales, J., Danner, F., & Crosby, R. (2011). Association between sexually transmitted diseases and young adults' self-reported abstinence. *Pediatrics, 127*(2), 208-213.

Dowling, N., Smith, D., Proeve, M., & Lee, J. (2000). The Multi-Phasic Sex Inventory: A comparison of American and Australian samples of sexual offenders. *Australian Psychologist, 35,* 244-248.

Esho, T. C., Muniu, S. K., Yussuf, M., Okondo, C., & Kabiru, C. W. (2019). Measurement of the sexual health and wellbeing of women who have undergone female genital mutilation/cutting: A scoping review. *International Journal of Sexual Health, 31*(1), 92-108. https://doi.org/10.1080/19317611.2019.1572687

Fenton, K., Johnson, A., McManus S, & Erens, B. (2001) Measuring sexual behaviour: Methodological challenges in survey research. *Sexually Transmitted Infections, 77,* 84-92.

Folch, C., Zohrabyan, L., Vagaitseva, N., Casabona, J., Toskin, I., & local REDAN Group. (2018). Measurement of sexual health outcomes among people who inject drugs: Pilot study in Catalonia, Spain and Barnaul, Russia. *BMC public health, 18*(1), 187. https://doi.org/10.1186/s12889-018-5065-x

Freund, K., & Watson, R. J. (1991). Assessment of the sensitivity and specificity of a phallometric test: An update of phallometric diagnosis of pedophilia. *Psychological Assessment: A Journal of Consulting and Clinical Psychology, 3*(2), 254-260. https://doi.org/10.1037/1040-3590.3.2.254

Goldfarb, S., Baron, S., & Tessler Lindau, S. (2013). Female sexuality and sexual function. In M. Goldman, R. Troisi, & K. Rexrode (Eds.), *Women and Health* (pp. 347-357). Academic Press. doi: 10.1016/B978-0-12-384978-6.00023-6

Grover, S. & Shouan, A. (2020). Assessment scales for sexual disorders - a review. *Journal of Psychosexual Health, 2*(2), 121-138. http://doi.org/10.1177/2631831820919581

Higgins, J. A., Mullinax, M., Trussell, J., Davidson, J. K., Sr, & Moore, N. B. (2011). Sexual satisfaction and sexual health among university students in the United States. *American Journal of Public Health, 101*(9), 1643-1654. https://doi.org/10.2105/AJPH.2011.300154

Houser, M. (2015). A history of antisocial personality disorder in the Diagnostic and Statistical Manual of Mental Illness and treatment from a rehabilitation perspective. *OpenSIUC,* Issue 4, May. https://opensiuc.lib.siu.edu/cgi/viewcontent.cgi?article=1795&context=gs_rp

Isidori, A. M., Pozza, C., Esposito, K., Giugliano, D., Morano, S., Vignozzi, L., Corona, G., Lenzi, A., & Jannini, E. A. (2010). Development and validation of a 6-item version of the female sexual function index (FSFI) as a diagnostic tool for female sexual dysfunction. *The Journal of Sexual Medicine, 7*(3), 1139-1146. https://doi.org/10.1111/j.1743-6109.2009.01635.x.

Kalichman, S., Henderson, M., Shealy, L., & Dwyer, M. (1992). Psychometric properties of the Multiphasic Sex Inventory in assessing sex *offenders. Criminal Justice and Behavior, 19*(4), 384-396. https://doi.org/10.1177/0093854892019004003

Langevin R., & Paitich D. (2002). *Clarke Sex History Questionnaire for Males-Revised (SHQ-R).* Multi-Health Systems.

Mackaronis, J., Strassberg, D., & Marcus, D. (2011). The latent structure of Multiphasic Sex Inventory-assessed pedophilic interest. *Psychological Assessment, 23,* 1017-1022.

Nichols, H. R., & Molinder, I. (1984). *Multiphasic Sex Inventory: A test to assess the psychosexual characteristics of the sexual offender*. Nichols and Molinder Assessments.

Paitich, D., Langevin, R., Freeman, R., Mann, K., & Handy, L. (1977). The Clarke SHQ: A clinical sex history questionnaire for males. *Archives of Sexual Behavior, 6,* 421-436. https://doi.org/10.1007/BF01541185.

Peterson, F. (2020). Measuring your sexual satisfaction. In F. Peterson, J. Bley, & R. Frabotta, *The gender revolution and new sexual health: Celebrating unlimited diversity of the Human Sexuality Hypercube* (pp. 31-50). Cognella Academic Press.

Peterson, F., Bley, J., & Frabotta, R. (2020). *The gender revolution and new sexual health: Celebrating unlimited diversity of the Human Sexuality Hypercube.* Cognella Academic Press.

Rosen, R., Brown, C., Heiman, J., Leiblum, S., Meston, C., Shabsigh, R., Ferguson, D., & D'Agostino, R. (2000). The Female Sexual Function Index (FSFI): A multidimensional self-report instrument for the assessment of female sexual function. *Journal of Sex & Marital Therapy, 26,* 191-208. https://doi.org/10.1080/009262300278597

Rosen, R., Cappelleri, J. C., & Gendrano, N. (2002) The International Index of Erectile Function (IIEF): A state-of-the-science review. *International Journal of Impotence Research, 14*(4), 226-244. https://doi.org/10.1038/sj.ijir.3900857

Rosen, R., Riley A., & Wagner G. (1997). The International Index of Erectile Function (IIEF): A multidimensional scale for assessment of erectile dysfunction. *Urology, 49,* 822-830. https://doi.org/10.1016/s0090-4295(97)00238-0.

Sanders, S., & Reinisch, J. (1999). Would you say you "had sex" if...? *Journal of the American Medical Association, 281,* 275-277. https://doi.org/10.1001/jama.281.3.275

Seto, M. C., &., Lalumière, M. L. (2001). A brief screening scale to identify pedophilic interests among child molesters. *Sexual Abuse: A Journal of Research and Treatment, 13,* 15-25. https://doi.org/10.1177/107906320101300103

Wiegel, M., Meston, C, & Rosen, R. (2005) The Female Sexual Function Index (FSFI): Cross-validation and development of clinical cutoff scores. *Journal of Sex & Marital Therapy, 31*(1), 1-20. https://doi.org/10.1080/00926230590475206

4

Senior Sexual Health: The Effects of Aging on Sexuality

Patricia Schiml and Emily Chriswell

Seminal work within the field of human sexuality has included the study of the effects of aging on sexuality. Kinsey described a precipitous decline in sexual activity with age in both men (Kinsey et al., 1948) and women (Kinsey et al., 1953) but found that there was considerable variation in the effects of age on sexual expression and that the shifts over the lifespan seemed to be sex-specific. Masters and Johnson's groundbreaking work describing the physiological sexual response cycle was, in part, initiated to explore negative age-related changes in male sexuality in order to determine effective ways of treating sexual dysfunction (Brecher, 1969; Masters & Johnson, 1966). Since those early days, much has changed in terms of the therapeutic (medical and psychological) treatment of sexual problems that emerge later in life, societal expectations and stereotypes about sexual activity in aged individuals, and internalized expectations about one's own sexuality over the course of life.

AGE-RELATED CHANGES IN SEXUALITY

The elderly are often stereotyped as asexual because of developmental declines in reproductive physiology and a societal emphasis on sexuality as existing within the realm of youth. The reality, however, is quite different. A majority of older adults say that sexual interaction is an important part of romantic relationships and their quality of life; they report being sexually active while participating in a wide variety of sexual behaviors (Solway et al., 2018). Data from the National Survey of Sexual Health and Behavior (Schick et al., 2010) indicate that approximately one fifth of older (50+) respondents reported masturbating and nearly one fourth engaged in penile-vaginal intercourse (PVI) a few times per month, with men generally reporting more solo and partnered sexual interaction than women, a trend also observed in younger individuals (Karraker et al., 2011). While older adults are sexually active and emotionally fulfilled by being so, nonetheless, the frequency with which older people are sexually active does decrease with age (Granville & Pregler, 2018; Gray et al., 2019; Karraker et al., 2011; Solway et al., 2018).

Aging and Sexuality in Men

As men age, sexual responses slow. The latency between erection and "penetrative readiness" is increased, and time to orgasm is prolonged. The refractory period increases in duration and can last up to several days in elderly men (Agronin, 2014). While these changes are normal, they may also be related to testosterone reductions that naturally occur with age (Vermeulen et al., 1972) and may be worse in those in poor health (Karraker et al., 2011). For men with clinically low levels of testosterone, androgen supplementation may boost sexual responses including erection, coitus, masturbation, and orgasm (Davidson et al., 1979; Vermeulen, 2000), as well as improve obesity parameters, muscle strength, and reduce age-related joint pain (Kazi et al., 2007; Yassin et al., 2014).

The most common sexual complaints by older men concern difficulties having or maintaining an erection that is firm enough for penetrative sex. Between 25% to 30% of older (45+) men report having problems or being formally diagnosed with erectile dysfunction, and as men age, a greater proportion of men experience this (Fisher, 2010; Laumann et al., 2007). Moreover, poor health can exacerbate age-related erectile dysfunction (Schick et al., 2010). Indeed, there is more research within the field of sexuality and aging in men on erectile problems and on erection-enhancing drugs than many other areas of male sexuality (Sinković & Towler, 2019).

Since the late 1990s, erection-enhancing drugs like sildenafil citrate (brand name Viagra) have been available to restore erectile responses in men, and that don't contraindicate with other medications they may be taking for cardiovascular disorders (Heidelbaugh, 2010; Tracqui et al., 2002). These medications bypass the typical emotional and behavioral factors that usually contribute to erection and produce one by directly modifying genital vasocongestion, increasing penile firmness. Erection-enhancing drugs are widely requested by aging men, and those who use such drugs report increased satisfaction with intercourse, orgasmic function, and improvements in sexual relationships and confidence (Lowy et al., 2007). Not all men, however, are good candidates for these drugs; men who take certain nitrate medications for cardiovascular function or those who have peripheral neuropathy because of diabetes, injury, or neurodegenerative disorders are not good candidates for these medications.

With sexual "performance" in men tied to erection and penetrative sex, the slowing of arousal responses, erection, and orgasm is likely to be distressing to men as they age. Indeed, sexual satisfaction decreases with age in men (Fisher, 2010), and this may be potentiated by the fact that men are more likely to hold negative sexual stigmas about sexuality and aging than are women (Syme & Cohn, 2016). Indeed, those who hold more negative views on aging and sexuality are substantially less satisfied with their sexual activity over time (Estill et al., 2018). Men may experience anxiety and doubts about their masculinity as a result of these changes, and it seems likely that following the introduction of erection-enhancing drugs, societal expectations of prolonged, pharmaceutically enhanced male sexual vigor into later adulthood became fixed (Loe, 2001). This expectation that a decline in sexual function need never occur may be damaging to men who are unable to take these medications. For such men, however, there are alternatives to PVI. Older men in poorer health who have more erectile difficulties and more discomfort during sex exhibit an increase in masturbation and may substitute PVI for other partnered behaviors, like frottage (sexual rubbing against a partner's body) or manual stimulation of or by a partner (Schick et al., 2010). An expansion of the definition of what it means to "have sex" (Schick et al., 2016) can open up new possibilities for interpersonal sexual interactions and can increase intimacy between partners in a way that does not rely on erection. Likewise, the slowing of sexual responses with age can open the door for the experience of intimacy and romance in a way that is markedly different, more languid, and sensual, relative to what younger men experience (Sandberg, 2013).

Aging and Sexuality in Women

Like men, women experience changes in physiology with age that may affect sexual behaviors and interactions. Following menopause, ovarian production of estrogen, progesterone, and testosterone ceases; these changes can result in reduced desire and frequency of sexual interactions in women (Avis et al., 2017; Cappelletti & Wallen, 2016), perhaps due to reduced vaginal elasticity and lubrication responses (Mernone et al., 2019) which are associated with pain during sex and reduced frequency of orgasm (Schick et al., 2010). Unlike the gradual reductions in testosterone that men experience as they age, the reduction in ovarian function occurs over a shorter time period of 2 to 3 years and once completed, the cessation is absolute.

Hormone replacement therapy (HRT) is frequently administered to women to reduce the negative consequences of menopause on sexuality. Estrogen may be prescribed to women for whom it does not pose a health risk based on personal history or genetic/familial factors, as HRT is associated with an increased risk of estrogen-dependent cancers and other health risks (Kumle, 2008). Off-label use of low doses of testosterone may also be prescribed as testosterone has been linked to increased desire and orgasm in women (Kingsberg, 2007; Mernone et al., 2019) and may produce improvements in the number of satisfying sexual events (Davis & Braunstein, 2012) when estrogen alone does not provide a woman with sufficient relief. However, there is concern that the doses of testosterone create circulating plasma levels that are above those typically found in periovulatory women and may produce negative side effects (Cappalletti & Walen, 2016) such as hirsutism or increased cardiovascular health risk. In 2015, flibanserin (brand name Addyi) was approved in the U.S. to treat hypoactive sexual desire in women, and this drug improves the number of sexual events and measures of desire in women (DeRogatis et al., 2012). The high cost of flibanserin and the lack of coverage by most insurance companies, along with limitations on alcohol consumption while using it, has limited its popularity among American women (Aftab et al., 2017).

These age-related changes in sexuality in women may be exacerbated by poor health (Schick et al., 2010). Type II diabetes can result in neuropathy that blunts genital responses (Enzlin et al., 1998; Kizilay et al., 2017), and cardiovascular disease can negatively impact sexual responsivity in women (Kaya et al., 2007). Maintenance of a healthy lifestyle, including managing weight and engaging in physical activity may not only promote better health overall, but may also have beneficial effects on the longevity of a woman's sexual response.

Whereas HRT is no longer prescribed ubiquitously, antidepressant use is quite common today, especially among older women. Nearly one out of four women over the age of 60 is on antidepressant medication, a proportion much higher than observed in men (Brody & Gu, 2020). One common side effect of antidepressant medication is orgasmic delay (Grover et al., 2012). Generally, women require a longer period of sexual stimulation before orgasm than do men; antidepressants may increase this duration.

It is important to note that not all the changes in women's sexuality with age are negative. Older women report more sexual satisfaction relative to younger women (Gray et al., 2019) as they become more sexually experienced and familiar with their own sexual responses and needs. Relationship quality can also affect this as women who report higher levels of emotional support from their partners have higher levels of sexual function (Mernone et al., 2019). Indeed, relationship, social, and cultural considerations can profoundly impact a woman's sexual desire and should be addressed when assessing dysfunction in women, particularly for those reporting distress with low sexual desire (Wood et al., 2006). Interestingly, the slowing of sexual responses in men with whom women are partnered may actually benefit women, as women require a prolonged period of sexual interaction before penetrative readiness, and this pattern reflects the age-related changes that are occurring in their male partners (for those in heterosexual relationships with men of a similar age).

PSYCHOSOCIAL CONSIDERATIONS

Partner Availability

In addition to the changes in sexual function that accompany an aging body, there are psychosocial changes that must also be considered. One obvious influence on sexual behavior is partner availability. With age, both men and women may lose partners to divorce or death. As men age, partner availability may predict their sexual behavior: single men report a greater frequency of masturbation than partnered men (Schick et al., 2010). In this case, masturbatory activity may be a substitute for partnered sex. Alternatively, older men may seek out new partners, but those who have sex with a new partner are less likely to have an orgasm than men who have sex with a long-term partner (Schick et al., 2010), indicating that familiarity may enhance certain aspects of an aged man's sexual response. Women who are divorced or widowed have less sex relative to married women whose husbands are alive (Karraker et al., 2011), and the relatively strong relationship between sexual frequency and happiness that is observable in younger women is weaker in older women. As women age, happiness becomes dissociated from sexual frequency, perhaps due to reduced levels of desire that occur with age. In contrast to what is observed in men, however, women who have sex with *new* partners report greater levels of sexual arousal and fewer problems with lubrication than do women who have sex with a long-term partner (Schick et al., 2010).

Sexual Health

While most older adults report feeling comfortable talking about sexual problems with a health care provider, less than 20% have done so within the past few years and if so, about half of those conversations were initiated by the provider and not the individual (Solway et al., 2018). Health care providers should include time in visits with older individuals to inquire about sexual health, making a point to note that changes in sexual function can reflect larger health issues (e.g., a man who is experiencing impaired erectile and ejaculatory function may be experiencing diabetic neuropathy due to long-term effects of poorly controlled blood glucose levels). Moreover, when sexual side effects are possible with new medications, providers should fully disclose this to their patients, as well as the possible medications that could treat those side effects and other forms of therapy that could be useful.

Interestingly, older Americans engage in risky sexual interactions and the likelihood of this varies between men and women, as well as between those with long-term partners versus those without. The National Survey of Sexual Health and Behavior (Schick et al., 2010) found that substance use prior to sex was fairly common (alcohol: 23% of men, 10% of women) and that the use of paid sexual partners was not uncommon, especially among men. While younger men and women are more likely than older men and women to use condoms during heterosexual sex (Reece et al., 2010), older men are more likely to use a condom with a paid sexual partner relative to other partners, but older women are more likely to use a condom when having sex with "a friend" relative to new dating partners (Schick et al., 2010). Race/ethnicity and educational status are also predictive of condom use (Reece et al., 2010). People of color report higher rates of condom use relative to whites, and those with post-high school education report more condom use than those without (Reece et al., 2010). These findings collectively illustrate the need for educating older, white, or less-educated individuals (who might be engaged in dating after leaving long-term partners or the death of partners) about the risks of sexually transmitted infections (STI), safer sex practices, and STI testing.

Long-term Care Facilities

With advanced age and poor health, some older adults require long-term care in nursing homes and long-term care facilities. In 2019, 1.3 million Americans resided in nursing homes, with greater demand for such care from adults 85 and older (Harris-Kojetin et al., 2019). Additionally, far more women than men reside in long-term care facilities; nearly 70% of residents are female. Lester et al. (2016) found that sexual activity (including partnered sexual interactions and masturbatory activity) between residents of long-term care facilities is often viewed as problematic by staff and administration, although only a minority of facilities have formal, written policies in place regulating sexual interactions. Interestingly, larger facilities, more so than smaller ones, may have such formal policies regulating residents' sexual activity, and they may include requiring physician approval or formal permission of the family; such large organizations may also provide private spaces that are designated for residents' sexual interactions. While sex between individuals who are cognitively sound is the most common type of sexual interaction reported by staff in nursing home, sexual interactions between individuals with dementia is also quite common (DiNapoli et al., 2013). Clearly, age-related decline in cognitive capacity directly impacts an individual's ability to seek or give consent to sexual engagement. Facilities in charge of the care of older adults should have clear policies in place regarding sexual interactions, and they must be communicated to family members and others involved with the aged adult's care.

Aging and Sexuality in the LGBT Population

In surveying aging Americans (weighted age range 50-94 years of age with median ages of 61.74 and 62.16 for men and women, respectively), Schick et al. (2010) found that 9% of men and 2% of women reported having a same-sex encounter during their most recent sexual interaction. Lifetime reporting (Gates, 2011) of *any* same-sex interaction (8.2%) is much higher than the number of individuals who *self-identify* as lesbian, gay, or bisexual (3.5%), and transgender identification is even more rare (0.3%). Still, when considered together, several million Americans fall under the LGBT umbrella (Gates, 2011; Houghton & Quartey, 2020).

There is a paucity of research done on the experiences of aging individuals who identify as sexual minorities, particularly for transgender folks. One finding that is apparent, however, is the finding that there are fundamental differences among age cohorts of LGBT (e.g., Generation Xers versus baby boomers) in terms of their lifelong experiences and how those experiences shape their expectations about relationships, aging, healthcare, and therapy. Older sexual minority individuals may worry more than younger folks about revealing their identities to therapists, doctors, or long-term care facilities because of previous experiences with discrimination, and may feel the need to "return to the closet" when approaching therapists and other healthcare professionals (DeLamater & Koepsel, 2015; Dentato et al., 2014).

In contrast, LGBT individuals may possess resources unique to their communities in terms of dealing with the challenges of aging. Because they have coped with the trials inherent to being a marginalized population, they may possess a greater degree of resilience relative to others (Dentato et al., 2014). This ability to adapt and seek help from unexpected places often leads to the formation of "chosen families" among sexual minority populations. "Chosen family" is a term that refers to accepting and affirming friends, colleagues, and community members that may serve to replace non-accepting family members or communities of origin, and this chosen family often includes partners and friends. Gay men are less likely to be in long-term relationships as they age relative to lesbian women, and most gay men feel less connected to accepting communities and chosen families relative to lesbians (Houghton & Quartey, 2020). Interestingly, trans-identified individuals report the lowest levels of familial support among aging sexual minority Americans (Houghton & Quartey, 2020). This is especially concerning given that with age, many elderly individuals seek help from family; among members of the LGBT community, this may not be an option. Therefore, having affirming and accepting mental health care providers, physicians, and extended care services is critically important. Providers should be vigilant about making their practices inclusive. From the language used on intake and assessment forms to the manner in which office staff interact with LGBT elderly clients and patients, education and thorough training can ensure an inclusive professional climate.

THERAPEUTIC CONSIDERATIONS

Redefining What it Means to "Have Sex"

Older people who define sex strictly as PVI paired with orgasm suffer more from the changes associated with sexual aging (Levin, 2015) relative to those who have a more expansive view of sexual expression. Interestingly, there are no universal definitions of what it means to "have sex" (Schick et al., 2016) and even among women who report "having sex" with both men and women, the inclusion of specific sexual acts in one's definition of "having sex" varies by the sex of their partners. Garcia et al. (2014) found that the rate of orgasm is highest for lesbian women relative to bisexual or heterosexual women, presumably because of qualitative differences in the way in which sexual interactions progress. Orgasm is more likely to occur in women if a greater number of sexual practices are incorporated into a sexual encounter (Richters et al., 2006), but for men, more satisfying sexual encounters occur with relationship partners relative to new partners (Herbenick et al., 2010). Broadening the definition of what it means to "have sex" may allow for couples to expand the ways in which they feel intimately connected. Indeed, studies of older married couples indicate that emotional connection stems more from nonpenetrative activities as they age (DeLamater & Koepsel, 2015).

Sexual intimacy, for younger people, can be tied to sexual performance in a way that is difficult with aged bodies. Aging can bring with it the need to have a more open definition to define closeness and physical intimacy. Therapists can help aged individuals appreciate the fact that sexual expression is a continuum of bodily and emotional experiences that includes PVI, but also encompasses non-coital interactions including kissing, holding one another and being physically close, sensual touch, massage, and anything that allows partners to connect emotionally (Granville & Pregler, 2018). Men, in particular, may need guidance in recognizing that a slowing of the biological sexual responses may allow for sensual and emotional intimacy that is noncoital (Sandberg, 2013).

Differences in Desire

As with younger couples, older couples may experience sexual conflicts when one partner feels stronger sexual desire than the other. As noted above, physiological changes that accompany aging may result in a reduced physical need for sex; when this occurs more so in one partner than another, it can result in relationship conflict. When couples with discrepant desire disengage from one another, rather than addressing the issues, relationship satisfaction is decreased (Vowels & Mark, 2020). Couples should be encouraged to share whatever limitations they feel regarding their own levels of desire, arousal, and ability to complete whatever the desired/typical interaction is for them. Individual knowledge limits about elements of anatomy, physiology, and aging concerns should be explored, and if necessary, corrected. Open and honest communication about the discrepancies experienced can be facilitated by a therapist, and alternatives to a couple's typical mode of sexual interaction can be explored (Brandon, 2016). Indeed, several strategies dealing with discrepancies in desire have been suggested including masturbation, engaging in alternative activities (other than PVI), or cuddling as an alternative to sex (Vowels & Mark, 2020). For instance, an individual may find that masturbating in the presence of their partner may allow one to have an orgasm and still feel intimately connected to the other. Individuals should be reminded that sexual satisfaction is everyone's right, no matter what their age. Other couples may explore options like consensual non-monogamy; this includes swinging, open relationships, and/or polyamory (Vowels & Mark, 2020). Such solutions may allow for the partner who feels more desire to explore sexual outlets outside of the primary relationship. Importantly, however, non-monogamy should be explored with full honestly and openness; such explorations may well be aided by a therapist.

CONCLUSION

While age-related changes in sexuality may be inevitable, being fully educated as to the limitations they might create as well as to the expansion of possibilities that can emerge for individuals or couples can allow clients to navigate aging in a less-distressful fashion. Satisfying sexual expression is possible throughout the lifespan, regardless of age, sexuality, or physical status.

REFERENCES

Aftab, A., Chen, C., & McBride, J. (2017). Flibanserin and its discontents. *Archives of Women's Mental Health, 20*, 243-247.

Agronin, M. E. (2014). Sexuality and aging. In Y. M. Binik & K. S. K. Hall (Eds.), *Principles and practice of sex therapy* (pp. 525-539). Guilford Press.

Avis, N. E., Colvin, A., Karlamangla, A. S., Crawford, S., Hess, R., Waetjen, L. E., Brooks, M., Tepper, P. G., & Greendale, G. A. (2017). Change in sexual functioning over the menopause transition: Results from the Study of Women's Health Across the Nation (SWAN). *Menopause, 24*, 379-390.

Brandon, M. (2016). Psychosocial aspects of sexuality with aging. *Topics in Geriatric Rehabilitation, 32*, 151-155.

Brecher, E. M. (1969). *The sex researchers*. Little, Brown and Company.

Brody, D. J., & Gu, Q. (2020). *Antidepressant use among adults: United States, 2015-2018.* National Center for Health Statistics Data Brief (No. 377). https://www.cdc.gov/nchs/data/databriefs/db377-H.pdf

Cappalletti, M., & Wallen, K. (2016). Increasing women's sexual desire: The comparative effectiveness of estrogens and androgens. *Hormones and Behavior, 78*, 178-193.

Davidson, J. M., Camargo, C. A., & Smith, E. R. (1979). Effects of androgen on sexual behavior in hypogonadal men. *Journal of Clinical Endocrinology and Metabolism, 48*, 955-958.

Davis, S. R., & Braunstein. G. D. (2012). Efficacy and safety of testosterone in the management of hypoactive sexual desire disorder in postmenopausal women. *Journal of Sexual Medicine, 9*(4), 1134-1148.

DeLamater, J., & Koepsel, E. (2015). Relationship and sexual expression later in life: A biopsychosocial perspective. *Sexual and Relationship Therapy, 30*, 37-59.

Dentato, M. P., Orwat, J., Spira, M., & Walker, B. (2014). Examining cohort differences and resilience among the aging LGBT community: Implications for education and practice among an expansively diverse population. *Journal of Human Behavior in the Social Environment, 24*, 316-328.

DeRogatis, L. R., Komer, L., Katz, M., Moreau, M., Kimura, T., Garcia, M., Wunderlich, G., & Pyke, R. (2012). Treatment of hypoactive sexual desire disorder in premenopausal women: Efficacy of flibanserin in the VIOLET study. *Journal of Sexual Medicine, 9*, 1074-1085.

DiNapoli, E. A., Breland, G. L., & Allen, R. S. (2013). Staff knowledge and perceptions of sexuality and dementia of older adults in nursing homes. *Journal of Aging and Health, 25*, 1087-1105.

Enzlin, P., Mathieu, C., Vanderschueren, D., & Demyttenaere, K. (1998). Diabetes mellitus and female sexuality: A review of 25 years' research. *Diabetic Medicine, 15*, 809-815.

Estill, A., Mock, S. E., Schryer, E., & Eibach, R. P. (2018). The effect of subjective age and aging attitudes on mid- to later-life sexuality. *The Journal of Sex Research, 55*, 146-151.

Fisher, L. L. (2010). *Sex, romance, and relationships: AARP survey of midlife and older adults* (Publication D19234). AARP. https://assets.aarp.org/rgcenter/general/srr_09.pdf

Garcia, J. R., Lloyd, E. A., Wallen, K., & Fisher, H. E. (2014). Variation in orgasm occurrence by sexual orientation in a sample of U.S. singles. *Journal of Sexual Medicine, 11*, 2645-2652.

Gates, G. J. (2011). *How many people are lesbian, gay, bisexual and transgender?* UCLA: The Williams Institute. https://escholarship.org/uc/item/09h684x2

Granville, L., & Pregler, J. (2018). Women sexual health and aging. *Journal of the American Geriatrics Society, 66*, 595-601.

Gray, P. B., Garcia, J. R., & Gesselman, A. N. (2019). Age-related patterns in sexual behaviors and attitude among single U.S. adults: An evolutionary approach. *Evolutionary Behavioral Sciences, 13*, 111-126.

Grover, S., Shah, R., Dutt, A., & Avasthi, A. (2012). Prevalence and pattern of sexual dysfunction in married females receiving antidepressants: An exploratory study. *Journal of Pharmacology and Pharmacotherapeutics, 3*, 259-265.

Harris-Kojetin L, Sengupta M, Lendon JP, Rome V, Valverde R, & Caffrey C. (2019). *Long-term care providers and services users in the United States, 2015-2016* (NIH Publication 2019-1427). National Center for Health Statistics. *Vital Health Statistics, 3*(43). https://www.cdc.gov/nchs/data/series/sr_03/sr03_43-508.pdf

Heidelbaugh, J. J. (2010). Management of erectile dysfunction. *American Family Physician, 81*, 305-312.

Herbenick, D., Reece, M., Schick, V., Sanders, S. A., Dodge, B., & Fortenberry, J. D. (2010). An event-level analysis of the sexual characteristics from a national probability sample in the United States. *The Journal of Sexual Medicine, 7*, 346-361.

Houghton, A., & Quartey, N. . (2020). *Maintaining dignity: Understanding and responding to the challenges facing older LGBT Americans*. AARP. https://doi.org/10.26419/res.00217.006

Karraker, A., DeLamater, J., & Schwartz, C. R. (2011). Sexual frequency decline from midlife to later life. *The Journals of Gerontology, Series B: Psychological Sciences and Social Sciences, 66*, 502-512.

Kaya, C., Yilmaz, G., Nurkalem, Z., Ilktac, A., & Karaman, M. I. (2007). Sexual function in women with coronary artery disease: A preliminary study. *International Journal of Impotence Research, 19*, 326-329.

Kazi, M., Geraci, S. A., & Koch, C. A. (2007). Considerations for the diagnosis and treatment of testosterone deficiency in elderly men. *The American Journal of Medicine, 120*, 835-840.

Kingsberg, S. (2007). Testosterone treatment for hypoactive sexual desire disorder in postmenopausal women. *Journal of Sexual Medicine, 4*, 227-234.

Kinsey, A. C., Pomeroy, W. B., & Martin, C. E. (1948). *Sexual behavior of the human male*. W. B. Saunders Company.

Kinsey, A. C., Pomeroy, W. B., Martin, C. E., & Gebhard, P. H. (1953). *Sexual behavior of the human female*. W. B. Saunders Company.

Kizilay, F., Gali, H. E., & Serefoglu, E. C. (2017). Diabetes and sexuality. *Sexual Medicine Reviews, 5*, 45-51.

Kumle, M. (2008). Declining breast cancer incidence and decreased HRT use. *The Lancet, 372*, 608-610.

Laumann, E. O., West, S., Glasser, D., Carson, C., Rosen, R., & Kang, J. (2007). Prevalence and correlates of erectile dysfunction by race and ethnicity among men aged 40 or older in the United States: From the Male Attitudes Regarding Sexual Health Survey. *Journal of Sexual Medicine, 4*, 57-65.

Lester, P. E., Kohen, I., Stefanacci, R. G., & Feuerman, M. (2016). Sex in nursing homes: A survey of nursing home policies governing resident sexual activity. *Journal of the American Medical Directors Association, 17*, 71-74.

Levin, R. J. (2015). Sexuality of the aging female–the underlying physiology. *Sexual and Relationship Therapy, 30*, 25-36.

Loe, M. (2001). Fixing broken masculinity: Viagra as a technology for the production of gender and sexuality. *Sexuality & Culture, 5*, 97-125.

Lowy, M., Collins, S., Bloch, M., Gillman, M., Lording, D., Sutherland, P., Wang, H., & Stecher, V. (2007). Quality of erection questionnaire correlates: Change in erection quality with erectile function, hardness, and psychosocial measures in men treated with sildenafil for erectile dysfunction. *Journal of Sexual Medicine, 4*, 83-92.

Masters, W. H., & Johnson, V. E. (1966). *Human sexual response*. Little, Brown, & Co.

Mernone, L., Fiacco, S., & Ehlert, U. (2019). Psychobiological factors of sexual functioning in aging women – findings from the women 40+ healthy aging study. *Frontiers in Psychology, 10*, 1-13.

Reece, M., Herbernick, D., Schick, V., Sanders, S. A., Dodge, B., & Fortenberry, J. D. (2010). Condom use rates in a national probability sample of males and females ages 14 to 94 in the United States. *Journal of Sexual Medicine, 7*, 266-276.

Richters, J., de Visser, R., Rissel, C., & Smith, A. (2006). Sexual practices at last heterosexual encounter and occurrence of orgasm in a national survey. *The Journal of Sex Research, 43*, 217-226.

Sandberg, L. (2013). Just feeling a naked body close to you: Men, sexuality and intimacy in later life. *Sexualities, 16*, 261-282.

Schick, V., Herbenick, D., Reece, M., Sanders, S. A., Dodge, B., Middlestadt, S. E., & Fortenberry, J. D. (2010). Sexual behaviors, condom use, and sexual health of Americans over 50: Implications for sexual health promotion of older adults. *Journal of Sexual Medicine, 7*, 315-329.

Schick, V., Rosenberger, J. G., Herbenick, D., Collazo, E., Sanders, S. A., & Reece, M. (2016). The behavioral definitions of "having sex with a man" and "having sex with a woman" identified by women who have engaged in sexual activity with both men and women. *The Journal of Sex Research, 53*, 578-587.

Sinković, M., & Towler, L. (2019). Sexual aging: A systematic review of qualitative research on the sexuality and sexual health of older adults. *Qualitative Health Research, 29*, 1239-1254.

Solway, E., Clark, S., Singer, D., Kirch, M., & Malani, P. (2018). *Let's talk about sex.* University of Michigan National Poll on Healthy Aging/ Institute for Healthcare Policy and Innovation. https://deepblue.lib.umich.edu/bitstream/handle/2027.42/143212/NPHA-Sexual-Health-Report_050118_final.pdf?sequence=1

Syme, M. L., & Cohn, T. J. (2016). Examining aging sexual stigma attitudes among adults by gender, age, and generational status. *Aging and Mental Health, 20*, 36-45.

Tracqui, A., Miras, A., Tabib, A., Raul, J. S., Ludes, B., & Malicier, D. (2002). Fatal overdose with sildenafil citrate (Viagra®): First report and review of the literature. *Human & Experimental Toxicology, 21*, 623-629.

Vermeulen, A. (2000). Andropause. *Maturitas, 34*, 5-15.

Vermeulen, A., Rubens, R., & Verdonck, L. (1972). Testosterone secretion and metabolism in male senescence. *Journal of Clinical Endocrinology, 34*, 730-735.

Vowels, L. M., & Mark, K. P. (2020). Strategies for mitigating sexual desire discrepancy in relationships. *Archives of Sexual Behavior, 49*, 1017-1028.

Wood, J. M., Koch, P. B., & Mansfield, P. K. (2006). Women's sexual desire: A feminist critique. *The Journal of Sex Research, 43*, 236-244.

Yassin, D. J., Doros, G., Hammerer, P. G., & Yassin, A. A. (2014). Long-term testosterone treatment in elderly men with hypogonadism and erectile dysfunction reduces obesity parameters and improves metabolic syndrome and health-related quality of life. *Journal of Sexual Medicine, 11*, 1567-1576.

5

Medications and Sexual Health*

Ruth A. Roa-Navarrete, Tonie Taft, and Timothy Pagano

During the past few decades both the incidence and treatment of mental illnesses have increased. Starting in the late 1980s, Serotonin Specific Reuptake Inhibitors (SSRIs) were introduced, followed by Second Generation Antipsychotics (SGAs) and other "safer" psychotropics. Pharmacotherapeutic treatment has also increased, with nonpsychiatry health care providers, including primary care physicians (and pediatricians) as well as nonphysician health professionals (physician assistants, nurse practitioners) being the primary prescribers of these agents in the United States. Issues related to sexual health have often been recognized as being both part of psychiatric disorders as well as a consequence of their treatment. Specifically, most psychiatric medications are known to induce sexual dysfunction in men and women. Patients with mental illness may also be predisposed to sexual dysfunction (e.g., as a result of sexual or other types of victimization). While estimates vary, a significant number of patients with depression and other mental illnesses exhibit sexual dysfunction as a baseline.

In this chapter, we will focus on the challenges associated with treatment of psychiatric disorders and sexual dysfunction. A reductionistic approach would have us simply describe the mechanisms by which psychotropic medication or psychiatric (and medical) illnesses can negatively affect sexual function, and ways to ameliorate the impact. Prior to Engel's seminal work on the biopsychosocial model of medicine (1992), psychologists recognized that manifestations of dysfunction and function and illness and health are the result of interactions among an individual's biological, psychological, and social world. This is an idea which is now widely acknowledged and integrated into the fields of medicine and psychology. We will then highlight the need to integrate both the psychological and the biological sources of dysfunction to the understanding of medication management and sexual health. Additionally, we affirm that it is critical to understand the experience from the patient's perspective and to partner with each patient to identify and address their specific source of distress, which may not be as simple as removing the offending agent (e.g., the antidepressant contributing to erectile dysfunction). Therapists are particularly well suited to assess and understand the intricacies of an individual's experience, and therefore, to assist them in facilitating targeted approaches.

Given their relative influence on sexual function, in this chapter we will address psychotropic medications, cardiovascular medications, endocrine and antineoplastic agents, as well as drugs of abuse. We will also provide guidance for the assessment and treatment of medication-induced sexual dysfunction, including with the use of nutraceuticals. Finally, we will address the potential value of genetic testing in decreasing the probability of sexual side effects secondary to medication trials, hence increasing medication tolerability and adherence.

*The opinions contained herein are the private views of the authors and should not be construed as the official policy or position of the U.S. Government, the Department of Defense, or the Department of the Air Force.

PSYCHOTROPIC MEDICATIONS

Antidepressant Medications

Throughout psychotherapeutic practice, antidepressants stand as the psychotropic medication most likely to be encountered. As of 2014, 8 of the top 50 medications prescribed throughout the United States were antidepressants (Fuentes et al., 2018). In recent years, the ubiquity of these medications has increased in large part due to improved toleration of side effects rather than improved efficacy. All antidepressants prove more beneficial than a placebo. However, small differences exist between medications with regard to symptom resolution (Cipriani et al., 2018; Gartlehner et al., 2011). Sexual dysfunction for men and women resulting from antidepressant pharmacotherapy is well documented. In one survey of men and women taking antidepressants long-term (3-15 years), 71.8% reported some level of sexual dysfunction with 18% reporting sexual dysfunction as "severe" (Cartwright et al., 2016).

The most widely prescribed antidepressants are SSRIs. The potential for sexual dysfunction stemming from this class of antidepressants in both men and women is well documented. In spite of this, it is common for medical professionals to overlook SSRI-induced sexual dysfunction (Atmaca, 2020). This may occur due to a provider's discomfort with discussing sex, and a lack of recognition sex and libido may play in depression. Upon assessing for SSRI-induced sexual dysfunction, providers are likely to experience difficulty discerning the origin of sexual dysfunction. In one study, both men (67%) and women (75%) reported instances of sexual dysfunction prior to initiating antidepressant treatment (Thakurta et al., 2012). Additionally, depression may yield a 50% to 70% increase in sexual dysfunction, while sexual dysfunction may increase rates of depression by 130% to 200% (Atlantis & Sullivan, 2012).

The most common sexual side effects of SSRIs are related to arousal, libido, and difficulty achieving orgasm for both men and women (Reichenpfader et al., 2014). Clayton et al. (2006) reported men are more likely than women to experience dysfunction related to desire (91.2% vs. 79.0%) and orgasm (81.5% vs. 45.4%). Women are more likely to report dysfunction during arousal (71.9% vs. 83.3%).

In men, though uncommon, it is possible for SSRIs to induce priapism. Rates of priapism, defined as a prolonged erection that often occurs without sexual arousal, increase for those men taking alpha blockers (Budzak et al., 2019). A common side effect of SSRIs in men is difficulty with ejaculation and achieving an erection. A Serotonin Antagonist and Reuptake Inhibitor (SARI), trazodone, is an antidepressant that is often prescribed in conjunction with other antidepressants in an effort to treat insomnia in patients with psychiatric comorbidities. Though numerous benefits of trazodone exist (no evidence of tolerance, dependence, or withdrawal), it may lead to priapism in men. As is the case with SSRIs, those men prescribed trazodone should be counseled regarding this risk (Stahl et al., 2018).

Though all SSRIs utilize the same mechanism of action to treat depression, their side effects may differ greatly. Women reported higher rates of sexual dysfunction with paroxetine compared to sertraline (Aberg-Wistedt et al., 2000). Jacobsen et al. (2015) reported reduced sexual dysfunction following transition from sertraline to escitalopram, both SSRIs.

A novel class of antidepressant medications are Serotonin Modulators and Stimulators (SMS). The most common SMS are vortioxetine and vilazodone. For males and females with well-controlled major depressive disorder via utilization of SSRIs, vortioxetine demonstrated significant reduction in sexual side effects while maintaining improvements in depressive symptoms (Jacobson et al., 2020).

Bupropion, a Norepinephrine-Dopamine Reuptake Inhibitor (NDRI), is another widely prescribed antidepressant. Though sexual side effects still exist with this medication, multiple meta analyses indicate reduced frequency and severity of sexual dysfunction compared to SSRIs (Fava et al., 2005; Patel et al., 2016; Reichenpfader et al., 2014).

Prior to the widespread proliferation of SSRIs and Serotonin-Norepinephrine Reuptake Inhibiters (SNRIs) in the 1990s, Tricyclics (TCAs) and Monoamine Oxidase Inhibitors (MAOIs) were the most widely prescribed antidepressant medications. Today, TCAs and MAOIs may be utilized should first-line antidepressants prove ineffective. Their lack of utilization in pharmacotherapy is a result of greater rates of adverse side effects, including sexual side effects, as well as significant adverse interactions with certain foods. Though SSRIs result in milder side effect profiles than TCAs, Wang et al. (2018) found no significant difference in rates of sexual dysfunction for men and women. For men, these side effects include decreased libido and delayed orgasm. Possible sexual side effects for women stemming from TCA treatment include decreased libido, delayed orgasm, and possible breast enlargement (Taylor et al., 2018).

Central Nervous System Stimulants

Central Nervous System (CNS) stimulants stand as commonly prescribed psychotropic medications throughout the western world. They are primarily utilized to treat attention-deficit/hyperactivity disorder and may be used, in limited settings, as a second-line treatment for depression. Six of the top 200 prescribed medications in the United States for 2014 were CNS stimulants. CNS stimulants such as amphetamine and methylphenidate commonly result in sexual dysfunction for men and women (Fuentes et al., 2018). Edvinsson and Ekselius (2018) found an approximately 17% reduction in sexual desire among men and women who were treated with methylphenidate for 6 years. In children and adolescent males, though uncommon, there is risk for priapism (Ekinci et al., 2019; Kelly et al., 2013).

CNS stimulants are also regularly utilized by adolescents and adults without a prescription. One study highlighted that approximately 12.5% of young adults utilize or have utilized CNS stimulants illicitly. Such illicit use was associated with numerous changes in sexual behavior. Those young adults were more likely to be sexually active, sexually active at a younger age, and forego the use of a prophylactic (Grant et al., 2018). Thus, assessing the use of psychostimulants should be an integral part of ascertaining accurate sexual health information from adolescents and young adults.

Anxiolytics/Benzodiazepines

Benzodiazepines, commonly prescribed for anxiety, have received much attention in recent years due to the prevalence rates of patients developing dependence. Olfson et al. (2015) reported those prescribed benzodiazepines varied from 2.6% (18- to 26-year-olds) to 8.7% (65- to 80-year-olds). As of 2014, 5 of the top 200 medications prescribed in the United States were benzodiazepines (Fuentes et al., 2018). In addition to concerns related to dependence, forgetfulness, and toxicity, sexual side effects exist. In both men and women, decreased libido and anorgasmia have been reported. Men may also experience erectile dysfunction, difficulty with ejaculation, and breast tissue enlargement (Procyshyn et al., 2019). Buspirone is an anxiolytic with lower rates of sexual side effects than benzodiazepines. The central drawback to buspirone is its inability to function as a remedy for acute anxiety (Wilson & Tripp, 2020).

Other Psychotropic Medications

For clients diagnosed with psychotic disorders, medication designed to mitigate symptoms may result in sexual dysfunction (Downing et al., 2019). Due to the negative symptoms that often accompany psychotic disorders, it may prove difficult to discern if sexual dysfunction is a result of medication or the psychotic disorder itself. There is a paucity of research pertaining to potential sexual side effects of mood stabilizing medications. Research that does exist largely focuses on lithium bicarbonate (Gómez Sánchez-Lafuente et al., 2017). Though lithium bicarbonate is well-researched, it is more common for SGAs to be utilized. This is punctuated by the fact that of the top 200 medications prescribed in the United States, 4 may be utilized to treat Bipolar Disorder, none of which are lithium bicarbonate. Grover et al. (2014) posit approximately 37% of patients treated with lithium experience some amount of sexual dysfunction. This dysfunction ultimately resulted in decreased medication adherence (Gómez Sánchez-Lafuente et al., 2017; Grover et al., 2014). One study (clients with bipolar disorder who had long-term stability on lithium) found that sustained, significant reduction in sexual desire and sexual function was ameliorated by the addition of benzodiazepines. Such medication augmentation posed new risks due to the addictive potential of new medications (García-Blanco et al., 2020).

All providers should be aware that pharmacotherapy consisting of a single psychiatric medication is uncommon. As a result, it may prove difficult to discern which medication(s) may prove to be causing the presenting sexual dysfunction.

Case Vignette

Paul is a 45-year-old cisgender European American male who was initially referred for pharmacotherapy after having experienced sexual dysfunction in response to trials of two SSRIs (sertraline and escitalopram), which were prescribed in order to target symptoms of anxiety secondary to previous experience of traumatic events. At the time of his initial visit to an outpatient mental health clinic, Paul reported he was in "fair" health with a history of allergies, gastrointestinal esophageal reflux, dizziness, and unspecified chest pain which were being addressed by his primary care physician. His laboratory exams resulted in no abnormal findings. He described a positive, loving relationship with his spouse of 17 years. He noted that she was supportive of his seeking treatment. Paul was ultimately diagnosed with Other Specified Trauma and Stressor Related Disorder and successfully participated in 18 sessions of Eye Movement Desensitization and Reprocessing, from which he derived significant success in resolving adult trauma, and partial success in resolving childhood sexual abuse. Pharmacotherapy involved switching to Venlafaxine XR 75 mg daily, which was beneficial in addressing his mood and anxiety symptoms and in resolving sexual dysfunction.

Discussion questions: How would you change the care of this patient? What psychosocial factors may need to be addressed? What other interventions may need to be addressed?

DRUGS OF ABUSE

Most drugs of abuse, including alcohol and nicotine, are commonly perceived to enhance sexual performance and/or activity, perhaps because of their disinhibiting effects. The drugs' effects on social and performance anxiety may also explain this widespread misconception. While much of the literature has focused on the relationship between illicit drug use and risky sexual behaviors, including the impact of both on sexually transmitted diseases such as HIV/AIDS, relatively few studies specifically focus on the effects of drug use on sexual health. Fewer studies have focused on the effect of substances on female sexual function. Despite this, there is clear evidence of negative effects of most commonly abused drugs.

The effects of alcohol on sexual function and reproduction have been well documented. Chronic cocaine use has been associated with delayed ejaculation in men and irregular menses in women (Carey, 2006; Macdonald et al., 1988; Palha & Esteves, 2008). In a comparison study of substance abusing men in Turkey, Dissiz (2019) found that 41.5% reported a sexual problem, with the cannabis use group reporting erectile dysfunction (ED) at a rate of 83.3%. Amphetamine use has also been associated with ED (Chou et al., 2015), as well as decreased libido and premature ejaculation (PE) (Dolatshahi et al., 2016). Chou et al. (2015) found that 62% of men who abused cocaine and alcohol reported sexual dysfunction. The use of anabolic steroids has been associated with ED especially at high doses, which may persist after the androgen is removed. Testicular atrophy may also occur, though it may be reversible (van Amsterdam & Hartgens, 2014).

The proliferation of opioid abuse, both prescription and nonprescription, in the United States and the world in the past years warrants specific attention. According to Hashim et al. (2020), heroin addicts report rates of ED, PE, orgasmic dysfunction, and decreased sexual interest at rates that are higher than the general population. Several studies have documented effects of chronic opioid use on the endocrine system, which can manifest in sexual dysfunction and reproductive changes (de Vries et al., 2020). The mechanism of action appears to be disruption or suppression of the hypothalamic-pituitary-gonadal axis as well as the hypothalamic-pituitary-adrenal axis (Gudin et al., 2015; Katz & Mazer, 2009; McWilliams et al., 2014; Rhodin et al., 2010). The resulting hypogonadism can manifest in decreased or nonexistent libido, ED, gynecomastia, irregularities or disappearance of menses, in addition to depression, fatigue, hot flashes, and night sweats. In one meta-analysis, authors found 63% of male patients showed hypogonadism related to chronic opioid use.

Longer acting opioids (e.g., fentanyl) had higher odds vs. shorter acting opioids (e.g., hydrocodone) (de Vries et al., 2020). There are conflicting reports about the utility of testosterone replacement therapy to address this. AminiLari et al. (2019) suggest the benefit on sexual functioning is "very low to low." A separate review showed a prevalence of amenorrhea in 23% to 71% of female chronic opioid users, along with decreased libido rates of 61% to 100% (Wersocki et al., 2017). These changes may be reversible after the opioid is withdrawn.

Sexual dysfunction is also associated with various substance use treatment agents. One study of methadone users found 52% reported sexual symptoms (Yee et al., 2014). The authors noted that buprenorphine may have lower risk of sexual dysfunction, however, more information is needed. Disulfiram (Antabuse) is associated with ED (Epocrates, 2020). The first author has also treated cases of ED and delayed ejaculation secondary to naltrexone use, though it is not currently listed as a "common" side effect.

CARDIOVASCULAR MEDICATIONS

Cardiovascular disease (CVD) encompasses coronary heart disease, heart failure, stroke, and hypertension. The prevalence of CVD in adults $\geq$20 years of age in the U.S. is 48.0% based on data from the 2013-2016 National Health and Nutrition Examination Survey (Benjamin et al., 2019). Heart disease is the leading cause of death for men and women across racial and ethnic groups in the United States (Heron, 2019). The utilization of blood pressure lowering medications as well as statin regimens has proven to decrease the relative risk of cardiovascular events and mortality. In 2014, lisinopril, an antihypertensive agent, was the number one medication prescribed throughout the United States and 10 of the top 20 prescriptions dispensed were cardiovascular agents (Fuentes et al., 2018). Sexual dysfunction is a potential side effect of cardiovascular medications. A majority of the studies conducted have evaluated the effects of antihypertensive medications on sexual dysfunction in men. The topic of sexual dysfunction in women has been underexplored. It is noteworthy to mention that the methodology, the operational definition of sexual dysfunction, survey methods and rating scales, as well as the findings have varied across studies (La Torre, 2015).

Alpha Blockers

Alpha-1 adrenergic blockers including alfuzosin, silodosin, doxazosin, prazosin, tamsulosin, and terazosin, have primarily been used in the treatment of hypertension and benign prostatic hyperplasia (BPH) (Wynne, 2012). Recent evidence from two systematic meta-analyses has shown that prazosin has been more effective than placebo in reducing nightmare frequency, improving sleep quality, and reducing overall illness symptoms in PTSD (DeBerardis et al., 2015; George et al., 2016). ED, ejaculatory difficulties, and reduced sexual desire are some reported sexual side effects of treatment of lower urinary tract symptoms (LUTS) with alpha blockers. Silodosin followed by tamsulosin appear to have the highest incidence of ejaculatory disorders. Alfuzosin, on the other hand, has shown not to have any negative effects on sexual function in men (La Torre et al., 2016). LUTS/BPH and ED are highly prevalent as men age and there is evidence to suggest that there is a strong relationship between these conditions independent of medication treatment (De Nunzio et al., 2017). Treatment with alpha blockers has not resulted in significant sexual dysfunction in hypertensive women (Choy et al., 2019).

Angiotensin II Receptor Blockers

There is evidence that angiotensin II receptor blockers (e.g., irbesartan, losartan, and valsartan) may improve sexual function in men and women compared to other antihypertensive medications. Placebo-controlled studies suggest that valsartan may actually improve overall sexual function in hypertensive men compared to beta blockers (atenolol and carvedilol) or placebo (Fogari et al., 2001, 2002, 2004; Fogari & Zoppa, 2004). Treatment with irbesartan or losartan alone, as well as in combination with hydrochlorothiazide (diuretic) was associated with increased sexual activity in patients with cardiovascular disease (Baumhäkel et al., 2008; Della Chiesa et al., 2003). Hypertensive male patients that received a 12-week treatment with losartan had a significant increase in sexual satisfaction and decrease in ED (Caro et al., 2001). Similar results have been reported in women. Women treated with valsartan in comparison to atenolol had improved sexual desire, sexual behavior, and sexual fantasies (Fogari et al., 2004).

Angiotensin-Converting Enzyme (ACE) Inhibitors

ACE inhibitors including benazepril, captopril, enalapril, fosinopril and lisinopril, to name a few, appear to have a neutral or possibly a beneficial effect on sexual function in men and women. Treatment with ACE inhibitors in several trials has not influenced erectile function (Baumhäkel et al., 2011). One study evaluated the effects of treatment with an ACE inhibitor in patients with ED compared to placebo. While there was a positive trend of improving ED with ACE inhibitors, results were not significant (Speel et al., 2005). Treatment with ACE inhibitors has not resulted in significant sexual dysfunction in hypertensive women (Choy et al., 2019). The use of antihypertensive medications including ACE inhibitors was not associated with sexual activity or sexual dysfunction in hypertensive women (Foy et al., 2016).

Beta Blockers

An international survey of men utilizing health care systems in the United States, Germany, United Kingdom, France, and Spain discovered that approximately 10% to 20% of men using beta blockers for hypertension had ED (Shabsigh et al., 2005). A meta-analysis performed in the early 2000s showed that beta blocker therapy was associated with a small but significant annual increase in risk of sexual dysfunction in cardiac patients compared with placebo (Ko et al., 2002). The literature has also demonstrated that the prevalence of sexual activity was lower among men taking beta blockers vs. those not taking beta blockers. However, there were no significant associations between beta blocker use and sexual problems in men or women. In addition, there were no differences in sexual activity of women taking beta blockers (Spatz et al., 2013).

The incidence of sexual problems including ED appears to be more likely with treatment with nonselective beta blockers as opposed to cardio selective beta blockers (Derby et al., 2001). Propranolol, a first-generation nonselective beta blocker, has been used in the treatment of hypertension and migraine headaches, as well as off-label uses to treat performance anxiety and antipsychotic drug-induced akathisias (Lexicomp, 2020). Propranolol is associated with a high incidence of erection problems in men and decreased sexual desire in both sexes (Due et al., 1986; Fogari & Zoppi, 2004; Stevenson & Umstead, 1984). Nebivolol, a third-generation beta blocker, appears to have a more favorable effect on ED in hypertensive men. One clinical trial demonstrated that switching treatment from atenolol, metoprolol, or bisoprolol to nebivolol, a highly selective beta blocker, improved ED in more than 69% of patients (Doumas et al., 2006). More recent research has challenged traditional findings proposing that sexual dysfunction is significantly more common in men and women with cardiovascular disease in comparison to nonaffected populations, and that sexual dysfunction is no more common with beta blockers than with other antihypertensive medications (Choy et al., 2019; Cordero, et al., 2010; Erdman, 2009).

Alpha 2 Agonists

Central acting alpha 2 agonists such as methyldopa, clonidine, and guanfacine are second line agents used in the treatment of resistant hypertension when other drugs are not effective. The exception is methyldopa which is a first line therapy for pregnant patients. Clonidine has been used off label to lessen unpleasant symptoms associated with withdrawal from alcohol and other substances. Both clonidine and guanfacine are also utilized in the management of attention-deficit/hyperactivity disorder (ADHD), Tourette's disorder, behavioral disturbances in children, and insomnia (Wynne, 2012). Some older research has correlated use of methyldopa with a high rate of ED (14%-36%), ejaculatory disorders (7%-19%), desire disorders (7%-14%), and gynecomastia (Aldridge, 1982; Duncan & Bateman, 1993; Hogan et al., 1980). Similar sexual side effects in men have also been reported with clonidine (Hogan et al., 1980; Stevenson & Umstead, 1984). While alpha 2 agonists may negatively affect sexual function in men, the quality of studies available to support this claim is limited. More recent research has not shown any significant associations between antihypertensive medication class and sexual activity or problems in men or women. However, it is noteworthy to mention that alpha agonists have not been included in these studies, likely due to their decreased use in the treatment of cardiovascular conditions (Foy et al., 2016; Spatz et al., 2013).

Calcium Channel Blockers

Calcium channel blocker medications including amlodipine, diltiazem, felodopine, nifedipine, and verapamil, do not seem to be associated with sexual dysfunction or are likely to have a neutral effect (La Torre et al., 2016). A placebo control study evaluating the safety of nifedipine in patients with stable angina noted more reports of impotence as a side effect in the treatment group compared with placebo (Poole-Wilson et al., 2006). However, this result must be interpreted cautiously considering there are no clinical trials that specifically evaluate the effect of calcium channel blockers on erectile function using validated assessments (Baumhäkel et al., 2011). Treatment with calcium channel blockers has not resulted in significant sexual dysfunction in hypertensive women (Choy et al., 2019). The use of antihypertensive medications including calcium channel blockers was not associated with prevalence of sexual activity or sexual dysfunction in hypertensive women (Foy et al., 2016).

Diuretics

Thiazide diuretics, including hydrochlorothiazide and chlorthalidone, have been associated with adverse side effects in men including decreased sexual desire, erectile dysfunction, and difficulty with ejaculation (Sica, 2003). Results in a multicenter randomized placebo-controlled trial comparing diets and pharmacological therapies in obese hypertensive patients indicated that a low dose of chlorthalidone negatively affected sexual function in men (Wassertheil-Smoller et al., 1991). It appears that combination treatment with a thiazide diuretic and an angiotensin receptor antagonist do not show negative effects. In fact, one study showed that combination treatment with irbesartan and hydrochlorothiazide improved sexual desire, frequency of sexual activity, and erectile function in patients with CVD (Baumhäkel et al., 2008).

One study demonstrated that the prevalence of sexual activity was lower among men taking diuretics vs. those not taking diuretics. However, there were no significant associations between diuretic use and sexual problems in men or women. In addition, there were no differences in sexual activity of women taking diuretics (Spatz et al., 2013).

Aldosterone Receptor Antagonists

Aldosterone inhibitors like spironolactone have been associated with untoward side effects including gynecomastia, mastodynia, and ED in men. Adding spironolactone has been helpful in treatment resistant hypertension. However, one study discovered that approximately 9.9% of patients developed adverse effects leading to treatment discontinuation. A total of 5.2% of the males developed gynecomastia and 1.3% experienced impotence (Engbaek et al., 2010).

Compared with spironolactone, eplerenone is a more selective androgen receptor antagonist used in the treatment of heart failure and hypertension, and has overall reduced likelihood of adverse effects including gynecomastia, mastodynia, or ED (Barnes & Howard, 2005; Parthasarathy et al., 2011). Lastly, there is some clinical evidence to suggest that spironolactone may be associated with vaginal pain and female sexual arousal disorder (L. Mitchell et al., 2019).

Statins

Statins including atorvastatin, rosuvastatin, simvastatin, and pravastatin are known to improve clinical outcomes in patients with atherosclerotic cardiovascular disease. Two recent meta-analyses have demonstrated that the use of statin medications is associated with better erectile function in men. It is possible that the mechanism of improvement of ED is associated with improved endothelial function and enhanced availability of nitric oxide (Cai et al., 2014; Kostis & Dobrzynski, 2014). Few studies have evaluated the clinical effects of statins on gonadal-sexual function in women. One retrospective cohort analysis demonstrated that statin use in women was not associated with sexual dysfunction, menstrual disorders, infertility, or ovarian dysfunction (Ali et al. 2015).

Case Vignette

> Jack is a 64-year-old married European American cisgender male who presented to an outpatient mental health clinic upon recommendation from his internist due to "Ativan overuse." His presenting concern was a lifelong history of anxiety manifested as panic episodes 1 to 3 times a day. Medical history was positive for Parkinson's disease (5 years), along with degenerative disc disease, esophageal reflux, BPH, asthma, seasonal allergies, and hypertension. He was on a regimen of sertraline 50 mg daily and lorazepam 1 mg every 6 to 8 hours, along with medications addressing all his medical conditions including finasteride 5 mg for BPH and lisinopril for hypertension. In addition to reported anxiety, Jack related distress secondary to

projected impairment associated with the progression of Parkinson's disease, as well as dissatisfaction with his sexual functioning. Given the complexity of his medical presentation as well as his medication regimen (finasteride alone is known to cause decreased libido, ED, and generalized sexual dysfunction; sertraline and lorazepam could also be contributors), psychoeducation and psychosocial interventions were necessary.

Discussion questions: What pharmacotherapeutic options would you consider, if any? What biopsychosocial factors may need to be addressed? What interventions would you offer this patient and their partner?

OTHER MEDICATIONS

Gender Affirming Treatments in Transgender Individuals

Not every transgender person suffers from gender dysphoria and the desire for gender affirming medical treatments including surgery and hormone therapy may vary (T'Sjoen et al., 2019). An increasing number of studies have demonstrated that gender affirming treatments improve mental and physical health of transgender people (Hayon & Stevenson, 2019; Kerckhof et al., 2019; Murad et al., 2010; T'Sjoen et al., 2019). A systemic review and meta-analysis evaluated quality of life and psychosocial outcomes in transgender persons that specifically received hormonal therapy. Their results indicated decreased gender dysphoria, improvement in psychological functioning with reduction of psychiatric symptoms, lower suicide rates, enhancement of quality of life, and improvement in sexual function (Murad et al., 2010).

Tables 1 and 2 (pp. 68-69) describe the various medication interventions used in transgender women and men as well as the mechanisms of action, desired clinical outcomes, clinical considerations, and sexual side effects.

Sexual dysfunctions among trans women and men are very common. The most frequent sexual concerns reported in both trans women and men is difficulty initiating and seeking sexual contact as well as difficulty achieving orgasm. Reports have indicated that trans women and men who receive both hormone therapy and genital surgery had the lowest number of sexual dysfunctions. The exception to this notion appears to be trans men who opt for a metoidioplasty and report more sexual dysfunction than trans men who had hormone therapy and a mastectomy (Kerckhof et al., 2019).

> LGBTQ is an acronym that includes various groups of sexual and gender minorities including lesbians, gay, bisexual, transgender, and queer questioning people.
>
> LGBTQ individuals have unique health needs and may qualitatively experience disturbances in sexual function differently when compared to a heterosexual population.

Table 1: Hormone Therapy for Transgender Women*

Medication	Mechanism of Action	Desired Clinical Outcomes	Clinical Considerations	Sexual Side Effects
Estrogen	1. Reduce testosterone levels 2. Promote formation of female sexual characteristics	1. Decrease body and facial hair 2. Decrease lean muscle mass and strength 3. Increase weight and redistribute fat mass 4. Breast growth 5. Increase softness of skin	1. Increase risk of thromboembolism 2. Increase LDL and triglycerides 3. Increase risk of breast cancer and endocrine gland cancers	1. Decrease penile erections, prostrate size, sperm quality, and sexual desire
Spironolactone	1. Inhibits testosterone secretion 2. Blocks androgen receptor binding 3. May have estrogenic activity	1. Suppress testosterone levels (adjunct agent taken with estrogen) 2. Decrease male pattern hair growth 3. Breast growth 4. Decrease acne	1. Monitor for electrolyte abnormalities	1. Decrease sexual desire, sperm production, erections, and testicular volume
Cyproterone acetate	1. Decrease testosterone levels	1. Suppress testosterone levels (adjunct agent taken with estrogen) 2. Decrease male pattern hair growth 3. Breast growth	1. Increase risk of meningioma, depression, and hyperprolactinemia 2. Risk for liver toxicity (not available in U.S.)	1. Decrease sexual desire, sperm production, erections, and testicular volume
GnRH agonists (i.e., leuprolide)	1. Suspend puberty 2. Inhibit gonadotropin secretion, and suppress testosterone secretion	1. Decrease serum testosterone and estrogen levels 2. Breast growth 3. Decrease hair growth	1. Expensive	1. Decrease sexual desire, sperm production, erections, and testicular volume
5 alpha reductase inhibitor (i.e., finasteride)	1. Inhibits conversion of testosterone to dihydrotestosterone	1. Improve hair loss	1. Increase risk for prostate cancer	1. Decrease libido and impotence

*Hayon & Stevenson (2019); T'Sjoen et al. (2019).

Table 2: Hormone Therapy for Transgender Men				
Medication	**Mechanism of Action**	**Desired Clinical Outcomes**	**Clinical Considerations**	**Sexual Side Effects**
Testosterone	1. Increase testosterone levels 2. Promote formation of male sexual characteristics	1. Amenorrhea 2. Develop male physical contours 3. Deepen voice 4. Increase facial and body hair 5. Increase muscle mass and strength 6. Prevent bone loss	1. Male pattern baldness may occur 2. Acne 3. Decrease HDL and increase LDL, and triglycerides 4. Increase systolic BP 5. Increase hemoglobin and hematocrit	1. Increase sexual desire 2. Clitoral growth

*Hayon & Stevenson (2019); T'Sjoen et al. (2019).

<u>Case Vignette</u>

Mitch is a 17-year-old transgender male whose preferred pronouns are he, him, and his. Mitch has a psychiatric history of borderline personality disorder, major depressive disorder, and generalized anxiety disorder with multiple inpatient admissions for suicidal ideations and nonsuicidal self-injuries (primarily cutting). His medical history includes asthma, obesity, and chronic pain related to a genetic disorder, Ehlers-Danlos Syndrome. Mitch's psychotropic medications include bupropion ER 300 mg daily, buspirone 15 mg twice a day, clonidine 0.2 mg at bedtime and 0.5 mg in the morning, sertraline 100 mg daily, and hydroxyzine 25 mg twice a day. Mitch mentioned in a recent therapy session that he has a new male sexual partner and asked whether any of his psychotropic medications could be contributing to his decreased energy and sexual desire.

Discussion questions: What are some additional questions you would want to ask Mitch in performing a holistic sexual assessment? What changes if any, would you make to his current medication regimen? What nonpharmacological recommendations would you provide?

Contraception

In 2019, oral contraceptives were used by over 20% of women of reproductive age in 27 countries worldwide with the highest prevalence in European countries. The majority of women living in the United States utilized either female sterilization (13.7%) or oral contraception (13.7%) over other methods of birth control, followed by male condom use (9.3%) and IUD (8.3%) (United Nations, 2019).

Hormonal contraceptives may influence female sexual function. Some literature suggests that women using hormonal methods of contraception including birth control pills, vaginal ring, implants, and levonorgestrel-releasing intrauterine device (IUD) experience more negative sexual side effects than women using nonhormonal methods including male and female condoms, copper IUD, and withdrawal method. Women who utilize hormonal methods of contraception may experience less frequent sexual arousal, pleasure, activity, and orgasm and report more difficulty with lubrication. Women who use nonhormonal methods have reported more frequent sexual activity, sexual arousal, and orgasms (Butt et al., 2019; Smith et al., 2014; Wallwiener et al., 2015).

There does not appear to be a significant association between sexual dysfunction and specific dosages of progestin or ethinyl estradiol (Wallwiener et al., 2015). However, there is conflicting data suggesting that hormonal contraceptives including combined oral contraception (COCs), Depot Medroxyprogesterone Acetate (DMPA), as well as the contraceptive ring and patch are libido neutral (Pastor et al., 2013; Wright & O'Connor, 2015). It is important to mention that, in addition to providing an effective form of contraception, COCs are also utilized to decrease pain associated with myriad gynecologic disorders including endometriosis, dysmenorrhea, and menorrhagia. All of these conditions can influence a female's sexual health (Burrows et al., 2012). In summary, there appears to be potential positive and negative effects of hormonal contraception on female sexuality.

Antineoplastic Agents

There is a high prevalence of sexual problems in female breast cancer patients receiving endocrine therapy. Fulvestrant, tamoxifen and aromatase inhibitors including anastrozole, letrozole, and exemestane have been associated with vaginal dryness, vaginitis, dyspareunia, hot flashes, and changes in sexual response including decreased desire and arousal (Baumgart et al., 2013; Falk & Dizon, 2013; Goldfarb et al., 2013). Administration of chemotherapy can result in systemic side effects that affect one's body image as well as diminish both sexual desire and arousal in both men and women (Cavalheiro et al., 2012; Falk & Dizon, 2013; Rudberg et al., 2002). Androgen deprivation therapy (ADT) including GnRH agonists (leuprorelin, goserelin, triptorelin, or histrelin), GnRH antagonists (degarelix), and anti-androgens including bicalutamide have been used as a primary or adjunct treatment in men with prostate cancer. ADT has been associated with decreased sexual desire, inability to achieve orgasm, and erectile dysfunction in men (Donovan et al., 2018; Nguyen et al., 2018; Wassersug, 2016; White et al., 2015).

Assessment of Sexual Side Effects

A strong functional assessment of medications' potential sexual side effects is critical to ensuring treatment adherence, patient satisfaction, and ultimately successful resolution of the patient's presenting mental health concerns. Assessment of the sexual implications of psychotropic medications may prove uncomfortable and intimidating at first (Nicolai et al., 2013). Mental health providers of various professional identities will find their skill sets translate well into this arena, as an open and impartial approach to discussing a topic that is potentially disconcerting for clients is important.

Assessment of sexual side effects stemming from pharmacotherapy should be based in a biopsychosocial approach, as sexual dysfunction may emanate from one or more geneses (Wincze & Weisberg, 2015). Utilizing a functional, biopsychosocial approach garners a nuanced understanding for sexual functioning across time and context. An assessment to discern one's baseline sexual functioning would ideally occur prior to initiating pharmacotherapy; however, a retrospective assessment may still be beneficial.

Objective measures provided at treatment initiation and regular intervals may provide valuable data as clients acclimate to medications. Such measures include the Arizona Sexual Experience Scale (ASEX; McGahuey et al., 2011) and the Psychotropic-Related Sexual Dysfunction Questionnaire (PRSexDQ; Montejo et al., 2000). To ensure appropriate assessment for males, the International Index for Erectile Function may prove efficacious (IIEF; Rosen et al., 1997). For female clients, clinicians may desire to utilize tailored questionnaires such as the Sexual Interest and Desire Inventory-Female

(SIDI-F; Clayton et al., 2006) and the Female Sexual Function Index (SFSI; Meston, 2003). Reviewing fluctuations in scores on such assessments may prove to be a valuable clinical tool as patients may not fully appreciate the often-gradual changes in sexual functioning.

Direct queries of clients should also take place to assess the impact of pharmacotherapy on sexual functioning (Montejo et al., 2019). Though possibly uncomfortable at first, if a provider makes assessment of sexual functioning a regular part of treatment, such discomfort should become more tolerable for the provider and patient alike. Examples of questions to begin such a discussion may include the following: "Have you noticed any changes in your sexual life since starting the medication?" and "Do any of those changes concern you?" Should such open-ended questions garner little information from clients, direct questions about specific potential side effects should be asked, such as, "Have there been any changes in your desire for sex since starting sertraline?" or "Have you noticed any changes in your ability to maintain an erection?" (Montejo et al., 2019). Scaling questions such as, "On a scale of 1 to10, with 1 indicating no concern and 10 indicating high concern, how concerning is your change in sexual desire?" may aid in this effort. It is important to note that although sexual dysfunction stemming from medications may persist in spite of various interventions, clients may find the dysfunction preferable to the mental health symptoms that prompted their seeking help. Like objective measures, reviewing fluctuations in scaling question results may assist with developing insight into symptom amelioration or exacerbation.

Intervention

From a biopsychosocial perspective, treatment of sexual dysfunction secondary to medication use should target interventions that fit into the patient's physical, psychological, and social (relationship) status. Treatment should include behavioral interventions common to most behavioral health providers. Psychoeducation regarding medication-induced sexual dysfunction may assist in normalizing such reactions as well as facilitate meaningful conversation which may result in nonbehavioral interventions. Exercise is well-validated to improve sexual functioning in both men (Jiannine, 2018) and women (Stanton et al., 2018). Behavioral health providers would do well to utilize common evidence-based interventions that include behavioral activation and Acceptance and Commitment Therapy (ACT). Behavioral activation can assist in development of regular exercise schedules and other healthy habits that may assist with sexual functioning concerns resulting from pharmacotherapy. Additionally, ACT can assist in developing other forms of intimacy with a romantic partner to minimize the impact of sexual dysfunction.

Regardless of diagnosis, intervention should:

- Set realistic expectations. Consider how the patient's primary illness (e.g., depression) may affect their self-view, confidence, communication, and openness with their partner with and without the impact of their sexual dysfunction.
- Normalize, reassure, offer hope. Provide psychoeducation to the patient (and if possible, their partner) about causal, contributing, and treatment factors, and how they may be resolved. Explain they are not alone and open communication with the healthcare provider is critical.
- Discuss the interplay of the multiple factors that may be contributing to dysfunction. Offer strategies to target in a systematic fashion. Identify (and address) comorbid medical conditions (obesity/metabolic syndrome, anemia, pain, urinary incontinence, thyroid problems) as well as psychiatric disorders. For men and women with cardiovascular disease, target lifestyle changes that may decrease the need for the offending medication(s). Address relationship conflict (or loss) if applicable.
- Engage in shared decision-making regarding options (e.g., continue pharmacotherapy, decrease dose, taper off, switch medication, add ameliorating agent).

- Wait and see. While other common side effects usually are short-lived, spontaneous remission of sexual dysfunction associated with psychotropic medication use can take several weeks. However, keep in mind that it is unlikely that remission will occur with *severe* sexual dysfunction, and 4 out of 5 patients will continue to experience it (Montejo-Gonzales et al., 1997).
- Decrease the dose if sexual impairment persists but therapeutic benefit is moderate. This may be better for patients on therapeutic maintenance or who are taking relatively high doses (e.g., Citalopram 40 mg or Sertraline 200 mg). Be mindful of loss of therapeutic benefit; therefore, recommend a slow taper (e.g., decrease 25-50 mg of Sertraline daily every 2-4 weeks) coupled with close monitoring of the patient's symptoms and level of function in other areas of their lives.
- Switch to bupropion or augment with bupropion on an as-needed basis, especially if therapeutic effect has been relatively low and sexual dysfunction is moderate to severe. Use of this medication for SSRI-induced sexual dysfunction is an off-label indication; however, several studies point to the decreased incidence of sexual dysfunction with this agent (Clayton et al., 2004; Gartlehner et al., 2011) .
- Switch to Mirtazapine. A meta-analysis of four randomized trials compared mirtazapine with three commonly used SSRIs (fluoxetine, paroxetine, and sertraline), and found that sexual dysfunction was less likely with mirtazapine (Watanabe et al., 2011)
- Switch to Vortioxetine. It appears to have a lower risk of sexual dysfunction compared to other antidepressants (Alam et al., 2014; Boulenger et al., 2012). In a head to head comparison, vortioxetine resulted in greater improvement of sexual dysfunction compared to escitalopram (Jacobsen et al., 2015).
- Switch to Monoamine Oxidase Inhibitors (MAOIs). Sexual dysfunction was found to be comparable between these agents in a pooled analysis of several randomized trials: agomelatine, moclobemide, selegiline, and placebo (Serretti & Chiesa, 2009). This being said, the risk of a hypertensive crisis when MAOIs interact with dietary sources of tyramine makes treatment with MAOIs risky and potentially impractical.
- Consider pharmacotherapeutic treatment of the specific sexual dysfunction. For men with ED, treatment with a phosphodiesterase-5 inhibitor (e.g., sildenafil, vardenafil) may be warranted. For women with low libido or anorgasmia, bupropion at therapeutic range (extended release 300 mg/day) may be warranted. Some have suggested phosphodiesterase-5 inhibitors for women with delayed orgasm or anorgasmia, but there is contradictory evidence. In a randomized study of almost 800 women with problems of low libido, arousal, orgasm, and/or dyspareunia, Basson et al. (2002) found that sildenafil did not result in improvements in sexual function or satisfaction. Nurnberg et al. (2008) found positive effects on sexual arousal and orgasm with the use of sildenafil with women with SSRI-induced sexual dysfunction.

At least one source recommends considering use of bupropion for women with sexual dysfunction *without* depression or anxiety. In a randomized trial of 75 premenopausal women without underlying depression, sustained release bupropion resulted in reported increased sexual pleasure, arousal, and orgasm (Segraves et al., 2004).

Some data suggest that buspirone (typically used as an antianxiety medication) may be helpful for decreased libido. Flibanserin was the first drug approved by the Federal Drug Administration (FDA) specifically for the treatment of female sexual dysfunction. However, women on SSRIs were specifically excluded from the clinical trials, therefore, safety and efficacy with this population is unclear (Joffe et al., 2016). In 2019, the FDA approved bremelanotide, an injection to be administered 45 minutes before anticipated sexual activity to address arousal disorders. In a randomized 24-week trial, 25% of women had an increase in their sexual desire score, while 35% had a decrease in a distress score, however, it is important to note that there was no difference with placebo with regards to number of satisfying sexual events (Food and Drug Administration, 2019).

In sum, all currently available pharmacotherapies for female sexual disorders are of limited efficacy, so a careful evaluation of potential benefits vs. risks is required. The decision to switch vs. augment psychotropic therapy should follow careful consideration (and shared decision-making) with regard to the unknown and known risks of polypharmacy, including increased adverse effects and difficulties with adherence (Osterberg & Blaschke, 2005; Zajecka, 2001), as well as the potential loss of therapeutic benefits (all of which may impact therapeutic alliance).

Table 3 below and on pages 74-75 describes the effects of several nutraceuticals on sexual dysfunction. It is important to highlight that studies of nutraceuticals generally lack the rigor required by the FDA for the approval of pharmaceuticals. Therefore, caution is advised in recommending the following.

Table 3: Nutraceuticals and Sexual Health

Name	Scientific Name	General Information	Effects on Sexual Health	Side Effects/ Precautions
Maca	Lepidium meyenii	Maca is a root vegetable rich in nitrates that is native to the Peruvian Andes.	1. Women taking Maca have had improvement in antidepressant induced sexual dysfunction. 2. Maca taken daily in healthy young men can increase semen volume, sperm count, and motility as well as sexual desire.	No adverse effects were noted in the studies. Maca does not have any known drugs, herbs, or food interactions.
Yohimbine	Pausinystalia yohimbe	Yohimbe is an evergreen tree that is native to countries in central and western Africa. The bark of this tree contains a chemical called yohimbine.	1. Yohimbine may improve sexual dysfunction associated with SSRIs. 2. Yohimbine appears to help men with various types of ED.	1. Yohimbine can cause hypertension, tachycardia, palpitations, anxiety, sweating, agitation, headache, and insomnia. 2. Yohimbine is contraindicated in patients taking many drugs including TCAs, MAOIs, phenothiazines, anticoagulants, antihypertensives and stimulants.

Table 3: Nutraceuticals and Sexual Health

Name	Scientific Name	General Information	Effects on Sexual Health	Side Effects/ Precautions
L-arginine	2-Amino-5-guanidinopentanoic acid	L-arginine is an amino acid that helps build protein in the body. It is found naturally in foods such as red meat, poultry, fish, and dairy products.	1. L-Arginine taking orally may improve ED. 2. L-Arginine taken orally in high doses seems to improve subjective measures of sexual functioning including intercourse satisfaction, desire, and orgasmic function.	1. May cause gastrointestinal distress including bloating, nausea, diarrhea, headache, and insomnia. 2. Precautions include potential drug/drug interactions with antihypertensive, anticoagulants, and oral hypoglycemic drugs.
Ginkgo	Ginkgo biloba	Ginkgo biloba is a large tree with fan shaped leaves native to Asian countries including China, Japan, and Korea.	1. There is mixed data on whether taking ginkgo leaf extract orally might help sexual dysfunction caused by antidepressant therapy. 2. Some evidence of improved sexual satisfaction in women with sexual dysfunction that have used ginkgo leaf extract in combination with other nutraceuticals.	Side effects include mild gastrointestinal upset, headache, dizziness, palpitations, constipation, and allergic skin reactions. Ginkgo may increase risk of bleeding in patients taking anticoagulants and affect blood glucose levels in diabetics.
Red Ginseng	Panax ginseng	Panax is a plant that grows in Korea, northern China, and far eastern Siberia.	Panax Ginseng taken daily seems to improve sexual function in men with ED as well as improve sexual arousal and satisfaction in postmenopausal women.	Side effects may include headaches, insomnia, gastric upset, rash, and constipation. May also cause hypoglycemia.

Table 3: Nutraceuticals and Sexual Health				
Name	**Scientific Name**	**General Information**	**Effects on Sexual Health**	**Side Effects/ Precautions**
Tribulis	bulis terrestris	Tribulis is a plant that produces fruit covered with spines. It grows in diverse climates. The fruit, leaf, and root are used as medicine.	Taking tribulis daily may improve sexual desire, arousal, satisfaction, orgasm and lubrication in women as well as sexual desire and intercourse satisfaction in men. There is conflicting data on whether tribulis can help ED	Seems to be well tolerated, though excitation, insomnia, and menorrhagia have been reported.
Saffron	Crocus sativus	Saffron is a spice and medicinal plant.	Saffron may help some but not all symptoms of fluoxetine-induced sexual dysfunction in men and women. Women taking saffron had improvement in sexual arousal, lubrication, and pain. Saffron was also an efficacious treatment for fluoxetine-related ED in men.	Typically well tolerated with minimal side effects at low doses (up to 30 mg). Orally saffron can be lethal when taken in doses of 12-20 grams.

<u>Case Vignette</u>

Amelia is a 25-year-old cisgender Latina female who was referred for pharmacotherapy to address symptoms of depression. At the time of her initial evaluation, she was 4 months postpartum and described what seemed like a painful and traumatic labor and delivery experience with medical complications and difficult recovery. She reported that the impact of her depression was evident in her relationship with both of her children (ages 2½ and 4 months), and her spouse of 3 years. She described their relationship as supportive. She described their sexual relationship as "strained," owing to multiple factors including her depression and postpartum recovery.

Amelia was initially trialed on sertraline 50 mg daily but could not tolerate symptoms of nausea and diaphoresis so was ultimately maintained on 37.5 mg daily with beneficial effects to her mood and overall functioning. However, she also experienced sexual dysfunction characterized by decreased libido, and inability to achieve orgasm despite what she described as acceptable stimulation. Given the positive effects on her mood, Amelia opted for continuation of pharmacotherapy and was counseled on communication and other behavioral means of addressing this issue.

Her dysfunction ultimately dissipated about 10 weeks after initiation of treatment, and she reported marked improvement in her quality of life.

Discussion questions: How would you change the care of this patient? What psychosocial factors that may need to be addressed? What other interventions would you consider?

PHARMACOGENETICS AND SEXUAL DYSFUNCTION

Perhaps the best intervention for medication-induced sexual dysfunction is prevention. Only 37% of patients with nonpsychotic major depression achieved remission on first line therapy with a selective serotonin reuptake inhibitor (SSRI) whereas another 16% withdrew completely from treatment because of drug intolerance in the now infamous STAR*D (Sequenced Treatment Alternatives to Relieve Depression; NIMH) trial. Similarly, over 74% of patients with schizophrenia discontinued their antipsychotic medication either because of lack of efficacy or tolerability in the Clinical Antipsychotic Trials of Intervention Effectiveness (CATIE). Finally, over 75% of patients with bipolar disorder experienced symptom relapse when treated with mood stabilizers and antidepressants in The Systematic Treatment Enhancement Program for Bipolar Disorder (STEP BD) trial. These landmark clinical trials emphasize the limited efficacy and undesirable side effects including weight gain, insomnia, and sexual dysfunction of psychotropic medications as well as the opportunity to improve psychiatric treatments (Zandi & Judy, 2010).

Pharmacogenetics is the study of how genetic variations can influence efficacy or tolerability of certain drug treatments. The identification of certain genetic biomarkers that could predict a therapeutic response as well as decreased likelihood of side effects would assist providers in determining the psychiatric care of patients. Most pharmacogenetics tests evaluate the gene variants of the most common Cytochrome P450 (CYP) pathways used in the metabolism of psychotropic drugs. Some individuals carry alleles that encode for inactive or no enzyme at all, whereas others have duplications of certain genes that result in high levels of enzyme activity and thus ultra-rapid metabolism of substrates. Pharmacogenetics will typically tell whether individuals are poor, intermediate, extensive, or ultra-rapid metabolizers. Theoretically, individuals that are poor metabolizers of a certain CYP pathway may be more likely to develop adverse side effects of medication therapy (Lohoff & Ferraro, 2010).

Sexual dysfunction is a major contributor to treatment discontinuation and nonadherence among patients treated with SSRIs and other psychotropics. Genetic polymorphisms of the serotonin and glutamate systems have been associated with sexual dysfunction in patients receiving antidepressant treatments. Of the 1,473 participants in the STAR*D trial, 799 (54%) reported decreased libido, 525 (36%) reported difficulty achieving an orgasm, and 211 of the 574 men (37%) reported erectile dysfunction. Their data showed that single nucleotide polymorphisms in glutamatergic genes were associated with decreased libido (GRIA 3; GRIK2), difficulty achieving orgasm (GRIA 1), and difficulty achieving erection (GRIN 3A) (Perlis et al., 2009).

The therapeutic action of antidepressants is also thought to be at least partially through serotonin neurotransmission. The serotonin transporter 5HTT, which codes for the presynaptic membrane-bound serotonin transporter protein that is the target of SSRIs has been widely studied. The long allele of the promoter polymorphism of 5HTT has been associated with a better response and remission rate as well as lower side effects (Zandi & Judy, 2010). Another possible pathway of sexual side effects from antidepressants may be mediated through serotonin 2A (5HT2A) receptors. Bishop and colleagues (2006) discovered that patients with a GG genotype of the 5HT2A-1438 single nucleotide polymorphisms (SNP) were significantly more likely to be categorized as having sexual dysfunction than persons with a GA or AA genotype. Moreover, the 5HT2A-1438 GG genotype was a significant predictor of lower arousal scores (Bishop et al., 2006).

In addition to genetics, demographic characteristics, diet, substance abuse, smoking, medical and psychological comorbidities, and concurrent drug treatments are other dynamics that may influence treatment response to psychotropic medications. While pharmacogenetics testing may be one strategy in personalizing the psychiatric care of patients, there is still a need for further research to substantiate and clarify how genetic factors can influence treatment response as well as the likelihood of side effects to psychotropic drug regimens. There are also inherent challenges in translating the results of research and pharmacogenetics tests into clinical practice. However, this is an area of practice that will likely grow in interest for patients and providers seeking an alternative to the conventional trial-and-error method of prescribing (Zandi & Judy, 2010).

REFERENCES

Åberg-Wistedt, A., Ågren, H., Ekselius, L., Bengtson, F., & Åkerblad, A. (2000). Sertraline versus Paroxetine in major depression: Clinical outcome after six months of continuous therapy. *Journal of Clinical Psychopharmacology, 20*(6), 645-652. https://doi: 10.1097/00004714-200012000-00010

Alam, M. Y., Jacobsen, P. L., Chen, Y., Serenko, M., & Mahableshwarkar, A. R. (2014). Safety, tolerability, and efficacy of vortioxetine (Lu AA21004) in major depressive disorder: Results of an open-label, flexible-dose, 52-week extension study. *International Clinical Psychopharmacology, 29*(1), 36-44. https://doi.org/10.1097/YIC.0000000000000010

Aldridge, S. A. (1982). Drug-induced sexual dysfunction. *Clinical Pharmacy, 1,* 141-147.

Ali, S. K., Reveles, K. R., Davis, R., Mortensen, E. M., Frei, C. R., & Mansi, I. (2015). The association of statin use and gonado-sexual function in women: A retrospective cohort analysis. *The Journal of Sexual Medicine, 12*(1), 83-92. https://doi.org/10.1111/jsm.12736

AminiLari, M., Manjoo, P., Craigie, S., Couban, R., Wang, L., & Busse, J. W. (2019). Hormone replacement therapy and opioid tapering for opioid-induced hypogonadism among patients with chronic noncancer pain: A systematic review. *Pain Medicine, 20*(2), 301-313. https://doi.org/10.1093/pm/pny040

Atlantis, E., & Sullivan, T. (2012). Bidirectional association between depression and sexual dysfunction: A systematic review and meta-analysis. *The Journal of Sexual Medicine, 9*(6), 1497-1507. https://doi.org/10.1111/j.1743-6109.2012.02709.x

Atmaca, M. (2020). Selective serotonin reuptake inhibitor-induced sexual dysfunction: Current management perspectives. *Neuropsychiatric Disease and Treatment, 16*, 1043-1050. https://doi.org/10.2147/NDT.S185757

Barnes, B. J., & Howard, P. A. (2005). Eplerenone: A selective aldosterone receptor antagonist for patients with heart failure. *The Annals of Pharmacotherapy, 39*(1), 68-76. https://doi.org/10.1345/aph.1E306

Basson R., McInnes R., Smith, M. D., Hodgson, G., & Koppiker, N. (2002). Efficacy and safety of sildenafil citrate in women with sexual dysfunction associated with female sexual arousal disorder. *Journal of Women's Health & Gender Based Medicine, 11*(4), 367-377. https://doi.org/10.1089/152460902317586001

Baumgart, J., Nilsson, K., Evers, A. S., Kallak, T. K., & Poromaa, I. S. (2013). Sexual dysfunction in women on adjuvant endocrine therapy after breast cancer. *Menopause, 20*(2), 162-168. https://doi.org/10.1097/gme.0b013e31826560da

Baumhäkel, M., Schlimmer, N., Böhm, M., & DO-IT Investigators. (2008). Effect of irbesartan on erectile function in patients with hypertension and metabolic syndrome. *International Journal of Impotence Research, 20*(5), 493-500. https://doi.org/10.1038/ijir.2008.28

Baumhäkel, M., Schlimmer, N., Kratz, M., Hackett, G., Jackson, G., & Böhm, M. (2011). Cardiovascular risk, drugs and erectile function--a systematic analysis. *International Journal of Clinical Practice, 65*(3), 289-298. https://doi.org/10.1111/j.1742-1241.2010.02563.x

Benjamin, E. J., Muntner, P., Alonso, A., Bittencourt, M. S., Callaway, C. W., Carson, A. P., Chamberlin, A. R., Chang, A. R., Cheng, S., Das, S. R., Francesca, N. D., Djousse, L., Elkind, M. S. V., Ferguson, J. F., Fornage, M., Jordan, L. C., Khan, S. S., Kissela., B. M., Knutson, K. L., . . . Virani, S. S. (2019). Heart disease and stroke statistics--2019 update: A report from the American Heart Association. *Circulation, 139*(10). E56-528. https://doi.org/10.1161/CIR.0000000000000659

Bishop, J. R., Moline, J., Ellingrod, V. L., Schultz, S. K., & Clayton, A. H. (2006). Serotonin 2A-1438 G/A and G-protein Beta3 subunit C825T polymorphisms in patients with depression and SSRI-associated sexual side-effects. *Neuropsychopharmacology: Official Publication of the American College of Neuropsychopharmacology*, *31*(10), 2281-2288. https://doi.org/10.1038/sj.npp.1301090

Blood Pressure Lowering Treatment Trialists' Collaboration. (2014). Blood pressure-lowering treatment based on cardiovascular risk: A meta-analysis of individual patient data. *Lancet*, *384*(9943), 591-598. https://doi.org/10.1016/S0140-6736(14)61212-5

Boulenger, J. P., Loft, H., & Florea, I. (2012). A randomized clinical study of Lu AA21004 in the prevention of relapse in patients with major depressive disorder. *Journal of Psychopharmacology*, *26*(11), 1408-1416. https://doi.org/10.1177/0269881112441866

Budzak, L. M., Yasin, W., & Mulhall, J. (2019). Raising more than moods: Escitalopram-associated priapism. *Federal Practitioner: For the Health Care Professionals of the VA, DOD, and PHS*, *36*(2), 94-96.

Burrows, L. J., Basha, M., & Goldstein, A. T. (2012). The effects of hormonal contraceptives on female sexuality: A review. *The Journal of Sexual Medicine*, *9*(9), 2213-2223. https://doi.org/10.1111/j.1743-6109.2012.02848.x

Butt, M. R., Lema, V., Mukaindo, A., Mohamoud, G., & Shabani, J. (2019). Prevalence of and factors associated with female sexual dysfunction among women using hormonal and non-hormonal contraception at the AGA Khan University Hospital Nairobi. *African Journal of Primary Health Care & Family Medicine*, *11*(1), e1-e9. https://doi.org/10.4102/phcfm.v11i1.1955

Cai, X., Tian, Y., Wu, T., Cao, C. X., Bu, S. Y., & Wang, K. J. (2014). The role of statins in erectile dysfunction: A systematic review and meta-analysis. *Asian Journal of Andrology*, *16*(3), 461-466. https://doi.org/10.4103/1008-682X.123678

Carey, J. C. (2006). Pharmacological effects on sexual function. *Obstetrics and Gynecology Clinics of North America*, *33*(4), 599-620. https://doi.org/10.1016/j.ogc.2006.10.005

Caro, J. L. L., Vidal, L., Roca, M. A., Bravo, C. P., Vicente, J. A., & Ferrario, C. M. (2001). Sexual dysfunction in hypertensive patients treated with losartan. *The American Journal of Medical Sciences,* 321(5), 336-341.

Cartwright, C., Gibson, K., Read, J., Cowan, O., & Dehar, T. (2016). Long-term antidepressant use: Patient perspectives of benefits and adverse effects. *Patient Preference and Adherence*, *10*, 1401-1407. https://doi.org/10.2147/PPA.S110632

Cavalheiro, J., Bittelbrunn, A., Menke, C., Biazús, J., Xavier, N., & Cericatto, R., Schuh, F., Pinheiro, C. V., & Passos, E. P. (2012). Sexual function and chemotherapy in postmenopausal women with breast cancer. *BMC Women's Health*, *12*(28), 1-8. https://doi.org/10.1186/1472-6874-12-28

Cholesterol Treatment Trialists' (CTT) Collaborators, Mihaylova, B., Emberson, J., Blackwell, L., Keech, A., Simes, J., Barnes, E. H., Voysey, M., Gray, A., Collins, R., & Baigent, C. (2012). The effects of lowering LDL cholesterol with statin therapy in people at low risk of vascular disease: Meta-analysis of individual data from 27 randomised trials. *Lancet*, *380*(9841), 581-590. https://doi.org/10.1016/S0140-6736(12)60367-5

Chou, N. H., Huang, Y. J., & Jiann, B. P. (2015). The impact of illicit use of amphetamine on male sexual functions. *The Journal of Sexual Medicine*, *12*(8), 1694-1702. https://doi.org/10.1111/jsm.12926

Choy, C. L., Sidi, H., Koon, C. S., Ming, O. S., Mohamed, I. N., Guan, N. C., & Alfonso, C. A. (2019). Systematic review and meta-analysis for sexual dysfunction in women with hypertension. *The Journal of Sexual Medicine*, *16*(7), 1029-1048. https://doi.org/10.1016/j.jsxm.2019.04.007

Cipriani, A., Furukawa, T., Salanti, G., Chaimani, A., Atkinson, L., Ogawa, Y., Leucht, S., Ruhe, H. G., Turner, E. H., Higgins, J. P. T., Egger, M., Takeshima, N., Hayasaka, Y., Imai, H., Shinohara, K., Tajika, A., Ioannidis, J. P. A., & Geddes, J. R. (2018). Comparative efficacy and acceptability of 21 antidepressant drugs for the acute treatment of adults with major depressive disorder: A systematic review and network meta-analysis. *The Lancet*, *391*(10128), 1357-1366. https://doi.org/10.1016/s0140-6736(17)32802-7

Clayton, A., Keller, A., & McGarvey, E. L. (2006). Burden of phase-specific sexual dysfunction with SSRIs. *Journal of Affective Disorders*, *91*(1), 27-32. https://doi.org/10.1016/j.jad.2005.12.007

Clayton, A. H., Segraves, R. T., Leiblum, S., Basson, R., Pyke, R., Cotton, D., Lewis-D'Agostino, D., Evans, K. R., Sills, T. L., & Wunderlich, G. R. (2006). Reliability and validity of the Sexual Interest and Desire Inventory-Female (SIDI-F), a scale designed to measure severity of female hypoactive sexual desire disorder. *Journal of Sex & Marital Therapy*, *32*(2), 115-135. https://doi.org/10.1080/00926230500442300

Clayton, A. H., Warnock, J. K., Kornstein, S. G., Pinkerton, R., Sheldon-Keller, A., & McGarvey, E. L. (2004). A placebo-controlled trial of bupropion SR as an antidote for selective serotonin reuptake inhibitor-induced sexual dysfunction. *The Journal of Clinical Psychiatry*, *65*(1), 62-67. https://doi.org/10.4088/jcp.v65n0110

Cordero, A., Bertomeu-Martinez, V., Mazon, P., Facila, L., Conthe, P., & Gonzalez-Juanatey, J. R. (2010). Erectile dysfunction in high risk hypertensive patients with beta blocked agents. *Cardiovascular Therapeutics, 28,* 15-22. https://doi.org/10.1111/j.1755-5922.2009.00123.x

Cui, T., Kovell, R. C., Brooks, D. C., & Terlecki, R. P. (2015). A urologist's guide to ingredients found in top-selling nutraceuticals for men's sexual health. *The Journal of Sexual Medicine, 12*(11), 2105-2117. https://doi.org/10.1111/jsm.13013

De Berardis, D., Marini, S., Serroni, N., Iasevoli, F., Tomasetti, C., de Bartolomeis, A., Mazza, M., Tempesta, D., Valchera, A., Fornaro, M., Pompili, M., Sepede, G., Vellante, F., Orsolini, L., Martinotti, G., & Di Giannantonio, M. (2015). Targeting the noradrenergic system in posttramatic stress disorder: A systematic review and meta-analysis of prazosin trials. *Current Drug Targets, 16*(10), 1094-1106. https://doi.org/10.2174/1389450116666150506114108

Della Chiesa, A., Pfiffner, D., Meier, B., & Hess, O. M. (2003). Sexual activity in hypertensive men. *Journal of Human Hypertension, 17*(8), 515-521. https://doi.org/10.1038/sj.jhh.1001580

De Nunzio, C., Roehrborn, C. G., Andersson, K. E., & McVary, K. T. (2017). Erectile dysfunction and lower urinary tract symptoms. *European Urology Focus, 3*(4-5), 352-363. https://doi.org/10.1016/j.euf.2017.11.004

Derby, C. A., Barbour, M. M., Hume, A. L., & McKinlay, J. B. (2001). Drug therapy and prevalence of erectile dysfunction in the Massachusetts Male Aging Study cohort. *Pharmacotherapy, 21*(6), 676-683. https://doi.org/10.1592/phco.21.7.676.34571

de Vries, F., Bruin, M., Lobatto, D. J., Dekkers, O. M., Schoones, J. W., van Furth, W. R., Pereira, A. M., Karavitaki, N., Biermasz, N. R., Zamanipoor, N., & Amir, H. (2020). Opioids and their endocrine effects: A systematic review and meta-analysis. *The Journal of Clinical Endocrinology & Metabolism, 105*(4). https://doi.org/10.1210/clinem/dgz022

Dissiz, M. (2019). Evaluation of sexual function in Turkish male individuals who are substance abusers: A descriptive study. *Addictive Disorders & Their Treatment 18*(3), 176-183. https://doi: 10.1097/ADT.0000000000000172

Dolatshahi, B., Farhoudian, A., Falahatdoost, M., Tavakoli, M., & Rezaie Dogahe, E. (2016). A qualitative study of the relationship between methamphetamine abuse and sexual dysfunction in male substance abusers. *International Journal of High Risk Behaviors & Addiction, 5*(3), https://doi: 10.5812/ijhrba.29640

Donovan, K. A., Gonzalez, B. D., Nelson, A. M., Fishman, M. N., Zachariah, B., & Jacobsen, P. B. (2018). Effect of androgen deprivation therapy on sexual function and bother in men with prostate cancer: A controlled comparison. *Psycho-oncology, 27*(1), 316-324. https://doi.org/10.1002/pon.4463

Dording, C. M., Schettler, P. J., Dalton, E. D., Parkin, S. R., Walker, R. S., Fehling, K. B., Fava, M., & Mischoulon, D. (2015). A double-blind placebo-controlled trial of maca root as treatment for antidepressant-induced sexual dysfunction in women. *Evidence-Based Complementary and Alternative Medicine, 2015*, 949036. https://doi.org/10.1155/2015/949036

Doumas, M., Tsakiris, A., Douma, S., Grigorakis, A., Papadopoulos, A., Hounta, A., Tsiodras, S., Dimitriou, D., & Giamarellou, H. (2006). Beneficial effects of switching from beta-blockers to nebivolol on the erectile function of hypertensive patients. *Asian Journal of Andrology, 8*(2), 177-182. https://doi.org/10.1111/j.1745-7262.2006.00076.x

Downing, L., Kim, D. D., Procyshyn, R., & Tibbo, P. (2019). Management of sexual adverse effects induced by atypical antipsychotic medication. *Journal of Psychiatry & Neuroscience, 44*(4), 287-288. https://doi.org/10.1503/jpn.190053

Due, D. L., Giguere, G. C., & Plachetka, J. R. (1986). Postmarketing comparison of labetalol and propranolol in hypertensive patients. *Clinical Therapeutics, 8*(6), 624-631.

Duncan, L., & Bateman, D. N. (1993). Sexual function in women. Do antihypertensive drugs have an impact? *Drug Safety, 8*(3), 225-234. https://doi.org/10.2165/00002018-199308030-00004

Edvinsson, D., & Ekselius, L. (2018). Long-term tolerability and safety of pharmacological treatment of adult attention-deficit/hyperactivity disorder: A 6-year prospective naturalistic study. *Journal of Clinical Psychopharmacology, 38*(4), 370-375. https://doi.org/10.1097/JCP.0000000000000917

Ekinci, O., Üstündağ, B., Tunali, B. D., Abdulrazzaq Al-Bayati, M. B., Demir, H., & Adak, İ. (2019). Priapism with methylphenidate use in a preschool-aged boy resolved with switching to atomoxetine. *Clinical Neuropharmacology, 42*(5), 184-185. https://doi.org/10.1097/WNF.0000000000000357

Engbaek, M., Hjerrild, M., Hallas, J., & Jacobsen, I. A. (2010). The effect of low-dose spironolactone on resistant hypertension. *Journal of the American Society of Hypertension, 4*(6), 290-294. https://doi.org/10.1016/j.jash.2010.10.001

Engel, G. L., (1992). The need for a new medical model: A challenge for biomedicine. *Family Systems Medicine, 10*(3), 317-331. http://dx.doi.org/10.1037/h0089260

Epocrates. (January, 2020). *Disulfiram* [Epocrates - online medical reference app]. https://online.epocrates.com/drugs/217705/Antabuse/Adverse-Reactions

Erdman, E. (2009). Safety and tolerability of beta-blockers: Prejudices and reality. *European Heart Journal Supplements.* Supplement A, A21-25. https://doi.org/10.1093/eurheartj/sup001

Ernst, E., & Pittler, M. H. (1998). Yohimbine for erectile dysfunction: A systematic review and meta-analysis of randomized clinical trials. *The Journal of Urology*, *159*(2), 433-436. https://doi.org/10.1016/s0022-5347(01)63942-9

Falk, S. J., & Dizon, D. S. (2013). Sexual dysfunction in women with cancer. *Fertility and Sterility, 100*(4), 916-921. https://doi.org/10.1016/j.fertnstert.2013.08.18

Fava, M., Rush, A. J., Thase, M. E., Clayton, A., Stahl, S. M., Pradko, J. F., & Johnston, J. A. (2005). 15 years of clinical experience with bupropion HCl: From bupropion to bupropion SR to bupropion XL. *Primary Care Companion to the Journal of Clinical Psychiatry, 7*(3), 106-113. https://doi.org/10.4088/pcc.v07n0305

Fogari, R., Preti, P., Derosa, G., Marasi, G., Zoppi, A., Rinaldi, A., & Mugellini, A. (2002). Effect of antihypertensive treatment with valsartan or atenolol on sexual activity and plasma testosterone in hypertensive men. *European Journal of Clinical Pharmacology*, *58*(3), 177-180. https://doi.org/10.1007/s00228-002-0456-3

Fogari, R., Preti, P., Zoppi, A., Corradi, L., Pasotti, C., Rinaldi, A. & Mugellini, A. (2004). Effect of Valsartan and Atenolol on sexual behavior in hypertensive postmenopausal women. *American Journal of Hypertension,* 17(1), 77-81. https://doi.org/10.1016/j.amjhyper.2003.08.016

Fogari, R., & Zoppi, A. (2004). Effect of antihypertensive agents on quality of life in the elderly. *Drugs & Aging*, *21*(6), 377-393. https://doi.org/10.2165/00002512-200421060-00003

Fogari, R., Zoppi, A., Poletti, L., Marasi, G., Mugellini, A., & Corradi, L. (2001). Sexual activity in hypertensive men treated with valsartan or carvedilol: A crossover study. *American Journal of Hypertension*, *14*(1), 27-31. https://doi.org/10.1016/s0895-7061(00)01214-0

Food and Drug Administration. (January, 2019). *FDA approves new treatment for hypoactive sexual desire disorder in premenopausal women* [FDA news release]. https://www.fda.gov/news-events/press-announcements/fda-approves-new-treatment-hypoactive-sexual-desire-disorder-premenopausal-women

Foy, C. G., Newman, J. C., Berlowitz, D. R., Russell, L. P., Kimmel, P. L., Wadley, V. G., Thomas, H. N., Lerner, A. J., Riley, W. T., & SPRINT Study Research Group. (2016). Blood pressure, sexual activity, and dysfunction in women with hypertension: Baseline findings from the systolic blood pressure intervention trial (SPRINT). *The Journal of Sexual Medicine*, *13*(9), 1333-1346. https://doi.org/10.1016/j.jsxm.2016.06.014

Fuentes, A. V., Pineda, M. D., & Venkata, K. (2018). Comprehension of top 200 prescribed drugs in the US as a resource for pharmacy teaching, training and practice. *Pharmacy, 6*(2), 43. https://doi.org/10.3390/pharmacy6020043

García-Blanco, A., García-Portilla, M. P., Fuente-Tomás, L., Batalla, M., Sánchez-Autet, M., Arranz, B., Safont, G., Arqués, S., Livianos, L., & Sierra, P. (2020). Sexual dysfunction and mood stabilizers in long-term stable patients with bipolar disorder. *The Journal of Sexual Medicine*, *17*(5), 930-940. https://doi.org/10.1016/j.jsxm.2020.01.032

Gartlehner, G., Hansen, R. A., Morgan, L. C., Thaler, K., Lux, L., Van Noord, M., Mager, U., Thieda, P., Gaynes, B. N., Wilkins, T., Strobelberger, M., Lloyd, S., Reichenpfader, U., & Lohr, K. N. (2011). Comparative benefits and harms of second-generation antidepressants for treating major depressive disorder: An updated meta-analysis. *Annals of Internal Medicine*, *155*(11), 772-785. https://doi.org/10.7326/0003-4819-155-11-201112060-00009

George, K. C., Kebejian, L., Ruth, L. J., Miller, C. W. T., & Himelhoch, S. (2016). Meta-analysis of the efficacy and safety of prazosin versus placebo for the treatment of nightmares and sleep disturbances in adults with posttraumatic stress disorder. *Journal of Trauma & Dissociation, 17*(4), 494-510. https://doi.org/10.1080/15299732.2016.1141150

Goldfarb, S., Mulhall, J., Nelson, C., Kelvin, J., Dickler, M., & Carter, J. (2013). Sexual and reproductive health in cancer survivors. *Seminars in Oncology*, *40*(6), 726-744. https://doi.org/10.1053/j.seminoncol.2013.09.002

Gómez Sánchez-Lafuente, C., Reina Gonzalez, R., & Hernandez Abellán, M. (2017). Sexual dysfunction and mood stabilizers in bipolar disorder: A review. *European Psychiatry*, *41*(S1), s849. https://doi.org/10.1016/j.eurpsy.2017.01.1682

Grant, J. E., Redden, S. A., Lust, K., & Chamberlain, S. R. (2018). Nonmedical use of stimulants is associated with riskier sexual practices and other forms of impulsivity. *Journal of Addiction Medicine*, *12*(6), 474-480. https://doi.org/10.1097/ADM.0000000000000448

Grover, S., Ghosh, A., Sarkar, S., Chakrabarti, S., & Avasthi, A. (2014). Sexual dysfunction in clinically stable patients with bipolar disorder receiving lithium. *Journal of Clinical Psychopharmacology*, *34*(4), 475-482. https://doi.org/10.1097/JCP.0000000000000131

Gudin, J. A., Laitman, A., & Nalamachu, S. (2015). Opioid related endocrinopathy. *Pain Medicine, 16*(1), S9-S15. https://doi.org/10.1111/pme.12926

Hashim, M. A., El Rasheed, A. H., Ismail, G., Awaad, M. I., El Habiby, M. M., Mohsen Ibrahim, N. M., & Abdeen, M. S. (2020). Sexual dysfunction in tramadol hydrochloride use disorder male patients: A case-control study. *International Clinical Psychopharmacology*, *35*(1), 42-48. https://doi.org/10.1097/YIC.0000000000000286

Hayon, R., & Stevenson, K. (2019). Hormonal, medical, and nonsurgical aspects of gender affirmation. *Facial Plastic Surgery Clinics of North America, 27*(2), 179-190. https://doi.org/10.1016/j.fsc.2018.12.001

Heron, M. (2019). Deaths: Leading causes for 2017. *National Vital Statistics Reports. 68*(6), 1-76. https://www.cdc.gov/nchs/data/nvsr/nvsr68/nvsr68_06-508.pdf.

Hogan, M. J., Wallin, J. D., & Baer, R. M. (1980). Antihypertensive therapy and male sexual dysfunction. *Psychosomatics, 21,* 234-237. https://doi.org/10.1016/S0033-3182(80)73698-8

Jacobsen, P. L., Mahableshwarkar, A. R., Chen, Y., Chrones, L., & Clayton, A. H. (2015). Effect of vortioxetine vs. escitalopram on sexual functioning in adults with well-treated major depressive disorder experiencing SSRI-induced sexual dysfunction. *The Journal of Sexual Medicine, 12*(10), 2036-2048. https://doi.org/10.1111/jsm.12980

Jacobson, P., Nomikos, G., Zhong, W., Cutler, A., Affinito, J., & Clayton, A. (2020). Clinical implications of directly switching antidepressants in well-treated depressed patients with treatment-emergent sexual dysfunction: A comparison between vortioxetine and escitalopram. *CNS Spectrums, 25*(1), 50-63. https://doi.org/10/1017/S1092852919000750

Jiannine, L. M. (2018). An investigation of the relationship between physical fitness, self-concept, and sexual functioning. *Journal of Education and Health Promotion, 7*, 57. https://doi.org/10.4103/jehp.jehp_157_17

Joffe, H. V., Chang, C., Sewell, C., Easley, O., Nguyen, C., Dunn, S., Lehrfeld, K., Lee, L., Kim, M. J., Slagle, A. F., & Beitz, J. (2016). FDA approval of Flibanserin--Treating hypoactive sexual desire disorder. *The New England Journal of Medicine, 374*(2), 101-104. https://www.nejm.org/doi/full/10.1056/NEJMp1513686

Kashani, L., Raisi, F., Saroukhani, S., Sohrabi, H., Modabbernia, A., Nasehi, A. A., Jamshidi, A., Ashrafi, M., Mansouri, P., Ghaeli, P., & Akhondzadeh, S. (2013). Saffron for treatment of fluoxetine-induced sexual dysfunction in women: Randomized double-blind placebo-controlled study. *Human Psychopharmacology, 28*(1), 54-60. https://doi.org/10.1002/hup.2282

Katz, N., & Mazer, N. A. (2009). The impact of opioids on the endocrine system. *The Clinical Journal of Pain, 25*(2), 170-175. https://doi.org/10.1097/AJP.0b013e3181850df6

Kelly, B. D., Lundon, D. J., McGuinness, D., & Brady, C. M. (2013). Methylphenidate-induced erections in a prepubertal child. *Journal of Pediatric Urology, 9*(1), e1-e2. https://doi.org/10.1016/j.jpurol.2012.03.017

Kerckhof, M. E., Kreukels, B., Nieder, T. O., Becker-Hébly, I., van de Grift, T. C., Staphorsius, A. S., Köhler, A., Heylens, G., & Elaut, E. (2019). Prevalence of sexual dysfunctions in transgender persons: Results from the ENIGI follow-up study. *The Journal of Sexual Medicine, 16*(12), 2018-2029. https://doi.org/10.1016/j.jsxm.2019.09.003

Ko, D. T., Hebert, P. R., Coffey, C. S., Sedrakyan, A., Curtis, J. P., & Krumholz, H. M. (2002). Beta-blocker therapy and symptoms of depression, fatigue, and sexual dysfunction. *JAMA, 288*(3), 351-357. https://doi.org/10.1001/jama.288.3.351

Kostis, J. B., & Dobrzynski, J. M. (2014). The effect of statins on erectile dysfunction: A meta-analysis of randomized trials. *The Journal of Sexual Medicine, 11*(7), 1626-1635. https://doi.org/10.1111/jsm.12521

La Torre, A., Giupponi, G., Duffy, D., Conca, A., Cai, T., & Scardigli, A. (2016). Sexual dysfunction related to drugs: A critical review. Part V: α-blocker and 5-ARI drugs. *Pharmacopsychiatry, 49*(1), 3-13. https://doi.org/10.1055/s-0035-1565100

Lexicomp. (March, 2020). *Propranolol* [Lexicomp – online medical reference site]. https://online.lexi.com/lco/action/home.

Lohoff, F. W., & Ferraro, T. N. (2010). Pharmacogenetic considerations in the treatment of psychiatric disorders. *Expert Opinion on Pharmacotherapy, 11*(3), 423-439. https://doi.org/10.1517/14656560903508762

Lorenz, T., Rullo, J., & Faubion, S. (2016). Antidepressant-induced female sexual dysfunction. *Mayo Clinic Proceedings, 91*(9), 1280-1286. https://doi.org/10.1016/j.mayocp.2016.04.033

Macdonald, P. T., Waldorf, D., Reinarman, C., & Murphy S. (1988). Heavy cocaine use and sexual behavior. *Journal of Drug Issues, 18*(3), 437-455. https://doi.org/10.1177/002204268801800309

McGahuey, C., Gelenberg, A., Laukes, C., Moreno, F., Delgado, P., McKnight, K., & Manber, R. (2000). The Arizona Sexual Experience Scale (ASEX): Reliability and validity. *Journal of Sex & Marital Therapy, 26*(1), 25-40. https://doi.org/10.1080/009262300278623

McWilliams, K., Simmons, C., Laird, B. J., & Fallon, M. T. (2014). A systematic review of opioid effects on the hypogonadal axis of cancer patients. *Supportive Care in Cancer, 22*(6), 1699-1704.

Meston, C. M. (2003). Validation of the Female Sexual Function Index (FSFI) in women with female orgasmic disorder and in women with hypoactive sexual desire disorder. *Journal of Sex & Marital Therapy, 29*(1), 39-46. https://doi.org/10.1080/713847100

Mitchell, K., Lewis, R. S., Satterfield, J., & Hong, B. A. (2016). The new Medical College Admission Test: Implications for teaching psychology. The American Psychologist, 71(2), 125-135. https://doi.org/10.1037/a0039975

Mitchell, L., Govind, V., Barela, K., & Goldstein, A. T. (2019). Spironolactone may be a cause of hormonally associated vestibulodynia and female sexual arousal disorder. *The Journal of Sexual Medicine*, *16*(9), 1481-1483. https://doi.org/10.1016/j.jsxm.2019.06.012

Modabbernia, A., Sohrabi, H., Nasehi, A. A., Raisi, F., Saroukhani, S., Jamshidi, A., Tabrizi, M., Ashrafi, M., & Akhondzadeh, S. (2012). Effect of saffron on fluoxetine-induced sexual impairment in men: Randomized double-blind placebo-controlled trial. *Psychopharmacology*, *223*(4), 381-388. https://doi.org/10.1007/s00213-012-2729-6

Montejo, A. L., García, M., Espada, M., Rico-Villademoros, F., Llorca, G., & Izquierdo, J. A. (2000). Propiedades psicométricas del cuestionario de disfunción sexual secundaria a psicofármacos. Grupo Español de trabajo para el estudio de las disfunciones sexuales secundarias a psicofármacos [Psychometric characteristics of the psychotropic-related sexual dysfunction questionnaire. Spanish work group for the study of psychotropic-related sexual dysfunctions]. *Actas Espanolas de Psiquiatria*, *28*(3), 141-150.

Montejo, A. L., Prieto, N., de Alarcón, R., Casado-Espada, N., de la Iglesia, J., & Montejo, L. (2019). Management strategies for antidepressant-related sexual dysfunction: A clinical approach. *Journal of Clinical Medicine*, *8*(10), 1640. https://doi.org/10.3390/jcm8101640

Montejo-González, A. L., Llorca, G., Izquierdo, J. A., Ledesma, A., Bousoño, M., Calcedo, A., Carrasco, J. L., Ciudad, J., Daniel, E., De la Gandara, J., Derecho, J., Franco, M., Gomez, M. J., Macias, J. A., Martin, T., Perez, V., Sanchez, J. M., Sanchez, S., & Vicens, E. (1997). SSRI-induced sexual dysfunction: Fluoxetine, paroxetine, sertraline, and fluvoxamine in a prospective, multicenter, and descriptive clinical study of 344 patients. *Journal of Sex & Marital Therapy, 23*(3), 176-194.

Morrissette, D. L., Skinner, M. H., Hoffman, B. B., Levine, R. E., & Davidson, J. M. (1993). Effects of antihypertensive drugs atenolol and nifedipine on sexual function in older men: A placebo-controlled, crossover study. *Archives of Sexual Behavior, 22,* 99-109. https://doi.org/10.1007/BF01542360

Murad, M. H., Elamin, M. B., Garcia, M. Z., Mullan, R. J., Murad, A., Erwin, P. J., & Montori, V. M. (2010). Hormonal therapy and sex reassignment: A systematic review and meta-analysis of quality of life and psychosocial outcomes. *Clinical Endocrinology*, *72*(2), 214-231. https://doi.org/10.1111/j.1365-2265.2009.03625.x

Nguyen, C., Lairson, D. R., Swartz, M. D., & Du, X. L. (2018). Risks of major long-term side effects associated with androgen-deprivation therapy in men with prostate cancer. *Pharmacotherapy*, *38*(10), 999-1009. https://doi.org/10.1002/phar.2168

Nicolai, M. P. J., Both, S., Liem, S. S., Pelger, R., Putter, H., Schalij, M., & Elzevier, H. (2013). Discussing sexual function in the cardiology practice. *Clinical Research in Cardiology, 102,* 329-336. https://doi.org/10.1007/s00392-013-0549-2

Nurnberg, H. G., Hensley, P. L., Heiman, J. R., Croft, H. A., Debattista, C., & Paine, S. (2008). Sildenafil treatment of women with antidepressant-associated sexual dysfunction: A randomized controlled trial. *JAMA*, *300*(4), 395-404. https://doi.org/10.1001/jama.300.4.395

Olfson, M., King, M., & Schoenbaum, M. (2015). Benzodiazepine use in the United States. *JAMA Psychiatry*, *72*(2), 136-142. http://doi.org/10.1001/jamapsychiatry.2014.1763

Osterberg, L., Blaschke T. (2005). Adherence to medication. *The New England Journal of Medicine, 353*(5), 487-497. https://www.nejm.org/doi/full/10.1056/nejmra050100

Palha, A. P., & Esteves, M. (2008). Drugs of abuse and sexual functioning. *Advances in Psychosomatic Medicine, 29,* 131-149. https://doi.org/10.1159/000126628

Parthasarathy, H. K., Ménard, J., White, W. B., Young, W. F., Jr, Williams, G. H., Williams, B., Ruilope, L. M., McInnes, G. T., Connell, J. M., & MacDonald, T. M. (2011). A double-blind, randomized study comparing the antihypertensive effect of eplerenone and spironolactone in patients with hypertension and evidence of primary aldosteronism. *Journal of Hypertension*, *29*(5), 980-990. https://doi.org/10.1097/HJH.0b013e3283455ca5

Pastor, Z., Holla, K., & Chmel, R. (2013). The influence of combined oral contraceptives on female sexual desire: A systematic review. *The European Journal of Contraception & Reproductive Health Care: The Official Journal of the European Society of Contraception, 18*(1), 27-43. https://doi.org/10.3109/13625187.2012.728643

Patel, K., Allen, S., Haque, M. N., Angelescu, I., Baumeister, D., & Tracy, D. K. (2016). Bupropion: A systematic review and meta-analysis of effectiveness as an antidepressant. *Therapeutic Advances in Psychopharmacology, 6*(2), 99-144. https://doi.org/10.1177/2045125316629071

Perlis, R. H., Laje, G., Smoller, J. W., Fava, M., Rush, A. J., & McMahon, F. J. (2009). Genetic and clinical predictors of sexual dysfunction in citalopram-treated depressed patients. *Neuropsychopharmacology: Official Publication of the American College of Neuropsychopharmacology, 34*(7), 1819-1828. https://doi.org/10.1038/npp.2009.4

Poole-Wilson, P. A., Kirwan, B. A., Vokó, Z., de Brouwer, S., van Dalen, F. J., Lubsen, J., & ACTION Investigators (2006). Safety of nifedipine GITS in stable angina: The ACTION trial. *Cardiovascular Drugs and Therapy, 20*(1), 45-54. https://doi.org/10.1007/s10557-006-6312-4

Procyshyn, R., Bezchlibnyk-Butler, K., & Jeffries, J. (Eds.). (2019). *Clinical Handbook of Psychotropic Drugs* (23rd ed.). Hogrefe.

Reichenpfader, U., Gartlehner, G., Morgan, L. C., Greenblatt, A., Nussbaumer, B., Hansen, R. A., Van Noord, M., Lux, L., & Gaynes, B. N. (2014). Sexual dysfunction associated with second-generation antidepressants in patients with major depressive disorder: Results from a systematic review with network meta-analysis. *Drug Safety, 37*(1), 19-31. https://doi.org/10.1007/s40264-013-0129-4

Rhim, H. C., Kim, M. S., Park, Y. J., Choi, W. S., Park, H. K., Kim, H. G., Kim, A., & Paick, S. H. (2019). The potential role of arginine supplements on erectile dysfunction: A systemic review and meta-analysis. *The Journal of Sexual Medicine, 16*(2), 223-234. https://doi.org/10.1016/j.jsxm.2018.12.002

Rhodin, A., Stridsberg, M., & Gordh, T. (2010). Opioid endocrinopathy: A clinical problem in patients with chronic pain and long-term oral opioid treatment. *The Clinical Journal of Pain, 26*(5), 374-380. https://doi.org/10.1097/AJP.0b013e3181d1059d

Rosen, R. C., Riley, A., Wagner, G., Osterloh, I. H., Kirkpatrick, J., & Mishra, A. (1997). The international index of erectile function (IIEF): A multidimensional scale for assessment of erectile dysfunction. *Urology*, *49*(6), 822-830. https://doi.org/10.1016/s0090-4295(97)00238-0

Rudberg, L., Carlsson, M., Nilsson, S., & Wikblad, K. (2002). Self-perceived physical, psychologic, and general symptoms in survivors of testicular cancer 3 to 13 years after treatment. *Cancer Nursing*, *25*(3), 187-195. https://doi.org/10.1097/00002820-200206000-00003

Segraves, R. T., Clayton, A., Croft, H., Wolf, A., & Warnock, J. (2004). Bupropion sustained release for the treatment of hypoactive sexual desire disorder in premenopausal women. *Journal of Clinical Psychopharmacology*, *24*(3), 339-342. https://doi.org/10.1097/01.jcp.0000125686.20338.c1

Serretti, A., & Chiesa, A. (2009). Treatment-emergent sexual dysfunction related to antidepressants: A meta-analysis. *Journal of Clinical Psychopharmacology*, *29*(3), 259-266. https://doi.org/10.1097/JCP.0b013e3181a5233f

Shabsigh, R., Perelman, M. A., Lockhart, D. C., Lue, T. F., & Broderick, G. A. (2005). Health issues of men: Prevalence and correlates of erectile dysfunction. *The Journal of Urology*, *174*(2), 662-667. https://doi.org/10.1097/01.ju.0000165389.73148.d1

Shamloul, R. (2009). Natural aphrodisiacs. *International Society for Sexual Medicine*, 7, 39-49. https://doi.org/10.1111/j.1743-6109.2009.01521.x

Sica, D. A. (2003). Diuretics. *Side Effects of Drugs Annual, 26,* 238-242. https://doi.org/10.1016/S0378-6080(03)80028-4

Smith, N. K., Jozkowski, K. N., & Sanders, S. A. (2014). Hormonal contraception and female pain, orgasm and sexual pleasure. *The Journal of Sexual Medicine*, *11*(2), 462-470. https://doi.org/10.1111/jsm.12409

Spatz, E. S., Canavan, M. E., Desai, M. M., Krumholz, H. M., & Lindau, S. T. (2013). Sexual activity and function among middle-aged and older men and women with hypertension. *Journal of Hypertension*, *31*(6), 1096-1105. https://doi.org/10.1097/HJH.0b013e32835fdefa

Speel, T. G., Kiemeney, L. A., Thien, T., Smits, P., & Meuleman, E. J. (2005). Long-term effect of inhibition of the angiotensin-converting enzyme (ACE) on cavernosal perfusion in men with atherosclerotic erectile dysfunction: A pilot study. *The Journal of Sexual Medicine*, *2*(2), 207-212. https://doi.org/10.1111/j.1743-6109.2005.20230.x

Stahl, S. M., Grady, M. M., & Muntner, N. (2018). *Stahl's Essential Psychopharmacology: Prescriber's Guide*. Cambridge University Press.

Stanton, A. M., Handy, A. B., & Meston, C. M. (2018). The effects of exercise on sexual function in women. *Sexual Medicine Reviews*, *6*(4), 548-557. https://doi.org/10.1016/j.sxmr.2018.02.004

Stevenson, J. G., & Umstead, G. S. (1984). Sexual dysfunction due to antihypertensive agents. *Drug Intelligence & Clinical Pharmacy*, *18*(2), 113-121. https://doi.org/10.1177/106002808401800204

Taylor, D., Young, A., & Barnes, T. (2018). *The Maudsley Prescribing Guidelines in Psychiatry* (13th ed.). Wiley-Blackwell.

Thakurta, R. G., Singh, O. P., Bhattacharya, A., Mallick, A. K., Ray, P., Sen, S., & Das, R. (2012). Nature of sexual dysfunctions in major depressive disorder and its impact on quality of life. *Indian Journal of Psychological Medicine*, *34*(4), 365-370. https://doi.org/10.4103/0253-7176.108222

Therapeutic Research Center. (March, 2020). *Natural Medicines Database*. TRC. https://naturalmedicines.therapeuticresearch.com/.

T'Sjoen, G., Arcelus, J., Gooren, L., Klink, D. T., & Tangpricha, V. (2019). Endocrinology of transgender medicine. *Endocrinology Review, 40*(1), 97-117. https://doi.org/10.1210/er.2018-00011

United Nations. Department of Economic and Social Affairs. (2019). *Contraceptive Use by Method 2019 – Data Booklet.* https://www.un.org/development/desa/pd/sites/www.un.org.development.desa.pd/files/files/documents/2020/Jan/un_2019_contraceptiveusebymethod_databooklet.pdf

van Amsterdam, J., & Hartgens, F. (2014). Acute and chronic adverse reaction of anabolic-androgenic steroids. *Adverse Drug Reaction Bulletin, 288*(1), 1111-1114. https://doi.org/10.1097/FAD.0000000000000006

Wallwiener, C. W., Wallwiener, L. M., Seeger, H., Schönfisch, B., Mueck, A. O., Bitzer, J., Zipfel, S., Brucker, S. Y., Taran, F. A., & Wallwiener, M. (2015). Are hormonal components of oral contraceptives associated with impaired female sexual function? A questionnaire-based online survey of medical students in Germany, Austria, and Switzerland. *Archives of Gynecology and Obstetrics*, *292*(4), 883-890. https://doi.org/10.1007/s00404-015-3726-x

Wang, S. M., Han, C., Bahk, W. M., Lee, S. J., Patkar, A. A., Masand, P. S., & Pae, C. U. (2018). Addressing the side effects of contemporary antidepressant drugs: A comprehensive review. *Chonnam Medical Journal*, *54*(2), 101-112. https://doi.org/10.4068/cmj.2018.54.2.101

Wassersug, R. J. (2016). Maintaining intimacy for prostate cancer patients on androgen deprivation therapy. *Current Opinion in Supportive and Palliative Care*, *10*(1), 55-65. https://doi.org/10.1097/SPC.0000000000000190

Wassertheil-Smoller, S., Blaufox, M. D., Oberman, A., Davis, B. R., Swencionis, C., Knerr, M. O., Hawkins, C. M., & Langford, H. G. (1991). Effect of antihypertensives on sexual function and quality of life: The TAIM Study. *Annals of Internal Medicine*, *114*(8), 613-620. https://doi.org/10.7326/0003-4819-114-8-613

Watanabe, N., Omori, I. M., Nakagawa, A., Cipriani, A., Barbui, C., Churchill, R., & Furukawa, T. A. (2011). Mirtazapine versus other antidepressive agents for depression. *The Cochrane Database of Systematic Reviews, 12,* CD006528. https://doi.org/10.1002/14651858.CD006528.pub2

Wersocki, E., Bedson, J., Chen, Y., LeResche, L., & Dunn, K. M. (2017). Comprehensive systematic review of long-term opioids in women with chronic noncancer pain and associated reproductive dysfunction (hypothalamic-pituitary-gonadal axis disruption). *Pain*, *158*(1), 8-16. https://doi.org/10.1097/j.pain.0000000000000691

White, I. D., Wilson, J., Aslet, P., Baxter, A. B., Birtle, A., Challacombe, B., Coe, J., Grover, L., Payne, H., Russell, S., Sangar, V., Van As, N., & Kirby, M. (2015). Development of UK guidance on the management of erectile dysfunction resulting from radical radiotherapy and androgen deprivation therapy for prostate cancer. *International Journal of Clinical Practice*, *69*(1), 106-123. https://doi.org/10.1111/ijcp.12512

Wilson, T. K., & Tripp, J. (2020). Buspirone. In *StatPearls* [Internet]. StatPearls Publishing.

Wincze, J. P., & Weisberg, R. B. (2015). *Sexual Dysfunction: A Guide for Assessment and Treatment* (3rd ed.). Guilford Press.

Wright, J. J., & O'Conner, K. M. (2015). Female sexual dysfunction. *Medical Clinics of North America, 99*(3), 607-628.

Wynne, A. L. (2012). Drugs affecting the autonomic system. In T. M. Woo & A. L. Wynne (Eds.), *Pharmacotherapeutics for Nurse Practitioner Prescribers* (pp. 167-231). F.A. Davis Company.

Yee, A., Loh, H. S., Hisham Hashim, H. M., & Ng, C. G. (2014). The prevalence of sexual dysfunction among male patients on methadone and buprenorphine treatments: A meta-analysis study. *The Journal of Sexual Medicine*, *11*(1), 22-32. https://doi.org/10.1111/jsm.12352

Zajecka, J. (2001). Strategies for the treatment of antidepressant-related sexual dysfunction. *The Journal of Clinical Psychiatry*, *62*(Suppl 3), 35-43.

Zandi, P. P., & Judy, J. T. (2010). The promise and reality of pharmacogenetics in psychiatry. *The Psychiatric Clinics of North America*, *33*(1), 181-224. https://doi.org/10.1016/j.psc.2009.12.001

6

Ethics in Sex Therapy*

Sarah Dalton

INTRODUCTION

Ethics is a discipline dealing with obligations and moral duty, a set of values or moral principles of conduct that govern the behaviors of an individual or group. Five main principles underpin ethical guidelines: truthfulness, confidentiality, autonomy, informed consent, and beneficence/non-maleficence. These principles set forth standards that should be followed by any professional intending to provide quality of service and maintain excellence in their field of practice (American Association of Sexuality Educators, Counselors and Therapists [AASECT], 2014a). But who determines what is right or wrong, moral or immoral, good or bad, proper or improper, and ethical or unethical, especially in the field of sexuality?

Within each culture, values and moral principles are often the outgrowths of a religious tradition that occasionally is incorporated into law. In the United States, our ethical standards are based primarily on the Judeo-Christian tradition, though the religious traditions within the United States are vast. Throughout history, religious beliefs have varied from strict moral positions to relaxed and open-minded perspectives. As moral views have been interpreted differently by religion, views on sexuality have changed.

The changes witnessed throughout time regarding sexuality and ethics have reshaped guidelines and professional conduct within the field of sexuality. The first decades of the 21st century brought to light rapid technological development, passionate acknowledgment of diversity, and an effervescent emphasis on social justice. Codes of ethics and professional conduct have followed these changes to ensure that guidelines for professional practice are up to date.

The General Principles within the American Psychological Association (APA) *Code of Ethics* broadly guide the clinician's practice to first do no harm to those seeking service, to practice within the limits of competence, to be truthful, to uphold the dignity of all people, and to not condone unjust practices and prejudice (American Psychological Association, 2017, General Principles A-E). Virtue ethics was originally formulated by Aristotle as a response to the perennial question of how people are to lead flourishing and happy lives. In the Good Lives Model, by Ward and Stewart (2003), clinicians are encouraged to give patients as many opportunities to enhance their life and make it worthwhile, as they also account for individual abilities, life situations, and opportunities.

*Portions of this chapter were adapted and updated from "Ethics in Sex Therapy" by Catherine Dailey Ravella in L. VandeCreek, F. L. Peterson, Jr., and J. W. Bley (Eds.), *Innovations in Clinical Practice: Focus on Sexual Health,* © 2007 by Professional Resource Press. Adapted with permission.

WHAT IS ETHICAL SEX THERAPY?

Who decides what is an ethical practice or the correct observance of standards for professional interactions in the field of sex therapy, especially in the media-enhanced, frequently emotionally charged area of human sexuality? How can we ensure ethical guidelines are followed in times where virtual connections and technology guide sex and relationships? Issues regarding professionalism and ethical practice can arise unexpectedly, leaving clinicians in potentially confusing and awkward situations. Ethical issues confront all therapists, which is why codes of ethics have been created in the helping professions. This contribution highlights some ethical issues that are within the realm of sex therapy, but the basic principles may also be applied to practice issues in general therapy. Understanding and adhering to the code of ethics prescribed by your specific profession offers the soundest guide. No one single code will ever be a complete guide for the conscientious therapist. Regular supervisor and/or peer consultation, in addition to referring to one's professional code of ethics, will help avoid many ethical pitfalls.

THE ROLE OF PROFESSIONAL ORGANIZATIONS

The American Association of Sexuality Educators, Counselors and Therapists (AASECT) *Code Conduct for Certified Members* is included in Section VI (pp. 529-538) of this book. This organization certifies psychologists, psychiatrists, psychiatric nurse specialists, clinical social workers, marriage and family therapists, and counselors; in other words, clinicians in varied therapeutic disciplines that have completed the additional training and supervision for certification in sex therapy, sex counseling, or sex education. An individual who maintains several professional roles will be bound by more than one code of ethics; therefore, it is advisable to abide by the most stringent or restrictive code or you risk ethical violations under that organization's code of ethics. It may be challenging as some professional codes conflict with one another.

Most mental health professionals have a working definition of ethics. Professional codes of ethics often emphasize words such as "enforce" and "professionalism" to define the importance of professional ethics. The *Code of Conduct for AASECT Certified Members*, for example, states: "Certified members of AASECT, in the conduct of all aspects of their life that relates to their professional work and identity, are expected to honor the Code, and AASECT certification is predicated upon adherence thereto" (AASECT, 2014, Article I). Professional codes of ethics have evolved to provide increased guidance to practitioners rather than disciplinary action and include helpful guidelines for both professional and personal actions.

No code can offer a clear guideline in every possible clinical situation, just as no law can always foresee every possible situation where its relevance may come to bear. An education that is commensurate with the type of practice the sex therapist performs goes without saying, yet nothing stops individuals in some states from inaccurately and unethically calling themselves a Sex Therapist. What is unethical is not always against the law.

THE ETHICAL NATURE OF ANY THERAPEUTIC RELATIONSHIP

Fundamental to the therapeutic contract is the issue of the expected vulnerability of the patient in the task of restoring the patient to a higher level of functioning and relieving symptoms of distress. The sex therapist may have special moral and ethical obligations that go beyond the care provided by general therapists due to the sexual topics regularly discussed in therapy.

The ethical delivery of service primarily focuses on the patient and therapist relationship and a strong therapeutic rapport. The use of the terms patient and consumer (client) provides an interesting and somewhat diverse view of the clinical relationship. The term patient is used most frequently by those who come from a medical model. The Merriam-Webster Dictionary (n.d.) tells us the patient is "an individual awaiting or under medical care and treatment" or "the recipient of any of various personal services," while client is the term applied to "a person who engages the professional advice or services of another." The consumer (client) is one who "utilizes economic goods." Each term may suggest a specific view of the clinical relationship, which is used in the various helping professions.

In the mental health field, the emergence of new modalities based on diverse theories and approaches have changed the relationship between therapists and patients, including in sex therapy. Boundaries are challenged by techniques of modalities that push therapists to constantly revisit the principles underpinning ethical guidelines. The interpretation of transference and countertransference is still relevant in therapist-patient interaction. The psychological concept of transference lies in the therapeutic relationship, and although it can be processed positively, transference may also be misused when the patient or couple are damaged by the therapist's use of the therapeutic relationship to gratify his or her own emotional, financial, or sexual needs (Blackshaw & Patterson, 1992).

The following vignette* should stimulate some thoughtful consideration for understanding and establishing professional boundaries in clinical practice:

> Bill is a 48-year-old, divorced, Catholic psychologist, in private practice. He presented for treatment in a sex therapy practice with a chief complaint of erectile dysfunction with his present partner, Nancy, age 44. Nancy is also divorced and is employed as a certified professional accountant. Nancy's ex-husband, Sean, was Bill's practice partner.
>
> While Nancy and Sean were going through their divorce, Nancy sought emotional support from Bill. During the time Bill was providing emotional support to Nancy, their sexual relationship began.
>
> Bill's primary ethical infraction was with Alyssa, a patient in treatment for depression. Alyssa had announced she was quitting therapy because she had lost her job and her health insurance. Bill had been wishing to hire a transcriptionist/secretary for some time and decided to offer the position to Alyssa, who accepted. She discontinued therapy and began work in Sean and Bill's office. Alyssa, as an employee, was rewarded with gifts from Bill, including shopping trips for clothing that was more "professional" in appearance. Bill suggested she "seduced (him) into sexual liaisons" in the office.
>
> Bill's practice partner Sean reported the sexual relationship to the psychology licensing board. Bill's license was suspended for 2 years for sexual misconduct with a recent patient. The partnership with Sean ended and eventually, so did the relationship with Alyssa.

---

*Names and characteristics in all case examples have been changed to protect privacy.

> The treatment issues in the present relationship between Nancy and Bill were intertwined with Bill's understanding of his ethical role as a therapist, his self-perception as a "rescuer" for both Alyssa the patient and Nancy the girlfriend, and his lack of professional boundaries. Bill sought and received the suggested counseling recommendation for his ethical infraction.

What role does the sex therapist have, if any, to further rehabilitate this patient as a psychologist? Should Bill's role as a psychologist be considered part of the present couple treatment?

Throughout therapy with a sex therapist, Bill made personal gains with Nancy. Understanding his own sexual needs and gender role socialization helped provide him with increased awareness of his patient issues, as well as his countertransference issues. His basic caring, warm, and sensitive personality were encouraged to incorporate respect for trustworthiness, honesty, and prudence in his professional as well as personal dealings. Ongoing peer supervision was recommended with a colleague as a way of dealing with his sexualized views of dependent, vulnerable female patients. The underlying issue, sexual activity with a patient, underscored the role and treatment focus of the sex therapist.

Acting on sexual attraction toward patients is strictly forbidden; "talking about any countertransference (including erotic countertransference) is definitely encouraged . . . 'desensitization' and greater openness [with a supervisor] are essential if the current situation is ever to change" (Blackshaw & Patterson, 1992, p. 353).

Peer supervision is essential in the field of sex therapy as all therapists can benefit from an outside opinion. However, clinicians are smart to avoid the personal opinions of friends and should see similarly credentialed professionals. A peer supervisor may have helped Bill in those first questionable choices: hiring an ex-patient (which was a questionable act for his colleague, Sean, as well), buying personal gifts, and eventually becoming involved in a sexual relationship with a former patient.

In the *Code of Conduct for AASECT Certified Members*, the therapist is restricted from any type of sexual contact with "a potential, current, or former consumer . . . whether the consumer consents to such behavior or not" (AASECT, 2014, Principle Three, Section 13). This clearly states that sexual relationships are never acceptable with potential, current, or former patients. However, this is distinctly different from the American Psychological Association's (APA) *Code of Ethics*, which states that "psychologists do not engage in sexual intimacies with former clients/patients for at least 2 years after cessation or termination of therapy" (American Psychological Association, 2017, Standard 10.08). An example of how professionals need to uphold the highest level of ethical standards is when a psychologist who is an AASECT-certified sex therapist would need to follow AASECT's ethical code.

Following ethical standards is essential to clinical practice because the therapist begins the therapeutic relationship in a position with higher power than the patient, inherently having trust within the relationship. We ask the patient to suspend the usual cultural defenses and reveal intensely personal material with the hope of being understood and helped. It is to be expected that some patients will develop intense feelings toward a therapist, which is the nature of transference. In sex therapy, the numerous explicit sexual discussions may arouse sexual feelings comingled with the normal attachments that take place in a therapeutic relationship. Sex therapists need to be aware of these potential feelings and trained in how to manage them ethically and professionally.

While the *Code of Conduct for AASECT Certified Members* is clear and specific regarding sexual relationships with patients, some clinicians still test this unethical boundary and attempt to have a patient and therapist romantic and/or sexual relationship. There is a blind spot in clinicians who argue that the patient is not harmed by sexual contact with a therapist or that it is the *right* of patients to choose a sexual relationship with whomever they wish. This blind spot points to the therapist's inability to move beyond the need for personal gratification by not recognizing that the change in the relationship is a betrayal of that initial trust and a misuse of the power inherent in the relationship. There is ample evidence that patients are harmed by sexual contact with a therapist (American Psychological Association, 2004; Capawana, 2016).

Prohibited sexual behaviors are spelled out in the AASECT's ethical codes and include kissing, sexual intercourse, and/or the touching by either party of breasts or genitals (Article VI, Principle Three, 13). Some therapists have even questioned if a "friendly hug" is ever allowed in the therapeutic relationship as it may stir up sexual feelings from either patient or therapist. In a 2014 position paper, AASECT outlines potential sexual touch and the AASECT-certified professional. This document prohibits all forms of sexual contact with patients except for professionals operating within the scope of their professional practice. The position paper offers the example of "physicians, nurses, physical therapists, occupational therapists, physicians assistants, and pelvic floor specialists [who] are licensed to provide a standard of care that includes manual contact for clinical purposes" (AASECT, 2014b). Overall, one helpful guideline for physical touch with a patient is: "Would you do 'it' in front of your clinical supervisor when you were a graduate student?" In other words, can your behavior stand up to another professional's scrutiny? If not, it would be best to avoid this situation and potential ethical dilemmas.

THERAPIST COMPETENCE AS A MEASURE OF SOCIAL RESPONSIBILITY

Understanding your personal boundaries, including limits of expertise, is part of the role of a professional. In the *Conference Report: Ethical Guidelines for Research and Clinical Perspectives on Human Sexuality* developed in March 1978 by the Reproductive Biology Research Foundation (later known as the famed Masters and Johnson Institute), it is clearly stated that it is unethical for any type of sexual relationship between patient and therapist (Kolodny, 1978). This paper was originally presented at a time when sex therapy was still emerging as a separate, specialized area of treatment. The timeliness of this document is still evident. The task force outlined five major areas of ethical concern: (a) competence and integrity of sex therapists, (b) confidentiality in sex therapist, (c) welfare of the patient, (d) welfare of students and trainees, and (e) welfare of research subjects. The substance of these five areas still stands in AASECT's ethical code.

Within the AASECT organization and other professional helping organizations, there is an opportunity for colleagues, patients, and/or supervisors to fill out ethical complaint forms when an ethical code has been broken by the professional. These complaints are then investigated by the ethics committee of that organization. The easily accessible option to report ethical violations helps hold professionals accountable for their actions, which is especially important in the field of sex therapy. One ethical issue that continues to present itself is professionals who claim to possess a title or degree that is unaccredited or credentials that are not possessed. Similarly, there are professionals who use an organization's certification credentials in an unclear manner, making it questionable who is an AASECT-certified professional (AASECT, 2014, Article VI, Principle One, Competence)

The 2014 *Code of Conduct for AASECT Certified Members* states that all certified members "shall be committed to maintaining high standards of scholarship and practice and shall be accountable as an individual to the AASECT Standards" (Article VI, Principle One, Competence). To claim to be an AASECT-certified sex therapist, one must hold a valid license in another discipline first and then submit to additional training and supervision to achieve competence and certification as a sex therapist. Holding a license in a therapeutic field is a prerequisite. Those trained in these disciplines bring their professional experience and insights to provide the foundation upon which sex therapy training is added.

Individuals who offer sexual treatments and use titles such as sex coach, life director, and personal sex educator frequently may not be licensed or hold valid membership in any professional organization that requires these individuals to be accountable to a prescribed code of ethics. These individuals may offer some valuable advice, but in seeking treatment for sexual problems, the patient should look for credentials where the clinician is required to follow a code of ethics, following applicable training and supervision.

AASECT members that are certified as Sex Educators or Sex Counselors are advised to follow the PLISSIT model, which has been implemented in sex-related fields for decades. The model involves the clinician assessing the need for permission, limited information, specific suggestion, and intensive therapy (Annon, 1976). PLISSIT is most applied when providers are triaging patients with complex sexual health concerns who need referrals to sex therapists. At the point in a counseling or educational interaction when it is recognized that intensive therapy is required beyond the more straightforward suggestions and/or support that may be offered in such initial interactions, a referral to a more qualified professional is deemed appropriate.

THE USE OF SURROGATES IN SEX THERAPY

The use of partner surrogates in sex therapy is a highly debated issue. This practice involves the use of a separate individual, not in a romantic partnership with the patient, who uses "hands-on adjunctive treatment services" with the patient (AASECT, 2018). Often, this practice is used to help patients overcome complex sexual issues that they cannot correct on their own or within their romantic partnership. It may be ethically permissible in establishing a therapeutic environment if conducted responsibly. If a surrogate is to be used at all, it is understood that the partner surrogate is not a sex therapist. Surrogates should understand that their role is never as a sex therapist or psychotherapist.

AASECT's ethical code, being national in scope, does not specifically prohibit the use of surrogates nor does it condone the practice. It states, "The Certified member shall not enter into association for professional practice . . . or promote in any manner the practice of an unqualified or incompetent person . . . [who] does not adhere to the Code or is in violation of any law" (AASECT, 2014, Article VI, Principle One, Aiding/Abetting Unqualified Practice). Several states and local attorneys have interpreted the use of surrogates as prostitution and therefore in violation of state law. Again, it is prudent to be aware of the local laws in the state in which a therapist is practicing.

A therapist who chooses to utilize the services of a surrogate must exercise caution in protecting the welfare of both the patient and the surrogate and be aware of the local laws governing this practice. In 2018, AASECT created a position paper titled "Position on FOSTA-SESTA and its Impact on Consensual Sex Work and the Chilling of Sexual Speech" in response to President Donald J. Trump's law, Fight Online Sex Trafficking Act and the Stop Enabling Sex Trafficking Act (FOSTA-SESTA). The law removed previously provided "safe harbor" provisions and forced "sites and platforms to remove or censor any user content that could, per the language of the law, promote and facilitate prostitution" (AASECT, 2018).

Within the position paper, AASECT clearly outlines that "sex workers, including sexological bodyworkers, surrogate partners, professional dominants, and lifestyle educators sometimes facilitate the work of sex educators, counselors, and therapists by providing hands-on adjunctive treatment services" (AASECT, 2018). Operating within ethical standards, surrogates can be used within the field of sex therapy. The primary question for a sex therapist would be if the practice breaks any laws within their jurisdiction.

The use of surrogates in couple's therapy also is questioned for therapeutic value due to the nature of couple's treatment. In couple's therapy, the focus is on assisting the couple to work out of their interpersonal issues and achieve a more fulfilling relationship, including sexual functioning, though it is not solely focused on sexual functioning. Virginia Johnson, of The Masters and Johnson Institute, described couple's sex therapy as a combination of sex education, communication skill training, and general marriage counseling. However, the addition of any other parties within the romantic couple can cause the partner issues to become more complicated, therefore, leading to questions about the effectiveness of surrogates in couple's therapy.

Yet the use of surrogates has continued in this country for decades. An interesting example of surrogate therapy for an individual was presented as a case conference at a national sex therapy meeting in the late 1970s.

> A sex therapist working in a correctional facility reported treating a 28-year-old man, described as a pedophile. His current *DSM-5* supported diagnosis would be Pedophilic Disorder (American Psychiatric Association, 2013b). He was arrested and convicted as a sex offender and served an 8-year jail term. The man was evaluated by the sex therapist and continued in therapy throughout his incarceration. The therapist continued to follow this individual in treatment for 4 years postdischarge. He was convicted for molesting 12- to 14-year-old boys. He met them in a boy's club where he worked, befriended them, and engaged in mutual masturbation and oral sex. He had not been prosecuted for his previous sexual activities that had begun at age 19, and now confided these to his therapist. He had never engaged in an adult sexual experience. His history included sexual experiences with a male cousin, 2 years older than himself, at approximately 10 years of age.
>
> During his incarceration, the therapist introduced an adult male surrogate to help the prisoner/patient gain comfort with his sexual orientation and to provide adult socialization and sexual experience opportunities. At the time of the case presentation, the individual had been out of prison for more than 4 years. He lived in a gay community, experiencing sexual contact only with adult partners. He continued in voluntary weekly outpatient therapy. He claims to have not involved adolescent boys in his sexual activities since his discharge from prison.

While this case study is decades old, similar surrogate work still exists. The ethics of this case present some interesting considerations. The jurisdiction of practice did not prohibit the use of surrogates since this was in a public facility, so we assume no actual laws were violated. Some will question the use of a male surrogate, since initially the prisoner denied his attraction to males. Little consideration is given to the patient's vulnerability as someone presenting for treatment against his will when the therapist is administering a state-ordered treatment, even though the therapist is attempting to restore some "normalcy" for the offender. The offender may not have perceived his behavior as maladaptive. This paradigm presents the sex therapist with a unique ethical role in treating a convicted sex offender.

The traditional patient-centered ethical guidelines may be breached when viewed in what has been called therapeutic jurisprudence (Glaser, 2003). In therapeutic jurisprudence, the rights of the community trump the rights of the individual. We attempt to force the views of the community agencies on offenders to promote an effective intervention. Yet to many in the community, the use of surrogates is not an acceptable practice, even when the outcome for community safety may appear to be more desirable.

The offense-free time of the preceding individual was offered as a symbol of success in an area that sees high recidivism. There was a suggestion that disregard for the offender's "autonomy and welfare" is not an exception to routine ethical guidelines (which would consider it a violation of his rights to confidentiality when he self-incriminated by admitting past offenses) or his right to have his perceived "best interests" protected.

Sex offender treatment may not promote the offender's "well-being" if the offender senses a lack of congruent behavior on the part of the therapist. It may be difficult for sex offenders to learn the virtue of honesty and congruent behavior if we as therapists are ethically conflicted between the needs and interests of society and the therapeutic needs of the offender. A sex therapist whose conflicted ethical loyalties may be breached must be clear from the onset about what can be offered to the individual who has violated community sexual norms, to prevent erratic and inconsistent trust. Advising the patient at the onset of therapy of the limits of the patient/therapist relationship in these circumstances at least will clarify the parameters of informed consent.

REPARATIVE/CONVERSION THERAPY

It has been a relatively short time since the American Psychiatric Association removed homosexuality as a diagnosis in the second edition of its *Diagnostic and Statistical Manual of Mental Disorders*, in 1973 (Drescher, 2015). Since that time, professional organizations like the American Counseling Association (ACA) have encouraged clinicians to educate themselves regarding the many different issues impacting the Lesbian, Gay, Bisexual, Transgender, Queer, and Questioning (LGBTQQ) communities. Several organizations have created competencies for working with these communities, covered under their codes of ethics.

If a clinician aims to cure or change the affectional orientation, previously called the "sexual orientation" of a patient, it is labeled "reparative therapy" or "conversion therapy." These terms are placed in quotation marks as they are terms most often used to imply that individuals within the LGBTQQ communities are "disordered," "broken," or need to be repaired (Gay & Lesbian Alliance Against Defamation [GLAAD], n.d.). This type of intervention is viewed by the American Psychological Association, American Counseling Association, American Academic of Child and Adolescent Psychiatry, American Academy of Pediatrics, American Association for Marriage and Family Therapy, American College of Physicians, American School Counselor Association, and many others as unethical and harmful to patients. "Reparative therapy" is not to be confused with a therapist who is offering counseling or therapy geared toward developing a better understanding of the patient's affectional orientation and ultimately developing a congruent lifestyle.

The American Psychiatric Association has created several position statements on "reparative therapy," strongly denouncing its practice. It states that attempting to alter one's affectional orientation through "reparative therapy" "represents a significant risk of harm by subjecting individuals to forms of treatment which have not been scientifically validated and by undermining self-esteem when sexual orientation fails to change" (American Psychiatric Association, 2013a, p.1). The American Counseling Association (ACA) has created competencies for counseling LGBTQQ Individuals and states that reparative therapy is "detrimental or may even be life-threatening . . . and must not be undertaken" (Association for Lesbian, Gay, Bisexual, and Transgender Issues in Counseling [ALGBTIC], n.d., p. 5). Similarly, the American Medical Association (AMA) and Health Professionals Advancing LGBTQ Equality (GLMA) created an Issue Brief, which states that efforts to convert a patient's affectional orientation "may cause significant psychological distress" and lists "depression, anxiety, low self-esteem, internalized homophobia, self-blame, intrusive imagery, and sexual dysfunction" as potential outcomes (American Medical Association, 2018).

Given the available scholarly literature that negates such a practice and the published ethical guidelines which assert that clinicians must support the affectional orientation of the patient, it is startling that some professionals are still trying to alter patients' affectional orientations. All professionals are required to follow the ethical guidelines put forth by their professional organization, however, those operating without a license or membership in a professional organization are not held to the professional codes of ethics. This is how some professionals are conducting "reparative therapy" with patients and risking harm to the patient.

Individuals who conduct "reparative therapy" often see this practice as their moral imperative, typically linked to strong religious beliefs. They claim that to help people live according to their religious beliefs and values they must alter their affectional attractions. Many therapists and organizations exist claiming the success stories of their "reparative therapy." One cannot help but question the possibility that these "successful" individuals may be closer to the midrange on the Kinsey scale of human sexuality (Kinsey et al., 1948) and that their sex drive and/or orientation may be less of an issue in their self-concept than their spiritual motivation and affiliation. The majority of anecdotal stories of attempted "reparative therapy" describe painful experiences of everything from rejection to physical abuse.

The personal and religious values of clinicians who engage in "reparative therapy" become increasingly dangerous when youth are forced to enroll, against their will, often by parents or religious leaders. Many jurisdictions have researched the potentially damaging effects on youth and have banned "reparative therapy" for underage youth. However, it continues to occur regularly in some areas of the country.

There is no longer an ethical dilemma regarding "reparative therapy" as ethical codes and competencies are clearly against the practice, however, this does not limit clinicians from acting outside of their code of ethics when they do not subscribe to their professional organization. These clinicians are breaking the code of ethics but if they do not belong to a professional organization, there is no organization to sanction the unethical practice.

FACILITATED SEX

The question of "facilitated sex" is not to be confused with the use of surrogates. A person with a disability who is unable to satisfy their own sexual needs may request the services of a caretaker or personal assistant to set up or assist with positioning and removing clothing to allow for partner activity or masturbation. The personal assistant facilitator is not participating in any sexual activity with the individual in treatment. For these individuals, this service may be no different from requesting a set up for feeding, bathing, toileting, or any activities of daily living.

According to Mitch Tepper, PhD, MPH, it is not easy assigning sexual preparation roles to personal assistants (Melby, 2003). Involving a sex therapist who is connected to a medical facility or who has a medical background may help with some of the preparation. Nursing facility staff members have long assumed maternalistic care of their parents and, as such, frequently do not see their charges as being independent adults with sexual needs.

Carolyn Livingston, ARNP, PhD, described the ethical questions regarding her role as a sex therapist for a cerebral palsy patient. She was told the patient wished to masturbate but needed assistance in removing her clothing, positioning her and providing an apparatus that the patient was capable of using independently. Some caregivers refused to assist in these activities. After Livingston attempted to educate the nursing staff, instructing and assisting the willing staff members, the patient was placed on a specifically designed board with a control for a vibrator near the head of her bed. Livingston was clear that she "never touch[ed] my patients, I sit down and talk to my patients. I don't want anything to be misinterpreted" (Melby, 2003). This instance seemed to offer no conflict for Livingston, who with the assistance of one of the caregivers, removed the clothing of the patient and helped position her, and then left the patient alone to engage in sexual pleasure.

In other instances, personal assistants of disabled persons have refused to assist a patient to act on sexual needs if it is acting outside of their professional boundaries. Often when nursing staff members are instructed about the sexual needs of patients, they will claim the information is "too personal." However, they do not find it inappropriate to manually remove a fecal impaction from a rectum or place a catheter in a urethra. These aspects of physical health are generally viewed as very personal, yet they are viewed as legitimate care needs for those who cannot provide for themselves. Therefore, it leaves a patient to wonder if their sexual needs are less important than the daily physical needs.

According to AASECT's ethical code, it is unethical for a sex therapist to engage in sexual activity with a patient and therefore, procedures generally involved with nudity or observation of sexual activity may go beyond the boundaries of established therapeutic practice (AASECT, 2014a, Article VI, Principle Three,13). However, when there is good evidence that the patient's best interests are being served and not the personal interest of the therapist, such activity falls within an ethical practice.

Establishing legitimacy in performing any function requires knowledge of what is needed, the development of personal comfort with the procedure, and the appropriate setting for the activity, all part of the purview of a skilled professional. Perhaps it is a misuse of ethical standards when we deny care to those who need assistance in providing sexual expression, a basic *need*, not just a *want*. Establishing legitimate functioning in our professional arena may be the most ethical behavior.

APPROPRIATE SETTING FOR SEX THERAPY: THE USE OF ELECTRONIC MEDIA

With the use of the internet, the issue of online therapy via chat, email, video, or other electronic media is a frequently used form of therapy. The American Psychological Association (APA) has stated that telepsychology is acceptable if the professional "strive[s] to take reasonable steps to ensure their competence with both the technologies used and the potential impact of the technologies on patient/patients" (American Psychological Association, 2013a, 2.01).

Similarly, the American Counseling Association (ACA) and American Mental Health Counselors Association (AMHCA) both have established guidelines surrounding telebehavioral health that focus on competency, the safety of the patient, confidentiality, and serving the needs of the patient (ACA, 2014; AMHCA, 2020). With sudden worldwide changes during the COVID-19 global pandemic in 2020, most organizations expedited telebehavioral health standards so patients could continue to receive care while self-quarantining and being out of physical contact with their therapist. While the lasting impact of these changes is yet to be seen, it is reasonable to say that most organizations providing professional codes of ethics will continue to allow telebehavioral health in some capacity.

Now that telebehavioral health is widely used, distinct ethical issues must be considered. Primarily, if telebehavioral health is an appropriate clinical fit for the patient. Therapists must assess the severity of the patient's presenting symptoms and might not engage in teletherapy if the patient has severe mental health concerns including suicidal or homicidal thoughts. Similarly, if the patient is not familiar with the use of required technologies, telebehavioral health might not be appropriate.

Therapists who engage in online distance therapy must be aware of the laws and regulations both in the therapist's physical location and the patient's location (ACA, 2014, Section H.1.a). In addition to the typical informed consent that a therapist reviews with a patient, the ACA requires additional ethical guidelines to be included in a telebehavioral health consent form that includes distance counseling credentials, always knowing the physical location, address, time zone of the patient, confidentiality, and informing the patient of the risks and benefits of distance counseling (ACA, 2014, Section H.2.a).

When the patient and therapist are not in the same physical location, the therapist must consider additional safety procedures. For example, if the patient was at risk of self-harm or a sudden emergency occurred, like choking, the therapist must know exactly how to dispatch emergency help. The local emergency address and phone numbers must be gathered before each distance therapy session in case use is required. The patient must also be aware of response times if the therapist is needed outside of regular appointments and what procedures to take for these issues.

Another essential ethical guideline for telebehavioral health is a protocol for technology failure. If the internet should fail on either the therapist or patient's end, both parties need to know an appropriate follow-up form of communication, like using the telephone. If the telephone should also fail, there would be another step, like rescheduling the appointment. Within the telebehavioral health consent form, all these procedures must be clearly outlined for the patient, to lessen the likelihood that the patient would be harmed through online therapy.

Though mental health organizations have incorporated telebehavioral health requirements into their ethical codes, the *Code of Conduct for AASECT Certified Members* does not specifically address online counseling, education, or therapy. However, AASECT's ethical code does require that Certified members always operate within their level of competence to best serve the patient. If there is ever a time when the therapist is operating outside of professional abilities, the patient should be referred to another clinician (AASECT, 2014, Article VI, Principle One, Informed Consent).

The most accurate location for official AASECT-certified professionals is via AASECT's webpage where you can find the name, contact information, and website of any AASECT-certified sex therapist. Google also provides the names of many individuals who have self-identified as sex educators or counselors, though these individuals might not be appropriately credentialed to provide services.

The range of information available to individuals surfing the internet suggests that most people have learned a fair amount of information about their perceived sexual problem before they contact a certified sex therapist. However, the wish for anonymity may still exist and patients may prefer online counseling or therapy to face-to-face services. Additional reasons for online therapy could be travel difficulties, the need for online consultation, and flexibility in scheduling throughout the patient's day. Plenty of patients benefit from online services, including sex therapy. This option could be appropriate if all ethical guidelines are followed, a specific consent form for online services is signed, and the therapist knows the patient's physical location. Essentially, all ethical codes must be followed with additional steps to ensure online safety and confidentiality.

One potential challenge with online counseling and therapy is the reimbursement procedures for insurance companies, who may not support online services. Fees for therapy are generally set in accord with a "standard allowable" (as set by an insurance company) or prevailing rate in the area of practice. However, if insurance does not support online services, the patient may need to consider face-to-face therapy or pay the full session fee. This may cause undue hardship to patients who cannot afford the entire session without the use of their insurance and for patients who experience shame or discomfort discussing sex-related topics in person.

Online communication is also used to benefit AASECT-certified members who engage in the AASECT list-serv to stay up to date on many issues about the field. Many sex therapists appear to benefit from using the AASECT list-serv for case discussion, consultation, and general information exchange. This illustrates a new form of peer consultation that can help to avoid some ethical entanglements as the field shifts to using the internet for therapy. While ethical issues will continue to exist with online therapy, the benefits are increasingly clear in the field of sex therapy.

CONCLUSIONS

Sexual ethics has presented several problems throughout history because the fundamental beliefs of each individual and society reflect our assumptions about the nature of sex. With the struggle for more self-determination and an increase in individual rights in the United States, our sexual rights as a society have changed. Our view of what is an ethical practice as a therapist has also changed with the flow of history. The illustrations in this contribution offer only some of the ethical dilemmas that modern sex therapists encounter. The general psychotherapist may confront some of these issues in varied forms as well.

All professionals are expected to follow the code of ethics of the most restrictive field of practice to most ethically serve the needs of patients. The ethical professional therapist is required to follow the code of ethics as set out by the individual's professional organization. Sex therapists follow the *Code of Conduct for AASECT Certified Members* as well as their professional codes for nursing, medicine, psychology, counseling, and the like. Not every potential ethical dilemma will be covered in any written code, and the good therapist is wise to consult with respected colleagues to avoid ethical violations. While it can be challenging to converse about practical, coherent sexual ethics related to professional codes, these ongoing discussions must continue to provide patients with the most competent and ethical sex therapy possible.

REFERENCES

American Association of Sexuality Educators, Counselors and Therapists. (2014a). *Code of conduct for AASECT certified members.* https://www.aasect.org/sites/default/files/documents/Code%20of%20Conduct-11.2020.pdf

American Association of Sexuality Educators, Counselors and Therapists. (2014b). *Touch and the AASECT certified professional* [Position Paper]. https://www.aasect.org/position-touch-and-aasect-certified-professional

American Association of Sexuality Educators, Counselors and Therapists. (2018). *Position on FOSTA-SESTA and its impact on consensual sex work and the chilling of sexual speech* [Position Paper]. https://www.aasect.org/position-fosta-sesta-and-its-impact-consensual-sex-work-and-chilling-sexual-speech

American Counseling Association. (2014). *2014 ACA code of ethics.* https://www.counseling.org/docs/default-source/default-document-library/2014-code-of-ethics-finaladdress.pdf

American Medical Association. (2018). *LGBTQ change efforts (so-called "conversion therapy"* [Issue brief by the American Medical Association and GLMA - Health Professionals Advancing LGBTQ Equality]. https://www.ama-assn.org/system/files/2019-12/conversion-therapy-issue-brief.pdf

American Mental Health Counseling Association. (2020). *AMHCA Code of Ethics* (revised 2015, 2020). https://www.amhca.org/HigherLogic/System/DownloadDocumentFile.ashx?DocumentFileKey=24a27502-196e-b763-ff57-490a12f7edb1&forceDialog=0

American Psychiatric Association. (2013a). *APA reiterates strong opposition to conversion therapy.* https://www.psychiatry.org/newsroom/news-releases/apa-reiterates-strong-opposition-to-conversion-therapy

American Psychiatric Association. (2013b). *Diagnostic and statistical manual of mental disorders* (5th ed.). https://doi.org/10.1176/appi.books.9780890425596

American Psychological Association. (2004, December). Sexual involvements with former patients: A delicate balance of core values. *Monitor on Psychology, 35*(11). http://www.apa.org/monitor/dec04/ethics

American Psychological Association. (2013a, December). *Guidelines for the practice of telepsychology.* https://www.apa.org/pubs/journals/features/amp-a0035001.pdf

American Psychological Association. (2013b, December). *Position statement on issues related to homosexuality.* [Position Paper]. https://www.psychiatry.org/newsroom/news-releases/apa-reiterates-strong-opposition-to-conversion-therapy

American Psychological Association. (2017). *Ethical principles of psychologists and code of conduct* (2002, amended effective June 1, 2010, and January 1, 2017). https://www.apa.org/ethics/code/ethics-code-2017.pdf

Annon, J. S. (1976). *Behavioral treatment of sexual problems: Brief therapy.* Harper & Row.

Association for Lesbian, Gay, Bisexual, and Transgender Issues in Counseling (ALGBTIC). (n.d.). *Competencies for counseling with lesbian, gay, bisexual, queer, questioning, intersex and ally individuals.* https://www.counseling.org/docs/ethics/algbtic-2012-07

Blackshaw, S. L., & Patterson, P. G. (1992). The prevention of sexual exploitation of patients: Educational issues. *The Canadian Journal of Psychiatry/La Revue Canadienne de Psychiatrie, 37*(5), 350-353.

Capawana, M. R. (2016). Intimate attractions and sexual misconduct in the therapeutic relationship: Implications for socially just practice. *Cogent Psychology*, *3*(1), Article 1194176. https://doi.org/10.1080/23311908.2016.1194176

Drescher J. (2015). Out of DSM: Depathologizing homosexuality. *Behavioral Sciences*, *5*(4), 565-575. https://doi.org/10.3390/bs5040565

GLAAD. (n.d.). *GLAAD media reference guide-in focus: "Conversion therapy."* https://www.glaad.org/reference/exgays

Glaser, B. (2003). Therapeutic jurisprudence: An ethical paradigm for therapists in sex offender treatment programs. *Western Criminology Review 4*(2), 143-154.

Kinsey, A. C., Pomeroy, W. B., & Martin, C. E. (1948). *Sexual behavior in the human male.* W. B. Saunders.

Kolodny, R. C. (1978). IV. CONFERENCE REPORT: Ethical guidelines for research and clinical perspectives on human sexuality. *Newsletter on Science, Technology & Human Values*, *3*(3), 17-22. https://doi.org/10.1177/016224397800300317

Melby, T. (2003). Facilitated sex. *Contemporary Sexuality, 37*(11), 1-6.

Merriam-Webster. (n.d.). *Merriam-Webster.com dictionary*. Retrieved June 27, 2020 from https://www.merriam-webster.com/

Ward, T., & Stewart, C. A. (2003). The treatment of sex offenders: Risk management and good lives. *Professional Psychology: Research and Practice, 34*(4), 353-360. https://doi.org/10.1037/0735-7028.34.4.353

Section II

Sexuality Models With Important Clinical Implications

7

Sexual Identity and Sexual Expression: An Empirical Reexamination

Frederick L. Peterson, Jr. and Ronald Skip Carter

INTRODUCTION

This chapter fundamentally challenges long-held traditional conceptualizations of both sexual identity and sexual/gender expression considered "understood and settled" definitions within psychiatry and psychological sciences.

The original title of this chapter was "Reconsidering Sexual Identity and Sexual Expression," but it turns out that "A Reexamination" is a more appropriate title because the literature is so varied in opinion that there is really no accepted single concept to reconsider and argue against. At this point in the development of the field of Sexual Health (also referred to in health care circles as Clinical Sexuality or Sexual Medicine), all thoughtful perspectives on the subject of sexuality, especially those developed from a multidisciplinary perspective, can contribute to better understanding of this most basic element of human existence.

That is the nature of the evolution of scientific advancement. Varied individual opinions are explored, models are developed, hypotheses are tested, results are discussed and debated, and gradually consensus is developed. A dominant perspective (paradigm) emerges over time and represents a widely accepted (not necessarily unanimous) collective hunch of what reality is, at least until counterarguments and evidence force reconsideration and modification of accepted definitions to better describe the new collective hunch of reality.

It is necessary to understand the many aspects of the broader concept of sexuality before we start poking around the notion of sexual identity and sexual/gender expression. As you will see, if science does not have consensus on the basic definition of sexuality, we can also expect varied opinions on the definition of sexual identity and expression.

WHAT IS SEXUALITY?

Most of us often think of "sex," but we seldom ponder "sexuality." People generally refer to sex as one of two things. Most often they use the term to refer to sexual intercourse. Sex also means a biological designation of being male or female. But what exactly is sexuality? Some authors who do define sexuality use all-encompassing descriptions of everything sexual about a person. McAnulty and Burnette (2003) define sexuality as "the sensations, emotions, and cognitions that are associated with physical sexual arousal and that usually give rise to sexual desire and/or behavior." Similarly, LeVay and Valente (2003) define the term as "the feelings, behaviors, and identities associated with sex." Greenberg et al. (2007) define human sexuality as "part of the total personality and involving the interrelationship of biological, psychological, and sociocultural dimensions."

These authors are well-respected authorities on the topic of sexuality, and their definitions vary considerably. Notice that the first one (McAnulty & Burnette, 2003) is focused solely on the individual whereas the last one (Greenberg et al., 2007) mentions both individual and societal dimensions. The second definition (LeVay & Valente, 2003) is the only one to refer to sexuality being associated to identity. That does not mean any of these authors are wrong, but because sexual science is relatively new, researchers are still working toward a consensus about many topics of sexuality, ranging from a basic definition of what sexuality means to more esoteric topics such as the G-spot, female ejaculation, and the mechanisms of orgasm. The bottom line, there is much more we do not know about sexuality than we definitively do know.

We could consult many other good sources such as the Kinsey Institute, the World Health Organization (WHO), and the American Association of Sex, Educators, Counselors and Therapists (AASECT); but let's not belabor the point any further. Instead, let's go to the people believed to be *the* authoritative source on all matters of human sexuality in America: The Sexuality Information and Education Council of the United States (SIECUS). It is their job to keep up with the latest research publications on sexuality and offer the best opinions available on sexual health topics as a valuable information service to the public.

SIECUS defines human sexuality comprehensively (brace yourself) as encompassing "the sexual knowledge, beliefs, attitudes, values, and behaviors of individuals. Its various dimensions involve the anatomy, physiology, and biochemistry of the sexual response system; identity, orientation, roles, and personality; and thoughts, feelings, and relationships. Sexuality is influenced by ethical, spiritual, cultural, and moral concerns" (2018, Para. 1). Wow! That is 20 different dimensions of being a sexual human mentioned in one definition!

WHAT IS SEXUAL IDENTITY? RESULTS OF A REVIEW OF COLLEGE TEXTBOOKS

About a decade ago, the authors reviewed all available publications that would be expected to contain a definition of sexuality and sexual identity. These publications included university textbooks used in courses of human sexuality, peer-reviewed journal articles, and other sources such as medical dictionaries. Considering only the textbooks, the majority (18 out of 27, or 66%) did not include the term "sexual identity" in the index and did not provide a definition of sexual identity in the body of the text. Nine texts (9 out of 27, or 33%) had definitions of sexual identity (Peterson & Carter, 2010). On the one hand, this finding astounded us as society looks to college textbooks as authoritative sources on any given topic. Surprisingly, the majority of the textbooks did not define what we considered a core concept of sexuality (sexual identity). On the other hand, this is the state of the field as the scientific study of sexuality is a little more than a century old and has been terribly hindered by social stigma, academic snobbery, and elusive research funding.

As expected, those textbooks providing definitions had significant variation. Variation among the definitions was measured in two ways: how many components of the definition were included and the specific nature of the definition's components. Besides the definitions found in textbooks, there are also definitions discussed by noted authors and leaders of the field (such as Coleman, Diamond, Levine, Hammack, and Bem discussed below) who are not necessarily authors of college textbooks. This gave a total of 15 definitions included in this review with varying numbers of components, including either two-dimensional, three-dimensional, or four-dimensional definitions.

Two-Dimensional Definitions

The texts defining sexual identity as two components basically use biological sex and sexual orientation as the two dimensions. These texts essentially state that sexual identity is synonymous with "sexual orientation." Examples include "One's self-label or self-identification as a heterosexual, homosexual or bisexual person" (Yarber et al., 2010) and "The terms sexual identity or sexual orientation refer to how people identify or classify themselves sexually" (Aulette et al., 2009). While using a limited definition of sexual identity is not considered adequate, both of these publications are excellent general sexuality textbooks that have been widely used in university classrooms (including courses taught by the authors). Also, to the credit of Yarber and Sayad, they updated their definition in their most recent (10th) edition: "Sexuality is one's self-label or self-identification as a heterosexual or LGBTQA person" (Yarber & Sayad, 2019).

` Although credit is deserved for these texts having a definition, two-dimensional definitions are inadequate because sexual identity is a more encompassing concept than sexual orientation. Sexual identity is not the same as sexual orientation, as sexual identity is a much broader concept. Said differently, two-dimensional definitions do not capture the diversity of how people identify themselves sexually. This is true of contemporary American culture and even more so regarding the greater diversity of cultures around the world.

Three-Dimensional Definitions

Three-dimensional definitions were the most common type (representing half of the definitions found) and varied in what factors comprised the third dimension. The first two dimensions already discussed are included in all the three-dimensional definitions (such as being a straight woman or gay man). Virtually all the definitions of sexual identity use the components of basic sex identification (sex orientation) and sexual attraction (sexual orientation) as the base to build upon as they expand beyond these two primary components. Regarding the nature of the third component, the additional dimensions referenced by several authors included factors such as an "inner sense of oneself," "specific sexual preferences," "group affiliation," "self-labeling," or "sex (gender) role." The most popular third factor referenced was sex (gender) role.

Four-Dimensional Definitions and Other Selected Scholars of Note

Two interesting definitions with four components were reviewed. The first is by McCammon et al. (2004). The second is by Coleman (2004). McCammon et al. (2004) describe sexual identity as "factors including one's biological sex, gender identity, gender role, and sexual orientation." Gender identity is incorporated into the "gender orientation" component of several of the three-dimensional definitions (including the Sexual Identity Cube, discussed later in this chapter). Now let us expand our consideration of sexual identity beyond college textbooks to include other leading voices is sexuality research.

Dr. Eli Coleman is the past president of several important organizations for the scientific study of sexuality, including the World Association for Sexology. Dr. Coleman has taken a lead on expanding and understanding the definitions of various forms of sexual identity, sexual compulsivity, and sexual health for several decades. He sees sexual identity as comprised of four basic components: *chromosomal sex/natal sex, gender identity, social sex-role,* and *sexual orientation* (Coleman, 2004). If the first two components are combined into one (chromosomal sex/natal sex and gender identity), then his definition is consistent with the three most common dimensions previously discussed (the three-dimensional model). As explained later, Coleman's first two components are combined into one (referred to as sex orientation) in the three-dimensional model of the Sexual Identity Cube.

Dr. Stephen Levine has been a steady and reasoned voice in care of patients with sexual health concerns as well as the training of health care professionals. Levine sees all sexual behavior (of any variety) as being constructed of four basic elements: biological, individual psychological, interpersonal, and cultural (Levine, 2007). Broadening his scope, he divides a person's sex life into three components: *sexual identity, sexual function,* and *sexual satisfaction.* He further subdivides sexual identity into gender identity, sexual orientation, and sexual intention. Sexual orientation is what you might expect (gay, straight, bi), but he defines gender identity as "the sense of the self as masculine or feminine" (not male or female or nonbinary). His third component of sexual intentions is interesting as he defines the concept as "what a person wants to do to his or her partner during sexual behavior and what the person wants to have done to him or her by the partner." Levine's notion of sexual intentions appears to address the issue of unusual (atypical) intentions expressed in a person's struggles with either gender identity, unusual types of sexual practices (such as fetishes, voyeurism, exhibitionism, and other paraphilia), and, according to Levine, even homosexuality when patients are struggling to balance their homeoerotic interests and participate in a traditional family life. While contributing a more nuanced definition, this conceptualization of both sexuality and sexual identity reflects a more traditional psychiatric perspective.

Dr. Lisa Diamond has been a strong voice of new insights into female sexuality, challenging the notion of rigid and lifelong sexual orientations (with what she calls "sexual fluidity"). Diamond has defined sexual identity as a "culturally organized conception of the self, usually 'lesbian/gay,' 'bisexual,' or 'heterosexual'" (2008). She introduces a new lexicon for people to describe themselves, preferring to use such terms as other-sex sexuality (for heterosexuality), same-sex sexuality (for homosexuality), and nonexclusive sexuality (instead of bisexuality). Diamond goes on to make distinctions between sexual identity and sexual orientation and argues for a more sophisticated understanding of sexual identity (Diamond, 2008). Her 10-year longitudinal data from studying adolescent girls turning into young women has shed light onto women's greater flexibility in their sexual expression in relationships (as compared with men).

The final two scholars noted here are Phillip Hammack and Daryl Bem. Both of these important voices have contributed a balanced perspective from an overall life-course human development framework, and both argue for an integrative view between the disparate opinions that attempt to explain all matters sexual by either biological essentialist models or by completely social constructionist models. Specifically related to our topic at hand, Hammack sees both biological factors (genes, hormones, and sexual desire) interacting with psychosocial factors (culture, history, personal development) to form sexual identity, which he clearly states is distinct from what we commonly refer to as sexual orientation (Hammack & Cohler, 2009). Bem has contributed a theory of how we direct our biologically based sexual interest toward others through a process he calls the "Exotic-Becomes-Erotic" (EBE) model of sexual attraction. This model is innovative, integrative, and attempts to explain the development of both heterosexuality and homosexuality by the same (EBE) process (D. Bem, 1996).

DEFINITIONS OF THE THREE BASIC COMPONENTS OF SEXUAL IDENTITY

Here is where the gender-bender mind-twist is about to start. Half the authors included in this review use three basic dimensions in their definitions of sexual identity. Therefore, it would be helpful to define these three primary components: Sex orientation (sex-designated status such as male, female, transgender), Sexual orientation (such as gay, straight, etc.), and Sex-role orientation (such as feminine, masculine, etc.). The following definitions may not make much sense until you read the sections below with the headings that start with "*How Are You So Sure That You Are . . .*" (which follow these definitions).

Sex Orientation (Designated Male/Female Spectrum Sex Status)

This refers to a person's fundamental status on a male-to-female continuum, which is composed of eight factors, both biological and psychosocial. Sex orientation is a person's most fundamental status of being human and is most often designated as male (having testicular or masculinized tissue present), female (having ovarian or feminized tissue present), or some combination of male-female sex traits referred to as transgender. People are typically considered transgender in one of two ways. Intersex transgender individuals have some combination of testicular (or masculinized) tissue and ovarian (or feminized) tissue present. The second type of transgender individuals are referred to as psychosocial transgender (not being intersex but having a psychological gender identity different from their socially assigned sex designation). Hence, there are four flexible types of sex orientation: male, female, intersex transgender, and psychosocial transgender individuals. These types of sex orientations are referred to as flexible because, while they remain constant for most people, they do change for a minority of individuals. It is important to note that the term *sex* has been primarily used in the literature to refer to biological characteristics of a person assigned to the status of male or female. However, "sex" is not that simple; as you will see, your sex status is mostly biological but also has psychological and social dimensions. It is important to note that sex orientation is on a spectrum with many variations and is not an "either/or" binary concept.

Sexual Orientation (Sexual Attraction Pattern)

This is a quality within you that describes to whom your sexual, affectionate, and/or love interests are directed. There are four primary points of the sexual orientation spectrum: gay, bi, straight, and asexual, but for the purposes of simplicity in this chapter, we are going to primarily use the first three types and respectfully defer the topic of asexuality for the time being. The word *orientation* has been challenged, and some authors choose to use different terms to describe a person's attraction to others, such as sexual attraction pattern, sexual desire, sexual pathways, sexual lifeways, and so on. The word *orientation* implies a static and inflexible trait that is inconsistent with many people's experience. However, because sexual orientation is the term understood by most people, it is used in this book acknowledging some debate about its use and the understanding that "orientation" is a malleable characteristic that can change over time (yet not simply considered a "choice"). As this book later argues, sexual orientation as well as sex orientation and sex-role orientation are all subject to change, and do for many people.

Sex-Role Orientation (Gender Role)

This refers to your personal response to role expectations that society associates with your designated sex and is manifest in your gender-role attitude and gender-role behavior. There are four basic primary points of sex-role orientation spectrum: traditionally masculine, traditionally feminine, androgynous, and undifferentiated. Again, for the purposes of simplicity in this chapter, we are going to primarily discuss the first three types and set aside the topic of undifferentiated sex role for the time being.

Sex orientation, sexual orientation, and sex-role orientation are the basic three components of sexual identity. It is necessary to make these terms clear before getting into the intersection of these concepts. Each of these three concepts can be a bit confusing themselves but will get more complex when we combine them in new ways. But before we do that, let us move to a deeper understanding of your sex, sexual, and sex-role orientations. To do so, there are three key questions for you: How are you so sure of your sex? How are you so sure of being gay, bi, or straight? How are you so sure of being masculine, feminine or androgynous? These questions can be considered irrelevant, provocative, silly, or even insulting. However, the explanations that follow reveal further details of what we take for granted.

BASIC SEX ORIENTATION: HOW ARE YOU SO SURE YOU ARE A MAN OR WOMAN?

In what ways do you identify your sex status as a male, female, or transgender individual (whether intersexed or psychosocially transgender)? Did you know there are at least five biological and three psychosocial variables to comprehensively classify your sex status? Most of the eight factors can be reasonably determined by you just by thinking about them. Also, most of them can be determined by a good developmental history, but a few factors always require physical examination by sexual health specialists. For example, one variable that always requires technical assessment is your chromosomal makeup.

The five biological variables include your chromosomes, prenatal hormone exposure, external genitalia, internal reproductive organs, and pubescent hormone development. Obviously, each of these factors has had a specific effect on your sexual development. But there are also three psychosocial variables, which include the sex you were medically assigned at birth (as designated on a birth certificate), the sex you were raised as in your family (this does not always match the sex assigned at birth), and the sex you believe you are (referred to as your gender identity), which may or may not match any of the other dimensions.

Hence, the "simple" question of your basic sex orientation (sex status) does not seem as simple as once thought. These eight dimensions of sex designation have been written about for decades, but they did not get put together into such nuanced relationships until the last few decades. The degree of complexity continues to increase when we focus on the significant variability within just one of the eight levels of biological sex status: chromosomal sex variations. Are you ready for this?

Traditionally, to have the status of "female," individuals have any of the following sex chromosomes (genotypes): XX (most typical female), XO (Turner syndrome – one X chromosome missing), XXX, or XXXX (see Table 1). In addition, individuals considered female can even have an XY sex chromosome combination (typically resulting in masculine development) if they have something called AIS – androgen insensitivity syndrome. Yes, that is right – XY chromosomal "males" can develop as women with a transgender orientation (whether they know of their chromosomal status or not). Individuals with AIS have an XY combination but did not experience the typical effects from the presence of prenatal androgens that flowed over the fetus and typically masculinize the developing sexual organs.

However, XY individuals with AIS (either partial or complete) may either have missing androgen receptors or ones that do not work well. Therefore, the fetus develops as a female anatomically, except they do not have a functional reproductive system. People with AIS can have happy and productive lives, such as Dr. Katie Baratz Dalke, who is a practicing psychiatrist. When she was young, she thought she was a typical girl until she was 6 years old and doubled over in pain. Her parents first thought she had a hernia, but her pain was actually caused by a descending testicle. She grew up as a beautiful woman, got married, adopted children and is an advocate for the civil rights of children born with variations of their sexual anatomy. The good doctor has also been an important health educator on the topic of AIS and been a board member of Advocates for Informed Choice, which works for empowering youth with intersex conditions and raising the visibility of intersex individuals (LeVay et al. 2015).

Now let's talk of "male" chromosomal variations. Traditionally, to have the status of "male," a person can have any of the following sex chromosomes (genotypes): XY (most typical male), XXY (Klinefelter syndrome), XYY, or other variations that include a Y sex chromosome (see Table 1 again). Similar to what was just described above, there are exceptions to the usual male sexual development as a fetus. There are XX chromosomal females that have a condition called CAH – congenital adrenal hyperplasia, which results in masculinization of fetal gonadal tissue. What happens during fetal growth is that the adrenal glands secrete an excessively large amount of androgens during the later stages of development. This results in a baby being born with either an enlarged clitoris (partial CAH) or penis structure if they experienced very significant masculinization (complete CAH).

Before we leave the area of females with gender variations, let's not forget the XY "males" who have developed a female gender identity. These chromosomal male individuals are also considered female and are classified as psychosocial transgender individuals. Many of these individuals pursue and complete sexual reassignment surgery, and many do not. They are sometimes referred to as male-to-female (M2F) transsexuals (an older term) or trans-women and do not have any (known) variation of sex chromosomes so are not included on the following table of chromosomal variations (Table 1). As with the XY women with female gender identity, let's not forgot the XX chromosomal females who develop male sexual identities. As with their gender counterparts, these individuals are considered to be male socially, but are classified as psychosocial transgender individuals. Many of these individuals pursue and complete sexual reassignment surgery, and many do not. They are sometimes referred to as female-to-male (F2M) transsexuals or trans-men and do not have any identifiable variations with their physical sexual development.

TABLE 1. Sex Chromosome Variations

Female Genotype Syndrome Prevalence and Male Genotype Syndrome Prevalence	
XX	Sex-typical and most common presentation of who we refer to as female
XY	Sex-typical and most common presentation of who we refer to as male
XO	Turner syndrome with estimated prevalence is 1:2000
XXY or XXXY	Klinefelter syndrome with estimated prevalence 1:500
XXX or XXXX	Triple-X syndrome with estimated prevalence 1:1000
XYY	Jacobs syndrome with estimated prevalence 1:1500
XX/XXX	Mosaic Unknown prevalence
XY/XXY	Mosaic Unknown prevalence

These variations occur naturally and regularly among all human births. When you add up their total estimated frequencies for atypical chromosomal variations in sexual development, it approximates a bit under 2% of all live births (see Table 2, p. 108), which represents estimated frequencies of selected sexual development variations within every 100 births (Fausto-Sterling, 2000). This discussion is not intended to turn you into a specialist in pediatric genetics but to drive home the point that there is a lot more to the "simple" assignment of sex status for many people – and we have talked only about chromosomal and hormonal variations. Those two variations add up to nearly two in every 100 people in the general population.

TABLE 2. Frequencies of Most Common Hormonal and Chromosomal Variations in Sexual Development (estimated frequencies per every 100 live births)*

XO	(Turner syndrome) 0.03690
XXY	(Klinefelter syndrome) 0.09220.
XY	(Androgen insensitivity syndrome – AIS full) 0.00760
XY	(Androgen insensitivity syndrome – AIS partial) 0.00076
XX	(Congenital adrenal hyperplasia – classic CAH) 0.00779
XX	(Congenital adrenal hyperplasia – late-onset CAH) 1.50000
XX	Vaginal agenesis (females born without a vagina) 0.01690
True hermaphroditism (both ovaries and testicles) 0.00120	
Idiopathic hermaphroditism 0.00090	
Non-XX or non-XY (except for Turner and Klinefelter syndromes) 0.06390	

****An estimation of the frequency for all hormonal and chromosomal variations equals 1.72815 births per 100 live births.***

That's a lot of stats. Let's take a real-life example to illustrate the numbers. Once there was a little girl who was assigned a female status at birth and raised as a girl by her family. She was considered feminine and grew up to be an attractive woman with a traditional bell-shaped figure (sizable breasts with a narrow waist and broader hips). She was athletic, had the strength of a woman, and did well in competition. So well, in fact, that during the 1980s she was Spain's best female hurdler, won international competitions, and planned to go to the Olympics. However, Maria Patiño of Spain was disqualified for participation in the female competition even though she always thought of herself as a woman. The problem the world-level athletic association had with this hurdler was that unbeknownst to her, she had a Y chromosome. She eventually was successful in overturning her disqualification and led a high-profile campaign to change the way the Olympics conducted testing for determining sex. There is an extensive list of such examples in athletics. Another notable and recent example is the case of the South African sprinter Caster Semenya, silver medal winner in the 2012 Olympics.

BASIC SEXUAL ORIENTATION: HOW ARE YOU SO SURE YOU ARE GAY, BI, OR STRAIGHT?

Sexual orientation is the quality within you that determines who your sexual, affectional, and/or love interests are directed toward and with whom you may choose to have sexual relations. Sexual orientation can be defined in many ways; no one definition is universally accepted. Most scholars understand that sexual orientation is much more complex than the traditional consideration of *with whom one chooses to have sexual relations*. Sexual orientation often (but not necessarily) has components of intense affection and/or love associated with sexual interest. A more common textbook definition is "the pattern of sexual and emotional attraction based on the gender of one's partner" (Hyde

& DeLamater, 2011). The American Psychological Association defines sexual orientation as "one's enduring sexual attraction to male partners, female partners, or both. Sexual orientation may be heterosexual, same sex (gay or lesbian), or bisexual" (*https://dictionary.apa.org/sexual-orientation*). Of course, this can include both males, females, and individuals of different transgender variations. How we think of sexual orientation today mostly stems from the groundbreaking work of Alfred Kinsey and colleagues (1948, 1953). The three types of sexual orientation that are generally accepted are represented on the famous Kinsey Scale continuum (see Figure 1). These three types of sexual orientation are heterosexuality, bisexuality, and homosexuality. Varying degrees and types of bisexuality are represented by categories 1-5.

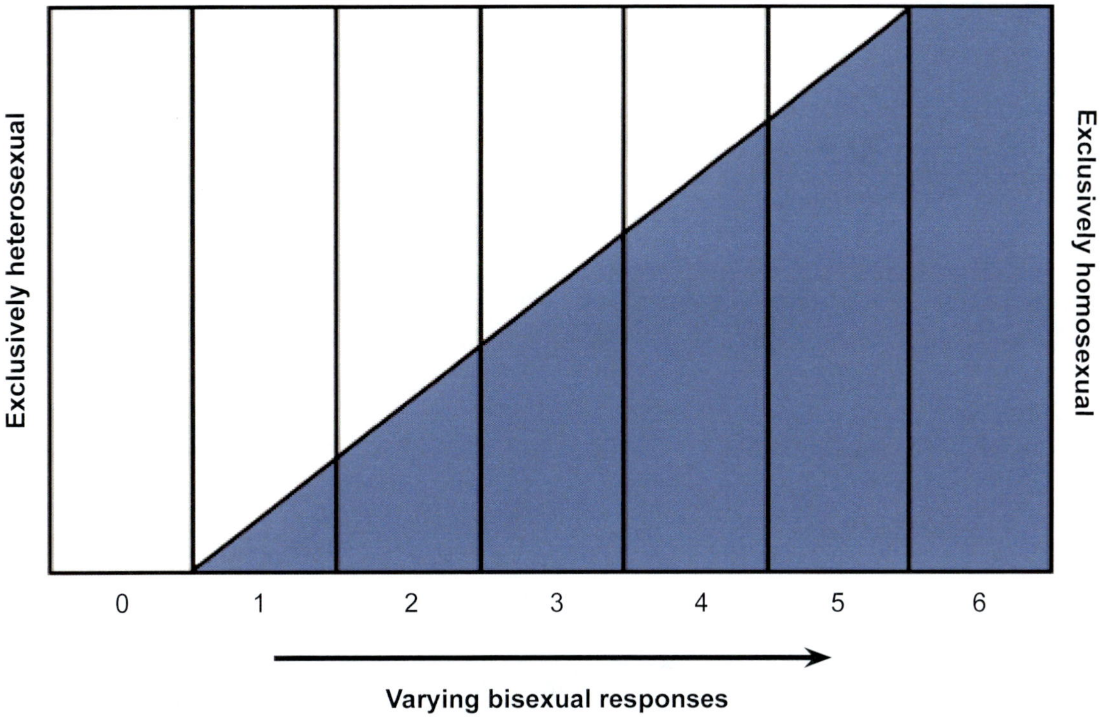

Figure 1. The Kinsey Scale of Heterosexuality-Homosexuality

From *Sexual Behavior in the Human Male* by A. C. Kinsey, W. P. Pomeroy, & C. E. Martin (1948).

This continuum represents the most common model of how we think of the relationship between heterosexuality and homosexuality in 21st-century American culture. However, there are still many people in this country (particularly members of conservative religious groups) who do not accept the Kinsey scale as factual, good science, and certainly not the dominant paradigm. Acknowledging anthropological studies of many same-sex practices around the world (at least where scholars are allowed to conduct such studies), there is a strong rejection of a normalized view of homosexuality outside America and Europe.

Indeed, homosexual behavior is still criminalized and reason for publicly sanctioned discrimination and persecution in many places around the world. However, another way of constructing the concept is to view sexual orientation not on a continuum, but as a 2 X 2 matrix. On one dimension is the variable of attraction to males (low or high). On the second dimension is attraction to females (low or high). This creates four quadrants within this 2 X 2 matrix of sexual orientation when crossing one axis of high attraction to women with low attraction to women and the high attraction to men with low attraction to men (see Table 3).

TABLE 3. Two-by-Two Matrix of Sexual Attraction

	High Attraction to Females	Low Attraction to Females
High Attraction to Males	**Bisexual attraction**	You are **gay** if a man You are **straight** if a woman
Low Attraction To Males	You are **straight** if a man You are **lesbian** if a woman	**Asexuality** (Low/no attraction to either)

Depending on the sex status of the person in question, two of the four quadrants of this 2 X 2 matrix represent heterosexuality or homosexuality. The first represents high attraction to women and low attraction to men (lower left quadrant). The second quadrant represents of low attraction to women and high attraction to men (upper right quadrant). However, there are two more quadrants for sexual orientation. The third category is "high attraction to both men and women" is the upper left quadrant and can be considered bisexuality. The fourth category (one not represented on the Kinsey Scale) is "low or no attraction to both men and women" (lower right quadrant) and can be considered asexuality.

Although there is not yet consensus that asexuality is a truly separate orientation or a lack of an orientation (Brotto & Yule, 2017), asexuality is defined as an individual having very low or no sexual interest in others as sexual partners. This is a definition supported by those who self-identify as asexual individuals. Considering the great diversity of human sexual behavior (as well as across the rest of the animal kingdom), it certainly makes sense that there are people who experience little to no sexual interest as there are those who report high interest in sex. A key point in this discussion is that asexual individuals typically have had little to no interest in sex as long as they can remember. Additionally, asexual people do not have an absence of sexual interest because of the effects of medical conditions, related medication side effects, depression, or a history of sexual abuse. Rather, they will likely say, "This is how I always have been."

How do asexual people differ from bisexual and pansexual individuals? Generally, bisexual individuals often report higher levels of sexual interest as well as a preference toward either males or females as sexual partners. Individuals identifying as pansexual are defined as those who are interested in and open to intimate relations with others regardless of gender (Yarber & Sayad, 2019), inclusive of others who see themselves as queer and/or transgender.

Asexual individuals, on the other hand, not only have little or no interest in sex but also have little or no preference for males or females as a sexual partner. Asexual individuals may abstain from sex, or they may have sex at times; but they typically do so for reasons other than sexual desire and/or sexual attraction. For example, they may report that they have sex for reasons such as wanting to be in a relationship for companionship, having children, or simply pleasing a partner.

The new sexual health paradigm includes an expanding range of normalcy, and asexual individuals should not be pathologized but accepted as another variation in the beautiful diversity of human sexuality. The descriptions for the four different quadrants of sexual orientation (reflected in Table 3) reflect dramatic changes in how we conceptualize what is normal in our society and the variations of sexual orientation across individuals. If you are old enough, you may remember that only 50 years ago, the consensus opinion in medicine was that all variations of sexual expression other than heterosexuality constituted pathological mental illness and resulted from an individual's choice of "lifestyle." The critical shift in perception occurred toward a significant expansion in what is considered "normal range" sexual expression. This shift in cultural perspective contributed to the declassification of homosexuality as a mental illness in 1973 and promoted greater self-acceptance among individuals who might otherwise criticize, reject, or even loathe themselves.

This reconceptualization has been accompanied by a shift away from the view of sexual expression simply as a moral "choice of lifestyle" and reflects a movement toward a view of sexual attraction being more biologically determined. However, some fascinating research over the past few decades supports a view that at least some aspects of sexual expression are socially constructed. Excellent examples of this view are the anthropological studies by Gilbert Herdt of the Sambian male rites of passage, where boys experience several years of same-sex sexual behavioral training to learn to be a man through ingestion of semen (from older boys and men). They are reported to then enter adulthood as heterosexual men who select a wife and raise a family (Herdt, 2005).

Sophisticated biosocial theories of the development of sexual attraction (such as Daryl Bem's "Exotic Becomes Erotic" theory) have replaced old (and artificial) "nature versus nurture" explanations. Bem combines well-researched traits such as child temperament and play preference (representing "nature") with factors such as the influence of social peer groups and who a child sees as different or the "exotic other." The exotic other becomes erotized during pubescent hormonal exposure (the exotic becomes erotic) resulting in either a heterosexual or homosexual orientation, depending on the sex designation of both the child and the eroticized other (D. Bem, 1996). Bisexuality could be conceptualized to be a variation of this biosocial process. What used to be called a "lifestyle choice" is now understood to be healthy and responsible sexual behavior. Research continues to develop and test new theories of sexual orientation, but the dramatic "societal rethink" of this basic component of sexuality in only a few decades is nothing short of revolutionary.

BASIC SEX-ROLE ORIENTATION: HOW ARE YOU SO SURE THAT YOU ARE AS MASCULINE, FEMININE, OR ANDROGYNOUS AS YOU BELIEVE?

As mentioned earlier in this chapter, sex-role orientation refers to your personal response to gender role expectations that culture places upon members of a particular gender. Your response is expressed in your sex-role attitude and sex-role behavior. What are gender-role attitude and gender-role behavior?

Sex-Role Behavior

Sex-role behavior is defined as specific acts or activities in which you engage according to your beliefs about your gender (based on your sex-role attitude). Hence, boys and men may choose (even though they may be unaware of making a choice) to act more aggressively and engage in socially sanctioned activities such as football. Girls and women may choose (even though they may be unaware of making a choice) to act more nurturing and engage in socially sanctioned activities such as selecting nursing as a career, as opposed to engineering (S. Bem, 1981a).

Let's go back to the definition of sex-role orientation (gender role). It is a combination of your personal attitudinal response to sex-role expectations (which go along with your sex status) and is expressed in your sex-role behavior. The key phrase is personal response, or how people choose (consciously at times, but mostly unconsciously) whether to accept or reject the cultural expectation for them to "swim with the current" and act in a socially sanctioned or expected manner. The boy footballer and female nurse are examples of "swimming with the current" via confluence with cultural expectations in America and would be considered a more traditional response to society's expectations. It is important to note that masculinity and femininity are not polar opposites on the same continuum. Masculinity and femininity are separate concepts on separate continuums, and they both exist within the same individual. For example, a particular person may have both a high degree of masculine traits and a high degree of feminine traits. This is what we refer to as androgyny (Carroll, 2016).

Androgyny is characterized by flexibility in one's response to sex-role expectations through the development of a combination of skills (what researchers call instrumental and expressive traits). The skills and traits we build are influenced by individual differences, historical situations, and our stage of the life cycle. Expressive traits are traditionally associated with females in many cultures, traits such as greater comfort showing affection and demonstrating nurturing behaviors. Instrumental traits are traditionally associated with males in many cultures, traits such as being more inclined to be analytical and more aggressive. This sounds like straight sex stereotyping, but remember, we are talking about very large and general trends on a societal level.

It is important to recognize that sexual orientation and sex-role orientation are independent of each other. What this means is that being gay or straight has little to do with being masculine or feminine. For example, stereotypes of gay men as effeminate florists or lesbians as motorcycle mamas are common. In reality, and in recognition of the great diversity of human experience, some gay men and lesbians do fit these stereotypes. However, the vast majority do not. Of course, the opposite of general sexual stereotyping may be true as well, such as the macho quarterback who identifies himself as gay.

Similar to the matrix involved with our discussion of sexual orientation, Dr. Sandra Lipsitz Bem introduced a 2 X 2 matrix several decades ago to use as a teaching tool about sex-role orientation (S. Bem, 1981b). Table 4 is created by intersecting the two variables of masculinity (low or high) and femininity (low or high). The left side of the matrix represents high masculinity, while the right side represents low masculinity. It is the same for femininity but "up and down" because femininity is on the side axis. Therefore, high femininity is on the top half of the matrix, whereas low femininity is represented on the lower half of the matrix.

Hence, this matrix results in four quadrants that represent four different sex-role orientations, and here is an important point: Each quadrant may represent an individual who identifies as a man or a woman. The four quadrants of sex-role orientation (gender role) are based on this 2 X 2 matrix and are as follows:

1. **Traditional masculinity** (high masculinity, low femininity). Examples could include a macho cowboy or a woman who mostly displays traditional masculine traits.
2. **Traditional femininity** (low masculinity, high femininity). Examples could include effeminate men (gay or straight) or a lipstick lesbian (a slang term for one who is feminine in manner or appearance, breaking any stereotype of female homosexuality being associated with masculine traits).
3. **Androgyny** (high masculinity, high femininity). Examples could include metrosexual men or assertive female executives.
4. **Undifferentiated** (low masculinity, low femininity). Examples could include men and women who are not easy at first to identify as male or female, and their appearance may be unintentional ("that's just the way I am") or intentionally attempting to generate a confusing presentation of gender (sometimes as a statement of protest against the standard heterosexual standard or against the "well-behaved" gay and lesbian stereotypes).

TABLE 4. Two-by-Two Matrix of Sex-Role Orientation (Gender Role) based on the work of Sandra Bem (1981b)

	High Traits of Masculinity	Low Traits of Masculinity
High Traits of Femininity	**Andronogy**	**Traditional Femininity**
Low Traits of Femininity	**Traditional Masculinity**	**Undifferentiated**

The category of "undifferentiated" is uncommon, and individuals who identify with this sex-role orientation are not well understood. As we did with "asexual" individuals, this type of sex-role orientation is being respectfully acknowledged, but detailed discussion of it is being set aside for the purposes of the brevity of this chapter. The last example (number 4 on page 112) of individuals who intentionally seek to create unique gender appearances sometimes self-identify as part of queer culture and deserve more discussion than they receive in this chapter.

NOW BACK TO THE CENTRAL QUESTION OF SEXUAL IDENTITY

So, Do You Know What Your Sexual Identity Is?

Even more basic, what exactly is identity? Using the big old *Webster's International Dictionary*, *identity* is defined as the "limit approached by increasing similarity" and the "sameness of all that constitutes the objective reality of a thing." Wow, that's cool. However, the most suitable meaning for our purposes is "unity and persistence of personality." Wow again – how we fit together and have a sense of persistence over time is what we call our identity.

To consider the subject of sexual identity, we also need to touch on Erik Erikson's stages of psychosocial development. Let us consider how Erikson conceived of the process by which we form our identity, which begins early in childhood but really blossoms in adolescence (ages 12-18). Teenagers often go through a crisis of who they are going to be as grown-ups. Erickson saw the central dynamics of this stage of identity formation involving a basic conflict between "identity vs. role confusion" (Kail & Cavanaugh, 2004). The developmental task for teens is to build a sense of self and personal identity (and to do that through exploration of social relationships). A central question about Erikson's theory on identity formation is "how is an adolescent realistically able to develop a sense of personal identity without developing a sexual identity as part of that overall identity as a person?" (Erikson, 1968).

Most kids do not wake up in the morning wondering if today is the day they figure out their identity in general and their sexual identity in particular. If they can think beyond breakfast, they might worry about how they are going to do their homework before they get to school or at least before they get to class. Any "big-picture thinking" is usually forced on them by an exceptional teacher who might engage the class in a stimulating discussion of "Who are we?" as girls and boys, as sons and daughters, as Americans, or even as human beings.

Identity has many aspects that each of us collectively call "me." Consider the roles of our ethnic, racial, and cultural backgrounds in the development of our overall identity. Many folks have identities closely tied to their religious training and beliefs. What we do for work and eventually as a career plays a significant part in how we respond to the question "Who are you?" When introducing themselves to a new person, few people start off their answer with "I am a lesbian" or "I am a heterosexual." The point is that your sexual identity is a part of your overall identity. Yet, for most people, sexual identity is a fundamental element of our identity.

This is why people are sometimes surprised to hear sexperts say "sex is not the most important thing in the world," yet at the same time, and quite paradoxically, it is very important. The evolutionists would say it is the most important element in life because perpetuation of the species is involved. If you don't think sex is so important, ask yourself the following questions. If you are gay, how would your life be different if you were straight? If you are straight, how would your world be different if you were gay? How about if you were another gender?

A NEW DEFINITION OF SEXUAL IDENTITY AND THE SEXUAL IDENTITY CUBE

Based on this chapter's discussion about all the significant variations across the many definitions of sexual identity, here are several conclusions:

1. If you are going to write a book, a journal article, or even present a lecture about sexuality, it would be good to define terms like sexuality and sexual identity.
2. Sexuality is a core experience of being human and can be generally considered all things about you as a sexual being. The formal definition of sexuality used in this chapter is from SIECUS: "Sexuality encompasses the sexual knowledge, beliefs, attitudes, values, and behaviors of individuals. Its various dimensions involve the anatomy, physiology, and biochemistry of the sexual response system; identity, orientation, roles and personality; and thoughts, feelings and relationships. Sexuality is influenced by ethical, spiritual, cultural, and moral concerns" (2018, Para 1). This is an excellent definition; our only suggestion is that it should include a reference to sexuality being a lifetime experience.
3. Sexuality can be broadly divided into your sexual identity and your sexual expression.
4. Sexual identity is not the same as sexual orientation, as sexual identity is a much broader term that encompasses sexual orientation. Sexual identity is part of one's overall identity as a person. SIECUS defines sexual identity as "an inner-sense of oneself as a sexual being, including how one identifies in terms of gender and sexual orientation" (2018).
5. Based on reviewing three dozen sources authored by leading authorities on human sexuality, there is a lack of consensus across these experts' attempts to define sexual identity. A new definition is needed; one that reflects the central elements most authors use yet reflects the great diversity of the human sexual experience.

The following definition of sexual identity is offered as a potential step toward the ultimate goal of developing a consensus of what sexual identity is (with further revisions expected). This definition is primarily based upon:

1. the three most commonly used components for definitions found in the review of sexuality and gender textbooks;

2. sex-role orientation (gender role) being the most commonly used "additional dimension" used in three- and four-dimensional definitions; and
3. the integration of key principles of leading scholars on the topic.

Sexual Identity – A New Definition

Sexual identity is the sense of who one is as a sexual being and is a fundamental human experience comprised of a person's sex orientation, sexual orientation, and sex-role orientation. Sexual identity is a central part of a person's sexuality and changes over the lifespan of an individual. The behavioral expression of sexual identity is different from the identity itself, encompasses a great diversity of expression transculturally, and is based on one's personal development of eroticism that is mediated by culturally and biologically based factors.

The first sentence above is the core definition of sexual identity, while all three sentences make up the full definition. This definition captures many key points made in the literature on sexual identity as well as the discussion presented in this chapter. As a visual representation of this definition, the Sexual Identity Cube (i-Cube for short) is presented as a conceptual teaching tool.

The i-Cube was originally developed to expand existing models beyond the limits of biological sex status and sexual orientation. This expansion is needed to more accurately reflect the complexity of sexuality in contemporary culture. However, the original version of the i-Cube was oversimplified (Peterson, 2007), and this revised version is expanded to be more inclusive, which is one of the goals of the i-Cube as a conceptual and teaching tool.

This new definition of sexual identity (and the i-Cube; see Figure 2 on the next page) is intended to more accurately describe the tremendous diversity of sexual identities among people that is well documented across the literature of anthropology, medicine, psychology, and sociology. This i-Cube model is designed to promote greater self-acceptance as well as acceptance of individual differences among us as people. Differences (in and by themselves) are often, especially historically, seen as a bad thing. Differences are actually a good thing, whether you are talking about sexual differences, different opinions, or biodiversity. As an evolving human culture, it is in our best interests to stop pathologizing variations in sexual identity and expression simply because they diverge from a cultural norm (Bley & Peterson, 2007). Oversimplified definitions of sexual identity limit the range of "what is normal" and therefore can limit a person's capacity for developing a positive self-worth. Consequently, they may contribute to some individuals concluding that they (as a person) do not fit the current definitions of healthy sexual identity and result in unnecessary self-perceptions of being abnormal and unacceptable.

The i-Cube is a pictorial reflection of what we have discussed in this chapter, only in the visual form of a 4 X 4 X 4 polygon. The i-Cube represents all four types of sex orientation (male, intersex transgender, psychosocial transgender, and female), all four types of sexual orientation (attracted to neither men nor women, attracted to both men and women, attracted to women, attracted to men), and all four types of sex-role orientation (traditional masculine, androgynous, traditional feminine, and undifferentiated).

This i-Cube has 64 "vector areas" representing many different sexual identities that range from common identities (like traditionally feminine heterosexual women and traditionally masculine heterosexual men; think Barbie and Ken) to vector areas (like the effeminate gay man and androgynous bisexual woman). The sexual identity of the aforementioned Olympian (Maria Patiño) is represented in the i-Cube by the vector area for androgynous heterosexual intersex transgender women. Before discussing "Joe, Cody, and Pam" in Figure 2, let me make some very important points about how to interpret what you see in the i-Cube (because what you *believe* you see can be very misleading).

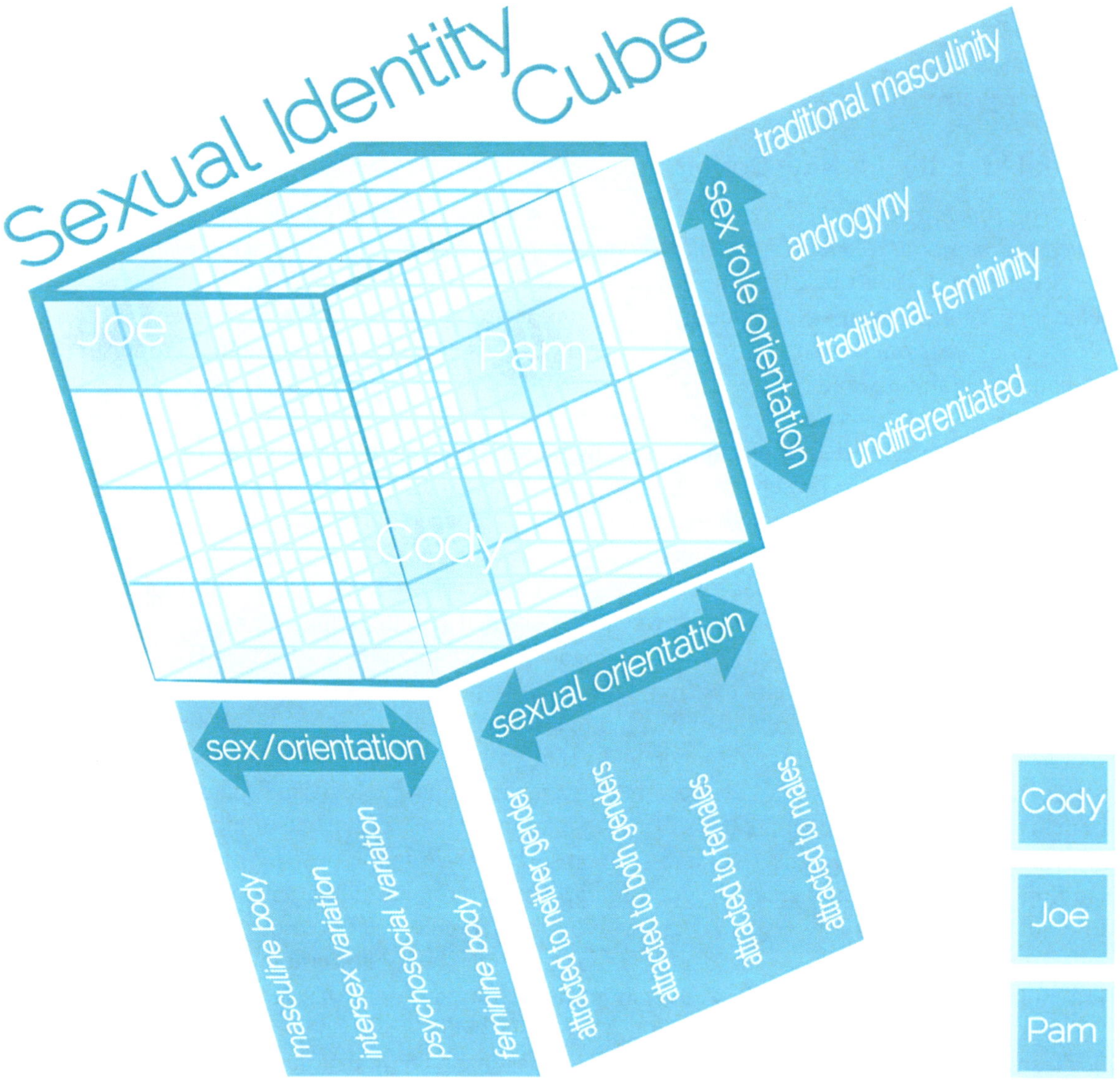

Figure 2. The Sexual Identity Cube (i-Cube).
Illustration by Max Fleishman.

Point 1
The directional *arrows* are much more important than what appears to be the smaller subunits of the i-Cube. The arrows represent a *continuum* or spectrum of characteristics as opposed to discrete categories within sex orientation, sexual orientation, and sex-role orientation. So, pay more attention to the continuum arrows as they are the most important visually.

Point 2
The smaller subunits within the i-Cube should be thought of as areas around a vector that represent the intersection of the three factors of sex orientation, sexual orientation, and sex-role orientation.

Point 3

Although our brain wants to see lines and squares as having firm boundaries between one side of a line and the other side (or the inside of a square and the outside), please inform your brain that all the lines of the i-Cube are diffuse and permeable. Think of the lines as being made of concentrated lines of fog as opposed to any solid boundary. Although the "lines" may be misleading, it is visually necessary to have the lines for teaching purposes to visually locate the vector area that is being discussed, such as Joe, Cody, and Pam.

Point 4

As mentioned, the "lines" within the i-Cube are permeable and do not represent discrete categorical states of sexual being, therefore representing the flexible nature of sexual identity and the possibility of change of self-identified sexual identity over time.

Point 5

Said differently, people can "move around" within the i-Cube from one stage of life to another, changing aspects of their sexual identity as they go (whether that is change in their sex orientation, sexual orientation, and/or sex-role orientation). As will be later argued, *most people do change* at least one of these three dimensions during their lifetime (most often sex-role orientation). Sometimes these changes are voluntary choices and sometimes they are not.

Back to Joe, Pam, and Cody (in that order). What does the vector area identified for Joe represent? Joe is in the upper-left corner of the i-Cube and represents an individual who identifies as a male with a masculinized body, displays traditional masculinity, and who is not attracted to either men or women (asexual). Get it?

The vector area directly behind Joe represents an individual who is a traditionally masculine man such as Joe but who happens to be bisexual. Pam represents a bit more common sexual identity than Cody. Pam identifies herself as an androgynous woman who is attracted to women. BOOM – that's how the i-Cube works.

Let's try Cody (this is an example of where the lines are very helpful for locating the vector area). If you follow the lines, Cody would be identified as an intersex transgender individual who is attracted to females and has an undifferentiated sex-role orientation. Depending on how Cody identifies as male/female/trans, he/she/they (using the singular "they") might also identify as a straight guy or identify herself as a lesbian. To be even more gender-nuanced, they may also identify their sexual orientation as something different (bi?) if they self-identify their sex orientation as *neither or both male and/or female.* Is your gender-bender brain spinning yet? Yes, please don't be discouraged. This can get complicated, but so is the nature of human sexual diversity. You'll get it.

Joe, Pam, and Cody are intended to help you get the basic idea of identifying different sexual identities with the i-Cube. While illustrative of how these three individuals identify themselves at a particular point in their life span, it is important to remember Point 5: That people can "move around" within the i-Cube across time by experiencing changes in their sex, sexual, or sex-role orientations. So, let's use some additional examples to reflect this movement.

Chapter 20 of this book introduces you to Alex, a former Navy Seal, who appeared to be a traditionally masculine, heterosexual male. However, through gender affirming surgery, Alex became an androgynous lesbian woman deeply in love with her wife. Chapter 20 will also introduce you to Gage, one of the best examples to "mobility" and gender fluidity you will ever meet. Gage's movement within the Sexual Identity Cube includes several vectors, including times in his life when he was: (a) a traditionally feminine, heterosexual girl (including birthing a son); (b) a masculine lesbian woman; (c) transitioning to a traditionally masculine transman in a heterosexual relationship; and (d) meeting and falling in love with a transman and living life as part of a gay couple.

This may be an unusual way to explain the i-Cube, but the point is this: We need a very large tepee to allow all human beings to feel like they belong to the tribe. To promote health and acceptance of your children and their children, we want to avoid teenagers feeling like they don't belong if they don't identify with the historically defined, socially sanctioned models of normalcy (traditionally masculine heterosexual men and traditionally feminine heterosexual women). If our children reject these traditional models and have few other socially sanctioned choices in which to relate, they are at increased risk for isolation, confusion, and possibly mental health problems. Many youths today reject the limited models offered them and therefore seek their own definition and style of expression, often assimilating with other alternative youth to become a "member of their own tribe" and sometimes doing so at great personal risk.

Although the i-Cube represents an expanded consideration of factors contributing to the formation of sexual identity, the new definition allows for consideration of important intersecting factors, which not only shape an individual's sense of sexual identity but partly determine the nature of their sexual expression. These cultural factors include, but are not limited to, such variables as ethnicity and racial identity, religious and nationality affiliations, historical context, disability status, age, personal sexual developmental factors, and familial factors. Many of these variables can come into play simultaneously. This is called "intersectionality" and refers to the accumulative influences on an individual as a result of identification with multiple cultural groups, especially those considered sexual minorities. For example, "African American women veterans who come from families that have been part of rural Appalachia for generations (referred to as Afrilachians) are more at risk for depression and other health care disparities (such as hypertension, diabetes, and obesity)" than white male heterosexual veterans (Cohen et al., 2013). Considering the interactive and intersecting nature of both sexual identity and expression, the number of permutations regarding cultural factors serving as influencing variables is virtually endless. Now THAT is the essence of human diversity! The definitions and interaction between sexual identity and expression are the focus of the rest of this chapter. So, let's focus on sexual expression.

Sexual Expression

There are a few central questions while exploring sexual expression. What exactly is sexual expression and what is the relationship between it and sexual identity? What are the primary forms of sexual expression? Why is the question regarding "Is it nature versus nurture" the wrong question? What are the most common themes among sexual fantasies and how are they directed by this thing called a "lovemap?" What are the types of sexual behaviors that result in orgasm, both through sex with yourself and sex with others? What are the biological and social factors that modify our sexual expression?

Like the first part of this chapter, exploring these questions will lead to several assertions, such as there is little consensus regarding a definition of sexual expression, let alone what constitutes healthy sexual expression. In the absence of consensus, the best scholarly opinions are brought to the forefront for your consideration. A second point is that there is a reciprocal relationship between sexual identity and sexual expression, with mutual influences going both ways. Third (and similar to the Sexual Identity Cube model), three major dimensions guide sexual expression and comprise a model referred to as the Sexual Expression Cube (e-Cube). The three dimensions, later discussed in detail, are sexual fantasies, sexual behaviors (that result in orgasm), and bio-culturally bound modifying factors.

WHAT IS SEXUAL EXPRESSION?

Let's go back to the new definition presented earlier in the chapter: Sexual identity is the sense of "who one is" as a sexual being based on one's sex orientation, sexual orientation, and sex-role orientation.

The behavioral expression of one's sexual identity is different from identity itself and is conceptually organized by culturally defined factors and one's personal development of eroticism.

This definition of sexual identity not only references sexual expression but also begins to define sexual expression. The purpose here is to emphasize the distinction between the two concepts. Of course, this description is not sufficient as a full definition unto itself. However, finding a definition for sexual expression is even more challenging than defining sexual identity, in part because sexual expression is an even more general notion than sexual identity. It is easier for most authors to define more specific concepts such as sexual desire, sexual intercourse, or masturbation.

If you go to commonly used dictionaries (e.g., *Merriam-Webster*, *Oxford*, or the *Free Online Dictionary*), you will not find an entry for sexual expression. Interestingly, you will find that dozens of definitions of different types of sexual expression use the phrase "sexual expression" within their definitions but give no specific definition of sexual expression itself. Of course, the same authors who have written college textbooks (and were referenced earlier in this chapter) were also reviewed again for further understanding of sexual expression. Of all the textbooks with a glossary, no definition of sexual expression was found. In reviewing the subject index of these textbooks, only two contained a specific reference to sexual expression. It is interesting to note that most all the textbooks on sexuality literally are full of descriptions of sexual expression but do not enumerate the basic building blocks of the concept. Of all the textbooks on sexuality, only two have chapters with titles using the term sexual expression.

The first one, *Human Sexuality: Diversity in Contemporary America* (Strong et al., 2005 up through the latest 10th edition by Yarber & Sayad, 2019) has a chapter simply entitled "Sexual Expression" describing theories of sexual attraction, different types of relationships, sexual desire, sexual fantasies, and masturbation. The second textbook, *Sexuality Now: Embracing Diversity* (Carroll, 2007) has two chapters using the term in chapter titles: "Sexual Expression: Arousal and Response" and "Varieties of Sexual Expression." Interestingly, this author includes physiological arousal and responses under the umbrella of sexual expression along with the many types of "external" sexual behaviors (like masturbation, different types of common sexual activity with others, unusual sexual practices with others, and safer sex behaviors). Carroll also addresses how our sexual expression changes as we age.

If you remember our definition of sexuality, only two of the meanings are useful for our purposes: "The expression of the sexual instinct" and "the condition, potential, or state of readiness of the organism in regard to sexual activity." The term *expression* can describe anything related to symbolism (one thing representing something else) as in artistic expression, musical expression, and sexual expression. The phrase "condition, potential, or state of readiness" is also all-encompassing when it comes to sexual activity and certainly includes not only the more obvious activities such as sexual behaviors, but also the less visible activities such as dreams, fantasies, and physiological responses. Essentially, sexual expression is the manifestation of your sexual self through your sexual thoughts, sexual feelings, and sexual behaviors; all of which are significantly mediated by bio-culturally bound modifiers. These modifiers include factors that influence (and can even completely inhibit) the overt expression of sexual identity. Some of the primary examples of these factors are your religious beliefs, the legal-political system you live within, disability status, ethnicity, and race.

Sexual expression has as its foundation your physical substructure and your sexual identity but is also interactive with both of them. Said differently, forget all those traditional and artificial divisions between biology and psychology, between behavior and hormones, and between nature and nurture. As noted, your "sex" has been historically defined as your biology (chromosomes, gonads, and hormones), but this view is limited and could be better described as one's "biological sex." And as described earlier in the chapter, put your biological sex together with these three psychosocial dimensions (sex assigned at birth, sex raised as, and gender identity) and you have your sex orientation. This is your real sex designation, and it is a more inclusive perspective of people's experience of being male, female, or transgender. It is much more demonstrative of the biopsychosocial approach that has been emerging as the dominant paradigm in the scientific study of sexuality.

NATURE VERSUS NURTURE? (THE WRONG QUESTION)

The influences in our lives that govern our sexual expression simply are not easily divided into strict categories of internal or external, cultural or physiological, or nature or nurture. Relative to sexual expression, "nature and nurture" are often equated with "internal and external." It can be argued that sexual fantasies and dreams are "internal" sexual activity (sexual behavior) as opposed to external behaviors that can be more easily observed and measured. Although dream activity can be measured and analyzed objectively (via sleep studies measuring rapid eye movement), the content is subjectively experienced. Both dreams and sexual fantasies can be considered "activities" and in a sense a behavior. However, we have less choice about dreams as behavior in terms of initiation, content, and termination of the activity. Fantasies are more under our control as we can willfully generate them as people often do during daydreaming and masturbation.

But what about your increased heartbeat, respiration, and pupil dilation when you meet someone you find sexually attractive? These are sexual arousal responses that are not under your control yet occur. They happen even if you don't want them to and even if you try to think your way out of your attraction. Are these "expressions of the sexual instinct" or "the condition, potential, or state of readiness" for sexual activity? The authors believe they are. In addition, they also defy any artificial division of nature or nurture because the physiological attraction you experience (increased heartbeat, respiration, and pupil dilation) is absolutely influenced by culturally defined notions of beauty.

Culture and biology have many interactive influences upon each other; some we are just understanding with the passing of time and development of further science. American culture during the early 20th century dictated that proper care of infants included a sterile environment and limited physical touch (beyond basic feeding and changing). The mild-to-moderate effects of this cultural "nurture" factor (or lack of it) led to stunted physical and intellectual growth for many children. Obviously, part of your sexual identity (either as a straight guy or lesbian, for example) will influence whom your sexual behavior is directed toward. That is an example of how sexual identity influences sexual expression. Influences can move in the reverse direction as well. When a person enjoys a new behavior that they were not "attracted" to do (such as a woman who identifies as heterosexual and accepts a kiss from her girlfriend and gets aroused), they subsequently may question or re-examine their sexual orientation.

A BRIEF NOTE ON NORMALCY

Before getting into the nuances of the many varieties of sexual expression, two questions need to be addressed as the leading concern for most people: "Am I normal?" and "What is unhealthy?" What some folks consider unhealthy is actually believed to be healthy for many others. There is a very wide range of sexual activity that is considered normal when sexual researchers employ the five dimensions of considering sexual behavior – the biological, psychosocial, behavioral, clinical, and cultural measures. Some sexual behaviors are considered atypical in terms of being statistically infrequent but do not really cause problems for people or their sexual partners. Examples of these types of behavior are people who want their earlobe gently sucked to the point of orgasm (eargasm) or rub their thighs together rhythmically to the point of orgasm (cricket orgasm). Both behaviors could be considered unusual but do not hurt anyone and can even be seen as exceptionally skilled sexual behavior. Now consider these behaviors as part of the sexual repertoire of individuals living with a severe physical disability, like quadriplegia or cerebral palsy. Exceptional indeed. Consider these behaviors as part of how people draw a line in their mind between what they believe is and is not normal. It is not as simple as we may think. It is a distinction that is often arbitrary and subjective based on many factors, including religious values, prevailing cultural norms, one's level of sexual literacy of sexual practices of other people within a culture, as well as sexual practices in other cultures. When the authors are asked by students or clients "Am I normal?" they usually give one or more of the following three responses:

1. Put the concern within the context of five dimensions of understanding sexuality and see what conclusions can be drawn. Again, these five dimensions are biological, psychological, behavioral, clinical, and statistical aspects of the sexual activity. How do these considerations change the question?
2. When a person is involved with sexual variations such as sadomasochism, sometimes it comes down to ensuring it is a consensual sexual exchange and whether there is tissue damage. If two adults freely engage in some bondage or sadomasochism and no one is seriously injured, that's up to them. Two commonly used bottom lines are: Sex needs to be consensual and not involve serious bleeding.
3. Look at the consequences of the behavior and ask if the typical person would feel it is worth the costs (consequences) of the behavior. As a popular pop psychology guru (Dr. Phil) famously asks, "So, how's that working for you?" Considerations of consequences include, but may not be limited to relational, emotional, financial, spiritual, vocational, health, and legal consequences.

For example, a young 20-something couple came to the clinic regarding his apparent "impotency." The fellow could not get an erection (first time ever) after a hard night of drinking. On the subsequent evening, he was not able to get it up again (most likely due to excessive worry this time – called performance anxiety). The couple was getting married in a couple of months and wanted to correct this problem before getting hitched. They were told to go home, not to have sex for 3 days, not to drink the third day (alcohol interferes with erectile ability), and try it again. They called the clinic after a week to report everything was fine again because they were "back to acting like rabbits." Let's apply the three guidelines to this scenario.

Their situation was understandable on a biological basis as his difficulty was due in part to heavy alcohol use (to be expected). From a psychosocial perspective, his anxiety regarding his failure to get erections for the first time with his girlfriend and subsequent worry during the second attempt also contributed to his dreaded surprise (but no real surprise as anxiety can override high attraction and erectile response anytime). Behaviorally, this is a very common experience for men: He was perhaps too young to know this and maybe expected that he could defy the laws of physics. Clinically, he certainly did not meet any diagnostic criteria and culturally he was very typical of young men (and many young women) who believe a man should always have an erection at the drop of a bra or boxer shorts.

An analysis of the consequences of his drinking could (one hopes) lead him to stay within recommended limits of alcohol use and avoid unnecessary frustration (such as the argument they had, his thinking that he was impotent, and her thinking she wasn't attractive enough to him). Finally, there were two consenting adults (only the penis was not) and no one was getting seriously hurt. Conclusion: This scenario and the couple's concerns were very normal (they just didn't know it). They may not have considered their experience as healthy, but it certainly was not a case of erection dysfunction.

LOVEMAPS, PARAPHILIAS, AND SEXUAL EXPRESSION

The three dimensions of the Sexual Expression Cube are sexual fantasies, sexual behaviors (that lead to arousal or orgasm), and bio-culturally bound modifying factors. For reasons explained below, the first two factors (fantasies and behaviors) are described as "ideoerotic." This does not mean we get turned on by idiots nor does it mean that we turn into idiots when we get turned on (although some of us may think back to when this latter meaning may have applied). Ideoerotic attraction and expression means each person has an individual pattern of what really gets their sexual motor running. The term *ideoerotic* comes from the concept of lovemaps developed by the late John Money, the noted medical psychologist at Johns Hopkins University. Money defined a lovemap as follows: "A developmental representation or template synchronously in the mind and in the brain depicting the idealized lover, the idealized love affair, and the idealized program of sexuoerotic activity projected in imagery or actually engaged in with that lover" (Money, 1994).

Money described lovemaps as the filter through which we see our sexual world, and one that dictates our sexual interests and behaviors. The development of our lovemap is directed by prenatal hormonal exposure and coded environmentally through sensual input to the brain via the senses, especially by tactile sensation through the skin and augmented by smell, taste, sight, and sounds. Money's notion of lovemaps is thought of as a cognitive and emotional guide for erotic interests that is developed at an early age and directs sexual behaviors in relationships later in adolescence and adulthood. Lovemaps can develop into heterosexual, homosexual, bisexual, asexual, or a paraphilic pattern. Although Money's ideas are helpful to accurately describe certain aspects of human sexuality, there is much we do not know about the specific neuropathic mechanisms by which lovemaps develop.

A paraphilia is an unusual form of sexual activity considered to be "alongside" (para) or outside the usual expression of love (philia) (American Psychiatric Association, 2013). Some paraphilias are private and may not cause distress to the paraphilic individual or a partner. An example is a man who sometimes cross-dresses with women's lingerie for sexual pleasure and spicing up his sex life with his wife but does so with his wife's knowledge and input as to what lingerie to buy (cross-dressing can also be done for fun, entertainment, or parody, not necessarily as a paraphilia). Some paraphilias are considered a crime, a mental illness, or both (e.g., when a person acts out a paraphilic disorder by victimizing a child).

People with paraphilic lovemaps tend to have fantasies and behaviors that are long-standing, compulsive in nature, and distressing to the individual (and their partners as well). One's lovemap usually serves as a guide to sexual enjoyment but does not prevent one from deciding to engage in other forms of sexual activity (via trying something new through sexual experimentation). However, a minority of people have a paraphilic lovemap that requires the compulsive use of unusual imagery or behavior (to the exclusion of all other forms of sexual gratification).

THE SEXUAL EXPRESSION CUBE: FANTASY AND BEHAVIOR

Similar to the Sexual Identity Cube visually representing the three primary components of the definition of sexual identity, the three primary dimensions of sexual expression are represented by the 3-D Sexual Expression Cube (e-Cube). These three primary dimensions are sexual fantasies, sexual behaviors (that may or may not result in orgasm), and bio-culturally bound mediating factors. The illustration of the e-Cube (Figure 3) is represented as a bit "wavy" compared with the i-Cube because sexual expression is less defined than sexual identity. As noted, the literature on sexual expression reflects this fact, although there seems to be an endless variety of specific sexual fantasies or behaviors that have been the focus of countless authors.

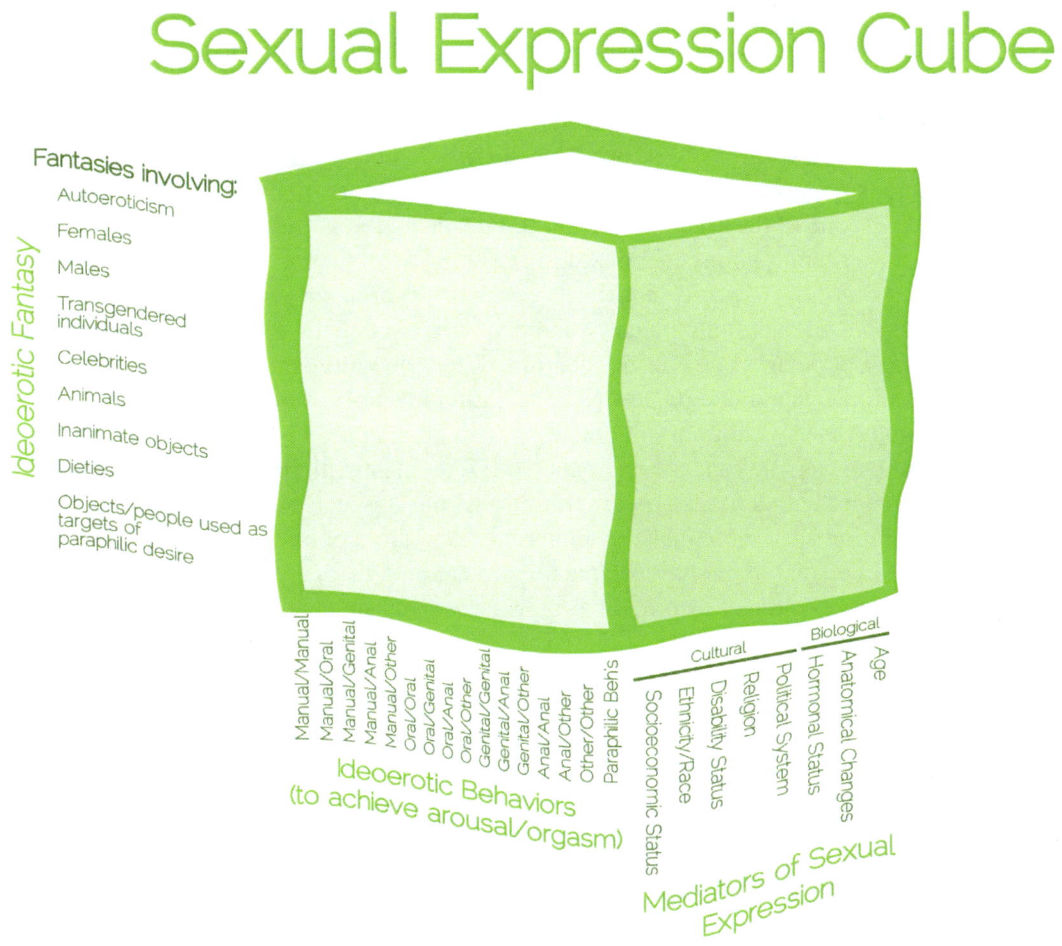

Figure 3. The Sexual Expression Cube (e-Cube).
Illustration by Max Fleishman.

This apparent paradox (less definition with endless description) also contributes to the reason the e-Cube appears "wavy." As will be discussed shortly, fantasies and behaviors (the latter to a lesser extent) leading to sexual arousal or orgasm cannot be easily enumerated precisely because of the extraordinary diversity of sexual expression among human beings. Therefore, the examples of sexual fantasies and behaviors listed in the e-Cube are representative of a larger set of fantasies and behaviors that people experience. The same is true for mediating factors of sexual expression.

Sexual Expression: Ideoerotic Fantasy

Sexual fantasy is defined as imagined sexual experiences while you are awake (as opposed to erotic dreams). A person's fantasies can be from an unlimited number of sources of erotic inspiration. If you can imagine it, someone somewhere likely takes erotic pleasure in the fantasized imagery of it (ranging from terrible pain and humiliation to corpses as sexual partners to eating animals alive or being eaten alive by an animal). Some fantasies are intentional and purposively created for sexual gratification, whereas others seem more "automatic" and repetitive. Both the variety and degree of intentional creation of sexual fantasies are heavily influenced by a person's individual lovemap.

The exact number of possible sexual fantasies can never be counted as evidenced by the endless supply and variety of erotica published every year. However, one can identify some categories of ideoerotic fantasies (resulting in a person experiencing arousal or orgasm) that are more popular than other varieties. Autoerotic fantasies are those enjoyed by people who fantasize about themselves, in part (like focusing upon their breasts) or whole (like making love to themselves). Others fantasize about the "generic male or female" (whole or part) or specialized types of individuals such as celebrities, transgender partners, or the newest hottie at the office. Others prefer to imagine themselves having sexual relations with (or having relations enhanced by) nature, deities, or mythological creatures and entities. Each one of these categories might be considered within a normal range of sexual fantasy and might have literally thousands of variations.

Paraphilic fantasy is also a world unto itself and can be divided generally into coercive and nonoercive. Descriptions of paraphilic imagery and behavior are beyond the scope of this chapter so only some of the most popular types will be mentioned. People with paraphilic lovemaps fantasize about animals (zoophilia), inanimate objects (fetish), individuals of a certain age (such as enduring sexual interest in prepubescent children), interactions with others involving domination and submission (sadomasochism, or S&M), bondage and pain (B&D), contact with body waste (coprophilia and urophilia), sexual contact with a corpse (necrophilia), making obscene phone calls (scatologia), exposing oneself (exhibitionism), secretively watching others undress or have sex (voyeurism), kissing or fondling a sleeping person (somnophilia), touching or rubbing up against a nonconsenting person (frotteurism), and sexual excitement from compulsive cross-dressing. These are just the most common paraphilic fantasies and there are many more varieties specific to ideoerotic paraphilic lovemaps (American Psychiatric Association, 2013; Money, 1986).

A general observation of individuals who disclose a capacity to enjoy sexual fantasies is that they are generally more sex-positive and able to share a greater capacity to explore and share sexual pleasure. Most people do report that they enjoy sexual fantasy, and it is a value-added aspect of their sexual life. There are many positive benefits to sexual fantasy, and it is a necessary step for women to learn when they come to the clinic with reports of not being able to become sexually aroused and/or climax. Research shows that people who place positive value on their sexual fantasies are more sexually assertive, regarding both the initiation of sex as well as the refusal of unwanted sex, than people who are negative about sexual fantasy (Santos-Iglesias et al., 2013). Men engage in fantasy more than women, but women have more frequent fantasies around the time of their ovulation (Dawson et al., 2012). Clinically, the only concerns masturbation sometimes cause is if an individual has guilt about experiencing pleasure, a person masturbates excessively (especially with pornography) to the reduction of interaction with a partner, or the small minority of men who become sexually compulsive with erotic fantasy to the point it becomes problematic with their behavior.

Of course, individuals can just fantasize about objects of desire, or they can also choose to express their interests behaviorally. Most any type of fantasy (paraphilic or nonparaphilic) can be acted out in behavior but certainly does not need to be acted out in every instance. For many reasons, people fantasize about sexual activity they never would act out in real life. That is one of the many functions of fantasy – to have sexual pleasure without explicit sexual behavior. Of course, very often the only explicit behavior that does accompany sexual fantasy is masturbation, as explained in the next section on ideoerotic behaviors.

The *Mayo Clinic Family Health Book* (Litin, 2009) has a section on "Teenage Sexuality" that makes the point when the author states: "It is normal to have sexual fantasies. Sexual fantasies may even be useful in the development of a teen's sexual identity because they allow exploration of sexual situations that would be inappropriate for the teen to act out." William Masters and Virginia Johnson studied the importance of fantasies as part of healthy sexual expression. Besides the function (just noted above) of a "safe alternative" to behavioral acting out with another person, Masters and Johnson enumerated several functions that sexual fantasy serves (Masters et al., 1995). The functions that fantasy serves include, but are not limited to:

1. inducing sexual arousal as an initial boost to get things underway;
2. enhancing arousal to help achieve orgasm during sexual relations;
3. allowing privacy that affords creativity without accountability;
4. improving our sexual self-image by fantasizing desired attributes;
5. reminiscing the joy of positive sexual experiences in the past when the partner is not available;
6. releasing anxiety/guilt by serving as psychological "safety valves"; and
7. allowing opportunity for controlled rehearsal in preparation of how to act in a future sexual encounter.

Sexual Expression: Ideoerotic Behaviors

Ideoerotic behaviors are what we do during sexual activities that lead to sexual arousal and/or orgasm. They are certainly more limited than the endless varieties of fantasy, yet there are scores (perhaps hundreds) of behavioral variations that result in orgasm and fall under numerous categories. As with fantasy, ideoerotic behaviors are also guided by Money's (1986) concept of lovemaps. One could argue that sexual fantasies can be included within a broad range of sexual behaviors and, if so, then sexual behaviors would need to be divided between external overt behaviors (such as intercourse) and internal "unobservable" behaviors (such as thinking of a sexual fantasy). In this chapter, fantasy is separated from behavior (into two categories) for teaching purposes of the Sexual Expression Cube and making the overall idea of sexual expression easier to communicate. Ideoerotic behaviors can be either solo (with yourself) or social (with others) as well as either nonparaphilic or paraphilic behaviors. They can also be relatively commonplace or can be relatively rare. The 2 X 4 matrix of these groupings generates four broad types of sexual behaviors as described in Table 5.

TABLE 5. Examples of Common and Uncommon Sexual Behaviors With Self and Others

	Common (Nonparaphilic)	Atypical (Paraphilic)
Common sexual acts with self	Masturbation	Shoe fetish
Uncommon sexual acts with self	Cricket orgasm	Autoerotic asphixiphilia
Common sexual acts with others	Intercourse	Voyeurism
Uncommon sexual acts with others	Eargasms	Lust murdering

Common Sexual Behaviors With Yourself

Common sexual behaviors with yourself (Table 6) include both direct and indirect stimulation of parts of your body that turn you on. Most of the time that involves touching the penis for men and the clitoris for women (but far from always). Women are believed to have a greater number of ways to arouse themselves to orgasm than men. However, many variations to stimulating body parts other than the genitals are common. Examples include touching your breasts, rubbing earlobes, stroking hair, and sensually stimulating your anus or perineum.

Just as common are indirect touching of the genital and anal areas with sexual aids of many different styles, including handheld (sometimes hand-mounted) vibrators for the clitoris or penis, vibrating and nonvibrating dildos for vaginal or anal insertion, vaginal and anal dilators, anal beads, and don't forget some common household items such as fruit (like a banana), vegetables (like a cucumber), or candles. People commonly smell body odors and/or taste body parts or fluids for arousal and orgasm.

Of course, there are the tried-and-true methods of rubbing the genitals against an object (humping), which may be more common to girls and women for masturbation but is also employed by boys and men. Humping is exceedingly common with preschoolers as a form of self-soothing and is often carried through childhood (and even adulthood) to cope with tension and/or emotional distress. Many types of sexual behavior displayed by children are fairly common (Friedrich et al., 1998) and cannot necessarily be considered as evidence that child abuse has occurred. Table 6 delineates many, not all, of the many variations of sexual self-pleasuring.

TABLE 6. Forms of Self-Pleasuring

Manual pleasuring (by hand)	Self-hand massage/touch
Oral pleasuring (by lips/tongue/teeth)	Touching lips, sucking fingers, licking, kissing, orbiting hands and biting own lips
Genital pleasuring (by vulva, penis, or scrotum)	Solo genital masturbation, self-fellatio, self-cunnilingus, indirect rubbing of genitals (humping), vaginal containment of animals and objects
Anal pleasuring (by anus, buttocks, perineum)	Solo anal masturbation, anal eroticism, prostate massage, rectal containment of animals and objects,
Other forms of pleasuring (by breasts, ears, neck, legs, feet, hair, etc.)	Self-seductive touch, sex toy use (dildos, vibrators, etc.), breast stimulation, licking/biting own breasts, use of fruit or other food, thigh contractions (cricket orgasms)

The category that usually raises most eyebrows is the oral-genital self-pleasuring behavior. Many people do not believe that this is possible, so additional explanation is needed here. A man who can essentially give himself his own "blow job" is very rare, but you can see how this is possible given a man with a high degree of flexibility combined with an unusually long penis. A woman who is physically able to contort her body into a position by which she can orally stimulate her own genitals is extraordinarily rare and harder to believe possible. However, there is some evidence to believe both these types of self-pleasuring are possible. The internet continues to surprise and shock viewers with things people will video themselves doing for the planet to watch. Any good skeptic would also acknowledge the possibility of trick photography and the imagery of self-oral-genital contact being faked. At the same time, the likelihood exists of rare individuals in our sexually diverse world that do possess such abilities.

Alfred Kinsey and his associates documented the phenomenon of "self-fellation" more than 70 years ago. While acknowledging "Self-fellation is an anatomic impossibility for most human males," Kinsey was aware as a biologist that "It is a common form of masturbation among rhesus monkeys, the macaque, mandrill, chimpanzees, and other primates. . . . It has taken special interviewing techniques to get adults to admit to such experiences, but a considerable portion of the population does record attempts at self-fellation, at least in early adolescence. Only two to three males in a thousand are able to achieve the objective" (Kinsey et al., 1948, p. 510). This estimate was based on a sample of 12,214 American men completing in-depth interviews that required several hours, including one 31-year-old man who depended on self-fellation as his chief masturbatory technique for most of his life (Kinsey et al., 1948).

Common Sexual Behaviors With Others

Common sexual behaviors with others (Table 7) include many forms of pleasuring that many people do not consider "sex." Sexual pleasuring behaviors that you might think of as minor foreplay may actually be a very important (if not essential) aspect of another person's formula for sexual satisfaction and orgasm.

TABLE 7. Common Sexual Behaviors With Others

Manual pleasuring (by hand)	Mutual petting, handholding
Oral pleasuring (by lips/tongue/teeth)	Touching lips, sucking fingers, kissing, licking or biting (mouth to mouth)
Genital pleasuring (by vulva, penis, or scrotum)	Genital masturbation (single or mutual); G-spot stimulation; ball play, fellatio, cunnilingus, oral ball play; penile-vaginal intercourse, vulva-vulva intercourse (tribadism/humping), sword fighting
Anal pleasuring (by anus, buttocks, perineum)	Anal masturbation, anal eroticism, prostate massage, analingus (rimming), anal/penile intercourse, interbuttock intercourse ("hot dog in the bun" without penetration), anal/clitoral intercourse (with a very large erect clitoris)
Other forms of pleasuring (by breasts, ears, neck, legs, feet, hair, etc.)	Seductive touch, sensuous massage; sex toy use (dildos, vibrators, etc.); breast stimulation; licking/biting any part of body; earlobe sucking (eargasms); use of knee, thigh, or other body part to stimulate genitals; intercourse; use of other body parts to stimulate anus; all forms of breast stimulation; thigh contractions (cricket orgasms); Interfemoral is intercourse by penis (or very large erect clitoris) between the thighs; interbreast is intercourse by penis (or very large erect clitoris) between the breasts.

For many people, these behaviors are *the* most important aspects of sexual satisfaction as opposed to sexual intercourse. These behaviors include simple things like holding hands, touching your partner's lips, stroking their hair, sensual massage, or sucking a finger! (Remember when holding hands was such a big deal?)

Usually when we think of sex with others, we immediately go to intercourse – what many believe to be the Holy Grail of Sex! There is a reason for this: Heterosexual Americans of all ethnic groups overwhelmingly prefer vaginal intercourse over all other forms of sexual pleasuring. Rumor has it that the Patron Saint of Procreation smiles every time penis meets vagina. Yet America's top preferences for the most appealing sexual relations also include giving/receiving oral sex and watching your partner undress.

Exceedingly popular as well are practices such as masturbating your partner, mutual masturbation, and use of sexual toys and aids. Less frequent but common forms of interpersonal sexual touch include anal eroticism, rubbing vulvas together (tribadism), rubbing boobs together (titty mashing), interfemoral intercourse (penis between the legs), interbreast intercourse ("titty fucking"), and inter-buttock intercourse (humping).

Uncommon Paraphilic Sexual Behaviors With the Self and Others

Uncommon paraphilic sexual behaviors with the self are a bit more complicated. Let's recall that paraphilias are unusual sexual behaviors often practiced by a person who may experience distress and compulsion about the activity. The official definition of paraphilia is a mental disorder that is characterized by recurrent, intense, sexually arousing fantasies, urges, or behaviors (lasting at least 6 months) that involve objects or animals, and the suffering or humiliation of oneself, a partner, children, or other nonconsenting individuals. Examples of uncommon paraphilic sexual behavior during masturbation include a person who requires either just the fantasy and/or the actual act of the paraphilic object, imagined lover, or activity. This may involve fantasies of (or actual activity) involving pain, fantasies of handling or wearing certain materials (such as lingerie or rubber), or fantasies of certain types of imagined sexual partners, such as a dead person (necrophilia).

Any type of paraphilia can manifest during masturbation through use of fantasy. This includes the many types of paraphilias that are not listed in the official *Diagnostic and Statistical Manual of Mental Disorders* (*DSM*), which is considered an authoritative guide to mental illnesses published by the American Psychiatric Association (2013). Another type of solitary paraphilic sexual behavior, which can be deadly, is called autoerotic asphyxia. This practice involves (partial) self-strangulation during masturbation to restrict oxygen supply to the brain to increase the intensity of the climax experience. The self-strangulation is accomplished by a number of mechanical methods (very often using ropes, chains, or cords for partial suspension or hanging) and involves great risk of losing consciousness during the act of masturbation. Estimates of approximately several hundred to about one thousand American youth die this way every year. But adults can die by this manner of asphyxia as well, as it has been reported the actor David Carradine (of *Kung Fu* fame) is thought to have died this way when his body was found hanging naked in a hotel with a rope around his neck and genitals (LeVay et al., 2015). The accuracy of these estimates is difficult to determine because of the varied accuracy of the reported cause of death. The cause of death may intentionally (or unintentionally) be ruled a suicide because of the greater stigma to the family of autoerotic asphyxia. What is more taboo than suicide? Suicide by (solo) sex.

Uncommon paraphilic sexual behaviors with others can overlap with the same activities one can do alone. The practice of restricting oxygen supply to the brain during sex can also occur between partners. Obviously, this practice is not recommended, and great caution is advised if you partake. You could die, and the other person could be charged with your murder, or the other person dies, and you go to jail! These are pretty heavy stakes for a few moments of feeling good. More typical of uncommon paraphilic sexual behaviors between partners is the fairly widespread (worldwide) practice of domination and submission (D/S) and its most common form of bondage and discipline (B&D). It is important to note that, as with cross-dressing, many couples engage in D/S or B&D activities as a lifestyle or to playfully spice up their sex lives (think pink furry handcuffs). These couples are not necessarily people with a paraphilia. It is the individual who has a strong and enduring preference for this type of sexual expression and has to do it compulsively (at least in fantasy if not in behavior) who is paraphilic.

An extremely damaging paraphilic behavior involving another person is pedophilic disorder because the object of this paraphilia is prepubescent children. It is considered so damaging because of the negative long-term effects on the victims and because of how common it is, with an estimated 1 of 4 females and 1 of 10 males reporting that they had been sexually molested by age 18 (American Psychiatric Association, 2013). Dr. Gene Abel of Emory University, one of the leading authorities on this subject, estimates that men with this one paraphilia (pedophilia) may account for up to a staggering 95% of child molestations (Abel et al., 2007). Hence, it is particularly important to understand this type of sexual expression, improve current practices of assessment and identification, and innovate better treatment approaches toward a goal of increased prevention of childhood sexual abuse.

Of course, the most dangerous and destructive type of paraphilic behavior involving others is the lust-murderer who serially kills people, in part for sexual gratification. Gary Ridgway, also known as the Green River serial killer, is such an example of this paraphilia. Over a period of 16 years, he killed 48 young women and girls in the Seattle area, mostly by strangling them during sexual encounters. Most of the victims were sex workers and Ridgway was under the delusion he was performing a community service and believed he could kill as many prostitutes as he wanted without getting caught. He avoided the death penalty by agreeing to give police information about the location of the victims' bodies. Fortunately, this type of paraphilia is rare (LeVay et al., 2015).

AS THIS CHAPTER CONCLUDES

Consider a fellow named Frank, who is a man that many of us know, yet we don't. He is the fellow that works in our school, business, or hospital that always keeps to himself, working quietly in building maintenance or janitorial services. If we knew Frank better, really talked to him, we might over time come to know Frank's self-description in both the Sexual Identity Cube (sex orientation of being designated as a man and sexual orientation of being attracted to men) as well as the Sexual Expression Cube (age, ethnicity or racial identification). Consider the three major dimensions of sexual identity and the three major dimensions of sexual expression. Do we really know Frank beyond stereotyped images and beliefs that come to mind? Do we know the most important questions to consider to really know Frank and appreciate him as a unique human sexual being? We might be wondering:

- Is Frank in or out of the closet?
- Is he single or married, and to whom?
- Does Frank have children or not?
- Does he live alone or with another person – man, woman, or both?
- Is Frank in an exclusive relationship or does he date multiple people?
- Does he live in a metropolitan city or in a small rural town?
- Is he middle class, working class, or poor?

Now consider that each of the basic factors contained within the i-Cube and e-Cube that are all interactive, and the number of possible interactions regarding how Frank expresses his sexual self is greatly expanded. There are now a few additional questions that arise that could help us get to know Frank better:

- How does Frank self-identify his sex orientation – is it different from male?
- How does he self-identify his sexual orientation – is it different from "gay?"
- How does Frank self-identify his sex-role orientation?
- Is he influenced by religious beliefs?
- Is there any conflict between Frank's spirituality and sexuality?
- What kind of sexual fantasy does he actively enjoy (if any)?
- How does Frank identify his ethnicity and race status?
- Does he have a light, medium, or dark complexion?
- What medical conditions does Frank get treated for by his health care system (which happens to be the Department of Veterans Affairs)?
- How does his amputation for combat injuries in Vietnam influence his sexual self-image?
- Does Frank use any sex-enhancement medications (such as Viagra), or aphrodisiac drugs intended to intensify his sexual experience?
- Does he have any adverse sexual side effects from any medications he is prescribed or recreational drugs he may use?
- Is Frank able to enjoy what he considers highly erotic stimulation and fantasy?

The list of questions goes on and on in terms of how to help oneself really appreciate the unique individual that people call Frank (as opposed to relying on stereotypes and assumptions). You see, Frank is a real man with real losses and dreams and people who love him. Most of the time, people see Frank and don't think too much about him. They just pass him on the street or in the hospital hallways and barely notice him except for his effort to be visible and simply be acknowledged by others. Folks don't know he was terribly misused as a child and grew up with so much chaos that he never learned to read and write past a sixth-grade level but joined the Army to serve his country. Most folks, even some of his family, don't know that he earned a Purple Heart from injuries carrying a fellow soldier out of a firefight. He doesn't like to talk about that. Most folks don't know he came back from Vietnam and started his own business to raise a family and at the same time hide his illiteracy. Most folks don't know how he truly loved a woman who was the mother of his children for decades before he lost her to cancer. Most folks don't know that, to Frank's surprise (and everybody else in his family), in time he fell in love again.

Mostly people see an old African American man shuffling past them, looking them in the eye, and tipping his head with a smile. Thanks Frank, you have served your country and had a full life. You can finally enjoy your retirement watching all the science shows you want about the universe and fourth dimension while tipping your hat in appreciation of your favorite astronomer, Carl Sagan. You have also led us to the Sexual Hypercube, the subject of the next chapter, where we explore the hundreds and even thousands of potential variations of Frank's sexual identity and sexual expression (Veh, 2017).

The Last Point – What is the Point?

This is a fair question about this whole matter of considering different points of view related to sexual identity and expression. There are several responses to this question as to why this chapter's discussion is necessary. First of all, one goal of this model is to more accurately understand sexuality based on emerging research findings and to stimulate further research questions. This may lead us a bit closer to consensus on the use of the terms *sexual identity* and *sexual expression*. As noted in this chapter, we are far from that. Exploring and discussing the concept and personal meanings of sexual identity and expression can be a value-added aspect of personal growth for anyone, and it also stimulates the possibility of advancing sexual science.

Better understanding the complexity of human sexuality helps us sort out commonly confused differences between sexual identity and sexual orientation as well as the differences between sexual identity and sexual expression. This chapter focused on identity and expression as core elements of the human experience. The authors' hopes are that we gain greater clarity for understanding two key points regarding the incredible complexity of human sexuality. The first is that the Sexual Identity Cube (i-Cube) has the potential to assist an individual to find a greater inner peace, increased self-understanding, and self-acceptance. Promoting greater self-understanding and self-acceptance of sexual identity minimizes internal conflict and negative self-image. So, on an individual basis, an expanded perspective of the full range of sexual identity may lead to less unnecessary stress (cultural press, as some authors define it) and more personal satisfaction.

The second key point is about interpersonal relations. The i-Cube and e-Cube are intended to promote greater tolerance of others as well as oneself. This can lessen the incidence of fear, prejudice, and violence toward those we *perceive* as different from us. The parent of violence is fear and the parent of fear is not understanding others. Both the i-Cube and e-Cube promote better understanding of ourselves as well as others. The next chapter illustrates the reciprocal relationship between the two cubes and how they dance together to contribute a fundamental understanding of ourselves as sexual beings.

REFERENCES

Abel, G., Wiegel, M., & Osborn, C. (2007). Pedophilia and other paraphilia. In L. VandeCreek, F. Peterson, & J. Bley (Eds.), *Innovations in clinical practice: Focus on sexual health* (pp. 157-175). Professional Resource Press.

American Psychiatric Association. (2013). *Diagnostic and statistical manual of mental disorders* (5th ed.). https://doi. Org/10.1176/appi.books.9780890425596

American Psychological Association. (2020). Sexual orientation. *APA dictionary of psychology.* https://dictionary.apa.org/browse/s

Aggrawal, A. (2009). *Forensic and medico-legal aspects of sexual crimes and unusual sexual practices*. CRC Press.

Aulette, J. R., Wittner, J. G., & Blakely, K. (2009). *Gendered worlds*. Oxford University Press.

Bem, D. (1996). Exotic becomes erotic: A developmental theory of sexual orientation. *Psychological Review*, *103*.

Bem, S. (1981a). Gender schema theory: A cognitive account of sex typing source. *Psychological Review*, *88*, 354.

Bem, S. (1981b). The BSRI and gender schema theory: A reply to Spence and Helmreich. *Psychological Review*, *88*, 369-371.

Benjamin, H. (1966). *The transsexual phenomenon.* Julian Press.

Bley, J., & Peterson, F. (2007). Making sexual health a part of your mental health practice. In L. VandeCreek, F. Peterson, & J. Bley (Eds.), *Innovations in clinical practice: Focus of sexual health* (pp. 5-17). Professional Resources Press.

Brutto, L., & Yule, M. (2017). Asexuality: Sexual orientation, paraphilia, sexual dysfunction, or none of the above? *Archives of Sexual Behavior*, *46*(3), 619-627.

Carroll, J. (2007). *Sexuality now: Embracing diversity* (2nd ed.). Thomson Wadsworth.

Carroll, J. (2016). *Sexuality now: Embracing diversity* (5th ed.). Cengage Learning.

Cohen, J., Peterson, F., Bottoms, J., Resch, W., Burgess, B., & Richards, M., (2013, March 28). *Healthcare in 21st century Appalachia: The arranged marriage of cultural competency training and relationship-based care approaches*. Paper presented at the Southwestern Social Science Association Annual Conference, New Orleans, Louisiana.

Coleman, E. (2004). *Bisexuality: Challenging our understanding of human sexuality and sexual orientation*. In E.E. Shelp (Ed.), *Sexuality and Medicine* (Vol. 1, pp. 225-242). Reidel.

Coleman, E. (2011). Assessment and treatment of impulsive and compulsive sexual behavior. In M. Grant & J. Potenza (Eds.), *Oxford handbook of impulse control disorders*. Oxford University Press.

Dawson, S., Suschinsky, K., & Lalumière, M. (2012). Sexual fantasies and viewing time across the menstrual cycle: A dairy study. *Archives of Sexual Behavior*, *41*, 173-183.

Diamond, L. (2008). *Sexual fluidity: Understanding women's love and desire*. Harvard University Press.

Erikson, E. (1968). *Youth: Identity and crisis*. Norton.

Fausto-Sterling, A. (2000). *Sexing the body: Gender politics and the construction of sexuality*. Basic Books.

Friedrich, W., Fisher, J., Broughton, D., Houston, M., & Shafran, C. (1998). Normative sexual behavior in children: A contemporary sample. *Pediatrics, 101*(4)e9. https://doi.org/10.1542/peds.101.4.e9

Greenberg, J., Bruess, C., & Conklin, S. (2007). *Exploring the dimensions of human sexuality*. Jones and Bartlett Learning.

Hammack, P., & Cohler, B. (2009). *The story of sexual identity: Narrative perspectives on the gay and lesbian life course*. Oxford University Press.

Herdt, G. (2005). *The Sambia: Ritual, sexuality, and change in Papua New Guinea*. Wadsworth.

Hyde, J., & DeLamater, J. (2011). *Understanding human sexuality*. McGraw-Hill.

Kail, R., & Cavanaugh, J. (2004). *Human development: A life-span view* (3rd ed.). Wadsworth/Thompson.

Kaplan, H. (1974). *The new sexual health*. Brunner/Mazel.

Kinsey, A., Pomeroy, W., & Martin, C. (1948). *Sexual behavior in the human male*. W.B. Saunders.

Kinsey, A., Pomeroy, W., Martin, C., & Gephard, P. (1953). *Sexual behavior in the human female*. W.B. Saunders.

Kupferman, I. (1991). Hypothalamus and limbic system motivation. In E. R. Kandel, J. Schwartz, & T. Jessell (Eds.), *Principle of neural science* (3rd ed.,). Elsevier.

LeVay, S., Baldwin, J., & Baldwin, J. (2015). *Discovering human sexuality* (3rd ed.). Sinauer Associates.

LeVay, S., & Valente, S. (2003). *Human sexuality*. W.H. Freeman.

Levine, S. (2007). *Demystifying love: Plain talk for the mental health professional*. Routledge.

Lips, H. (2005). *Sex and gender*. McGraw-Hill.

Litin, S. (2009). *Mayo Clinic family health book*. Time Home Entertainment.

Masters, W., Johnson, V., & Kolodny, R. (1995). *Human sexuality* (5th ed.). Harper-Collins.

McAnulty, R., & Burnette, M. (2003). *Exploring human sexuality: Making healthy decisions*. Pearson Education.

McCammon, S., Knox, D., & Schacht, C. (2004). *Choices in sexuality*. Atomic Dog.

Merriam-Webster. (1986). Identity. In *Merriam-Webster's third new international dictionary of the English language*. Merriam-Webster, Inc.

Money, J. (1986). *Lovemaps: Clinical concepts of sexual/erotic health and pathology, paraphilia, and gender transposition in childhood, adolescence, and maturity*. Irvington.

Money, J. (1994). *Reinterpreting the unspeakable*. Continuum.

Perelman, M. (2014). The history of sexual medicine. In *APA history of sexuality and psychology, Vol. II: Contextual approaches* (pp. 137-179). American Psychological Association. https://doi.org/10.1037/14194-005.

Peterson, F. (2007). *The complexity of sexual diversity: Sexual identity cube and self-awareness exercise*. In L. VandeCreek, F. Peterson, & J. Bley (Eds.), *Innovations in clinical practice: Focus on sexual health* (pp. 297-300). Professional Resource Press.

Peterson, F., Bley J., & Frabotta, R. (2020). *The gender revolution & new sexual health: Celebrating unlimited diversity of the human sexuality hypercube.* Cognella Academic Publishing.

Peterson, F., & Carter, R. (2010, October 8). *Re-defining sexual identity and introduction to the Sexual Health and Wellness Satisfaction Scale* (paper presentation). Annual Conference of the Ohio Psychological Association, Columbus, Ohio.

Peterson, F., & Peterson, C. (2007). A health care professional's guide to contemporary sexual myths. In L. VandeCreek, F. Peterson, & J. Bley (Eds.), *Innovations in clinical practice: Focus on sexual health* (pp. 323-325). Professional Resource Press.

Santos-Iglesias, P., Sierra, J. C., & Vallejo-Medina, P. (2013). Predictors of sexual assertiveness: The role of sexual desire, arousal, attitudes, and partner abuse. *Archives of Sexual Behavior*, *42*, 1043-1052.

Sexuality Information & Education Council for the United States (SIECUS). (2001). *SIECUS Report*, Vols. 30-31. https://siecus.org/resources/the-siecus-report/

Sexuality Information & Education Council for the United States (SIECUS). (2018). *Position statements*. https://siecus.org/wp-content/uploads/2018/07/Position-Statements-2018.pdf

Strong, B., DeVault, S., Sayad, B., & Yarber, W. (2005). *Human sexuality: Diversity in contemporary America* (5th ed.). McGraw-Hill.

Veh, V. (2017). *Statistical consultation report* (Appendix A). Ohio University.

Yarber, W., & Sayad, B. (2019). *Human sexuality: Diversity in contemporary society* (10th ed.). McGraw-Hill Education.

Yarber, W., Sayad, B., & Strong, B. (2010). *Human sexuality: Diversity in contemporary America* (7th ed.). McGraw-Hill.

8

Sex and the Fourth Dimension: The Sexual Hypercube

Frederick L. Peterson, Jr. and Jon Dembski

INTRODUCTION

Before explaining the hypercube as a model, it is important to understand the two major components that can be broken down into their own three-dimensional models. These models were described in detail in the last chapter; the Sexual Identity Cube (i-Cube) and the Sexual Expression Cube (e-Cube). If you read Chapter 7, skip this paragraph and the next. If you did not, here is a cursory review. The i-Cube model demonstrates the relationship between sex orientation (male, intersex transgender, psychosocial transgender, female), sexual orientation (attracted to neither men nor women, attracted to both men and women, attracted to women, attracted to men), and four types of sex-role orientations (androgynous, traditional feminine, traditional masculine, and undifferentiated; undifferentiated includes queer, non-binary, and gender nonconforming). The i-Cube allows for fluidity among any of these subsets, as each of the three orientations is on a continuum and models these orientations within a cube to demonstrate the complex intersectionality of the relationships between these orientations across the life span. If Figure 1 on the next page makes little sense to you, please review Chapter 7 of this text and/or for a more detailed explanation, please refer to Chapter 11 in *The Gender Revolution and New Sexual Health* (Peterson et al., 2020).

The e-Cube is similar in style to the i-Cube (albeit a bit more varied), but models sexual expression. In this cube, one axis represents ideoerotic fantasy, which when broken down is a limitless continuum, but some examples of the fantasy "object of desire" include autoeroticism, females, males, transgender individuals, animals, inanimate objects, and so forth. Another axis of the e-Cube is ideoerotic behavior, which is more limited than fantasies, but still too numerous in variation to completely cover here. Examples include any direct or indirect stimulation of parts of your body that turn you on. The final axis of the e-Cube represents the continuum of mediators of sexual expression, which are cultural and biological. Examples on the cultural mediator continuum are things such as socioeconomic status, ethnicity/race, disability status, religion, or political systems. The biological mediators of expression include things such as age, anatomical changes, hormonal status, all of which again affect sexual expression in different ways. All the variations of fantasy, behavior, and mediators affect how one expresses their sexuality. The e-Cube is a comprehensive model for expression, which is why there is such an endless number of points on each continuum for sexual fantasy, sexual behavior, and biocultural mediators of sexual expression. Similarly, if Figure 2 on page 135 makes little sense to you, please review Chapter 7 of this text and/or for a more detailed explanation, please refer to Chapter 12 in *The Gender Revolution and New Sexual Health* (Peterson et al., 2020).

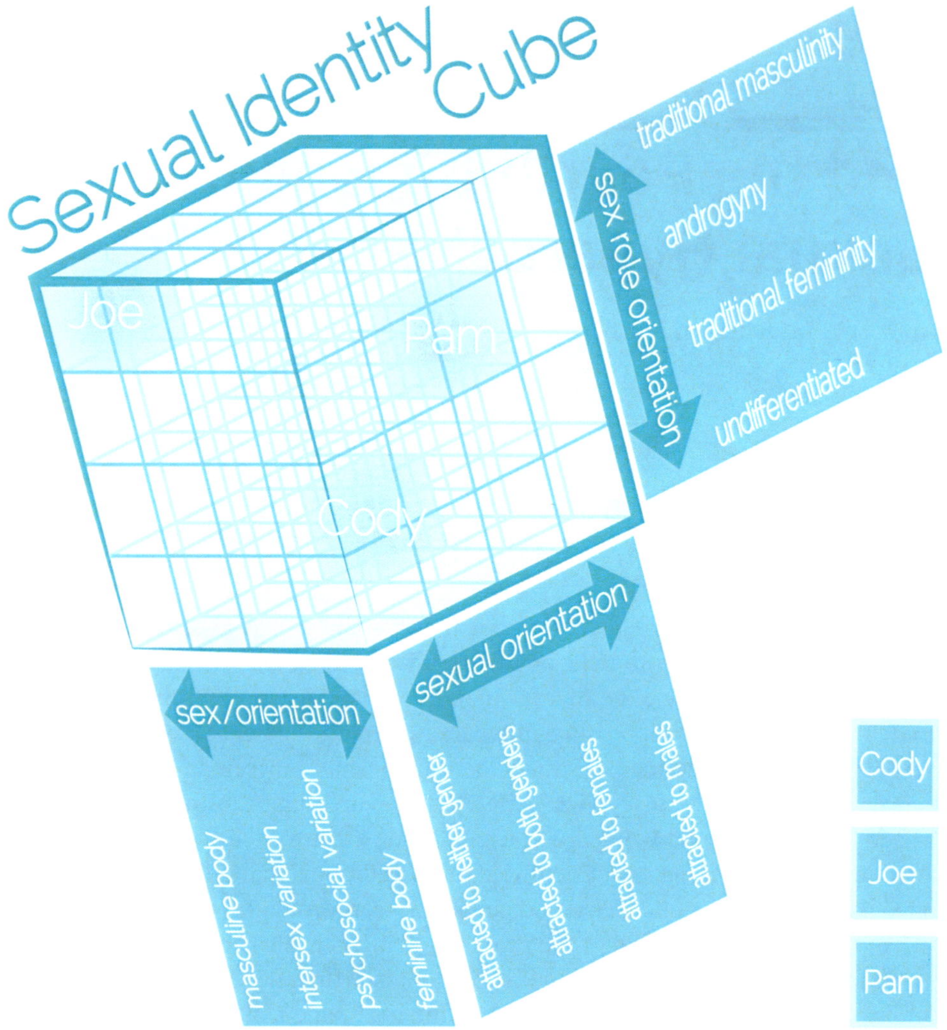

Figure 1. The Sexual Identity Cube (i-Cube).
Illustrated by Max Fleishman.

If we combine the three-dimensional Sexual Identity Cube (i-Cube) with the three-dimensional Sexual Expression Cube (e-Cube), then you have a model of sexual interaction describing much of human sexuality! This world of sexual possibilities is captured within a model called the "Sexual Hypercube" (hypercube, or h-Cube), illustrating an incredible mutually influencing relationship between sexual identity and sexual expression. The Sexual Hypercube is a theoretical model that accounts for the amazing diversity of human sexuality and as argued in this chapter, helps explain why and how we humans change our sexual identity and expression from one stage of life to another.

As you read this chapter, please consider a key question: Will your life seem unfulfilled without expanding your knowledge about the Sexual Hypercube? Probably not. By now, it is fair if you have concluded that the authors are either wannabe mad scientists or clinicians with a far different perspective on this whole sexuality thing. You could be correct on each count. After all, a hypercube model borrowed from the fourth dimension does sound a bit nutty. Valid criticisms could be: Can't you just explain human sexuality in the same three dimensions that we live in? How do you expect to explain a four-dimensional concept within a three-dimensional world, especially in two-dimensional representation (print)?

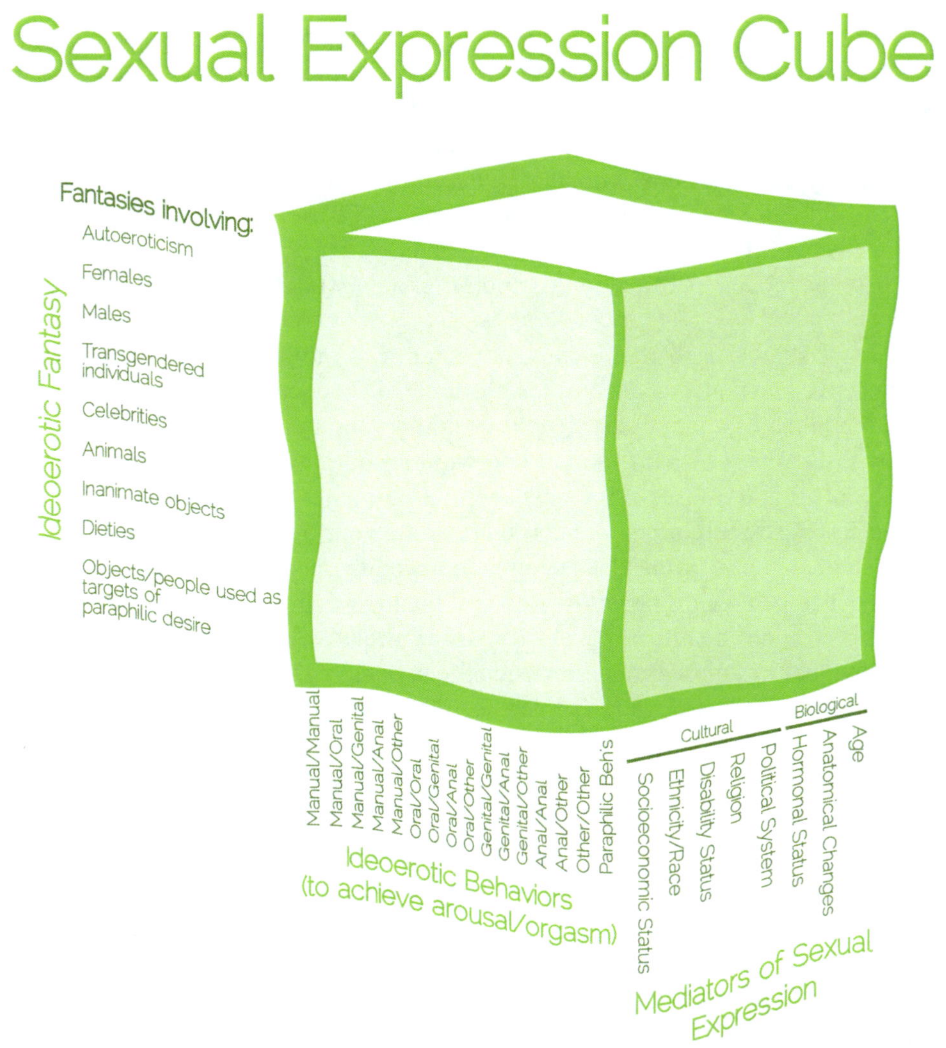

Figure 2. The Sexual Expression Cube (e-Cube).

Illustrated by Max Fleishman.

Before getting into the details of the Sexual Hypercube, let's make a few clarifications. The model has evolved from the fields of anthropology, biology, medicine, psychology, and clinical sexual health. The model has also been formed from sitting and listening to thousands of people's sexual stories. We are not by any means mathematicians, research scientists, or Rhodes Scholars. Fortunately, you do not need to be any of those specialists to understand human sexuality from the different perspectives presented in this chapter. Secondly, there will not be any attempts to teach everything there is about hypercubes as this is a book about sex, not geometric modeling.

The hypercube as a model is employed for its ability to visually represent concepts and relationships that have been discussed in Chapter 7 and this chapter. There will be no attempt to explain the connectivity of every human sexual possibility. That will be left to academic scholars whose dissertations compete for the Stephen Hawking of Sexuality Award. Therefore, with all due respect (and apologies) to my colleagues in the math and physics departments, the rules of applied mathematics have little bearing on the forthcoming explanation of the hypercube, just as the ordinary laws of physics do not apply either (at least in a three-dimensional world).

Having said that, there is a little background on this thing called "the fourth dimension" that is both interesting and helpful to our discussion of using a hypercube as a model for sexuality. Back to the question: *Can't you just explain human sexuality in the same three dimensions that we live in?* Why a hypercube as the model? It just comes down to this: There may be sexual science scholars who have the knowledge and/or creativity to know and/or imagine a different three-dimensional model that comprehensively describes how sexual identity and sexual expression relate to each other. We are not them. The closest three-dimensional model that may be useful is the concept of organic symbiosis, but it has its own limitations, which illustrates an earlier point that is worth repeating again. The sexual hypercube model presented in this book is certainly not the only general model of human sexuality.

However, as we shall see, there are some advantages of moving to higher dimensions to gain additional perspective and understand complex phenomena. Take combat of yesteryear, for example. Say you are in the midst of a bloody battlefield wielding your sword or ax. Perhaps you have your closest friend with you back-to-back, a man you would (and may) die to defend. While he covers what is behind you, all you can see is the next enemy running toward you with a spear or saber and all you have are seconds to kill or be killed. You are doing your best to survive the battle; you really do not have much of an idea of what else is going on beyond your immediate proximity. And so, one of the first rules developed regarding war was to win the higher ground (when available). In a sense, the higher ground provides a shift in perspective from a relatively two-dimensional "flat" fighting space for the individual to a more three-dimensional perspective the general has who is safely sitting on his horse on the hilltop. The elevation of perspective gives distinct advantage to allow movement of troops for a decisive win or make retreat to fight another day. Even though we may not be able to travel to the fourth dimension physically (at least in the foreseeable future), borrowing concepts from higher dimensions can (and often does in math and physics) provide additional and valuable perspectives to explain the phenomena that we do see in our three-dimensional world. Before diving deep into the sexual hypercube concept, let us take a brief look at alternative models to comprehensively describe human sexuality.

Sexual Modeling Literature Review

In today's world, people are becoming more accepting and aware of a broader range of self-identities and expressions. It is up to mental health clinicians counseling these people to be understanding of this and made aware of these ideas to better serve their clients. Sexual identity and expression have proven to be more complex subjects than once thought, and clinicians should be cognizant of the impact these ideas/interactions have on people's overall identities and perceptions of others. And of utmost importance, is that healthcare professionals do not judge or dismiss a client's lived experience and self-identity regardless of the variation from the provider's perception of typical norms.

Identity and expression have shown to work off each other, forming and shaping each other over people's life cycles. This has led to the topics being researched with many attempts to define variations in the last century. These attempts usually have resulted in the overpathologizing of individual expression. What has been demonstrated in a century of research is how deeply complex and fluid these two ideas (sexual identity and expression) can be when defining or measuring. As time has passed, many of the early models and definitions have proven to be biased, are not supported by data, and/or have not encompassed the wide diversity that is found when researching the sexuality of humans. Still, some of these past models have laid the groundwork to reaching a better understanding of human sexuality and have led to the formation of a more encompassing model presented in this chapter. Before talking about the hypercube (h-Cube), it can help to examine some of the past models.

Dr. Alfred Kinsey is credited with one of the first and most well-known models of sexual expression. Through his research, Kinsey developed the "Heterosexual-Homosexual Rating Scale," also known as the Kinsey Scale (Kinsey et al., 1948). The seven-point scale (0 being exclusively heterosexual, 6 meaning exclusively homosexual) has less relevance today as a tool for practitioners but was a pivotal development in treating and understanding people of different sexual orientations. Arguing that expression of sexual orientation was not binary (it could be fluid through someone's lifespan, it was not necessarily pathological) was a scientific groundbreaking moment for the study of human sexuality.

The sexual revolution in the 1960s and 1970s led to greater freedom of expression and a desire to better understand the LGBT communities. At the end of the 1970s, a researcher named Vivienne Cass developed "The Cass Identity Model" to better understand what was then referred to as the "homosexual population." "The Cass Identity Model" described homosexual identity formation as a six-stage process wherein homosexual individuals developed their homosexuality over their lifespan (Cass, 1979). The six stages included Identity Confusion, Identity Comparison, Identity Tolerance, Identity Acceptance, Identity Pride, and Identity Synthesis (Cass, 1979). A follow-up study in 1983 tested and found strong support for her theory in terms of stages of homosexual identity being formed through the lifespan. However, the data supported a four-stage model rather than her previously theorized six-stage model (Cass, 1983). Criticisms of Cass' model are demonstrated by Kaufman and Johnson in their 2005 work titled *Stigmatized Individuals and the Process of Identity.* Their arguments against the Cass model are threefold: the model ignores specific sociocultural factors which should not be overlooked, the model is dated in the way it looks at social stigma of homosexuality, and the model can assume if a homosexual individual doesn't experience each stage they may not be considered a "well-adjusted" homosexual (Kaufman & Johnson, 2004). While the Cass model is a dated view of identity formation, it was a giant step forward in understanding homosexuality as an identity and not as a problem to be fixed.

Fassinger's Model of Gay and Lesbian Identity Development, in the mid-1990s, proposed a broadening of the models to better encapsulate people and their preferences. Fassinger's model focused on the idea of identity being formed in the self as well as in the group (Fassinger & Miller, 1997; McCarn & Fassinger, 1996). Through several studies with lesbian and then gay populations, Fassinger began to formulate the model which has two separate processes (self and group), both comprised of four phases, and an individual may be in a different phase of each process (Fassinger & Miller, 1997). The four stages are "awareness, exploration, commitment, and synthesis," which reflect individual identity in one process and "group membership identity" in the other. The model allows for individuals to move to any of the phases because of cultural or environmental factors (Fassinger & Miller, 1997).

The mid-1990s also saw the publishing of Daryl Bem's "Exotic becomes Erotic" theory, which aimed to illuminate the complex relationship between one's biological makeup and their environment in forming patterns of sexual attraction. Bem notes certain factors (e.g., child temperament and play styles, along with social peer group influences) affect who the child sees as similar and those the child sees as different or the "exotic other." He then argues this "exotic other" becomes eroticized through the hormonal and social development resulting in a heterosexual or homosexual orientation depending on the sex designation of both the child and the eroticized other (Bem, 1996). Bem's theory shows a more nuanced understanding and approach to explain the development of sexual attraction, rather than the age-old (and artificial) dichotomy of nature vs. nurture debate about what the predominant influences are for the development of sexual orientation. Bem's "Exotic becomes Erotic" theory exemplifies the complexity and uniqueness of the interchange of biologic and psychosocial factors. This theory also allows for variations in development for each individual including bisexuality and children with play preferences more typical of gender expectations of another sex.

Contemporary models have expanded the scope of human sexuality into more complex and comprehensive guides of sexual identity development and/or expression. In 2011, Dillon et al. proposed a model which they hoped would be more "universal" (as Bem's model) as opposed to the earlier identity models which mostly focused on LGBT sexual identity formations. This particular model is influenced heavily by Fassinger's model in the sense that there are two separate processes of identity formation for individuals to go through: "an individual sexual identity development process," and "a social identity process" (Dillon et al., 2011). The two processes are comprised of five "nonlinear, flexible, and fluid" statuses: "compulsory heterosexuality, active exploration, diffusion, deepening and commitment, and synthesis" (Dillon et al., 2011). This model is a comprehensive and well laid out model that explains a lot about sexual identity development and expression. However, the model does not seem to address the great diversity in people's identities/expressions.

One final model that must be noted is the Sexual Tipping Point (STP) model, which describes how individuals initiate or suppress their own sexual behavior. The STP model and its history was mentioned in Chapter 2 and will be discussed in more detail in Chapter 9 of this book. However, it is worth mentioning here because of its great value as a complimentary model to the sexual hypercube. The model has nearly a 50-year history starting with sexologist Helen Kaplan and her first book, *The New Sex Therapy* (Kaplan, 1974). Kaplan made the case that sexual desire (motivation) played a bigger role in sexual activity than was being considered at the time, as opposed to purely physiological factors included in the Masters and Johnson four-stage model of sexual response. Kaplan continued her work on this topic until her last book in 1995, where she built on this premise with the ideas of a dual-control (mind-body) model of sexual motivation, the basis of which was "inhibition/excitation." Kaplan and her chief successor (Perelman, 2009) have built the STP model into a sophisticated model that envelopes interpersonal and intrapersonal mechanisms which fuel or suppress sexual expression at the individual level. The combination of the STP model (demonstrating the potential for sexual behavior being initiated in any specific situation) and the Sexual Hypercube (demonstrating the general influences for sexual expression across most all sexual situations) allows for the most overall explanation of human sexuality that currently exists.

Models of sexual identity and expression have come a long way in the last century as they have attempted to describe, explain, and predict human sexual behavior. However, as sexual science evolves and our understanding expands, these models will become outdated. The explosion of diversity in sexuality and gender have shown that modeling can be difficult as there are so many identities and expressions for which to account. For this reason, a newer more encompassing model must be brought forward, one that will evolve as society does. Perhaps one not bound by three dimensional constraints may serve as useful for a time. The Sexual Hypercube (h-Cube) model proposed in this chapter may do just that.

THE FOURTH DIMENSION, HYPERSPACE, AND THE SEXUAL HYPERCUBE

Some Interesting Background

The idea of a fourth dimension has been around for over a century and, for purposes of discussion here, does not refer to the notion of time being the fourth dimension. In our three-dimensional world (beyond length, width, and height), height refers to how *high* or *low* we consider the third dimension, which is *vertical*. When looking for an address of a friend, we typically think of a two-dimensional grid by which we can find a location (a map is a representation of this two-dimensional grid). But what if the friend you are seeking does not live on a farm but lives in a condo on the 35th floor of a skyscraper. Then we need to operate in a three-dimensional concept of the world. Of course, we need not only physical coordinates to locate our friend but *temporal* coordinates as well. We need to be in the same physical space as well as the same temporal space to enjoy lunch with our friend (excluding virtual hangouts here). In some ways, this all seems so commonsense. But until the beginning of the 20th century (1905, to be precise), time and space were considered separate scientific entities.

The notion of time as the fourth dimension was most notably employed by Albert Einstein, to link time and space together within his model of the space-time continuum. His theory of special relativity and discovery of the mathematical equation ($E = mc^2$) to explain the space-time continuum is widely considered the most important scientific advancement of the 20th century. However, time is not what we are talking about here. When using the term *fourth dimension* in the title of this chapter, we are referring to a spatial concept that our three-dimensional brains have great difficulty visualizing. Yes, Einstein forever integrated space and time together scientifically. Hence, some consider time the fourth dimension and any additional spatial dimension the fifth dimension. But for the purposes of this chapter, when you read *fourth dimension*, reference is being made to the fourth spatial dimension.

Can you imagine the mind of a person who was the first to come up with the idea that there are additional visual and geometric dimensions beyond what our perception allows? This was the mind of Charles Hinton, a British mathematician and science-fiction writer who came to the United States to teach mathematics and later worked at the U.S. Naval Observatory. Like Einstein, Hinton was also a mathematician who also worked at the patent office. He was an eccentric and fascinating character who was jailed at one time for bigamy and, while teaching mathematics at Princeton University, invented the first pitching machine for the college baseball team. Hinton is credited for coining the term *tesseract* as another name for a hypercube in his book *A New Era of Thought* (1888). It is fascinating when something old becomes forgotten in popular culture and then resurfaces again to enjoy another period of popularity. This is actually the case with the concept of the fourth dimension. After Hinton's publication, many authors started to jump on the "fourth-dimensional bandwagon" and the topic began to be a matter of general speculation and discussion at social gatherings for a 25-year period between 1890 and around World War I. People exchanged ideas about the fourth dimension possibly being the location of heaven, angels, demons, extraterrestrials, and so on.

One century later, the fourth dimension is popular again. Haven't heard anyone talking about it lately? Try doing an internet search for scientific articles and books about the fourth dimension. You will find Michio Kaku, who is a leading theoretical physicist based at the City College of New York and has written much to popularize the concept of the fourth dimension in recent years. In his book *Hyperspace* (1994), he explains the history of the late 19th-century popular fascination with the fourth dimension, claiming it was very influential in literature and the arts. In literature and especially science fiction, Kaku cites the significant impact the fourth dimension had on author H. G. Wells. In the arts, the fourth dimension had significant impact on expressionism and cubism, including Pablo Picasso and Salvador Dali.

Admittedly, hypercubes and higher dimensions are not typically part of common public discourse these days. For example, I was on my way to give a lecture at an institute of technology a while back and I had dinner with my daughter Mackenzie the night before. She is an amazing elementary school teacher with an advanced degree dedicated to public school Montessori education but was not familiar with the fourth dimension. After she inquired about the next day's address and hearing my explanation, she responded with some constructive feedback by saying, "That sounds really interesting, Dad. I am sure you will be a hit but maybe you ought to reconsider including that last part." I asked, "What last part – the hypercube and the fourth dimension?" "Right!" she said. "I wouldn't want them to disregard all the good information you are sharing by hearing about that higher dimensional stuff and think you're a kook! I responded, "Wow – that is very helpful! Remember my audience – they are at an institute of technology. Let's do an experiment. Do you know any friends who are mathematicians or physicists?" I asked. She did and agreed to ask the husband of her girlfriend about the fourth dimension (the husband was getting his doctorate in physics). A few days later, I called her up and asked what the physicist had to say. She laughed and responded, "He said, fourth dimension? Boring! We are already working on the eleventh!"

THE SEXUAL HYPERCUBE MODEL

The Sexual Hypercube (h-Cube) is a four-dimensional conceptual model of human sexuality that combines the three-dimensional Sexual Identity Cube (i-Cube) with the three-dimensional Sexual Expression Cube (e-Cube) to describe the reciprocal influences between the two, and provide a foundation for understanding the wide-ranging diversity inherent in human sexuality. A hypercube is one type of many geometrical models in the fourth dimension and can theoretically exist in other higher dimensions as well. So far, what we have discussed regarding "cubes" is a Sexual Identity Cube (i-Cube) and a Sexual Expression Cube (e-Cube). As you will see, the hypercube of the fourth dimension is a model that puts these two cubes in relationship to each other in a very dynamic and animated way.

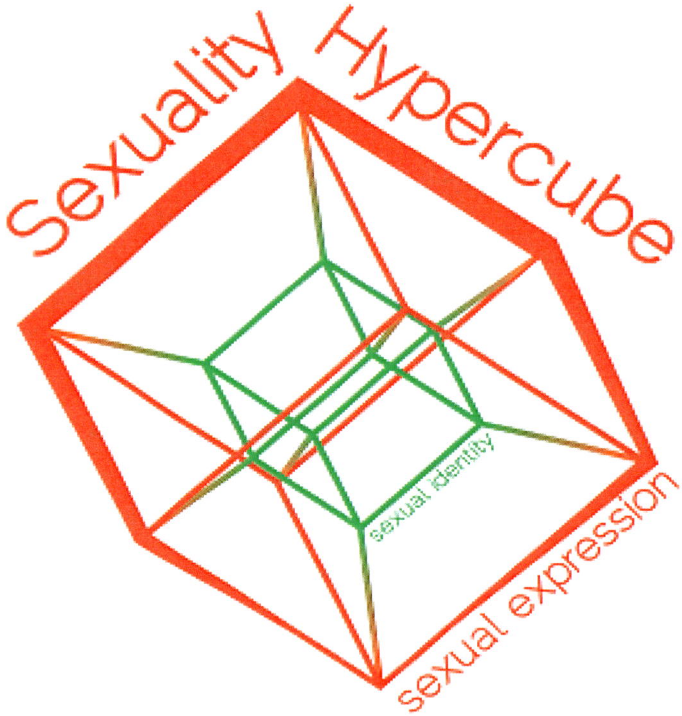

Figure 3. The Sexual Hypercube (h-Cube).
Illustrated by Max Fleishman.

At its core, the h-Cube is a teaching tool; its utility is as an aid to communication about sexuality in general and sexual health in particular. As previously noted, there is much to discover in understanding basic concepts of human sexuality. The h-Cube is one model that defines these basic concepts, describes their relationship to each other, and in doing so, gives a snapshot of the "big picture" representing the complexity of sexuality. Based on discussions with students, the h-Cube is relatively easy for most people to grasp (after all, we are not talking about the Higgs boson of particle physics).

However, the h-Cube model is a bit different from what most of us have been exposed to because it is a four-dimensional model and we live in a three-dimensional world. As a result of its unfamiliarity, it may seem a bit mind-blowing the first time you see a hypercube in action. However, the potential benefit of applying such a model to sexuality is that it can help those struggling to understand their sexuality find where they fit in the world, assist them in becoming more accepting of themselves, and feel more comfortable with their sexuality as well as the sexuality of others. As noted, the h-Cube is simply one model (among others) to help us figure out this whole sex thing. Enough clarification; let's get into the details.

The h-Cube we are going to focus on is a four-dimensional model (analog) of the regular three-dimensional cube. To better understand the whole four-dimensional aspect of this, please consider the following relationship. *The hypercube is to a regular cube as a regular cube is to the square.* In a sense, a square (in two dimensions of length and width) can simply be expanded or "folded out" into a cube of three dimensions (length, width, and height). In turn, the three-dimensional cube can be expanded (folded out) to a four-dimensional hypercube (length, width, height, and kata – the last term is described below).

If we were an animal that perceived the world only in two dimensions (say, like protozoa), then we would only consider moving left, right, diagonally, forward, or backward. If we could consider it though, we (as protozoa) would never think, "Hey everybody, let's go up there!" Living in a world in which we see three dimensions, humans have similar difficulty thinking about additional dimensions in which to see the world. For example, few people have ever heard of the word *kata* used as a spatial dimension or direction and would not understand instructions to "move kata" like most people would understand instructions to "duck" or "come up here." Kata and anana are names of two additional directions in the fourth dimension (also described by Hinton [1888] in *A New Era of Thought*).

Hypercubes can theoretically exist in many dimensions, and some astrophysicists believe the cosmos needs at least four spatial dimensions to be described accurately. Some cosmologists (especially those who subscribe to string theory) believe there must be more than three dimensions; otherwise, their mathematical equations of the universe do not work. Four-dimensional hypercubes are referred to by several names; probably the most common is *tesseract*. Essentially, the four-dimensional hypercube is an equal-sided cube within another equal-sided cube that has correlating and parallel lines (as in Figure 3). Notice that each corner (or vertex) of the outer cube is connected to the corresponding corner of the inner cube. To the three-dimensional human brain, this type of illustration causes an optical illusion of shifting perspectives.

The purpose of this brief technical description of the hypercube is to build an analog model of how the components of the sexual identity and expression cubes relate to one another. An analog model represents data by means of one or more physical properties and can express any value along a continuous scale (much like the positions of the hands on a clock are considered an analog representation of time). Time is a continuous scale that can be divided by many different units of measurement, such as 3,600 seconds in an hour or by the convention of 12 numbers around the face of a traditional clock representing 12 units of 5 minutes, each equaling an hour. These two units of analog measurement (3,600 seconds and one hour) are considered equal in quantity of time. This point is particularly important relative to the sexual cubes. The Sexual Identity Cube appears to be divided into 4X4X4 line segments limited to four sections. These divisions are artificial, as each dimension can be organized on a continuum, with points on the continuum designating four or a million units of measurement (just like the analog of the clock measuring an hour by 3,600 seconds or by one movement of the hour hand). So, the "four" designations of sex orientation (male, female, transgender intersex, or transgender psychosocial) could alternatively be measured by one thousand points ranging from a completely masculinized body to a completely feminized body.

The same can be said for the Sexual Expression Cube (e-Cube); it's all how you divide it up. Let's use another brief example: *your pinky finger*. If you bend it, you see it divides into three sections between the base knuckle (this first large knuckle closest to the palm of your hand) and the tip of the digit. So, you could say these sections represent three different parts of your finger. You could also count the number of skin cells in a straight line between your base knuckle and the tip of your pinky. This second form of measurement renders thousands of points along a continuum. Both measurements are accurate, and they represent the same length of space.

Where the expression cube looks like a fuzzy cube, consider it as the same dimensions as the identity cube. Consider the lengths of corresponding and parallel line segments in the expression cube and the identity cube to be equal. For example, the line in the identity cube representing sex orientation (divided into four segments) would be considered the same dimensions of the line in the Sexual Expression Cube representing sexual fantasy, even if the latter line segment may have thousands of points representing different varieties of sexual fantasy.

Therefore, there are three important considerations to remember in understanding the Sexual Hypercube (Figure 3, p. 140). First, as just described, any given line in either the identity cube or the expression cube can be measured differently but represents equal dimensions. The line can be measured using few divisions (four segments, as with sex orientation) or thousands of divisions (as with sexual fantasy) yet are equal. This is the concept of measuring the pinky by sections of the finger or number of skin cells.

Second, each line in both the identity cube and expression cube can expand or contract depending on a multitude of factors. Staying with the anatomical metaphor, you can extend your pinky finger or pull its tip back to touch the base of the finger. When your pinky is fully extended, it is about three times the length as when it is contracted. Perhaps better anatomical symbols would be erectile tissue, such as erectile bodies found within the clitoris and penis.

Third, this is the wild thing. Are you ready for the wild thing? The wild thing is that the hypercube moves! Imagine turning a flip book of the h-Cube and watching it create a simulation of perpetual movement. As the h-Cube moves, the smaller inner cube of the hypercube (identity) expands outward and envelops the once-larger outer cube (expression). Now the inner cube of identity becomes the outer, and the former outer cube (expression) becomes the smaller one in the center of the hypercube! Then the process continues with constant reversals. The movement represents how the h-Cube is dynamic, interactive, and synergistic.

Instead of a flip-book simulation taking up the next 30 pages, another engaging way to demonstrate the reciprocal nature of the h-Cube (that is also beyond the present publishing possibilities) is to imagine the scene from *Star Wars* when the Rebellion leaders assemble in their War Room around a rotating hologram to plan an attack against the Death Star. Someday, it would be useful to have a similar hologram of the Sexual Hypercube to rotate and peer inside to explain to students the many sexual identities contained within. Until then, the next best option is to view a sophisticated simulation of hypercube movement by googling any of the readily available "animated hypercube" videos on the internet. It is a very cool visual experience of your 3-D brain viewing a representation from the fourth dimension. *That* is the wild thing!

APPLICATION OF THE SEXUAL HYPERCUBE MODEL

The detailed explanations of terms and concepts discussed in this book so far were all necessary to get to this point: How the h-Cube works! Conceptually, the dynamic interactive nature of the movement of the h-Cube reflects how the elements of the i-Cube and the e-Cube influence each other. For practical application of the inter-workings of the h-Cube, we will examine the sexual development process during two stages of life, adolescence/young adulthood and later life.

The Sexual Hypercube Feedback Loop in Adolescence/Young Adulthood

One of the two major tasks of adolescence is establishing a sexual identity, which usually (but not always) involves initiating sexual experiences with others (expression). The other major developmental task is establishing autonomy and independence from parents. For the fortunate few, forming a sexual identity and establishing sexual activity seems to be completely programmed, is accomplished without any conscious planning, and takes as much effort as breathing. For the rest of us, adolescence is a struggle with major insecurities and paralyzing confusion over what the whole sex thing is about. Most adolescents essentially fumble their way through this stage of life trying to preserve any shred of dignity. Alas, many of us did well simply not to succumb to our private anxieties (or the sheer terror) of being the gangly awkward creatures we were.

Therefore, the key processes involved in adolescent sexual development are sexual maturation (involving physical changes of puberty), psychological processing of changes to the body (involving emotional responses to physical changes), sexual experimentation (involving masturbation and often sexual behaviors with others), and self-identification (involving the beginnings of self-attribution and self-labeling). The process of sexual identity development is complex (as reflected in the many influencing factors of the i-Cube) and can occur over the course of 1 or 2 decades. Sexual identity results from the biological, psychological, and social variables but is strongly influenced by the other two key processes of adolescent sexual development: self-exploration and sexual experimentation.

Self-exploration is confusing regarding the sexual metamorphosis of our bodies and, of course, also occurs over a long course of time. The process of sexual experimentation and expression with others can be confusing because of the process of trial-and-error. The key point here is that the feedback loop between our sexual identity and our sexual expression is a core and essential part of the developmental growth process. Of course, our developing sexual identity has strong and direct influence on how we express ourselves sexually and to whom. However, the way we see ourselves sexually (identity) is also determined, at least in part, by our self-exploration and the sexual experiences we have with others (expression).

Let's use a person's identification as being lesbian or gay, for example (as a reminder, this is not a person's full sexual identity, just a pattern of sexual attraction). In retrospect, many individuals who identify as lesbian or gay knew from a very early age that they were not attracted heterosexually. Many closeted themselves for protection and self-preservation (depending on the environment). Other individuals took years to develop a self-awareness of being lesbian or gay (bisexual as well) and slowly came to the conclusion through different sexual experiences.

In her book *Sexual Fluidity: Understanding Women's Love and Desire*, Lisa Diamond describes the greater fluidity of female sexuality when she found that one of four young women she studied (over a period of 10 years) spent some time in same-sex relationships. She described popular terms to capture these developmental explorations, such as "heteroflexibility," "has-bian," and "LUG" (lesbian until graduation) (Diamond, 2008). Sometimes after periods of same-sex experimentation, individuals settle into long-term heterosexual patterns. One way to understand these phenomena is to consider them a reflection of a feedback loop process with interactive influences between sexual identity and sexual expression.

The lack of sexual expression (both solo and socially) can essentially disable the feedback loop during the developmental stages of youth and slow down the movement of the Sexual Hypercube. Consequently, the delay (especially absence) of sexual expression handicaps the development of a confident sense of sexual identity and may make achieving sexual satisfaction more challenging (especially interpersonally). As seen in the sexual health clinic, individuals with the least amount of experience with masturbation (and especially a complete lack of it) tend to have the most difficulty achieving personal sexual satisfaction in relationships. It is very common for women with problems of sexual desire, arousal, and climax with their partner to report that they seldom or never masturbate. This scenario most often represents a lack of effective feedback looping within the dimensions of sexual expression, and on occasion reflects a lack of feedback looping between identity and expression as well.

The Sexual Hypercube Feedback Loop in Later Adulthood

Another reflection of feedback looping between identity and expression is the process of the changes to sexual identity and expression over the course of the lifespan, especially culminating in changes during later adulthood. For some, a variant version of the process described in Diamond's work with young women also occurs at the other end of the developmental process with older men and women. When we are young, we are much more cognizant of traditional sex-role expectations and generally more compliant (sex-typed) in our behavior. It is common for people to do so because they believe it is necessary for the purposes of courting and mate selection. After several decades of "swimming with the current" of the more traditional sex-role orientation, men and women essentially become more relaxed and less concerned about meeting sex-role expectations. In a sense, they give themselves the gift of being more authentic. This change was described in detail by Carl Jung's theory of sex-role convergence (Jung, 1960).

This process is a gradual and, for the most part, unconscious shift in the Sexual Identity Cube for some individuals, moving from the more traditional sex-role behavior (whether masculine or feminine) to more of an androgynous expression of the self. The mechanisms by which this shift occurs are biological (hormonal shift), psychosocial (changing priorities), and behavioral ("forget that macho shit"). They can be described as the long-term workings of feedback looping between the Sexual Identity and Sexual Expression Cubes within the hypercube across the lifespan.

The intent of the hypercube model is to provide an alternative means of understanding the complex and confusing world of sexuality; to promote greater opportunities for individual self-acceptance and "finding oneself" within a model of diverse sexual experiences; and finally, to facilitate movement toward higher levels of sexual health on individual, family, and community levels. The hypercube model is based on a multidisciplinary perspective (biological, psychosocial, behavioral, clinical, and cultural dimensions) that is interwoven into the human experience of sexuality. It is not meant to be an all-encompassing model for explanation of all things sexual, but rather another tool for those attempting to help themselves (or others) answer questions about sexuality or overcome challenges to personal sexual health.

WHAT EVIDENCE IS THERE THAT SEXUAL IDENTITY AND EXPRESSION CHANGE OVER TIME? ANIMAL MODELS OF CHANGES IN BIOLOGICAL SEX AND EXPRESSION

A Fish, Worm, Lizard, and Mole are a Few of a Thousand Examples

To help one think about more complex ways to conceive sexual identity and expression, examples are offered here of many types of change that occur across the lifespan as well as in the animal kingdom. There is evidence, in both animal and human models, that creatures small and large make transitions in their sexual status. Using the three-dimensional model of identity, changes in *sex orientation, sexual orientation,* and *sex-role orientation* among people are presented. But first, let us examine a few animal models as a reminder of how biological sex can change naturally in the wild.

There are actually hundreds of examples of species that change their sex status, especially if one looks at insects and fish. Only a few of the more celebrated examples of dramatic sex transitions are presented in this section. Interestingly, animals can make changes to their sex status on a "species-specific" basis (the individual member changes from female to male) or on a "species-wide" basis (such as when a species has "eliminated" an entire sex status category). The question is: If fish can do it, can people?

The Blue-Headed Wrasse (Thalassoma bifasciatum)

These fish live in harems of 10 to 12 females jealously guarded by a single male. If the male is killed (by another fish) or removed from the group (say by a researcher), the largest female (and she alone) literally changes into a male in terms of appearance and behavior. "He" now runs the harem and, in time (about 2 weeks) starts to fertilize the eggs of females with sperm this "new male" is now able to produce (Piper, 2007; Schärer & Vizoso, 2003).

The Green Spoonworm (Bonellia veridis).

This marine worm lives on the sea floor (10 to 100 meters deep) and is sexually undifferentiated until its larval stage. Then, the larvae move to the top of their little mud pile. The females then use a long proboscis (arm-like nose) to sweep the sea floor for other larvae. If a larva is not touched by the proboscis, then the female remains female. If a larva is touched by the hormones on the proboscis, then it develops into a male. The new male worm remains small in size and crawls inside the body of the larger female, where it spends the rest of its life supplying sperm to the female (from inside her). So, the sex of a Green Spoonworm is thus determined by external, environmental factors (the presence or absence of bonellin), not by internal, genetic factors (Berec et al., 2005).

The Desert Grassland Whiptail Lizard (Aspidoscelis uniparens)

One of the most well-known examples of animals making a "species-wide" change in sex status is the sex-free reproduction of the Whiptail lizard, which has managed to find a way to eliminate the male version of itself. Females simply lay eggs that hatch only daughters via a cloning process. Although there are scores of examples of animals that reproduce asexually (especially insects and fish), until recently the Whiptail lizard was the most complex animal to do so in the wild (Harmon, 2010).

The Transcaucasian Mole Vole (Ellobius lutescens)

In 1995, researchers discovered that the males of this mammal species do not have a Y chromosome or have even an SRY gene (sex-determining region). In fact, it is believed that all mole voles (both males and females) have a single X chromosome, making for an XO sex chromosome set. They are born, live, have babies, and die – all without the disadvantages of a Y chromosome (Starr, 2008). This rodent species found a way to activate the masculinization of its males by activating a "gene relay" a couple of stages down the line from SRY gene – thereby saving the species from the need to carry a Y chromosome and providing protection from all the inherited generic flaws that come with it. Hence, the mole vole is the only mammal known to have successfully escaped the inevitability of a Y-chromosome-driven extinction (Starr, 2008).

You might think these animal models are interesting but don't have much relevance to us. But according to Oxford University's top geneticist, Bryan Sykes, the human race is also vulnerable to Y chromosome-driven extinction that eventually will lead to a future of *humans without men*. However, in his book *Adam's Curse*, Sykes explains that a human race without men will not bring an end to the human species – that is, if we can go the way of the mole vole. Because of Y-chromosome decay in humans and the resulting decline in male fertility (0.1% decline each generation), it will take about 5,000 generations before "XY men" become extinct (Sykes, 2003). Holy cow! If you consider a generation to be 20 to 25 years, that's only 100,000 to 125,000 years from now! (Somebody better start working on a plan here!)

Other scholars don't believe male extinction will take that long because there has been a dramatic decline in male fertility measured over the 50-year span from 1940 to 1990. Ryan and Jetha (authors of *Sex at Dawn*) note that the decline has been measured in both sperm concentration and total sperm count. Average sperm concentration declined approximately 42% from 1940 to 1990 (from 1133106/mL to 663106/mL), and the average total sperm count declined approximately 42% during the same period from about 480 million sperm per ejaculate to about 280 million sperm per ejaculate (Ryan & Jetha, 2010).

What is going on here, and what reasons are there for the Y-chromosome deterioration and the decline in male fertility? The speculations are many and their exploration is fascinating yet beyond the focus of this chapter. Fortunately, women have always served as the cradle of civilization in human history and women's creativity may assist future men to continue their existence in a new form of masculinized "XX men or XO men," if, that is, women choose to still have us around by then (guys, I wouldn't count on it based on how things are at present).

HUMAN MODELS OF MOVEMENT ACROSS THE SEXUAL HYPERCUBE

Human beings also experience sexual transitions across the lifespan, which most frequently and dramatically involve changes in sexual expression. Changes also regularly occur in sexual identity and on a regular basis with many (but not all) people. Of course, animals are not believed to be influenced by the same kind of culture as humans and are not pressed upon by cultural scripts as we are. Again, if we use the three-dimensional model of the Sexual Identity Cube, we can examine changes in sexual identity as they occur within sex orientation, sexual orientation, and sex-role orientation.

Movement Across the Sexual Identity Cube: Sex Orientation

The examples of changes in sex orientation are divided into those that are voluntary and those that are not, because that is how these changes are experienced by people (see Table 1). Let's discuss the voluntary changes first. Adult gender-affirming surgeries started in the late 1920s in Europe upon the request of the patients (voluntary). The first recorded sex change was that of a Danish painter named Einar Wegener, who believed he developed a feminine personality named Lili Elbe and requested surgical reassignment (Hoyer, 1933). This story is the basis of the movie *The Danish Girl*

(Chasin et al., 2015). Today, accounts of these procedures are fairly commonplace, such as the several featured stories in this text as well as *The Gender Revolution and New Sexual Health* (Peterson et al., 2020).

Culturally sanctioned gender transitions involve cultures that allow space in their society for individuals to change sex designation from male to female (or vice versa). This category of voluntary transition is considered a "cultural" change of sex status and usually does not involve surgical change to anatomy. Transculturally, the most commonly known examples include the Hijra of India and the Two-Spirited of North America; the latter have been documented in many Native American tribes (LeVay et al., 2015; Masters et al., 1995; Yarber et al., 2010).

TABLE 1. Voluntary / Involuntary Changes in Human Sex Orientation
Voluntary
Adult gender-affirming surgery Adult hormonal sex transition (nonsurgical)
Involuntary
Infant/child sex reassignment surgery, Genetic/hormonal variations (XX males, XY females) Embryonic SRY injection (animal models currently) Culturally sanctioned gender transition (two-spirited)

In many communities across America (as well as most large international cities), one can find individuals living as an alternative sex (alternative to their sex designated at birth) as a permanent lifestyle (with or without hormonal or surgical intervention). These examples are all considered voluntary transitions in sex orientation. Examples of involuntary transition are when some of the same surgical procedures with adults just referenced are performed on children and babies who cannot make their own health care decisions. Similarly, people with genetic and hormonal variations (including XX males, XY females) are considered to have involuntary transitions because they also did not make a choice about their sex orientation. Injections of embryonic SRY (sex-determining region on the Y chromosome) are currently performed on animals only and so cannot be used for evidence of human transition of sex orientation at this time. If they are ever performed with human fetuses, then they would, of course, also be considered involuntary.

Movement Across the Sexual Identity Cube: Sexual Orientation

Changes in sex orientation are more dramatic and rare compared with changes in sexual orientation. Like sex orientation, examples of changes in sexual orientation are also divided into those that are voluntary and those that are not (see Table 2 on the next page). Again, let's discuss the voluntary changes first. As mentioned earlier, Diamond (2008) described what she calls "greater sexual fluidity" when she studied young women who had spent some time in both heterosexual and same-sex relationships. Her data suggest that some women experiment with lesbian relationships before settling into a heterosexual pattern. A key question is whether periods of demonstrated sexual fluidity do or do not represent actual changes in what we consider sexual orientation. It is complicated, and the jury is still out, but certainly it is an important line of research. Students and clients of the authors report that they, and many people they know, not only experiment with same-sex relations as adolescents (which is not considered unusual) but also go back and forth "switching teams" (sometimes several times) over the course of adulthood.

Not as many studies support similar sexual flexibility among males. Yet, there are volumes of reports regarding men being sexual with other men before, during, and after heterosexual relationships. It appears that there is less visibility regarding sexual fluidity among men, in part because of the higher social stigma associated with man-to-man sex than with lesbian relationships. In fact, many men do not consider their sexual contact with other men as "relationships," such as those associated with the colloquial phrase "down-low."

TABLE 2. Voluntary / Involuntary Changes in Human Sexual Orientation Status

Voluntary

Studies of "sexual fluidity" among women
Celebrity cases (Anne Heche, Julie Cypher)
Clinical case studies

Involuntary

Childhood cultural scripting (studies of Sambian boys)
Case studies of partners to M2F trans women (like Alex and his partner discussed in Chapters 7 and 20)

This disparity of social acceptance between gay and lesbian relationships also plays out in the world of celebrity. High-profile couples such as Ellen DeGeneres and Anne Heche (who were together for nearly 4 years) garnered much attention when their relationship ended and when Heche then had a child with Coleman Laffoon during their 5-year marriage. Throughout history, there are many more celebrity examples of women taking female partners in long-term relationships and then entering into heterosexual marriages. There are not as many corresponding celebrity examples of men transitioning from long-term gay relationships to heterosexual marriages. Historically, married men who identified as gay or bisexual were more likely to keep same-sex relations out of the public view (such as many celebrities, including Hollywood leading-man Rock Hudson).

However, it is not uncommon for men who have been married to women and then divorced to have long-term gay relationships (including marriages, more recently). These types of relationships do not come out of clinical files but are easily found in most LGBTQA communities. Whether gay or lesbian, these individuals are often considered to be finally accepting their "true" orientation of sexual attraction. However, this assumption is challenged when they later "switch teams" again and take up heterosexual partners. This raises the question of "serial bisexuality" as well. Of course, many relationships of similar nature can be drawn from clinical cases when questions and stress increase significantly to a point where mental health consultation is sought. I believe this latter scenario is the exception, as most people with questions about their sexual orientation never seek counsel from health care professionals for a multitude of reasons (the least of which are that many health care professionals do not feel comfortable or competent in addressing the sexual health concerns of their patients).

When discussed by university students, the particular matter of involuntary changes of sexual orientation is typically considered even more controversial than voluntary changes. This may be related to the fact that involuntary changes sometimes involve children in particular and that the topic of cultural relativity is almost always a decidedly controversial area within academics. Case in point is the cultural scripting ritual of Sambian boys (Herdt, 2005). As described in Chapter 7, these prepubescent boys leave their family hut, join a male-only communal hut, and engage in several years of sexual maturing by means of ingesting the semen of older boys. This is not a voluntary choice; it would be nearly impossible for these boys to refuse this developmental process that is culturally defined as the essential path to manhood and eventually the ability to select a bride and raise a family. It could be also argued that this form of sexual development does not necessarily involve a change of sexual orientation.

Similarly (and finally), the matter of sexual orientation of partners of post-op transsexual or transgender individuals may also not be considered any kind of change of sexual orientation. However, many partners do have significant concerns not only about the changes occurring with their trans spouses, but also what these changes mean in terms of their own sexual orientation "category." For example, if you are a woman who married a man who later becomes a woman, does that make you a lesbian? The common refrain is, "I didn't sign up for this." Some spouses don't see it like that, and some do. The point is, besides the stress related to the change of their trans spouse's sex orientation, they are often stressed about their own sexual status. Alex's wife (discussed in Chapters 7 and 20) is a wonderful example of a supportive spouse who did not allow questions of "categories" to interfere with a loving and successful relationship. Of course, if there is any type of categorical change in the sexual orientation status of the spouse, it could be considered a "definitional change" with the partner as opposed to an actual anatomical change with the transsexual or transgender individual.

Of course, none of this applies if both you and your spouse are transsexual and essentially switch roles as husband and wife. While exceedingly rare, this does happen (as evidenced by the story of Devin and Gage discussed in Chapters 7 and 20). I once co-presented at Psychiatry Grand Rounds with such an individual. He is a trans man psychiatrist who used to be the female in his marriage. His present wife used to be the male husband in the same marriage. Although very rare, the internet draws these stories together from around the world under the rubric "double sex change couples." A web search will render multiple such couples, including an article entitled "Seven Unique Double Sex Change Couples" (Murano, 2013).

Movement Across the Sexual Identity Cube: Sex-Role Orientation

Although changes in sex orientation are the least frequent (followed in frequency by changes in sexual orientation), the changes that occur in sex-role orientation are very common. One could argue that they are unavoidable for a majority of people. Although changes in the previous two categories (sex and sexual orientations) are fairly distinguishable, the distinction regarding changes in sex-role orientation is much more blurred. For example, if people choose to make voluntary changes about anything in their lives, there is an inherent assumption that they are conscious of their options and conscious of deciding to make the change. Involuntary changes may be made with or without conscious awareness. The Sambian boys are old enough, certainly, to be aware of what happens to them, but they are also not conscious of the overall cultural process that strongly directs their sexual development rituals. It is exceedingly unlikely that any Sambian boy is going to forsake the cultural press upon him and say, "That's okay – I'll just skip this whole ritual thing about becoming a man."

The same is true of Jung's sex-role convergence theory. If you are old enough, you probably know people who seem to have significantly "mellowed out" over the course of several decades. Some of these individuals are cognizant of the changes they have made and others are not. Did they mellow out as a result of reflection and conscious choice, gradual changes in metabolism and hormonal levels, or social expectations of how older folks should behave? The answer is probably "yes" as the underlying process is multicausal and, as previously mentioned, a result of the interactive feedback looping within the Sexual Hypercube.

Hence, the distinction between voluntary and involuntary is not as important related to changes in sex-role orientation. Regarding Table 3, personal observations of the authors (anecdotal evidence) and Jung's sex-role convergence theory have been briefly discussed. At the same time, there are examples of changes that more reflect a voluntary status. Two will be mentioned here. The first is evidence from clinical case studies involving individuals who identify themselves as female-to male (F2M) trans men. Simply stated, these cases involve individuals who are planning to, or who have already accomplished, gender-affirming surgery and they seek consultation in terms of how to appear to others as more masculine. They voluntarily undergo surgery (which changes their sex orientation) and they voluntarily seek counsel in an effort to masculinize themselves (to change their sex-role orientation). Of course, the same is true for male-to-female (M2F) trans women who seek counsel on feminizing their appearance and behavior. Both types of consultation are provided through many sexual health and gender clinics as well as many transgender-oriented support groups.

TABLE 3. Voluntary / Involuntary Changes in Human Sex-Role Orientation Status
<u>**Voluntary**</u>
Clinical case studies (F2M trans men) Personal anecdotal observations
<u>**Involuntary**</u>
C. Jung's theory of sex-role convergence Change in sex-role reference group

WHAT GUIDELINES GOVERN CHANGES IN SEXUAL IDENTITY AND EXPRESSION?

1. Sexual identity (along with sexual expression) does change over time and cannot always be considered a constant fixed trait of development for many people.
2. These changes in status appear to occur by choice in some instances (voluntary) and, in other instances, without choice or even the awareness of the individual (involuntary). These transitions in sexual status appear to occur by various means but include three broad types:
   a. Physical (direct physical transitions in an individual involving genetic, anatomical, hormonal, or surgical change)
   b. Cultural (direct transition in an individual involving sexual scripting and, in many cases, socially sanctioned changes)
   c. Definitional (indirect transition based on relationship to another person, such as a partner's specific change of status)
3. Changes in sexual status are commonly believed to be based on an artificially separated set of influences involving apparent "biological" aspects of sexuality ("nature") and the apparent environmental aspects of sexuality ("nurture"). In reality, both types of factors influence each other in mutually reciprocal ways, facilitating continuous development and changes throughout the lifespan.

4. Within the model of the Sexual Hypercube, these changes can be seen as resulting from a multitude of causal factors related to interactive influences between the Sexual Identity Cube and the Sexual Expression Cube.

What Other Guidelines Might Emerge, and What Is the Point?

It is difficult to project what other trends will emerge that guide changes in the development of sexual identity and expression. If the Sexual Hypercube serves as a model of human sexuality, then the few principles listed in this exploratory discussion will be corrected, amended, or expanded upon. What are the benefits of considering different points of view about sexual identity and expression reflected by the Sexual Hypercube model? The benefits are:

- to more accurately understand sexuality through a general model based upon existing research findings and to stimulate further research questions, which may lead to more of a consensus on the use of the term "sexual identity." As noted, we are far from a consensus opinion.
- to have a broader perception of the complexity and diversity of human sexuality in modern culture, including the difference between sexual identity and sexual expression. This chapter focuses on the complexity of a person's identity as a sexual being. This is different from how individuals have a predisposition to, and/or choice to, manifest their sexual identity in terms of behavioral expression.
- to assert an empirical basis for considering sexual identity to be of a flexible (fluid) nature for many individuals over the course of their lifetime (a normalizing effect) and not a fixed trait as has been traditionally assumed.
- to promote greater self-acceptance of one's sexual identity and thereby minimize negative sexual self-image. On an individual basis, an expanded perspective of the full range of sexual identity and its correlated sexual expression may lead to a greater sense of self-worth and personal satisfaction.
- to use the model as a conceptual learning tool to promote greater tolerance of others as well as lessen the incidence of prejudice and violence toward those who appear different from ourselves.

All the human examples of human sexuality used to formulate the Sexual Hypercube model are drawn from real-world lives of people trying to do what most people want to do. They want to have a sense of health, self-worth and purpose, and have healthy relationships. The h-Cube is designed as a conceptual tool but has significant clinical and personal implications, especially related to promoting greater self-acceptance, a positive sexual self-image, and greater tolerance within which the human tribe can peacefully and cooperatively coexist.

REFERENCES

Bem, D. J. (1996). Exotic becomes erotic: A developmental theory of sexual orientation. *Psychological Review, 103(2), 320-335.*

Berec, L., Schembri, P., & Boukal, D. (2005). Sex determination in *Bonellia viridis* (Echiura: Bonelliidea): Population dynamics and evolution. *Oikos Journal: Synthesizing Ecology*, *108*(3), 473-484.

Cass, V. C. (1979). Homosexual identity formation: A theoretical model. *Journal of Homosexuality*, *4*(3), 219-235.

Cass, V. C. (1983). Homosexual identity formation: Testing a theoretical model. *The Journal of Sex Research, 20*(2), 143-167.

Chasin, L., Israel, U., Morgan, K., Reisman, L. (Producers), & Hooper, T. (Director). (2015). *The Danish Girl* [Film]. Focus Feature Films.
Diamond, L. (2008). *Sexual fluidity: Understanding women's love and desire*. Harvard University Press.
Dillon, F. R., Worthington, R. L., & Moradi, B. (2011). In S. J. Schwartz, K. Luyckx, & V. L. Vignoles (Eds.), *Handbook of identity theory and research* (pp. 649-670). Springer Science + Business Media. https://doi.org/10.1007/978-1-4419-7988-9_27
Fassinger, R. E., & Miller, B. A. (1997). Validation of an inclusive model of sexual minority identity formation on a sample of gay men. *Journal of Homosexuality*, *32*(2), 53-78.
Harmon, K. (2010). No sex needed: All-female lizard species cross their chromosomes to make babies. *Scientific American*. https://www.scientificamerican.com/article/asexual-lizards/
Herdt, G. (2005). *The Sambia: Ritual, sexuality, and change in Papua New Guinea*. Wadsworth.
Hinton, C. (1888). *A new era of thought.* Swan Sonnenschein.
Hoyer, N. (1933). *Man into woman: An authentic record of a change of sex*. E.P. Dutton.
Jung, C. (1960). The stages of life. In G. Adler, M. Fordham, & H. Reads (Eds.), *The collected works of C. G. Jung: Vol. 8. The structure and dynamics of the psyche*. Routledge.
Kaku, M. (1994). *Hyperspace: A scientific odyssey through parallel universes, time warps and the tenth dimension*. Oxford University Press.
Kaplan, H. S. (1974). *The new sex therapy: Active treatment of sexual dysfunctions.* Brunner/Mazel
Kaufman, J., & Johnson, C. (2005). Stigmatized individuals and the process of identity *Sociological Quarterly, 45*(4), 807-833. https://doi.org/10.1111/j.1533-8525.2004.tb02315.x
Kinsey, A. C., Pomeroy, W. B., & Martin, C. E. (1948). *Sexual behavior in the human male.* Saunders.
LeVay, S., Baldwin, J., & Baldwin, J. (2015). *Discovering human sexuality* (3rd ed.). Sinauer Associates.
Masters, W., Johnson, V., & Kolodny, R. (1995). *Human sexuality* (5th ed.). HarperCollins.
McCarn, S. R., & Fassinger, R. E. (1996). Revisioning sexual minority identity formation: A new model of lesbian identity and its implications for counseling and research. *The Counseling Psychologist, 24*(3), 508-534. https://doi.org/10.1177/0011000096243011
Murano, G. (2013). Seven unique double sex change couples. *Odde* [entertainment blog]. www.oddee.com/item_98756.aspx
Perelman, M. (2009). The Sexual Tipping Point®: A mind/body model for sexual medicine. *The Journal of Sexual Medicine, 6*(3), 629-632. https://doi.org/10.1111/j.1743-6109.2008.01177.x
Peterson, F., Bley, J. & Frabotta, R. (2020). *The gender revolution and new sexual health.* Cognella Academic Publishing.
Piper, R. (2007). *Extraordinary animals: An encyclopedia of curious and unusual animals*. Greenwood Press.
Ryan, C., & Jetha, C. (2010). *Sex at dawn*. HarperCollins.
Schärer, L., & Vizoso, D. B. (2003). Earlier sex change in infected individuals of the protogynous reef fish *Thalassoma bifasciatum*. *Behavioral Ecology and Sociobiology*, *55*(2), 137-143.
Starr, B. (2008). Why no Y? Gender-bending transcaucasian mole voles. *KQED*. https://www.kqed.org/quest/687/why-no-y-gender-bending-transcaucasian-mole-voles
Sykes, B. (2003). *Adam's curse: A story of sex, genetics, and the extinction of men*. Oxford University Press.
Yarber, W., & Sayad, B. (2019). *Human sexuality: Diversity in contemporary society* (10th ed.). McGraw-Hill.
Yarber, W., Sayad, B., & Strong, B. (2010). *Human sexuality: Diversity in contemporary society* (7th ed.). McGraw Hill.

9

The Sexual Tipping Point Model

Danielle M. F. Dockery, Zane Ferguson, Stacy Leet, Sallie N. Henderson, David Miller, and Meghan M. Bailey

INTRODUCTION

Discussion of sexual expression (and unexpected things that can go wrong) would be incomplete without including an explanation of the Sexual Tipping Point (STP) model, which is an amazingly sophisticated description of how individuals either initiate or suppress their own sexual behavior. Therefore, the STP model will be thoroughly examined within this chapter, as it utilizes a systems-type approach to identify and label influences which result in a predisposition to either engage, not engage, or discontinue a sexual behavior (Perelman, 2009).

The STP model helps to illustrate whether a person is "hot" or "not" through an examination of multiple determining factors, both physiological and psychological. Inciting factors that lead to more sexual desire in individuals include, but are not limited to, adequate testosterone levels in males, utilization of aphrodisiac-like drugs, genital stimulation, positive attraction to another partner, and the overall feeling of love one might have towards a partner (Peterson et al., 2020). Conversely, suppressant factors may include, but are not limited to, many of the inhibiting variables just mentioned but with inadequate or negative factors associated with them. Examples include low hormone disorders (causing low libido), the side-effects from medications, or the absence of attraction to another individual (Peterson et al., 2020).

Within the STP model, the aforementioned factors can be active against each other within the hypothalamic and limbic sexual-regulating centers of the brain (think of the effect of a person driving with one foot on the accelerator and the other foot on the brake pedal). This traditionally facilitates one of three possible outcomes determining an individual's level of sexual motivation in any given situation: (a) an excitation state of being that results in a form of optimal sexual readiness, (b) an inhibited state of sexual readiness that leads to resistance, or (c) an overall form of neutrality (Perelman, 2009).

In addition to illustrating this "sexual balance act" within an individual (thus leading to an awareness of one's overall sexual readiness), the STP model is predominantly useful in treatment when discussing options for patients with sexual disorders. The application of this model has much utility in reducing negative emotions such as blame and frustration with a client or couple, while simultaneously providing hope through clarification on diagnosis and overall treatment planning (Peterson et al., 2020).

Also included in this chapter are a literature review on the STP model and several examples of the STP model being applied to individuals (including individuals with Autism Spectrum Disorder). A clinical vignette is provided to demonstrate the clinical utility of the STP model with a middle-aged woman who was referred by her gynecologist for counseling services regarding complaints of low libido. Finally, an example is provided of how a one-page summary of the STP model was utilized to increase the sexual health literacy of a group of men in treatment for compulsive sexual behaviors.

A BRIEF HISTORY OF STP

The STP model was developed over the past 4 decades beginning with the pioneer sexologist Helen Kaplan in her first book, *The New Sex Therapy* (Kaplan, 1974). Kaplan was a contemporary of William Masters and Virginia Johnson and, as a psychoanalytic psychiatrist, had a different perspective from Masters' point of view as an obstetrician, gynecologist, and reproductive researcher. Masters and Johnson pioneered a couple-based, 2-week residential behavioral treatment program for sexual disorders that demonstrated very positive outcomes (Masters & Johnson, 1966). Kaplan modified the Masters and Johnson approach to make it more accessible to clients as an outpatient treatment and her book became the standard text for many students across several disciplines. As a result, it had a national impact on where and how people were treated for sexual problems for several decades (Peterson et al., 2020).

Kaplan was known for expanding the role that sexual desire (motivation) plays in sexual interaction – something thought-lacking in the more physiological four-stage model of Masters and Johnson. Kaplan expanded their model by emphasizing multilevel causality in sex therapy and popularized her "Kaplan model" by collaboration with many of her students, who later became leaders in the field of clinical sex therapy (Perelman, 2014). In her final book (1995), Kaplan described a psychosomatic (mind-body) dual-control model of sexual motivation emphasizing "inhibition/excitation" processes that is the heart of the STP model. She acknowledged borrowing from the work of Kupferman (1991), who wrote, "All examples of physiological motivational control seem to involve dual effects – inhibitory and excitatory – which function together to adjust the system" (p. 751).

Similar to the dual sets of inhibiting and stimulating mechanisms that regulate body temperature, Kaplan (and her collaborators) applied this perspective to the STP model in a sort of force-field analysis with the "let's get it on" factors on one side and "I'd rather not" factors on the other. These factors can actually be the same factors (such as testosterone) but differing levels of the hormone, with sufficient or high levels promoting a "let's get it on" state of mind and insufficient (low) levels effecting the "I'd rather not" inhibiting influence.

Aside from its clinical utility assisting those with sexual health concerns, the graphics of the STP model have evolved to very sophisticated visuals that have contributed to popularizing the model over the past 20 years. In 2013, the STP trademark registration was assigned to the MAP Education & Research Foundation so that STP resources could be distributed worldwide for free. Today's more sophisticated and nuanced figures feature "building blocks" that can be used to assemble unique representations of any given individual's STP at a particular moment in time.

Key STP images as well as fully narrated video descriptions of the STP model can be found on YouTube and Vimeo channels. You are encouraged to pursue any curiosity regarding the STP model and learn more about this important model by visiting YouTube and searching for "Sexual Tipping Point Model" or reading noted references by Michael Perelman at the end of this chapter.

LITERATURE REVIEW OF SEXUAL TIPPING POINT (STP) MODEL

Both mental health and medical professionals have struggled to assist individuals with many types of sexual dysfunction due to misunderstanding the many factors that are often involved, especially in those disorders that are often less reported to medical professionals. This is especially true of less frequently reported disorders such as retarded ejaculation (RE), delayed ejaculation (DE), as well as female sexual dysfunction involving dyspareunia (sexual pain) and vaginismus (involuntary contraction of the vagina). Having a common language and the ability to clearly articulate the mental health treatments that can coincide with medical treatments (e.g., medication options) can better assist clinicians and patients to make the best decisions for care. Cultivating a biopsychosocial-behavioral and cultural perspective allows for a straightforward approach that allows clinicians and their patients to understand presenting sexual problems as well as the potential solutions available (Perelman, 2016a).

The STP model endeavors to alleviate sexual dissatisfaction in the most common-sense manner possible. Approaching sexual dysfunction with the STP model allows for a mutual language to assist patients and clinicians in correcting inaccurate communication and assists clinicians lacking in-depth human sexuality education and/or the comfort level to engage in sexual health education with their patients. The STP concept is particularly useful in providing an explanation of benefits and risks for those individual patients that are not faring well with their sexual disorders. Therefore, the STP model explanation is used to help reduce client anger and despair while providing hope for a solution for clients with sexual concerns (Peterson et al., 2020).

CONNECTION BETWEEN STP AND CLINICAL APPLICATION AND CONCEPTUALIZATION

Retarded ejaculation (RE) and delayed ejaculation (DE) are often considered hard to treat by many healthcare clinicians because these providers are notoriously thought of as lacking in the grasp of the "interpersonal and psychological distress" (Perelman, 2016a) these disorders can often cause. Per the *DSM-5* (American Psychiatric Association, 2013), retarded ejaculation (RE) and delayed ejaculation (DE) are two of several sexual disorders considered under the diminished ejaculatory disorders (DED), a subset of male orgasmic disorders (MOD). Both RE and DE are considered to be uncommon, ranging in frequency of 1% to 4% of the male population for DE (Perelman & Rowland, 2006) and less than 3% of the male population documented for RE (Perelman, 2016a).

These disorders are widely documented as being difficult to treat, mainly due to the amount of time practitioners (such as urologists) would need to spend on patients who present with RE or DE versus patients who present with erectile dysfunction (ED), which is a more commonly treated disorder. DE and RE patients normally can achieve erectile capacity, however they are reported to suffer from the inability to ejaculate or they present with marked delayed ejaculation or diminished ability to ejaculate, including a reduction in volume of the ejaculation. However, RE and DE can often improve from a combined treatment approach (mind and body), including introducing mental health treatments in conjunction with pharmacological treatments. To successfully treat these elusive sexual disorders, it would be beneficial to clearly articulate an understanding of the patient's sexual disorder and what options are available.

The STP model allows clinicians to easily interpret and understand various sexual disorders. It provides the ability to clearly articulate treatment options to patients, particularly sexual disorders that are not easily treated. This model not only allows a clear method to present sexual disorders; it also takes into account sexual capacity, biopsychosocial-behavioral factors, and various cultural factors that could represent the patient as a whole (Perelman, 2016b). Use of the STP model with patients and their intimate partners allows for the education of the multiple problems accompanying DE and RE, and taught in a way that promotes understanding, including understanding that these disorders are neither the fault of the patient nor their intimate partner (Perelman, 2016b).

Although there continues to be a lack of larger controlled studies, it is documented that sex therapists have had a success rate of 70% to 80% for the treatment of RE compared to the urologist community that widely reports RE and DE as "difficult-to-treat" conditions (Perelman, 2016a, p. 574). This disproportionate rate of success, in and of itself, points to a greater need for the approach that the STP model provides.

According to many studies, sexual dysfunction in women is a common experience but prevalence varies according to definition and sampling (Laumann et al., 1999; Mercer et al., 2003). However, because the definitions of problems vary widely, distinguishing between sexual concerns, difficulties, disorders, and dysfunctions may be helpful (Wylie, 2007). Such a differentiation can be useful and is often important when assessing and looking at how to help them further. The STP model offers a way to help understand and distinguish between sexual concerns, difficulties, disorders, and dysfunction by using its multifactor approach to break down the many factors that contribute to inhibitor and excitatory responses. The STP also allows for multiple providers to utilize this same model when approaching female sexual dysfunction, and this multidisciplinary approach is important for the greatest level of success (Mimoun & Wylie, 2009).

APPLICATION OF STP MODEL WITH AUTISM SPECTRUM DISORDERS

One robust risk factor for Autism Spectrum Disorder (ASD) is the person's sex: for every female with ASD in the United States, there are 4.5 affected males, and a male bias in prevalence is consistent across countries and across diagnostic criteria (Developmental Disabilities Monitoring Network Surveillance Year 2010 Principal Investigators, & Centers for Disease Control and Prevention [CDC], 2014). In the past, Applied Behavioral Analysis (ABA) was the primary treatment for people diagnosed with ASD. The use of ABA helped therapists to challenge behaviors and to target skill acquisition. Applied Behavioral Analysis has also been useful in treating sexual behaviors in people with ASD, including hypermasturbation, public masturbation, and inappropriate romantic advances towards others (Beddows & Brooks, 2015; Visser et al., 2017).

In a survey of people with ASD aged 9 to 38 years, it was observed that 65% engaged in public masturbation and almost 20% engaged in inappropriate touching of the opposite sex (Visser et al., 2017). These behaviors can result in social consequences and legal ramifications, which could restrict the independence of individuals with ASD as a result of the symptoms of ASD rather than the intent to harm others (Berryessa, 2014). It is important that this education is provided for individuals with ASD both for their protection and for the protection of those individuals they may encounter.

It is important to recognize that the STP model is individually based, and therefore requires identification of person-specific positive and negative influences on their sexual behavior; these can be based on culture, upbringing, and biological variations from person to person. While the STP model emphasizes the necessity for pharmaceutical and cognitive therapy for undesired sexual behavior, Perelman (2009) also emphasizes the need for behavioral intervention. This notion is also supported by the statement from Laura Moen, PhD, of the National Institute of Health: "There is always a psychosocial, behavioral, and cultural balance to the sexual medicine equation."

Previous models for educating individuals with ASD about sex, such as the TEACCH model (Sullivan & Caterino, 2008) have various levels or degrees of education based on general impairment. While tiering education based on degree of impairment seems intuitive, in order to appropriately educate and respect the reproductive rights of individuals with disabilities, comprehensive education for all levels of impairment based on behavioral need seems to be an appropriate way to proceed with sex education. This need is further supported by Perelman (2009) indicating that factors increasing the likelihood of sexual behavior are person-specific and have the potential to be socially invalid or problematic. Limiting or reducing the degree of sexual education to this population assumes that they are asexual or unable to appropriately engage in sexual behaviors, thus hindering the potential for an individual with ASD, or other cognitive impairments, to experience healthy sexual behavior. Perelman (2009) makes this observation while describing the model for sexual activity in both neurotypical and neurodiverse (intellectual disabilities or illness) individuals.

Connection Between STP and Applied Behavioral Analysis

Applied Behavioral Analysis (ABA) is a practice founded on the principles of Radical Behaviorism, which conceptualizes both observable actions and internal behaviors (such as thoughts) as behaviors that can be targeted and modified. When applying this approach to the STP model, ABA can be used to target maladaptive or inappropriate thoughts and actions while also providing appropriate behavior replacements that can be reinforced using common ABA interventions. When considering modification of behavior, ABA targets behaviors that will be shaped to become more socially valid behavior replacements that are reinforced or punished using person-specific consequences. The STP model in conjunction with ABA create a comprehensive and communicable method and purpose for targeting influences that result in inappropriate sexual behavior while also providing an archetype for identifying and conceptualizing why sexual behavior occurs. While there is significant overlap between ABA and the STP model, Sullivan and Caterino (2008) identify the need for attention to the gender identity and sexual orientation of individuals with ASD, which may be better served using a more cognitive model such as the Sexual Hypercube (Peterson et al., 2020).

Clinical Vignette

Carolyn is a 47-year-old woman who was referred to the outpatient mental health clinic by her gynecologist after expressing her concerns of low libido. Carolyn attributes her low libido to perimenopause. She stated that she is experiencing symptoms such as irregular periods, hot flashes, night sweats, and lack of lubrication/elasticity in her vaginal tissue. During her appointment she became tearful, and said that she wanted to speak to a mental health professional about her concerns of low libido but did not want to go on medication. During the history and physical portion of her appointment she disclosed the following: she has been cohabitating with her current partner for 5 years. She stated that at the beginning of her relationship they had a healthy sex life. They had sex one to two times a week for the first 2 years of their relationship. She reported that her sex life gradually decreased over the course of the relationship as her symptoms of perimenopause worsened. Carolyn reported that her sex life was, at that time, nonexistent. She self-identifies as a Latino/Caucasian female. She reported that she was adopted at an early age and raised in a predominantly Caucasian household by her adopted parents. Carolyn's adoptive parents raised her in a nondenominational Christian household. She now attends church on major holidays but does not engage in religious practices regularly. She has no children but enjoys spending time with her partner's 15-year-old son.

Carolyn has a close relationship with her parents who live 4 hours away. She disclosed that her parents are supportive of her career, but she speculates that they wish she had fulfilled their wishes of having a family of her own. Carolyn feels fulfilled in the role of being a "mother figure" by being able to take care of her partner's son when he stays with them every other weekend. She denies any regret regarding not having her own children. Carolyn's main social support comes from her (female) childhood friend who lives close in proximity. They see each other monthly for social outings.

Carolyn has a Master's degree in Business Administration, with a minor in English. She runs and owns a small publishing company in the town in which she grew up in Utah. She works on average 60 to 70 hours each week. Her partner is a 35-year-old male who works in accounting, and recently was diagnosed with erectile dysfunction (ED). Due to the age difference, Carolyn compared herself to her partner's ex-wife and feels like she is beginning to look older. She often will tell herself she "isn't desired" by her partner. Carolyn reports that she feels tired more than half the days each week due to returning home from work late each night. She described symptoms that fit the diagnosis of anhedonia. Over the past 2 years, Carolyn has gained 20 pounds which has negatively impacted her self-image. She reports feeling uncomfortable in her own body.

During her intake appointment at the local outpatient mental health clinic, Carolyn disclosed the following: She attributed her low libido to perimenopause, negative self-image (due to weight gain and getting older), feeling exhausted due to working long hours, and symptoms of ongoing depression. In the beginning of her relationship with her partner, Carolyn described a healthy sex life, and had sex one to two times a week for the first 2 years of their relationship. Carolyn found sex enjoyable. During intimacy with her partner, she would orgasm each night through foreplay and penetration. Carolyn reported feeling desirable with her partner, who would express verbally that she was "desirable and beautiful." She reported that those types of positive messages have declined in frequency of late. She admitted to fears of her partner leaving because of her lower self-image and because he may desire a younger woman. Carolyn has continued to engage in sex although she has feelings of sadness when her partner takes Cialis 20 mg so that he can have an erection.

During sexual encounters, she finds her mind wandering due to feeling pain caused by vaginal dryness and vaginal discomfort. To negate the vaginal discomfort, Carolyn disclosed she will moan in fake-pleasure to help her partner achieve an orgasm since they do not engage in foreplay. She stated that she misses the closeness she used to experience with her partner from sexual intimacy, feelings of being desired, and feeling feminine. She is unsure of how to get these emotions back.

During her intake appointment, Carolyn reported having moderately severe depressive symptoms. There was no previous history of mental health symptoms. Based upon her presenting symptoms and screening measures, Carolyn was diagnosed with premenstrual dysphoric disorder. After her intake appointment she decided to make a follow-up appointment with her gynecologist about her new diagnosis. Her gynecologist recommended she take daily vitamins such as Vitamin B6, calcium, magnesium supplements, and start on a daily aerobic exercises schedule (biking/swimming/walking). After speaking to her gynecologist, she spoke to her Primary Care Manager who started her on a low dose of Celexa (20 mg daily).

Carolyn was treated using Cognitive Behavioral Therapy which helped to address her ongoing depressive symptoms. She was taught different exercises to address her problematic thoughts. She also engaged in role plays to help increase communication with her partner, and to learn the importance of setting boundaries with herself as it relates to a work/life balance. Through the combination of medication, therapy, and patient health education which employed the STP model (see the Sexual Tipping Point "Balance Sheet" at the end of this chapter), Carolyn decreased her scores from her baseline measures (representing symptom improvement). She also reported an increase in positive self-image which she attributes to going back to the gym while in treatment. In turn, Carolyn was able to lose some weight and began to wear more figure-fitting clothes.

After improving communication skills with her partner, he agreed to speak about utilizing lubrication during sex to help with Carolyn's vaginal dryness as well as focus more on foreplay and intimacy-building exercises. This included showing affection each day in numerous ways and speaking about how their bodies respond to different physical sensations during intimacy. The couple utilized a 1 to 5 number system during intimacy and when the other hit an area on the body that was a 4-5 on the number system (in pleasure), the partner provided feedback to the other partner. Through this, Carolyn and her partner begin to grow a stronger emotional connection. The couple began to use foreplay before intercourse. As a result, Carolyn began to feel more feminine and more desired again by her partner.

Carolyn remained on her SSRI and the vitamins that were recommended by her gynecologist as she began to taper back on the frequency of her therapy sessions. Carolyn was able to taper down the frequency of her appointments over a duration of 6 months, going from weekly appointments to a monthly basis. Carolyn was able to build closeness again with her partner and enjoy sex on a frequent basis. She reported much higher sexual satisfaction and no more faking of orgasms.

Reviewing Carolyn's experience, the STP model was used to help her understand the "hot" and "not" factors involved with her presenting low libido. It helped her in removing self-blame as well as blaming her partner, both of which are counterproductive to positive treatment outcome. The use of the STP model allowed Carolyn to understand the inhibiting factors of hormonal imbalance, a medication condition, her partner needing to use Cialis, low energy, physical pain during intercourse, lack of genital stimulation, depressive symptoms, negative self-talk, negative sexual self-image, and low attribution. Overall and put in simpler terms of the STP model, Carolyn became more balanced as her "not" (suppressing) factors were turned to "hot" (inciting) factors through patient health education (using the STP point-of-view), individual therapy, and medication management.

DISCUSSION

The STP point-of-view has been successfully employed for patient health education in individual, couples, and group treatment. For example, the simplified version of the STP model (the "Balance Sheet" as described at the end of this chapter) was used by service men who were in group treatment for sexually compulsive behaviors. The participants recognized and discussed several "hot" and "not" factors, both physical and psychological, that affected their health and recovery. Several men in that group were taking SSRIs (Serotonin Selective Reuptake Inhibitors) to lower their symptoms of anxiety and/or depression. They also welcomed the "usually unwelcomed" side effects of inhibited sexual responsiveness. For example, some men reported that the medication "tapped-down" their obsessive thoughts about their compulsive behavior, even when they experienced "the flag going up the flagpole but not waving" (inhibited or delayed ejaculation). The STP model helped them understand the "balancing act" that their treatment interventions would temporarily create but would not be a long-lasting effect. The men accepted that the medications were to be employed until their depressive and anxious symptoms diminished (Mood or Emotions in Situation), and while they developed the skill set (Self-Talk) to avoid old patterns of obsessive thinking and behaviors that trigger cycles of compulsive behavior. The STP model demonstrated utility as a means of client understanding and acceptance of aspects of their therapy which contribute to positive treatment outcomes.

The STP model serves as an individual example of sexual expression that complements the general model presented in the Sexual Expression Cube (or e-Cube) and Sexual Hypercube (h-Cube) that are described in the last two chapters. The STP model details the specific mechanisms (both intrapersonal and interpersonal) that result in the sexual behaviors represented in the e-Cube. The e-Cube and h-Cube emphasize the diversity of sexual fantasy and potential variations of human sexual behavior. However, the cubes do not delineate the specific mechanisms which dictate whether sexual behavior will or will not occur in any situation. The STP model is more descriptive of the specific means by which sexual expression is accomplished (more so than the e-Cube and h-Cube). In addition, the STP model includes much overlap with the biocultural mediators of sexual expression, which are referred to as biosocial-cultural factors that can either promote sexual expression (such as accepting an invitation to an orgy) or suppress sexual expression (not holding hands because one is living in a political system that criminalizes same-sex expression).

Therefore, the combination of the identity and expression cubes (represented by the hypercube model and emphasizing the incredible diversity of human sexuality) are complemented by the STP model, which represents what is happening on an individual basis. Each model alone is based on the leading sexual science research of the past several decades and together, the STP and h-Cube represent the most comprehensive explanation of human sexual diversity and interaction.

The Sexual Tipping Point*
"Balancing Sheet"

"Hot" (Inciting) Factors (Excitatory Influences) (More Sexual Potential)	*versus*	"Not" (Suppressing) Factors (Inhibitory Influences) (More Sexual Avoidance)
	Biological Factors	
Normal/High Libido	**Hormones** (such as testosterone)	Low Libido
No Influence if Absent	**Medical Conditions** (DM, PD, MS, HIV)	High Influence if Present
No Influence if Absent	**Medication Effects** (Heart, HTN, Psychotropic)	Lowering Response if Present
Excitation	**PDE5 Inhibitor Medications** (such as Viagra, Cialis, Levitra)	No Influence if Absent
Rested/Energetic	**Energy/Vitality** (Caffein, Stimulants)	Tired/Fatigued
No Influence if Absent	**Pain/Nausea** (Physical Pain/Feeling Sick)	Inhibiting if Present
Arousing if Sufficient/High	**Physical/Genital Stimulation** (Stimulation of Penis/Clitoris)	Inhibiting if Absent/Low
	Psychological Factors	
Facilitating if High	**Safety** (Absence of threat/coercion/ trauma triggers)	Inhibiting if Absent/Low
Happy/Excited/Love	**Mood** (Emotions in Situation)	Sad/Fearful/Disgust
Positive	**Self-Talk** (Beliefs/Thoughts/Expectations)	Negative
Positive/Celebrating	**Sexual Self-Talk** (Acceptance of One's Body)	Negative/Rejecting
High Erotic Match	**Fantasy** (Love Map)	Absent/Low Erotic Match
High Attraction	**Erotic Attraction** (Degree of Excitement)	Low Attraction

*Modified by Dr. Frederick Peterson for sexual health education. The original material was provided courtesy of Michael A. Perelman, PhD, and is based on the Sexual Tipping Point Model®, owned by and used with the permission of the MAP Education & Research Foundation (mapedfund.org).

REFERENCES

American Psychiatric Association. (2013). *Diagnostic and statistical manual of mental disorders* (5th ed.). https://doi.org/10.1176/appi.books.9780890425596

Beddows, N., & Brooks, R. (2015). Inappropriate sexual behaviour in adolescents with autism spectrum disorder: What education is recommended and why. *Early Intervention in Psychiatry, 10*(4), 282-289. https://doi.org/10.1111/eip.12265

Berryessa, C. M. (2014). Judiciary views on criminal behaviour and intention of offenders with high-functioning autism. *Journal of intellectual disabilities and offending behaviour*, *5*(2), 97-106. https://doi.org/10.1108/JIDOB-02-2014-0002

Cooper, J., Heron, T., & Heward, W. (2020). *Applied Behavior Analysis* (3rd ed.). Pearson.

Coshway, L., Broussard, J., Acharya, K., Fried, K., Msall, M. E., Lantos, J. D., & Nahata, L. (2016). Medical therapy for inappropriate sexual behaviors in a teen with autism spectrum disorder. *Pediatrics, 137*(4). https://doi.org/10.1542/peds.2015-4366

Developmental Disabilities Monitoring Network Surveillance Year 2010 Principal Investigators, & Centers for Disease Control and Prevention (CDC). (2014). Prevalence of autism spectrum disorder among children aged 8 years - autism and developmental disabilities monitoring network, 11 sites, United States, 2010. *Morbidity and mortality weekly report. Surveillance summaries (Washington, D.C.: 2002)*, *63*(2), 1-21.

Kaplan, H. (1974). *The new sex therapy: Active treatment of sexual dysfunctions*. Brunner/Mazel.

Kaplan, H. (1995). *The sexual desire disorders: Dysfunctional regulation of sexual motivations*. Brunner/Mazel.

Kupferman, I. (1991). Hypothalamus and limbic system motivation. In E. R. Kandel, J. H. Schwartz, & T. M. Jessell (Eds.), *Principles of neural science* (3rd ed.). Elsevier.

Laumann, E. O., Paik, A., & Rosen, R. (1999). Sexual dysfunction in the United States: Prevalence and predictors. *JAMA, 281*(6), 537-544. https://doi.org/10.1001/jama.281.6.537

Masters, W., & Johnson, V. (1966). *Human sexual response.* Little, Brown.

Mercer, C. H., Fenton, K. A., Johnson, A. M., Wellings, K., MacDowall, W., McManus, S., Nanchahal, K., & Erens, B. (2003). Sexual function problems and help seeking behaviour in Britain: National probability sample survey. *British Medical Journal, 327*(7412), 426-427. https://doi.org/10.1136/bmj.327.7412.426

Mimoun, S., & Wylie, K. (2009). Female sexual dysfunctions: Definitions and classification. *Maturitas,* 63(2), 116-118. https://doi.org/10.1016/j.maturitas.2009.04.003

Perelman, M. A. (2009). The Sexual Tipping Point®: A mind/body model for sexual medicine. *The Journal of Sexual Medicine, 6*(3), 629-632. https://doi.org/10.1111/j.1743-6109.2008.01177.x

Perelman, M. A. (2014). The history of sexual medicine. In D. L. Tolman, L. M. Diamond, J. A. Bauermeister, W. H. George, J. G. Pfaus, & L. M. Ward (Eds.), *APA handbook of sexuality and psychology, Volume 2: Contextual approaches* (pp. 137-179). American Psychological association. https://doi.org/10.1037/14194-005

Perelman M. A. (2016a). Psychosexual therapy for delayed ejaculation based on the Sexual Tipping Point model. *Translational Andrology and Urology*, *5*(4), 563-575. https://doi.org/10.21037/tau.2016.07.05

Perelman, M.A. (2016b). Why the Sexual Tipping Point® Model? *Current Sexual Health Reports, 8,* 39-46. https://doi.org/10.1007/s11930-018-0148-3

Perelman, M. A., & Rowland, D. L. (2006). Retarded ejaculation. *World Journal of Urology*, *24*(6), 645-652. https://doi.org/10.1007/s00345-006-0127-6

Peterson, F. L., Bley, J. W., & Frabotta, R. (2020). *The gender revolution & new sexual health: Celebrating unlimited diversity of the human sexuality hypercube*. Cognella Academic Press.

Sullivan, A., & Caterino, L. C. (2008). Addressing the sexuality and sex education of individuals with autism spectrum disorders. *Education and Treatment of Children, 31*(1), 381-394. https://doi.org/10.1353/etc.0.0001

Visser, K., Greaves-Lord, K., Tick, N. T., Verhulst, F. C., Maras, A., & Vegt, E. J. (2017). An exploration of the judgement of sexual situations by adolescents with autism spectrum disorders versus typically developing adolescents. *Research in Autism Spectrum Disorders, 36*, 35-43. https://doi.org/10.1016/j.rasd.2017.01.004

Wylie, K. (2007). Assessment and management of sexual problems in women. *Journal of the Royal Society of Medicine, 100*(12), 547-550. https://doi.org/10.1177/014107680710001201

10

Sex and the Cortisoaked™ Brain

Sarah E. Wright and Kylie Sheaffer

INTRODUCTION

Human beings are no strangers to stress. Whether it be the impact of working tirelessly to support a family, dealing with loss or unexpected hardship (like a pandemic), or feeling constantly concerned about judgment or rejection from others, people know stress. Some have even faced more dire circumstances and can relate to the toll that having safety threatened may take.

With some variation, based on the degree of control (Grimm et al., 2014) and impact to the physical body (Whiteman et al., 2019), our brains tend to respond to stressful events in a predictable way. The brain's functioning changes as it is increasingly doused with stress hormones like cortisol and is forced to continually interpret the degree of threat (freeze) and choose an appropriate reaction (fight or flight) (Roelofs, 2017). It is important to note that people may evaluate the stressfulness of similar events differently (Lancaster et al., 2014; Lukaschek et al., 2013) depending on past experiences, the triggering event, and others' reactions or judgments. Some may not even see the event as stressful. By focusing on the reaction of the brain instead of the perceived severity of what happened, people can begin to better understand their own reactions to stress and how to best mitigate these when needed.

This becomes especially relevant in the realm of sex and sexuality. Despite being inundated with sexual messages and imagery, American culture is not the greatest at talking openly about such "taboo" topics. For some, even saying the word "sex" can elicit a stress response! This chapter will explore a new way to understand intense stress and trauma, the impact these can have in the brain, and the effect they can have in our sexual worlds. How to make use of this knowledge when crafting clinical interventions will be discussed.

REDEFINING "TRAUMA"

"Trauma" and "stress" are terms frequently used without much thought into their meaning. One often describes an event (*That was so traumatic!*) while the other tends to represent a feeling (*I'm feeling super stressed this week*). Rarely do people think about what degree of stress is needed before something is traumatic, or whether something can have a trauma-like impact when there was no real threat to safety.

"Trauma" is defined in the *DSM-5* (American Psychiatric Association, 2013) as experiencing, witnessing, or having knowledge of a loved one enduring a life-threatening event. This definition feels limiting, though. Not everyone who faces the same life-threatening event will experience the same levels of stress, and some people who meet non-life-threatening stressful situations may feel immense measures of anxiety (Anders et al., 2014; Lancaster et al., 2014; Mol et al., 2005; Scott & Stradling, 1994). "Trauma" is typically seen as an extreme word, and its use may put more emphasis on the triggering event over the brain's physical response to the situation. People are likely to assume that "trauma" means life is in jeopardy, as this is the message perpetuated by the mental health field. This definition overlooks the daily struggles and horrific incidents that people endure regularly, which can potentially result in the same state of brain as a threat to life.

There is power in putting a name to our feelings and experiences. By identifying a continuum for stress levels, we may be able to help facilitate the stress recovery process. Labeling stress as positive, bearable, or destructive can help individuals better interpret how they are feeling, recognize the effect stress may play on their life, and navigate their recovery. They may begin to better identify and manage stressful triggers with recognition, mindfulness, and acceptance. Direct and intentional communication may help others better understand how someone is being impacted.

In the book *Redefining Trauma: Understanding and Coping With a Cortisoaked Brain* (Wright, 2020), the case is made to introduce a new set of terms: **Cortisprinkled**, **Cortisaturated**, and **Cortisoaked**. It is vital that we, as mental health professionals, have a way to understand life events that leave us feeling more than "overwhelmed" but do not actually threaten our lives.

> **Cortisprinkled** refers to a brain working as it does on a daily basis – being sprinkled with sufficient cortisol for adequate function and motivation, then returning to a state of balance. **Cortisaturated** alludes to a brain saturated with cortisol resulting in the activation of more protective responses while still being able to maintain some degree of daily operations. A slower return to baseline from this state is expected. **Cortisoaked** speaks to a brain soaked with cortisol (and other stress hormones) that it does not function as it does on a routine basis. This flooding of cortisol essentially puts the brain into emergency management mode, where the primary focus is on survival. Recovery from this state often includes the establishment of a new baseline altogether. (Wright, 2020, p. 4)

Using these terms, we refocus attention on the brain's reaction under intense duress instead of focusing on what happened and whether it was "bad enough" to warrant a trauma-like response. Better understanding the processes underway in the cortisol-doused brain allows us to better tailor coping responses to target specific areas or actions that may be hindering daily life. This lexicon does not intend to compare hardship or negate experiences. It simply recognizes that one brain may react to a potentially life-ending situation, like getting chased by a tiger, similarly to someone who suffers from repeated humiliation or ostracization by their peers due to their skin color, gender identity, or other factors (Finke et al., 2018). Cortisoaking can occur even though no immediate threat to life is present. People endure significant and horrific daily traumas, and this system of classification recognizes that "stress," especially mounting stress that builds up over time, can have a considerable effect on the brain (Chetty et al., 2014; Grimm et al., 2014; Lupien et al., 2018).

Cortisprinkled

Most people anticipate average stresses that could happen on any given day. Deadlines at work, family responsibilities, getting taxes paid; all these examples can apply. A cortisprinkled brain is the low-level stress response our brains produce every day to tackle our daily tasks (Gilbert et al., 2017). It can be thought of as positive stress; it is manageable and can even serve as a strong motivator. A cortisprinkled brain can look into the future, see the big picture, and take action to accomplish goals. Memory systems are functional and allow memories to be retained in a story-like fashion, with a beginning, middle, and end (Eichenbaum, 2014).

A cortisprinkled brain is readily able to stay in tune with partners, can read and respond appropriately to the emotions of others, and sexually engage as desired. The brain is alert and responsive but not flush with stress hormones.

Cortisaturated

A cortisaturated brain is a step up on the stress reaction scale. A person experiencing cortisaturation may feel on the verge of becoming overwhelmed. This individual may suffer from brief amounts of memory impairment or struggle with concentration. They may feel their mind is a little "foggy," or they may find their thoughts continuing to return to the stressful event or its impact. Sleep is likely to be affected (Selcuk et al., 2017), as this is a brain wary of potential danger, making rest challenging. There may be increased restlessness or waking throughout the night. This lack of rejuvenating sleep is apt to leave people feeling lethargic or unmotivated to get out of bed.

Emotional processing may become more challenging, and fear or anxiety tend to predominate. These effects may understandably take a toll on relationships and sexuality. People in this state of brain are more likely to interpret their environment as dangerous, which could make them less trusting of others. They may be more likely to misinterpret cues from a partner or assume hostility when it is absent. Distress tolerance begins to shrink, and it could make them appear short-tempered, visibly frustrated, or combative. It is not unusual for people in this state to seek out partners or trusted companions for comfort and support, especially if these relationships have been established as healthy and trusting.

Ultimately, despite their struggle, this is still a manageable level of stress. It is tolerable, yet likely not sustainable for long.

Cortisoaked

A brain continuously overwhelmed by cortisol and other stress hormones will likely become cortisoaked, reverting to an emergency management mode with the main goal being survival. Memory, focus, and concentration are all homed in on immediate safety, and any long-term or big-picture planning becomes irrelevant. This can leave people feeling stuck or that the future is hopeless because they cannot see a path forward. They likely feel unsafe, on edge, or constantly under threat.

Relationships are prone to be highly strained. It can be difficult to focus on the needs of a partner when a person believes their life may be in danger. Feelings of shame and guilt may arise (Aakvaag et al., 2016), which can further impede the ability to share one's experiences, further fueling isolation. Cortisol can wreak havoc on sexual response (Hamilton & Meston, 2013), limiting access to a viable means of connection for many couples.

This level is the toxic, unmanageable, and unsustainable degree of distress many people know as trauma.

Vignette: Sex and Stress

> While fishing on the lake one early morning, George and his son, Jacob, talked about school, baseball, and Jacob's friends, when Jacob suddenly announced that he asked someone to be his girlfriend. George, caught off-guard by the disclosure, was initially excited for his son but began to feel his heart rate pick up. Jacob was 14 after all; was it too early for "the talk?" Or worse, too late?! George had never discussed girls in the context of relationships with his son before. Feeling pressured to say anything, George began clumsily giving his son the "birds and the bees" talk. Jacob, unaware that he was opening the door for the "sex talk," felt immediately uncomfortable. His father was also noticeably uneasy. Jacob, wanting to get the whole conversation over with, shut down. He stopped listening to his father and tried to

focus on the water instead. He didn't even try to think about questions, knowing he could find anything he needed to know online. He had already stumbled on several porn-adjacent accounts on social media and was confident he knew how sex worked. George, feeling stressed by his son's silence, glossed over details and focused on how pregnancy or STIs could negatively affect his young life. He didn't even realize that Jacob had stopped listening to him. Both were relieved when the talk ended, and neither had any intention of bringing it up again.

POVERTY OF SEX EDUCATION

Sexual health is ever-changing and multifaceted. It encompasses physical health, romantic or sexual interests, gender identity, reproductive decisions, sexual fantasies and values, and more (World Health Organization, 2010). It's quite a robust concept! Having sex can be a form of self-expression, help cultivate an intimate bond with a partner, serve as a de-stressor, or be an overall pleasurable experience – which are the primary reasons why most people have sex (Meston & Buss, 2007). Despite sex being a potentially healthy, connecting, and pleasurable part of being human, it can also be incredibly stressful, even aside from complicating events. We often struggle to talk about it plainly and may even inflict shame on others for talking about it, having it, or not having enough of it!

How we collectively talk about sex plays a significant role in how readily accepted such discussions are in our society. This can be seen in the conversation between George and Jacob; they did not discuss body parts, how to give or ask for someone's consent, the mechanics of sex, how to communicate with one's partner, or anything beyond the fear-based consequences of having sex, similar to many ineffective sex education programs. Jacob is likely to perceive sex as a thing to be ashamed of or not talked about.

Sex education that is not as equally robust as sexual health itself does a disservice to everyone (Lindberg & Maddow-Zimet, 2012). Young adults are left on their own to self-educate, understand their evolving identity, engage in relationships, figure out how to have sex, and much more. Restricted sex education creates a negative cycle: Older generations may feel unprepared to talk about healthy sex, identity, or intimate relationships with younger generations, sending the message that these topics are shameful. This, in turn, may increase the young adults' tendencies to learn from friends or find answers online, both being of questionable validity. How can we ask parents or guardians to engage in comfortable conversation about sex if they themselves were never taught how?

This lackluster sex education is also typically absent of any information on queer identities and expressions, which can lend to more shame or fear-based conversations regarding sex, or zero sex talk at all. When shame and fear are used to control the conversation around sex, or used to judge others for their sexual activities, people are taught to associate sexual interactions with shameful behavior. These feelings of shame can release cortisol within the brain, triggering further stress responses (Aakvaag et al., 2016).

WHEN FEAR DOMINATES

Beyond being ill-informed, there are numerous reasons why someone may be fearful of having sex. One person may anticipate that it will hurt and they're afraid of the pain; another may feel scared of getting rejected by peers because their body isn't entirely "porn-perfect;" Someone else may feel overwhelmed because they don't know how one is "supposed" to behave during sex, and they don't want to appear unsexy. There can be excessive fear of judgment or rejection, and anxiety is a boner killer! When stress dominates one's awareness, sexual desire (Raisanen et al., 2018) and orgasmic responses (Rowland et al., 2018) can suffer. The brain is no longer engaged or prepared for sex; instead, it is in a state of readiness to address potential threat.

Cortisaturated or cortisoaked brains may particularly struggle to engage in sex because of anxiety's cyclical nature. The more one continues to stress out, the more difficult sex could be. And if the sex is lacking, relationships could become strained. If the couple is not having safe, productive conversations about their expectations or limitations with sex, the relationship could continue to spiral. Learning how to identify stress triggers, putting a name to feelings, and understanding our brain's reactions could help stop the buildup of stress and potentially help a person re-engage with their sex life.

SEXUAL AND GENDER IDENTITY

Being a queer person in today's society may be more accepted than in the past, but that does not make it easy. Identifying as anything other than cisgender (the gender identity that is aligned with sex assigned at birth) and heterosexual has been found to be associated with greater physical and mental health risks (Borgogna et al., 2019; Frost et al., 2015; Meyer, 2003), which is further exacerbated for people of color who are sexual minorities (Ouch & Moradi, 2019). Having a sense of community is invaluable to humans and is seen by our brains as necessary for survival. The ongoing doses of cortisol from stares, ignorant or hurtful comments, and very real threats of violence take a toll on those exposed to them. Add to this the impact of potentially having minimal opportunities for support and connection to buffer that cortisol, and the effects begin to quickly compound.

In addition to the stress of the many people who identify as a sexual minority experience, there is the extra burden of an even greater poverty of sex education. In the rare instance that sex education includes information about sexual and romantic orientation and gender identity and expression, it is still unlikely that information about the myriad ways queer people engage physically in sex will be addressed. So many young people are left thinking something is wrong with them since they are burdened with the notion that sex is supposed to be "natural" (i.e., insert tab A into slot B). Not only is this incredibly narrow, but it is also very heterocentric and hurtful to the understanding of the beautiful array of sexualities, gender identities, and sexual practices that exist.

WHEN STRESS TAINTS SEX

"A cortisoaked brain has difficulty staying in the present, maintaining awareness of what's happening in the here-and-now, establishing calm in the face of perceived danger, and persisting in feeling safe based on cognitive appraisal over emotional reaction" (Wright, 2020, p. 161).

A person overwhelmed by distress may struggle with any number of the characteristics described in the sentence above. Sexual health may understandably take a back seat if someone's everyday well-being is compromised. If that individual cannot feel present enough, comfortable enough, or safe enough in most environments, it would be tough to engage in any sexual behavior. Sex tends to be a vulnerable state of being. People are often naked, exposed, and open for judgment. Even if sex has never been directly associated with cortisol, the simple exposure of one's most basic self can be enough to elicit a burst of stress, which can be harmful to the sexual health of someone who is already struggling.

Sex under stress can lead to pain or displeasure. Feelings of pain may increase because anxiety can drive muscle tension (Brotto, 2013). Vaginal walls may tense up and natural lubrication may decrease due to distress. Sex may not be pleasurable because, for female-bodied people, the brain has to cognitively quiet and loosen its thinking to orgasm (Meston et al., 2004). It can be challenging to calm one's brain if it does not feel safe. Sex can quickly lose its appeal under these cortisoaked conditions.

LESS-THAN-IDEAL REACTIONS FROM OTHERS

Talking about distress if it is closely linked to sex can feel nearly impossible for some. Many people perceive talking about sex in any capacity as a way of being "sexy." If a person associates all conversations about sex as sexy, talking to a trusted adult or family member about an unwanted event can be difficult. Some individuals will go to measurable lengths to avoid their family learning about their sexual history, especially if they feel their family may interpret these events as shameful. It is a taboo conversation, and many people do not have comfortable communication skills (as previously displayed in the conversation between George and Jacob) or the terminology to name what happened to them, sometimes even to themselves.

How one's family, peers, community, and popular culture react to sex can significantly impact that person's comfort level when talking about it. For example, victim-blaming has historically been a frequent tool for silencing victims of sexual harassment or assault. If all one person sees culturally are victims being harassed or negated after speaking up about assault, that individual may struggle to bring up their own questions about sex or share intimate details about a nonconsensual sexual encounter for fear of being blamed or shamed.

There is also strong consideration to be given to the power and effect of "dismissal" concerning stress and sex on one's mental health (Relyea & Ullman, 2015). If a person's thoughts or fears are easily dismissed by their loved ones, confidants, or trusted doctors, it can instill a sense of unworthiness or shame. It potentially diminishes an individual's concerns and could leave them feeling confused or disregarded in their feelings, making it less likely they will share again.

This blame, shame, and dismissal, when linked to sexual health, could lead a person to internalize several harmful ideas about themselves and sex. *I'm only good for sex; Sex is going to hurt; I'm not likely to feel pleasure during sex; Sex is an obligation; There's something wrong with me for enjoying sex so much.* These are all beliefs a person can internalize from limited education, unwanted events, or communication that is not rooted in empathy regarding sex. This is especially true for people who have endured repeated childhood traumas, independent of their connection to sex (Krammer et al., 2018).

CORTISOAKED SEX

Unfortunately for many people, some stress triggers are directly linked to sex and sexuality. Sexual assault, frightening sexual encounters, or repeated harassment over one's gender and identity can leave a person feeling overwhelmed or in a state of terror when thinking about or engaging in sex. The brain may struggle to distinguish the triggering event from future healthy, consensual, and wanted sexual engagements.

After the idea of sex and stress have become inextricably linked, the act of sex itself could further trigger a cortisol response from the brain. A familiar touch, kiss, or specific position may force the person to remember painful conversations or events, and lead to a stress spiral. Even sensual sensations can elicit a reaction from a cortisoaked brain: a particular smell or even a single word may set off a cascade of cortisol.

A cortisoaked person may retreat from sex altogether. If they cannot associate sex with a secure, pleasurable experience, it may feel safest to avoid it completely (O'Callaghan et al., 2018). Avoidance of sex may be especially likely for people whose first sexual experiences were negative. If their first exposure to anything sexual was not consensual, inappropriate, or dangerous, that person might struggle to link sex with safety or comfort. Their brain may develop a mistrust, disgust, or complete avoidance of sex to ensure protection. That connection complicates one's awareness of their sexual health and sexual selves. One may find themselves accepting that they are only "good for sex," they're "damaged goods," or assume no one will ever want them because of their first introductions to sex. They have no other template to challenge those beliefs on their own and being unable to talk about it limits the opportunity for this to be challenged.

While some may retreat from sex in response to enduring unwanted events, others may engage in overt or increased sexual behavior. "For some people, the threshold for what is exciting gets raised after their brain has been cortisoaked" (Wright, 2020, p. 172). Changes in the prefrontal cortex may cause someone to think that their life is short and participating in higher amounts or riskier sex may be necessary to feel aroused and alive again. They may also participate in more frequent sexual behavior to combat feelings of distress, regain a sense of control over one's body, or feel connected or wanted by a partner.

This reaction may also be a way to regain an illusion of control over one's world. "Sexualizing something can be a way to take control and gain power over it – which is one of the reasons women are objectified and sexualized" (Wright, 2020. p. 171). The hallmark of unwanted sexual events is the loss of control. By recreating similar experiences with the goal of a different outcome, the brain tries to prove that the survivor's actions directly influenced that outcome (Herman, 1997). It is tempting to believe we are the masters of our own fate.

Engaging in fantasy is another potential way for people to correct parts of their reality that feel unsatisfactory. It can be a way to imagine control over a situation or allow for the replaying of an unwanted event with a different outcome. We must acknowledge that, because it is often used in public discourse, "rape fantasy" is a fallacy. "There is no such thing as rape fantasy from the perspective of the attacked person. This concept has been used to perpetuate blame on women for unwanted sexual events. Women are made to feel guilty if they fantasize about force and control, and then must contend with the question of whether certain events were wanted, or if it was really as bad as they thought. Rape is a crime of power, not a crime of sex" (Wright, 2020, p. 172). Fantasy is the brain's ultimate form of control and is not necessarily indicative of what someone wants to have happen in real life. If a person experiences more aggressive fantasies, it is a way for the brain to establish power and dominance over a situation. An aggressive fantasy is typical. Rape, however, is not. Rape is an atrocity – it is out-of-control, and it is devastating. The idea of "rape fantasy" diminishes the abomination of rape and vilifies women for their sexual wants and desires.

BEST PRACTICES: INDIVIDUAL AND PARTNER INTERVENTIONS

Speak With Intention

When beginning to work with someone around issues of sexuality, it is imperative to include some key information in the informed consent. Letting people know that direct questions about sex and sexuality will be asked brings the topic directly into the room without hesitation, ideally creating a sense of comfort and trust in the ability of a therapist. Let people know that clear sexual language will be used, and that if they prefer alternate words, this can be named and will be respected. People also need to have permission to question the therapist, especially if questions feel overly personal or probing. If a therapist cannot offer an explanation for why a question is being asked, then it probably does not need to be asked! Finally, let people know that they may feel a bit exposed after leaving the appointment. Most people are not accustomed to talking about sex. Divulging their innermost thoughts and feelings, while relieving, can also be anxiety provoking. Preparing people for this feeling can help combat assumptions they make about continuing or the potential benefit of therapy.

Consider the weight of using the word "you" during clinical practice. When confronted with the word "you" (*Why are you doing this? What were you thinking?*), people will instinctively turn inwards and reflect on themselves, creating the potential for self-blame. Use questions that center more on the event itself than the person's direct involvement in the event. Instead of *Were you drinking?*, ask *Was there alcohol involved?* and *Did you tell anyone?* becomes *Does anyone else know?* The more people feel like an event is their fault, the more they may be inclined to hide themselves.

Provide Education

For best clinical practice, do not assume sexual literacy. Check in on a person's basic understanding of anatomy and sexual response, as well as preferred terminology. Establishing a mutual language for talking about sex may make it easier for a client to name feelings or events. It can help them separate what happened previously from healthy physical connections. See if there is a stigma or negative thoughts linked to self-exploration or masturbation as well.

Help fill in the gaps of any lacking sex education. Talking about what is "normal" can help people understand their experience and build a framework for healthy sexual connections. Acknowledge and validate that insufficient sex education can fuel feelings of stress.

Foster Awareness

By explaining the brain's neurobiological response to stressful situations, trauma, or prolonged anxiety, a person can begin to understand how their body reacts to triggers and recognize panic. That can help them learn to identify precisely what stresses them and tailor specific coping mechanisms for handling anxiety. Learning the nuances behind stress and the tiers of cortisprinkled, cortisaturated, and cortisoaked brains can also help individuals understand how their stress levels may affect their lives. Exercises in mindfulness (Brotto, 2013) can be a wonderful way to facilitate this awareness.

Normalize their body's reactions, especially concerning sex and distress. That person may be better able to communicate needs to their partner or practice mindfulness in preparation for sex. Sex drive could increase unexpectedly, preferences could change, or a complete aversion to sex could develop under a cortisoaked or threatened brain (O'Callaghan et al., 2018). These reactions are normal.

As a clinician, be sure to recognize and validate the impact and influence an entire culture may have on a person's cortisoaked brain. Race, sexual identity, sexual preferences, and gender expression are potential stressors for an individual if not embraced by the broader society (Borgogna et al., 2019; Pachankis et al., 2020), and especially so if they don't feel connected to a community (Wilson & Liss, 2020). Therapists would benefit from learning to talk about culture in all of its facets, independent of the notion of "diversity." Culture is about more than just differences!

Address Cognitions

Research has shown that therapeutic interventions aimed at deconstructing the beliefs resulting from unwanted sexual events can be hugely successful in improving sexual satisfaction, sexual function, and overall relationship satisfaction (Trudel et al., 2001; Wells et al., 2019). Trauma-focused cognitive behavioral therapy (Smith et al., 2007) and cognitive processing therapy (Resick et al., 2017) are two of the most known treatments for addressing impacts of unwanted sexual events. Both of these approaches aim to process and aid in the understanding of thoughts, feelings, beliefs, and behaviors impacted by or resulting from cortisoaking events.

Communication is Key

Help clients start conversations about sex that are not "sexy." By discussing sexual experiences in objective ways with trusted others, a person may begin to understand the mechanics of sex, how to have better sex, and how to have productive conversations about sex. A deficit of language around sex can limit one's ability to explore their own sexual identity and desires.

"Don't push me in a pool and tell me I went swimming! Distinguishing unwanted events from healthy sexual expression is fundamental in reclaiming sexuality as a part of one's life" (Wright, 2020, p. 163). By giving unwanted sexual experiences a name, a person can begin to view the situation objectively and separate their identity from the event. Learning from one's experiences, grasping the extent of their physical and mental limits, and understanding how to communicate those events and boundaries to partners can help set a person up for safe sex.

Share tools on how best to talk to partners about sex and sensitive topics. Advise that people have important conversations about sex in a neutral territory. If emotional or painful subjects are discussed in the bedroom, the next time the couple is intimate, memories of the conversation may invade and make intimacy difficult. Partners should discuss sex before actually having sex, so both can be on the same page about expectations, limitations, concerns, and desires. Waiting until sex is underway can make rational conversation difficult. When using safe words, it is important to practice them in a nonsexual setting until all parties can trust the word will be respected when used.

Sexual Embodiment

Discuss masturbation as a tool for learning to become comfortable with and aware of one's sexuality. Sensual touching can help a person become present, orient themselves with their surroundings, and connect positive feelings with sex. Emphasize how important it is to reject self-judgment. Masturbation is a safe, normal way for people to figure out what feels good. It is a de-stressor and a way to reclaim one's sexual experience.

Targeting sexual dysfunction may reduce other mental health concerns (DiMauro et al., 2018). Sexual dysfunction such as arousal and orgasm issues can significantly affect people's overall quality of life. It may be tempting to focus solely on addressing unwanted or traumatic events and their impact, and this can sometimes be time and labor intensive. Many people may benefit from some directive interventions focused on reestablishing sexual function. The book *Principles and Practice of Sex Therapy* (6th ed.; Hall & Binik, 2020) is a must-have for any clinician engaging in the provision of sex therapy and contains explicit guidance for addressing a range of sexuality and sexual health concerns.

Staying present in the moment is a vital part of enjoying sex. It helps a person feel safe and allows the brain to manage its overwhelming cortisol levels. We are better able to trust our sexual selves if we are aware of what is happening. Practicing mindfulness regularly during sex leads to less discomfort and greater pleasure (Newcombe & Weaver, 2016). Mindfulness can be more challenging for some than others, but there are small actions one can take to implement even a bit of grounding in their daily lives. Consider the acronyms F.I.N.E. or F.U.C.K (the latter for those who favor a more adult version) to remember grounding actions during tense moments.

F – **F**reeze!
I – understand **I**ntent of what is happening
N – **N**otice surroundings with all senses
E – **E**valuate options and choose with intention

Or

F – **F**reeze!
U – **U**nderstand the intention of the warning
C – **C**oncentrate on the present using your senses
K – **K**now the reality and choose with intention (Wright, 2020, p. 182)

This method is a tool for evaluating why a brain may be on alert, determining the level of safety in a given situation, and then deciding whether one feels safe enough to move forward using all senses.

To enact FINE, be sure the sex partner(s) is on board. Identify and practice a safe word, like "Freeze," in nonsexual settings. As soon as anxiety starts bubbling up during sex, use the safe word. Both partners should freeze immediately and assess the situation. Validate why stressful feelings may have come up and allow some space to appreciate the intention of the brain; It is just trying to stay safe. Then reorient the body and brain to its surroundings. Notice the environment using all five senses while remaining frozen. By acknowledging what they can see, sounds they may hear, different smells in the room, the taste on their tongue, and the feel of their fingertips on their sheets, skin, or surroundings, a person can become grounded in the present moment (instead of lost in a cortisoaked memory). That action both retunes the brain to reality and allows stress levels to begin to return to normal. Finally, evaluate whether the environment is safe or comfortable enough to continue. Both partners can now choose how to move forward with the situation. That may result in continuing sex or opting to stop for the moment. Anyone can decide to end sex at any point. The point is for each partner to choose what would make them feel most comfortable. This grounding method is truly about acknowledging the brain and deciding an intentional and safe path forward instead of reacting to fear.

Whole Body Integration

Whole-body healing is an essential part of becoming comfortable in one's sexual skin. Some of this can be practiced as an individual intervention, and some may be more appropriate and important to do with partners.

Sensate focus is a guided touching exercise that can be practiced on its own or with a partner. It was first created by Masters and Johnson (1970) and was later updated to become more usable and accessible (Weiner & Avery-Clark, 2014). It is essentially a no-pressure way of tuning in to the feeling of touch. Partners are asked to eliminate sex as an outcome; Instead, focus solely on being touched or touching, and the sensations that may develop during the exercise. It opens the door for a more present, sensual experience and eliminates self-judgment or fear of what may happen next.

Movement is another tool for full-body healing (van der Kolk, 2014). Dance, yoga, or other forms of physical expression help connect the mind with the body. A cortisoaked brain may lead to physical effects on the body. Learning to appreciate and move the body in ways that feel enjoyable and challenging can help a person reclaim their healing and treat their stressed-out brain.

The idea of best practice is not always one-size-fits-all. Curating a response based on a person's stress levels, experience, and boundaries is essential – as seen in the following vignette.

Kiesha – a full-time, Black, queer graduate student, decided to spend an evening out with a few friends at a bar. The stress of recent political events had taken a toll on her, and she struggled to find a place she felt she could fully be herself. After some much needed genuine conversation, Kiesha left to go home, and one of her friends hopped in the rideshare with her. They had been flirting throughout the night, but she was still surprised when he jumped in the car. It had been several months since she had done anything sexual with a man and figured a hot make-out session would do her good. The pair went back to her place, and the situation escalated quickly. What started as kissing and touching turned into more aggressive behavior that Kiesha had not consented to. She realized she didn't know how to get him to stop and struggled to say "No." As the situation carried on, Kiesha became increasingly uneasy and no longer wanted to continue. She felt paralyzed, so she closed her eyes and waited for it to end.

Afterward, Kiesha tried to brush it under the rug. She was confused about the events and wondered if she had made it up. After all, wasn't he her friend? Hadn't he supported her coming out and encouraged her being herself? Kiesha began questioning the extent to which she could trust any of their mutual friends and worried they would blame her. She began to isolate and struggled to talk to anyone about the situation because she was afraid they wouldn't believe her, would shame her, or question why she just didn't ask him to stop. She felt the whole situation would be so much easier if it hadn't happened the way she knows it did.

After some time, Kiesha's family finally convinced her to connect with a therapist. They knew something was wrong, and assumed it was the stress of school. The therapist recognized how quickly she became tearful when asked about her romantic and sexual life. Her therapist soon realized that Kiesha was likely experiencing a cortisoaked brain. Through calm conversation, the therapist explained the nuanced stress Kiesha was feeling. She explained how the brain operates under distress and how different triggers or prolonged exposure can push a brain to a cortisoaked state. Kiesha learned the importance of language and found a way to name what happened to her. By labeling the triggering event, she began to separate it from her life and eventually, from healthy sex. It opened the door to vulnerable conversations that didn't feel full of judgment or shame. The pair discussed practicing mindfulness as a tool for staying grounded in moments of struggle or panic. Kiesha implemented that practice to stay present in her own life and eventually with a partner when she felt ready for sex again. The therapist also suggested she join a running or walking group, which helped Kiesha find a support network of people who also encouraged her to get her body moving regularly. The combined intervention – linking education, awareness, communication, sexual embodiment, and whole-body integration – helped Kiesha to process what happened and intentionally move forward in her life.

DISCUSSION AND CONCLUSIONS

This chapter discusses the interconnections between two highly repressed topics in our society: sexuality and trauma. By providing a framework for understanding the impact of extreme stress on the brain, clinicians are better equipped to provide needed education in a concrete and scientific manner. Through identifying the nuanced differences between cortisprinkled, cortisaturated, and cortisoaked, a person may better understand how and why their body reacts to triggering events and the impacts that prolonged stress can have on a person's life and health.

Sex can be stressful for anyone; it is a vulnerable position to be in and it can trigger a significant distress reaction for many, especially if clear communication and respect for boundaries are not practiced between partners. In a cortisoaked state, an individual may be incapable of engaging in sex comfortably or may find themselves taking part in significantly more or riskier sex. Fantasies, sexual drive and preferences, and the threshold for excitement all can change under a state of extreme stress. These reactions are common ways for the brain to attempt to regain control over a situation or event that may have made them feel out of control.

When a person's cortisoaked state is caused by sex (be it through humiliation, shame, fear, or violence), they may be unable to separate the painful event from future sexual engagements. Specific movements, sounds, or gestures may remind the individual of previous trauma, and trigger a flooding of cortisol in the brain.

How family, friends, educators, doctors, and popular culture approach conversations about sex, combined with judgments on sexual health, can leave lasting impacts on a person and their relationship to sex. An individual could internalize negative messages if they are made to feel ashamed for their sexual preferences, identity, or sex history. If a partner dismisses their significant other's struggles or belittles them, it could leave them feeling stressed out and gaslit into thinking their relationship and experience with sex must be "normal." A parent who mainly teaches their child that sex makes them impure could force them to link sex with anxiety, dirtiness, or guilt in later years. A cortisoaked brain may accept bad, harmful, or dangerous sex at face value; the person could believe that all sex is unpleasurable or that touching oneself is disgraceful.

Binary beliefs and conversations about sex (it's wrong or it's right; it's shameful or acceptable) make sharing one's thoughts seem precarious. It becomes risky to have essential conversations because no one wants to be rejected or humiliated by their community. Until people have permission to share their experiences and feelings safely, communication may feel more like judgment. It can all add to the cumulative effects of stress on the brain.

Approach a cortisoaked brain with a robust treatment plan. Educate on how stress physically operates in the brain and how a heightened distress state can impact multiple facets of an individual's life. Fill in the gaps of sexual education and encourage conversations about sex that are not "sexy." As a clinician, recognize how culture and identity could play a significant role in one's state of stress, as well as their sexual self, and learn how to talk about it. Give people the language to name what happened to them and open the door to talk about difficult events or memories in vulnerable but objective ways. Readily address sexual dysfunction as an early intervention to foster relationships and create hope. Create a recovery plan that is rooted in clear communication, cognitive processing, grounding during moments of stress, and whole-body integration. When this is done within a context of cultural respect and understanding, it is possible to reclaim sex from stress!

REFERENCES

Aakvaag, H. F., Thoresen, S., Wentzel-Larsen, T., Dyb, G., Røysamb, E., & Olff, M. (2016). Broken and guilty since it happened: A population study of trauma-related shame and guilt after violence and sexual abuse. *Journal of Affective Disorders, 204*, 16-23. https://doi.org/10.1016/j.jad.2016.06.004

American Psychiatric Association. (2013). *Diagnostic and statistical manual of mental disorders* (5th ed.). https://doi.org/10.1176/appi.books.9780890425596

Anders, S. L., Frazier, P. A., & Shallcross, S. L. (2014). Changes in functioning following potentially traumatic life events in college students. *Psychological Trauma: Theory, Research, Practice, and Policy, 6*(Suppl 1), S99-S106. https://doi.org/10.1037/a0033835

Borgogna, N. C., Mcdermott, R. C., Aita, S. L., & Kridel, M. M. (2019). Anxiety and depression across gender and sexual minorities: Implications for transgender, gender nonconforming, pansexual, demisexual, asexual, queer, and questioning individuals. *Psychology of Sexual Orientation and Gender Diversity, 6*(1), 54-63. https://doi.org/10.1037/sgd0000306

Brotto, L. A. (2013). Mindful sex. *Canadian Journal of Human Sexuality, 22*(2), 63-68. https://doi.org/10.3138/cjhs.2013.2132

Chetty, S., Friedman, A. R., Taravosh-Lahn, K., Kirby, E. D., Mirescu, C., Guo, F., Krupik, D., Nicholas, A., Geraghty, A. C., Krishnamurthy, A., Tsai, M-K., Covarrubias, D., Wong, A. T., Francis, D. D., Sapolsky, R. M., Palmer, T. D., Pleasure, D., & Kaufer, D. (2014). Stress and glucocorticoids promote oligodendrogenesis in the adult hippocampus. *Molecular Psychiatry, 19*(12), 1275-1283. https://doi.org/10.1038/mp.2013.190

Dimauro, J., Renshaw, K. D., & Blais, R. K. (2018). Sexual vs. non-sexual trauma, sexual satisfaction and function, and mental health in female veterans. *Journal of Trauma & Dissociation, 19*(4), 403-416. https://doi.org/10.1080/15299732.2018.1451975

Eichenbaum, H. (2014). Time cells in the hippocampus: A new dimension for mapping memories. *Nature Reviews Neuroscience, 15*(11), 732-744. https://doi.org/10.1038/nrn3827

Finke, J. B., Behrje, A., & Schächinger, H. (2018). Acute stress enhances pupillary responses to erotic nudes: Evidence for differential effects of sympathetic activation and cortisol. *Biological Psychology, 137*, 73-82. https://doi.org/10.1016/j.biopsycho.2018.07.005

Frost, D., Lehavot, K., & Meyer, I. (2015). Minority stress and physical health among sexual minority individuals. *Journal of Behavioral Medicine, 38*(1), 1-8. https://doi-org.pallas2.tcl.sc.edu/10.1007s10865-013-9523-8

Géonet, M., Sutter, P. D., & Zech, E. (2018). Do stressful life events impact women's sexual desire? *Sexologies, 27*(4). https://doi.org/10.1016/j.sexol.2017.09.012

Gilbert, K., Mineka, S., Zinbarg, R. E., Craske, M. G., & Adam, E. K. (2017). Emotion regulation regulates more than emotion: Associations of momentary emotion regulation with diurnal cortisol in current and past depression and anxiety. *Clinical Psychological Science, 5*(1), 37-51. https://doi.org/10.1177/2167702616654437

Grimm, S., Pestke, K., Feeser, M., Aust, S., Weigand, A., Wang, J., Wingenfeld, K., Pruessner, J. C., La Marca, R., Boker, H., & Bajbouj, M. (2014). Early life stress modulates oxytocin effects on limbic system during acute psychosocial stress. *Social Cognitive & Affective Neuroscience, 9*(11), 1828-1835. https://doi.org/10.1093/scan/nsu020

Hall, K. S. K., & Binik, Y. M. (Eds.). (2020). *Principles and practice of sex therapy* (6th ed.). Guilford Press.

Hamilton, L. D., & Meston, C. M. (2013). Chronic stress and sexual function in women. *Journal of Sexual Medicine, 10*(10), 2443-2454. https://doi.org/10.1111/jsm.12249

Herman, J. L. (1997). *Trauma and recovery: The aftermath of violence--from domestic abuse to political terror.* BasicBooks.

Krammer, S., Holtforth, M. G., Burri, A., Soyka, M., Gamma, A., & Liebrenz, M. (2017). Interpersonal sensitivity as a mediator between cumulative childhood traumatic events and adult sexual disturbance. *Journal of Sex & Marital Therapy, 44*(2), 213-220. https://doi.org/10.1080/0092623x.2017.1354343

Lancaster, S. L., Melka, S. E., Rodriguez, B. F., & Bryant, A. R. (2014). PTSD symptom patterns following traumatic and nontraumatic events. *Journal of Aggression, Maltreatment & Trauma, 23*(4), 414-429. https://doi.org/10.1080/10926771.2014.893276

Lindberg, L. D., & Maddow-Zimet, I. (2012). Consequences of sex education on teen and young adult sexual behaviors and outcomes. *Journal of Adolescent Health, 51*(4), 332-338. https://doi-org.pallas2.tcl.sc.edu/10.1016/j.jadohealth.2011.12.028

Lukaschek, K., Kruse, J., Emeny, R., Lacruz, M., Eisenhart Rothe, A., & Ladwig, K.-H. (2013). Lifetime traumatic experiences and their impact on PTSD: A general population study. *Social Psychiatry & Psychiatric Epidemiology, 48*(4), 525-532. https://doi.org/10.1007/s00127-012-0585-7

Lupien, S. J., Juster, R.-P., Raymond, C., & Marin, M.-F. (2018). The effects of chronic stress on the human brain: From neurotoxicity, to vulnerability, to opportunity. *Frontiers in Neuroendocrinology, 49,* 91-105. https://doi.org/10.1016/j.yfrne.2018.02.001

Masters, W., & Johnson, V.E. (1970). *Human sexual inadequacy*. Little, Brown and Company.

Meston, C. M., & Buss, D. M. (2007). Why humans have sex. *Archives of Sexual Behavior, 36*(4), 477-507. https://doi.org/10.1007/s10508-007-9175-2

Meston, C. M., Levin, R. J., Sipski, M. L., Hull, E. M., & Heiman, J. R. (2004). Women's orgasm. *Annual Review of Sex Research, 15*, 173-257.

Meyer, I. H. (2003). Prejudice, social stress, and mental health in lesbian, gay, and bisexual populations: Conceptual issues and research evidence. *Psychology of Sexual Orientation and Gender Diversity, 1*(S), 3-26. https://doi-org.pallas2.tcl.sc.edu/10.1037/2329-0382.1.S3

Mol, S. S. L., Arntz, A., Metsemakers, J. F. M., Dinant, G.-J., Vilters-Van Montfort, P. A. P., & Knottnerus, J. A. (2005). Symptoms of post-traumatic stress disorder after non-traumatic events: Evidence from an open population study. *The British Journal of Psychiatry, 186*(6), 494-499. https://doi.org/10.1192/bjp.186.6.494

Newcombe, B. C., & Weaver, A. D. (2016). Mindfulness, cognitive distraction, and sexual well-being in women. *Canadian Journal of Human Sexuality, 25*(2), 99-108. https://doi.org/10.3138/cjhs.252-A3

O'Callaghan, E., Shepp, V., Ullman, S. E., & Kirkner, A. (2018). Navigating sex and sexuality after sexual assault: A qualitative study of survivors and informal support providers. *The Journal of Sex Research, 56*(8), 1045-1057. https://doi.org/10.1080/00224499.2018.1506731

Ouch, S., & Moradi, B. (2019). Cognitive and affective expectation of stigma, coping efficacy, and psychological distress among sexual minority people of color. *Journal of Counseling Psychology, 66*(4), 424-436. https://doi.org/10.1037/cou0000360

Pachankis, J. E., Mahon, C. P., Jackson, S. D., Fetzner, B. K., & Bränström, R. (2020). Sexual orientation concealment and mental health: A conceptual and meta-analytic review. *Psychological Bulletin, 146*(10), 831-871. https://doi.org/10.1037/bul0000271

Raisanen, J. C., Chadwick, S. B., Michalak, N., & van Anders, S. M. (2018). Average associations between sexual desire, testosterone, and stress in women and men over time. *Archives of Sexual Behavior, 47*(6), 1613-1631. https://doi.org/10.1007/s10508-018-1231-6

Relyea, M., & Ullman, S. E. (2015). Unsupported or turned against: Understanding how two types of negative social reactions to sexual assault relate to postassault outcomes. *Psychology of Women Quarterly, 39*(1), 37-52. https://doi.org/10.1177/0361684313512610

Resick, P. A., Monson, C. M., & Chard, K. M. (2017). *Cognitive processing therapy for PTSD: A comprehensive manual.* Guilford Press.

Roelofs, K. (2017). Freeze for action: Neurobiological mechanisms in animal and human freezing. *Philosophical Transactions of the Royal Society B: Biological Sciences, 372*(1718), 1-10. https://doi.org/10.1098/rstb.2016.0206

Rowland, D. L., Cempel, L. M., & Tempel, A. R. (2018). Women's attributions regarding why they have difficulty reaching orgasm. *Journal of Sex & Marital Therapy, 44*(5), 475-484. https://doi.org/10.1080/0092623x.2017.1408046

Scott, M. J., & Stradling, S. G. (1994). Post-traumatic stress disorder without the trauma. *British Journal of Clinical Psychology, 33*(Pt 1), 71-74. https://doi.org/10.1111/j.2044-8260.1994.tb01095.x

Selcuk, E., Stanton, S. C. E., Slatcher, R. B., & Ong, A. D. (2017). Perceived partner responsiveness predicts better sleep quality through lower anxiety. *Social Psychological and Personality Science, 8*(1), 83-92. https://doi.org/10.1177/1948550616662128

Smith, P., Yule, W., Perrin, S., Tranah, T., Dalgleish, T., & Clark, D. M. (2007). Cognitive-behavioral therapy for PTSD in children and adolescents: A preliminary randomized controlled trial. *Journal of the American Academy of Child and Adolescent Psychiatry, 46*(8), 1051-1061. https://doi-org.pallas2.tcl.sc.edu/10.1097/CHI.0b013e318067e288

Trudel, G., Marchand, A., Ravart, M., Aubin, S., Turgeon, L., & Fortier, P. (2001). The effect of a cognitive-behavioral group treatment program on hypoactive sexual desire in women. *Sexual and Relationship Therapy, 16*(2), 145-164. https://doi.org/10.1080/14681990120040078

van der Kolk, B. (2014). *The body keeps the score: Mind, brain and body in the transformation of trauma.* Penguin Books.

Weiner, L., & Avery-Clark C. (2014). Sensate focus: Clarifying the Masters and Johnson's model. *Sexual and Relationship Therapy. 29*(3), 307-319. https://doi.org/10.1080/14681994.2014.892920

Wells, S. Y., Glassman, L. H., Talkovsky, A. M., Chatfield, M. A., Sohn, M. J., Morland, L. A., & Mackintosh, M.-A. (2019). Examining changes in sexual functioning after cognitive processing therapy in a sample of women trauma survivors. *Women's Health Issues, 29*(1), 72-79. https://doi.org/10.1016/j.whi.2018.10.003

Whiteman, S. E., Kramer, L. B., Petri, J. M., & Weathers, F. W. (2019). Trauma type and suicidal ideation: The mediating effect of cognitive distortions. *Traumatology, 25*(4), 262-268. https://doi.org/10.1037/trm0000192

Wilson, L. C., & Liss, M. (2020). Safety and belonging as explanations for mental health disparities among sexual minority college students. *Psychology of Sexual Orientation and Gender Diversity.* https://doi.org/10.1037/sgd0000421

World Health Organization. (2010). *Developing sexual health programmes: A framework for action* (No. WHO/RHR/HRP/10.22). World Health Organization. https://apps.who.int/iris/handle/10665/70501

Wright, S. E. (2020). *Redefining trauma: Understanding and coping with a cortisoaked brain.* Routledge.

11

Mindfulness and Sexuality

R. Brian Denton

There has been a boom throughout the last few decades in both professional literature and the acceptance of mindfulness as a supported practice in the mental health field, with the past 10 years being of particularly rapid growth. While mindfulness has been integrated into many theoretical models to this date, it is most widely seen applied to cognitive behavioral models, so much so that many consider the derivations as the "third wave" of cognitive behavioral therapy (Williams & Kabat-Zinn, 2011). These derivations include modalities such as Mindfulness-Based Cognitive Therapy for Depression (MBCT), Dialectical Behavioral Therapy (DBT), Acceptance and Commitment Therapy (ACT), and more. For many approaches, like MBCT, mindfulness was incorporated into existing models of cognitive therapy, and the approach was modified to incorporate this addition. For other approaches, like ACT, the development of the model itself had mindfulness featured as a core process. However, with the incorporation that happened, the resulting benefits made way for further study and utilization as a therapeutic inclusion. It was only a matter of time before the benefits of a mindfulness practice would make its way into the realm of professional sexology, and sex therapy specifically.

With continued growth in empirical support for a wide variety of mental health concerns like stress reduction, alleviation of anxiety, and depression, this expansion into the field of sexual health is a natural extension. Let's think about it for a moment. Stress, anxiety, depression, all of which can impact sexual health and functioning, seem to show some improvements through mindfulness practice. Would the benefits extend into the realm of the sexual? Current research trends and applied work in the field suggest that this is the case. This chapter will offer several suggestions on how to apply some principles of mindfulness into your sexuality-focused work, drawing from both literature and from my own experience and practice in applying those principles with real case examples (some details altered to protect the confidentiality of clients). But first, let's talk a bit about what mindfulness "is."

WHAT IS MINDFULNESS?

First off, let us understand that what Mindfulness "is" can take many definitions. The roots of what we commonly call mindfulness can be found throughout many cultures, with the methods most commonly utilized being housed within the framework of Buddhist thought and practice. Professionally speaking, the term Mindfulness has a particular circumscribed role in intervention strategies and is a method to cultivate certain helpful skills. It is not meant to replace other treatment modalities and/or techniques, but rather to potentiate those intervention strategies as an adjunctive practice.

Mindfulness itself is not a technique, but rather a process of cultivating awareness through repeated practice. There are common practice strategies that may very well look like a "technique." However, mechanical application of these practices often yields frustration because of the tendency to mistakenly view the practice as a "fix."

> . . . the teaching is merely a vehicle to describe the truth. Don't mistake it for the truth itself. A finger pointing at the moon is not the moon. The finger is needed to know where to look for the moon, but if you mistake the finger for the moon itself, you will never know the real moon. (Nhat Hanh, 1987)

While the practices that have been adopted in the clinical realm have roots in Asian meditative tradition, there is no need to relegate it simply to that history and tradition. If we think of mindfulness as an approach or framework for guiding actions, this moves us away from overly simplifying the process to mechanical applications.

So how can we define Mindfulness? Again, this is not a quick answer. If you spend some time looking through the many definitions of mindfulness you can see that there is no singular agreement between Buddhist scholars, researchers studying mindfulness process, and therapists who have incorporated mindfulness into their practice (Williams & Kabat-Zinn, 2011). For some historical context, the term mindfulness brought into the western world sphere is derived from the Pali word Sati (सति) and Sanskrit corresponding word Smrti (स्मृति) (Sharf, 2014). These words can be roughly translated into the phrase "to bear in mind" or "a remembrance." As it has come through Buddhist literature, the Chinese translation word Nian (pictured below) is from where our word mindfulness in English is more directly translated.

念

This Chinese character has a combination of a top half that means "now" or "present moment," and a bottom half means "heart" (referring to the emotional quality, not the physical organ) or "mind." Put these together and you get "Now Mind," or "Present Emotion." So, to culminate our understanding of this historical view, mindfulness encompasses a great many things that could imply the remembrance to stay present with our thoughts, emotions, and experiences. This is very different than the often-held mistake in early practice of mindfulness meditation that we need to "clear our mind." Rather, the implication is that we tune into our lives with full intention. To explore this further, let's look at a few other examples of how mindfulness has been defined.

Mindfulness is also:

> Paying attention in a particular way: on purpose, in the present moment, and nonjudgmentally. (Kabat-Zinn, 2003)

> The defused, accepting, open contact with the present moment and the private events it contains, as a conscious human being, experientially distinct from the content being noticed. (Hayes et al., 1999)

> Bringing one's complete attention to the present experience on a moment-to-moment basis. (Marlatt & Kristeller, 1999)

The nonjudgmental observation of the ongoing stream of internal and external stimuli as they arise. (Baer, 2006)

Awareness of present experience with acceptance. (Germer et al., 2013)

As you can clearly see, there is similar language across definitions. The focal point across each is a present focused attention to events that occur in our lives in a manner that does not get one stuck in thoughts and assumptions. To further expound upon the conceptual definition, this chapter will utilize the definition Jon Kabat-Zinn developed. This choice is certainly not to say this is the "best" definition, but simply because it is one of the more widely chosen definitions within the literature base.

Kabat-Zinn defines Mindfulness as "the awareness that emerges through paying attention on purpose, in the present moment, and nonjudgmentally to the unfolding of experience moment to moment" (Kabat-Zinn, 2003, p. 145). This definition has a few components to it that deserve some specific discussion before applying it to this chapter's focus topic. Whether you are new to the topic of mindfulness in clinical application, or someone that has been using it for some time, my goal is to offer some considerations to this definition that can enhance your understanding.

The definition starts off by discussing an emergent awareness. What differentiates an emergent awareness from simply "awareness?" Mindfulness specifically targets the ongoing experiential nature of awareness, and a shift from "automatic pilot" to being more in the driver's seat of engagement. In other language, it is about "waking up" to our experiences in real time. So often we can get pulled out of this awareness because of our anxieties about what will be coming down the road, or by getting stuck on thoughts about the past. The tools of mindfulness work to deliberately turn our attention to the emergent experiences of the "now."

The second section of our working definition emphasizes the notion of paying attention "on purpose." Have you ever paid attention on accident? Think about a time when you realized that you were paying attention to something other than what you were working on. Imagine a scenario where you are studying for a test and realizing that you have been listening to the people a table over discuss their recent trip to Hawaii. This distraction in attention was out of your awareness for a bit, until you caught yourself! What is paying attention on purpose then? We are talking about cultivating intentional focus. Mindfulness aims to develop skill in deliberate, conscious direction of our attention. As referred to earlier, we are stepping out of "automatic pilot" that takes over and directs our attention and patterns of behavior. This skill is really about helping to understand how our minds become distracted so that we can make a deliberate return to what the most important focus at that time is. This is not to say that we will free ourselves from distraction. To be distracted is to be human. In fact, our survival sometimes depends on it and is a useful feature when an unexpected danger presents itself. The problem is that the human brain can fall into patterns that are less helpful due to a perception of threat based on past experiences or for future threat mitigation. This brings us to the next part of our definition. The "present moment."

Present moment here can be a tricky thing to pin down. In fact, when you try to pin it, it is gone! What we are referring to as "present moment" in mindfulness really is about the engagement of what is present right in front of us. Often, the thoughts we have may be future minded or past reminiscent. If we become fused to these thoughts as truths, as Hayes et al. (1999) alluded to in their definition, we can often confuse or impose our cognitive experiences on the present time as though it were an actuality. The invitation of mindfulness is to realize that while we are having thoughts and emotions about the past and future in the present moment, we are able to observe those thoughts and feelings without getting as caught up in them to the point that we miss what may be occurring. One way that I remind people of this truth is by asking the question, "When can you make changes in your life?" The interesting thing is that this often sets up an answer about a future time. My response is, "show me!," and they can't do it! Through this dialogue, I point out that we can set up plans, but action only exists in present moment time. Present moment is really the only time we have. Once we are able to understand this, then we can be more conscious of what we choose to do during those times.

The inclusion of "nonjudgment" in Kabat-Zinn's definition is one that is of significant portion when we discuss sexuality, but certainly important in other arenas as well. One of the reasons why paying attention "nonjudgmentally" is difficult is because we habitually make comparisons. This is a natural process by which we create categories for future decision-making. This helps us in many ways but can become problematic when we start to categorize in ways that invalidate our experience. Additionally complex is the ability for our minds to take what we hear from others and treat those messages as truth. By placing these arbitrary judgmental standards like, "If I have had multiple partners, that makes me a slut," or "Masturbation is the sad default when you can't have sex with a partner," these thoughts can cause a lot of distress and reduces the availability of behaviors that may otherwise be valid. By learning to let go of judgment, we can find a place of acceptance.

There is a bit of a tricky reversal when talking about using acceptance and mindfulness-based interventions. We likely operate in a symptom reduction model system where clients are wanting to create changes. Acceptance and mindfulness asks clients to accept their thoughts, feelings, and experiences as they are. This can create a bit of a trap and can lead to "pseudo-acceptance." Pseudo-acceptance sounds a bit like this, "I'm willing to accept feeling my anxiety, as long as it helps it go away." If mindfulness strategies are being used to make something go away, this is avoidance in disguise! One thing to keep in mind in your own work with clients/patients is that when they start to allow feelings of anxiety from a mindful perspective, symptom reduction is likely to occur as a side effect. This is neither bad nor good from a mindfulness standpoint, but rather an experience to be observed. When this is being reported, a response that may be given could be something like "That is an interesting observation of your experience. Isn't it curious that by allowing anxiety to be present, it seems to take less of a lasting hold on your life?"

This leads us to the final component of our definition, the "unfolding of experience moment to moment." We have already discussed a bit about "present moment," and now we are expanding out to imply that this is an active process. We want to engage our awareness throughout our lived lives. Through practice of the micro-skills of mindful attention, individuals start to become more likely to get out of their own way to create lasting change in their lives. Now that I have described a "recipe" for what mindfulness is, let's take a moment to "eat the meal." That is, one of the best ways to get a sense of what mindfulness is rests on the actual practice. For that purpose, I invite you to take a moment to practice the following:

> *Start by drawing attention to your physical position, and shift your body as needed to find a comfortable position that will allow you to be still for a few minutes.*
>
> *Once settled, bring your awareness to your breathing. Notice how your body brings air in and out of your body. If you feel yourself attempting to control your breath, see if you can let go of that and let your body breath naturally without guidance for about 5 to 10 breath cycles.*
>
> *Expand your awareness out from your breath and check in with your physical body, noticing any physical sensations and/or the presence of tension or relaxation. Spend some time on each area of your body and just let yourself be aware of your experience of physical sensations. No need to change anything, just simply observe what is present.*
>
> *Bring your awareness back to your breath and spend another few minutes observing your breath, settling into this observation. During this time, you will likely notice that your mind*

> *will find some kind of distraction. This may be a thought, attending to a noise in the room, or some other momentary distraction. This is the natural process of observing the mind. When you observe that your mind has wandered, just notice this tendency, and bring your awareness back to your breath. Remember that we are not trying to control the mind, but rather observe the process of distraction and return to the present moment.*
>
> *After you have completed this exercise for a few minutes, take this process of awareness into the rest of your day.*

Ask yourself what this process was like. What did you observe? There are a few components to this process, that we can look at. First, we make a conscious choice to be present, calling attention to our breath and our body to anchor the process. Second, we choose a point of focus. In this case the choice was to stick with the breath. Third, we observe how we become distracted. Fourth, we make the choice to return. Through practices such as these, one can become more aware of their experiences in the present time.

That being said, cultivating this ability in all aspects of our lives brings the process alive and rather than a separate exercise, it becomes an active process of living. Let's discuss how to bring this awareness into the bedroom.

MINDFULNESS AND SEX

To date, the literature on incorporating mindfulness specifically into sex therapy is relatively limited. Despite this, the studies that have been done suggest benefit from the addition of mindfulness practice in the treatment of sexual difficulties. Anecdotally, I have seen great success in applying the principles and practices of mindfulness in the patients that I treat in my private practice. Like most of the current literature on mindfulness-based treatment approaches, the studies done in sexuality have been predominately within the cognitive behavioral therapy (CBT) approach.

One of the most prominent names when searching for mindfulness-based sex therapy approaches is Lori Brotto. She has several studies that suggest that mindfulness-based intervention is a helpful approach to working with female sexuality (Brotto, 2011, 2018; Brotto & Barker, 2014; Brotto et al., 2008; Brotto, Erskine et al., 2012; Brotto, Seal et al., 2012). Brotto et al. (2008) have developed a mindfulness group for women that has shown evidence to suggest improvements in desire, arousal, orgasm, and satisfaction for women who have been diagnosed with cancer, have histories of sexual trauma, and general difficulties accessing sexual desire. The Mindfulness-Based Sex Therapy groups were constructed to include mindfulness-based skills with sex therapy and psychosexual education. These groups were structured similarly to other cognitive-behavioral influenced programs like Mindfulness-Based Cognitive Therapy for Depression (Teasdale et al., 2000). Each group developed skill over time from engaging mindful practice in absence of a sexual situation, to the implementation of mindfulness skills during solo sex and then moving to partnered sexual experiences. There has been some study of utilizing mindfulness practice with men experiencing erectile dysfunction that suggests that by increasing dispositional mindfulness, it has a positive effect on mediating the psychological factors involved in situational erectile dysfunction (Déziel et al., 2017).

While the need for additional literature investigating the contribution of mindfulness in the specific context of sex therapy and sexuality-related work is certainly needed, we can extrapolate from the literature on psychological care regarding depression, anxiety, stress reduction, body image, and others that mediate sexual functioning (Baer, 2006). How then would we construct a mindfulness-based contribution to working with sexual difficulties? The remaining parts of this chapter will focus on applications to consider in your own work, based partly on the current literature and including examples that I have found useful in my own clinical work with clients and their partners.

Sex is an activity that includes the sensual, and where connection between two participants can be brought to life through physical and emotional experience. Difficulties can often occur when individuals become disengaged in those participatory qualities and become more of a spectator, getting caught up in thoughts, anxieties, shame, and other disruptive patterns. Masters and Johnson (1970) described this shift from fully engaged participant to observer or "spectator."

They associated this cognitive shift as a contributor to many sexual difficulties. Their groundbreaking therapeutic intervention, the "sensate focus," was developed to help individuals and partners to counteract this spectator role and to be more engaged in the process of giving and receiving touch. While "sensate focus" was not identified as a mindfulness intervention, the process of focusing in-the-moment on the pleasure of getting and giving touch is very much a mindful activity!

Given that mindfulness practice hits at the root of the tendency for individuals to become distracted, we can naturally incorporate these practices within the context of sexuality. One principle that we can examine is the nature of craving and aversion. Mindfulness practice teaches us that the dynamic tension created through attempts to push away unwanted and unpleasant experiences and grasping for the wanted pleasant experiences is part of the problem that keeps people distracted from their lives. To illustrate this concept, consider the following conversation between myself and two partners who have been in a decade-long relationship that (at the time we met) was absent of sexual encounters for approximately 6 years.

Therapist: Both of you are telling me that you have a wonderfully supportive and close emotional relationship, and that the times you have had sex in the past were wonderful. Tell me a bit about what keeps the both of you in a pattern of avoiding sexual intimacy.

Bill: Well, I absolutely love having sex with James the times that we have. But I also don't want to force him to do anything that he doesn't want to or that makes him feel uncomfortable.

James: Yes, that is true, probably to a fault. For me, the times that we have had sex in the past, things fell into place in such a way that it just worked, and it was beautiful.

Therapist: It sounds to me like there is some hesitancy to approach a new experience that may cause some uncomfortable feelings for the both of you. Do either of you think that is a possibility?

Bill: Yes! I am very hesitant to ask James to do something that makes him feel uncomfortable. He has had some really bad experiences in his life, and I am fine being patient to wait for him. We have a wonderful relationship in so many other ways.

James: See, that is part of the problem. Bill is so patient with me, and I feel such enormous pressure for things to work just right. If I start any kind of physical encounter, I worry so much about what I'm going to have to do next if he gets excited, and then if we go further, I worry about whether I can recreate those wonderful moments we had in the past.

Therapist: Ah, I see. So, part of the pattern here is that Bill, you don't initiate or ask for physical intimacy because it feels intolerable to have James be uncomfortable. And for you James, you get stuck in the unknown future of what may come, and the impossible recreation of a past event.

Bill & James:	(unanimously) Yes!
Therapist:	What if, instead of being stuck in the past and future, you were able to be present with what you were doing now without jumping to "what's next," and were able to create a new moment, whatever that may be, instead of feeling pressured to recreate the past?
James:	That would be wonderful.
Therapist:	Let's talk about how that can possibly happen.

In this dialogue, you can clearly see how Bill and James have gotten stuck in a pattern of avoidance, and very likely become pulled from their present experience with each other and caught up in the thoughts of past, future, and avoidance of discomfort. This pattern is exactly what mindfulness aims to learn to disrupt.

When it comes to sexuality and particularly the presence of sexual difficulties, there is often a dance between the desired and the feared. For example, the desire to get and maintain an erection for both the pleasurable aspects of sexual engagement and orgasm may be coupled with the fear of losing that erection and feeling shame or embarrassment in front of a partner. This tension between the desire and aversion can create a great deal of anxiety for the individual, which as you men know, effects the ability to get and maintain an erection. One way that we can counteract this is to develop skills around recognizing when we get caught in these cognitive traps and to pull ourselves back to the present moment of experience. We can teach clients a successive set of activities that allow for development of basic mindfulness skills in a nonsexual situation. This is followed up with implementing mindful touch, both nonsexual at first and moving towards sexual touch, and potentially both solo (masturbation) and partnered sexual experiences. The invitation given to both individuals and partnered systems we work with is to take the focus off of outcomes-based sex (e.g., "I need to have an orgasm"), and more towards process-focused sex that does not base satisfaction off of any specific outcome (e.g., "I am allowed to enjoy each moment with my partner[s] regardless of what happens").

One reason this is vitally important is that we do not want to set up the individual and/or their partners for a belief that mindful sex will "fix a problem" with them. Rather, mindful sex will allow them to connect fully with whatever the sexual moment they share with their partner(s) brings. Another vital importance to this process is that we are likely working with a diverse set of people in our office. We get a great deal of messages about what sex is "supposed to be." Whether straight, gay, pansexual, cisgender, transgender, Asian, Latinx, and more, these internalized messages influence how we think sex "should" happen. Mindfulness invites people to find satisfaction in the intimacy and sexual experiences that they and their partner(s) create through willingness to experience, nonjudgment, and presence. Our goal in working with a mindfulness framework is that we can help to counteract the effects of those patterns by accepting their presence and shifting focus towards what we can do to engage the moment. Individuals can let go of trying to control intrusive thoughts and difficult emotions and to stay with the physical sensations and relational engagement of their partner(s).

Mindfulness may be considered a strategy of approach, and one mechanism for creating change is thought to be the experience of exposure (Sears et al., 2011). Whereas many individuals attempt to avoid that which is uncomfortable, mindfulness invites us to sit with and observe thoughts and feelings that are uncomfortable to help understand that we can create behavioral change even in the presence of discomfort. Cognitive rumination in essence may be considered a form of avoidance to counteract feelings of anxiety. It gives the illusion that we are "doing something about it" by thinking through all the possibilities of what could go wrong. Meanwhile, we aren't really doing much at all but trying to avoid an unpleasant expectation. The challenge is that our attempts at avoidance work to some degree, which creates some reinforcement for the behavior. These attempts to control lead to solution-generated dilemmas.

Frasier (1998) discusses a process view of crisis points that lead to these solution-generated problems such as:

> [individuals] with the sexual problems of not being able to attain an erection or to have an orgasm, respectively, often engage in such deliberate and focused solution attempts that their attention is directed away from the sensuality of the sexual interaction, which itself tends to lead to excitement and release. . . .

These kinds of patterns set up a cycle in that the more the individual (or partners) attempt to solve their difficulty through thinking, avoidance, and attempts to make change through the same patterns that got them there, the more elusive the desired outcome seems to be. Mindfulness can be a useful tool in this struggle because we are disrupting that loop.

Consider for a moment this question: "How do you stand up?" What is your answer? Chances are, like many of the clients I ask this question to, you answered through thinking about how you have to activate the muscles in your legs, shift your balance, and apply some kind of pushing force up out of your chair, all while you remained seated. On a cognitive level, you are not wrong in your answer. This isn't an exercise in being right and wrong, but rather a recognition that we often default to thinking. Another very viable and active answer would be to simply stand up and demonstrate. This process can be likened to the thinking bias that occurs during sexual difficulties and the spectatoring that can pull an individual out of their experience and into problem-solving cognition. In order to do this, one must have the ability to observe how they are becoming pulled into these patterns and allowing a different possibility to exist. In ACT, this process of creating some flexibility and not getting so stuck in our thought process is called "defusing" (Hayes et al., 1999). One hallmark of a mindfulness-based approach is that we spend less time challenging these thought processes, instead recognizing that thoughts are not necessarily facts but are mental events that we can observe.

From an ACT perspective, this choice in exposure is the creation of psychological flexibility (Hayes & Smith, 2005). For example, if an individual is afraid of partner judgment for how their body looks, and they want to avoid the experience of judgment, their behavioral choices are somewhat limited. They may try to control this experience through things like keeping clothing on, having sex with the lights off, or avoiding sex altogether. The cost of this is that they are also limiting the ability for their partner to respond in a different way to their body, and the intimacy developed through acceptance of vulnerability. By choiceful exposure to the vulnerable state of being viewed unclothed by a partner, this allows a much greater range of choice, and while the initial feeling of anxiety may be present, it is no longer dictating behavioral choice. Over time, this can open up the experience to include greater feelings of connection, and the strength of the anxiety may dissipate.

Let's consider Bill and James once more. They were stuck in a loop of avoidance because their love for each other was such that neither of them wanted the other to feel uncomfortable, nor did they want to disappoint each other. This led to a gridlock that reduced their choices down to avoidance of sex and physical intimacy. Both of them very much wanted to engage their physical lives and to connect sexually, but their belief that it would end up poorly was so strong that they were not willing to risk the vulnerability. So, what do we do as mindful clinicians?

CLINICAL APPLICATIONS OF MINDFUL SEX

One of our jobs as a clinician is to help our clients get unstuck from the unhelpful patterns they have created. From a mindfulness perspective, we apply a compassionate view to the difficulties. By recognizing that these patterns were likely created from a place of protection and/or from modeling and experience, we can help the client(s) recognize that they themselves are not "broken" or "dysfunctional." Taking a good history with clients helps us understand their sexual story and an understanding of the rules and patterns that are currently present (see Chapter 2 on how to do a great sexual health assessment). From a mindfulness stance, we bear witness to the client's struggle and help them to settle into compassion for where they are starting from. We can encourage and help to shift their thinking from "I have to fix me," to include "I am working on learning new ways to go about addressing my difficulties because the way I have been doing it hasn't worked well."

MINDFULNESS OF THE BODY

Getting individuals (and partnered systems) to shift out of their thinking minds is one of the initial processes that I like to engage. As stated previously, the pull of "spectatoring" is so strong and such a common experience for individuals having difficulties that I want to have them actively going back into their bodily experiences as soon as possible. To do so, they need a tool to recognize when they are getting pulled out of bodily experience and into cognitive thought. When we talk about the physical body, we are bringing awareness to things like sensory experience. Bring awareness to the many ways in which a person can connect with a sexual moment, sight, sound, taste, touch, and smell, as well as the changing physical sensations such as body position and movement.

There are a few specific exercises that I ask individuals to practice that bring themselves into greater contact with the physical body. One of these is an adaptation on a body scan, similar to Jon Kabat-Zinn's (1990) book on Mindfulness Based Stress Reduction. In this body scan, I start with general body awareness in a similar fashion, and then also introduce an awareness of any physiological sensations related to sexual arousal and desire. My goal in doing this is to introduce the awareness of subtle changes in sexual energy and to tune into the body's sexual response. If partnered, I encourage doing a version of the body scan also as a pre- or postsexual experience exercise to ground them in body awareness. Similarly, this exercise can be deliberately bridged into the Sensate Focus exercises as outlined by Masters and Johnson.

Sexual Body Scan

Find a comfortable place to lie down or sit in a chair that allows your body to relax with its weight supported. Shift your body in a deliberate manner to find a settled spot and relax into that place.

In this settled space, shift your attention to your breathing, allowing your breath to find a natural rhythm without attempting to control it.

As you breathe in, bring awareness to your whole body and set an intention to simply observe the physical sensations you have, without judgment. If at any time you find yourself becoming distracted by thoughts or other experiences, simply note those experiences and return attention to your body.

Bring awareness to the feeling of your body as it comes in contact with the bed, floor, or chair you are in. With each breath, scan through your body, noticing how each section of your body feels. Spend some time on each section of your body: Feet, legs, hands, arms, torso, and head. Use the following for each area:

As you breathe in, become aware of your feet (legs, hands, arms, torso, and head). Notice any physical sensations that are present and observe what that experience is like. See if you can observe without judgment, or have the need to control your experience. After a few moments of observation, shift your awareness to the next body area with a breath cycle.

After going through your body's experience, bring awareness to your body as a sexual being. Scan throughout your body, recognizing that sexuality does not simply exist in the genitals, noticing any physical sensations of pleasure and/or arousal. Allow yourself to notice what feels good, without judgment, and simply enjoy any pleasurable experiences that may be present.

Finally, bring your awareness back to your breathing, and give yourself some permission to extend that sense of body awareness throughout your day, and into any future sexual experiences.

Bridging the sexual body scan to more direct sexual engagement, I will often bring in the idea of using solo sex (masturbation) as a form of sexual body meditation. One hurdle that may be present for some is to address internalized shame messages. This is particularly true for individuals who have never masturbated prior to engaging in this therapeutic work. I find that a bit of psychosexual education regarding the masturbation as a healthy aspect of sexual expression can go a long way. From a mindfulness perspective, I try to not get into arguments with clients, nor do I term these thoughts as "maladaptive" or "negative." Rather, I try to offer an invitation or suggestion to look at their thoughts openly as mental noise that may have less to do with truth and more to do with internalized shame messages from a sex negative culture. I offer the following scripts for individuals to use to help frame the mindful masturbation meditation. For partnered systems, there can be an added component of watching each other masturbate to view how their partners touch themselves to feel good. This can offer insights into what each partner enjoys, as well as further stepping into the exposure of intimacy and vulnerability.

Mindful Vulvar Masturbation

1. *Find space where you can have some uninterrupted time.*
2. *Begin by setting an intention to be with your own sexual self and body.*
3. *Begin touching your body, exploring what feels good to touch for you. Masturbation does not have to be focused on genitals, so feel free to touch any part of your body you find arousing.*
4. *Start exploring the exterior of your vulva, paying close attention to the feeling as you start to apply stimulation, and the response you have to different types of touch.*
5. *While exploring, find the clitoris. This will be easier to do as the clitoris becomes engorged with blood flow. Applying some pressure above the clitoris to pull back the clitoral hood may be helpful. (Lube can be quite helpful by creating less friction to the skin of the vulva.)*
6. *Once you locate the clitoris, begin to give some indirect stimulation to help increase blood flow. Exploration of stimulating the labia, pressure around the glans of the clitoris, and gentle rocking and/or circular motions to the surrounding areas can be stimulating. Find what feels good to you.*
7. *If it feels good to you, move to more direct stimulation of the clitoris, touching the head of the clitoris with back and forth or circular motions.*

8. *Explore various amounts of pressure, speed, and motions to see what feels good to you.*
9. *Insertion into the vaginal area can feel good, explore this if you enjoy the sensation of penetration (or "containment" if you prefer). Internal stimulation of the vagina may be pleasurable but is not necessary for arousal or orgasm.*
10. *Notice how your body responds to different amounts of touch, and notice any sense of building pressure or pleasure. Enjoy this, and try to not "make something happen."*
11. *If orgasm comes, enjoy this too.*
12. *At the end of your exploration, spend some moments resting in the conclusion of your self-pleasure.*

Mindful Penile Masturbation

1. *Find space where you can have some uninterrupted time.*
2. *Begin by setting an intention to be with your own sexual self and body.*
3. *Begin touching your body, exploring what feels good to touch for you. Masturbation does not have to be focused on genitals, so feel free to touch any part of your body you find arousing.*
4. *Start exploring the feeling of your nonerect penis, paying close attention to the feeling as you start to apply stimulation, and the response you have to different types of touch.*
5. *While exploring, explore different areas of the penis, from stimulation to the scrotum, the shaft, frenulum, and glans of the penis. As the penis becomes engorged with blood flow and if erection occurs, you can begin to apply more pressure and may be able to use your hand in a stroking motion. (Lube can be quite helpful by creating less friction to the skin of the penis.)*
6. *Explore various amounts of pressure, speed, and motions to see what feels good to you. You can also change hands or hand positions to explore different sensations and pressure.*
7. *Notice how your body responds to different amounts of touch, and notice any felt sense of building pressure or pleasure. Enjoy this, and try to not "make something happen."*
8. *If orgasm comes, enjoy this too.*
9. *At the end of your exploration, spend some moments resting in the conclusion of your self-pleasure.*

MINDFULNESS OF THOUGHTS AND EMOTIONS

In conjunction with the shift towards a greater body awareness, there is a recognition that thoughts and messages regarding sexuality and sexual expression are very present for people. As stated previously, we have countless messages that we accumulate through family of origin, peers, cultural influences, and direct experience. These messages in our thoughts can come at a price, and often pulls individuals out of direct experience and into their head. By bringing direct attention to how thoughts pull our attention out of the present moment and into past or future thinking, we can help to catch this tendency earlier and return to the current experience. One thing that we want to emphasize here is that thinking is not a "bad thing." We may have thoughts that we want to have, like "This feels so good," "I am so excited to be doing this with you," and we may have thoughts that we do not want to have, like "I hope that I look attractive," "I hope I can get an erection," and so forth.

The point here is not to make attempts to have more of the "good ones" and get rid of the "bad ones," but simply to point out that thoughts come and go throughout an experience. One way that I respond to discussions about sexual anxiety is that our brain attempts to solve problems around important things. This may be to prevent the loss of something important, or to try to gain something that is important. So, responding to thoughts in a mindful way could be to meet the thought, "I hope that I look attractive," with a recognition that it is important to us to connect with our partner and to be seen affectionately.

Specific ways to engage mindfulness of thoughts is by helping the clients recognize the ways in which thoughts are generated, and how this can narrow down into a rigid belief. One simple exercise I like to do is to repeat the phrase "Mary had a little . . ." with a pause to check in with the person I am working with. Most often, for individuals born into a culture that utilizes this nursery rhyme, they will respond with "Lamb." My follow-up is to point out how quickly they came up with this as the possibility because of repetition, and that it is equally plausible that Mary had a little motorcycle, or ice cream, or a cheery disposition, and so forth. Extending this tendency out to their internal thought process with sexuality, we can see how our minds do a similar process of selection based on past messages and experience. Engaging our clients in a bit of thought tracking regarding sex can be helpful to gain some awareness of persistent themes and/or patterns of thinking. Additionally, the simple act of tracking creates a bit of space between the thoughts running away versus pausing for reflection to write it down. This process is a bit of a mindful writing exercise! More formally, we can engage our clients in a process of learning to watch thoughts.

Mindful Thought Watching

Sit down with the intention of watching your thoughts, beginning with a moment to center yourself with your breath.

As you sit, begin to watch your thoughts come and go as though you were watching clouds pass by in the clear sky. Notice what these thoughts consist of, viewing your thoughts as mental events to be observed rather than as facts . . .

. . . relating to thoughts in the same way that you would to sound, for our thoughts are often internalized language made up of sounds.

You may invite a specific topic of reflection, to watch your associations and in an effort to identify particular thought patterns that are recurring old mental grooves. As you become more experienced, you can introduce topics that have previously felt difficult to address. This includes topics of sex and sexuality.

Gently ask yourself, "Am I jumping to conclusions? Am I thinking in black-and-white or judgmental terms? Am I expecting perfection? Are these old thought patterns keeping me from enjoying pleasure in my sexuality?"

As individuals get more able to recognize their own thought patterns and cognitive traps, we as professionals can help to expand out their options in responding. In essence, *mindful awareness of thoughts gives individuals options where they thought they had none before.*

FINAL THOUGHT

My sincerest hope is that this chapter gives some initial information regarding the application of a mindfulness approach to working with sexuality. While there is more research to be done in this area, there is evidence to support the inclusion of mindfulness-based principles in treatment strategies. I do believe that the interest in applying mindfulness to the enrichment of partnered relationships and sexual intimacy is fertile ground for moving and heartfelt clinical work and for future study.

The final closing point is that through the development of mindfulness skills, there is the possibility of a major shift. Rather than mindfulness being applied to help clients find more satisfaction in their sexual lives and to help alleviate the distress they feel in their sexual lives, sexuality can actually be applied as a way to increase their mindfulness!

REFERENCES

Baer, R. (Ed.). (2006). *Mindfulness-based treatment approaches: Clinician's guide to evidence base and applications.* Academic Press.

Basson, R. (2000). The female sexual response: A different model. *Journal of Sex and Marital Therapy, 26,* 51-65.

Brotto, L. A. (2011). Non-judgmental, present-moment, sex . . . as if your life depended on it. *Sexual and Relationship Therapy, 26,* 215-216.

Brotto, L. A. (2018). *Better sex through mindfulness: How women can cultivate desire.* Greystone Books.

Brotto, L. A., & Barker, M. (Eds.). (2014). *Mindfulness in sexual and relationship therapy.* Taylor & Francis.

Brotto, L. A., Basson, R., & Luria, M. (2008). A mindfulness-based group psychoeducational intervention targeting sexual arousal disorder in women. *Journal of Sexual Medicine, 5,* 1646-1659.

Brotto, L. A., Erskine, Y., Carey, M., Ehlen, T., Finlayson, S., Heywood, M., . . . Miller, D. (2012). A brief mindfulness-based cognitive behavioral intervention improves sexual functioning versus wait-list control in women treated for gynecologic cancer. *Gynecologic Oncology, 125,* 320-325. https://www.gynecologiconcology-online.net/article/S0090-8258(12)00067-4/ppt

Brotto, L. A., Seal, B. N., & Rellini, A. (2012). Pilot study of a brief cognitive behavioral versus mindfulness-based intervention for women with sexual distress and a history of childhood sexual abuse. *Journal of Sex & Marital Therapy, 38,* 1-27.

Déziel, J., Godbout, N., & Hébert, M. (2017): Anxiety, dispositional mindfulness, and sexual desire in men consulting in clinical sexology: A mediational model. *Journal of Sex & Marital Therapy, 44*(5), 513-520. https://doi.org/10.1080/0092623X.2017.1405308

Frasier (1998). A process view of crisis and crisis intervention: Critique and reformulation. *Crisis Intervention and Time-Limited Treatment, 4*(2-3), 124-144.

Germer, C. K. (2013). Mindfulness: What is it? What does it matter? In C. K. Germer, R. D. Siegel, & P. R. Fulton (Eds.), *Mindfulness and psychotherapy* (pp. 3-27). Guilford Press.

Hayes, S. C., & Smith, S. (2005). *Get out of your mind and into your life.* New Harbinger Publications.

Hayes, S. C., Strosahl, K. D., & Wilson, K. G. (1999). *Acceptance and commitment therapy: An experiential approach to behavior change.* Guilford Press.

Kabat-Zinn, J. (1990). *Full catastrophe living: Using the wisdom of your body and mind to face stress, pain, and illness.* Dell.

Kabat-Zinn, J. (2003). Mindfulness-based interventions in context: Past, present, and future. *Clinical Psychology: Science and Practice, 10*(2), 144-156.

Marlatt, G. A., & Kristeller, J. L. (1999). Mindfulness and meditation. In W. R. Miller (Ed.), *Integrating spirituality into treatment: Resources for practitioners* (pp. 67-84). American Psychological Association.

Masters, W. H., & Johnson, V. E. (1970). *Human sexual inadequacy.* Little, Brown and Company.

Nhat Hanh, T. (1987). *Old path, white clouds: Walking in the footsteps of the Buddha.* Parallax Press.

Sears, R. W., Tirsch, D., & Denton, R. B. (2011). *Mindfulness in clinical practice.* Professional Resource Press.

Sharf, R. (2014). Mindfulness and mindlessness in early Chan. *Philosophy East and West, 64*(4), 933-964.

Teasdale, J. D., Segal, Z. V., Williams, J. M. G., Ridgeway, V. A., Soulsby, J. M., & Lau, M. A. (2000). Prevention of relapse/recurrence in major depression by mindfulness-based cognitive therapy. *Journal of Consulting and Clinical Psychology, 68*(4), 615-623. https://doi.org/10.1037/0022-006X.68.4.615

Williams, J. M. G., & Kabat-Zinn, J. (Eds.). (2011). Mindfulness [Special issue]. *Contemporary Buddhism, 12*(1).

Section III

Sexual Dysfunctions and Disorders

12

The Treatment of Desire Disorders: The Intersystem Approach

Katherine M. Hertlein, Gerald R. Weeks, and Nicole Feno

INTRODUCTION

Hypoactive sexual desire disorder (HSDD) and Female Sexual Interest/Arousal Disorder (FSI-AD) are the two of the most common problems appearing in the practice of couples and sex therapy, affecting approximately 20% of men and 15% of women (Meana & Steiner, 2014; Meston & Stanton, 2017) and 27.9% men and 50.2% of women over the course of one's lifetime (Briken et al., 2020). Although HSDD and FSIAD are prevalent, they are also among the most complex and difficult sexual problems to treat.

Desire disorders are usually informed by several factors, from biological contributors to societal messages and everything in between (Goldstein et al., 2017; Malary et al., 2015; Weeks et al., 2020). Some treatment models focus on the identified partner and overlook the contribution of the partner and relationship dynamic in the development, maintenance, and treatment of the difficulty (Weeks & Gambescia, 2002). In such cases, a treatment that is grounded by an individualistic perspective is not systemic and therefore inadequate (Weeks, 1987, 1994, 2004).

The Intersystem approach is our preferred method for treating the complex systemic factors that are typically seen in desire disorder cases. The Intersystem approach was developed by Gerald Weeks (1987; 1994). Originally, the model outlined three domains as contributing to sexual desire issues: individual factors (e.g., personality), interactional factors (the relationship), and intergenerational factors (messages from family-of-origin). Weeks used this three-factor approach to inform his treatment of hypoactive sexual desire disorder in a text coauthored with Nancy Gambescia (2002). As the model developed, these three factors were further delineated into five and described in *Innovations in Clinical Practice: Focus on Sexual Health* (Hertlein et al., 2007). Since that time, the five-factor approach has been used by Weeks and colleagues in their application of the model to sex and couple therapy (i.e., Gambescia et al., 2021; Hertlein et al., 2009; Weeks & Fife, 2014). The five factors are listed below:

1. *Individual biological:* Therapists must understand what biological, physiological, and genetic factors might be present and influencing desire.
2. *Individual psychological:* This includes one's values, attitudes, psychological makeup, development, and intelligence. This is an important area to assess in desire disorders, as one's values and attitudes regarding sexuality and sexual behavior often affect one's level of desire.
3. *Dyadic:* The therapist must work from a systemic perspective because numerous relational factors influence the extent of sexual problems within the couple, including communication issues, power issues, and fears of intimacy (Abdo, 2013; Weeks & Gambescia, 2002).
4. *Family-of-origin:* Families have a profound impact on attitudes, values, and expectations toward sex. Some families, for example, might remain tight-lipped about sexuality, communicating to their children that sex is "bad." These feelings might often result in sex guilt and contribute to desire disorders (Gambescia & Weeks, 2020; Hall, 2020; Weeks & Gambescia, 2002).

5. *Sociocultural/environmental:* This includes societal, cultural, religious, and historical factors that can influence decision-making and judgments about behavior. Further, as times change, couples reinterpret their sexual behavior through other lenses (Weeks & Gambescia, 2002).

In this chapter, we review basic assessment and treatment procedures for desire disorders meeting *Diagnostic and Statistical Manual of Mental Disorders* (5th ed.; *DSM-5*; American Psychiatric Association, 2013) criteria based on the Intersystem approach (Weeks, 1987, 1994; Weeks & Gambescia, 2002). The treatment principles encompass an integrative approach to treating desire disorders in couples therapy (Schwartz & Southern, 2018). The foundation of this model is the Intersystem approach (Weeks, 1987, 1994) in that we view this problem to have individual, interactional, and intergenerational components. Our treatment strategy reflects our belief that desire disorders typically result from a convergence of intersystem factors and that it becomes embedded in the couple's dynamics (Weeks, 1987; Weeks & Gambescia, 2002).

DEFINING DESIRE DISORDERS

The overlap between HSDD and other conditions that result in impaired desire affects a therapist's ability to effectively intervene. To appropriately diagnose HSDD, there are criteria that must be met per the *DSM-5* (American Psychiatric Association, 2013). They include the lack of sexual fantasy or thoughts along with a lack of desire for sexual activity. The lack of sexual fantasy and desire for sexual activity must be accompanied by clinically significant distress for a duration of at least 6 months (APA, 2013; Hall, 2020). On the other hand, for a diagnosis of FSIAD, women must exhibit a deficiency or absence in at least three of six factors surrounding sexual cues and encounters, including absent or reduced interest to sexual cues and being unreceptive to their partner's advances (APA, 2013; Gambescia & Weeks, 2020). These may include a reduction in interest, sexual thoughts or fantasies, sexual initiation, sexual pleasure (in 75-100% of encounters), sexual arousal, and genital or nongenital sensations (APA, 2013; Gambescia & Weeks, 2020). In both conditions, a key component is the experience of subjective distress; without it, there is no diagnosable disorder. The longer people have these conditions, the less likelihood that it will be stressing them, thus dropping the prevalence rate (Gambescia & Weeks, 2020).

Sexual incompatibility, which is a very different issue with different treatment implications, is often confused for HSDD or FSIAD (Hall, 2020; Malary et al., 2015; Offman & Matheson, 2005). In addition, it is important to distinguish desire disorders from those who are asexual (Foster & Scherrer, 2014; Steelman & Hertlein, 2016). Foster and Scherrer (2014) cited "concern for dismissal" (p. 426) as one form of practitioner bias that they might encounter in a therapy room. In their qualitative study on bias in treatment for asexual individuals, a common theme emerged that those who identified as asexual; they were concerned their therapist "would try to treat his lack of sexual attraction and that he would be unable to advocate for himself in the interactions" (p. 426).

As if it was not challenging enough to separate lack of desire form FSIAD and HSDD, another complication with treating desire disorders is that HSDD and FSIAD can occur in conjunction with other sexual dysfunctions in either partner (Gambescia & Weeks, 2020; Hall, 2020). Therapists must be knowledgeable in how each dysfunction could be created by or maintained by another dysfunction and triage treatment accordingly (Gambescia et al., 2021). For example, desire discrepancy in a relationship may cause dyadic issues, internalization of poor messages regarding sexual performance or body image, and results in increasingly problematic sexual functioning over time (Hall, 2020). Likewise, there is significant comorbidity between HSDD and FSIAD despite being different conditions (Brotto & Basson, 2014; Gambescia & Weeks, 2020; Hall, 2020).

ASSESSMENT OF DESIRE DISORDERS

Etiology of Desire Disorders

Physiological

The etiology of sexual desire disorders can be a confluence of factors, including individual biology, individual psychology, relational factors, family of origin factors, and sociocultural factors (Gambecia & Weeks, 2020; Hall, 2020; Weeks & Gambescia, 2002). For example, normative physiological factors that fluctuate arousal and desire in women include fatigue, hormone imbalances during phases of the menstrual cycle, and breastfeeding (Chadwick et al., 2017; Malmborg et al., 2016; Thorton et al., 2015). Even though lack of sexual interest is less persistent with these normative physiological factors, medical risks such as postmenopausal estrogen deficiency, persistently low testosterone levels, diabetes, and thyroid dysfunctions can play a more constant role in interference (Costa et al., 2018; Shizari et al., 2019). Physiological factors that have a direct effect on sexual desire for men include endocrine disorders that effect prolactin and testosterone levels, hypothyroidism, vascular diseases, and cancer (Bhasin et al., 2007; Lara et al., 2012). The iatrogenic effects of many commonly used prescription medications can contribute to both HSDD and FSIAD (Taylor et al., 2013).

Psychological

Certain psychological characteristics in individual partners can be expressed within the context of sexual intimacy, thus giving rise to the development of FSIAD and HSDD. These include anxiety, depression, negative cognitive distortions, inaccurate beliefs about sex, a poor body image, a tendency to fuse sex and affection, career overload, and other sexual problems (Gambescia & Weeks, 2020; Offman & Matheson, 2005; Quinn-Nilas et al., 2016; Weeks & Gambescia, 2002). Psychiatric factors such as anxiety, depression, obsessive-compulsive disorder, and sexual orientation conflicts can contribute to the development of desire disorders (Gambescia & Weeks, 2020; Hall, 2020; Johnson et al., 2010; Kalmbach et al., 2014; Offman & Matheson, 2005; Trovão & Serefoglu, 2018). Stress tends to have different effects for men and women, where it seems to inhibit desire for women and increase desire for men (Hall, 2020). Further, physical and emotional trauma – and even vicarious trauma – can inhibit desire (Branson et al., 2014; O'Loughlin & Brotto, 2020; Pulverman & Creech, 2021).

The experience of fear also contributes to development and maintenance of a sexual desire disorder (Kalmbach & Pillai, 2014). These include fear of anger, fear of losing control, fear of feelings, fear of dependency, and fear of intimacy (Gambescia et al., 2021; Neilson et al., 2022; Weeks & Gambescia, 2002; Weeks & Treat, 2001; Weeks & Fife, 2014). The fear of intimacy, for example, might stem from the fact that emotional and physical intimacies are closely related. This means that working on sexual desire may be hampered by one partner's fear of being emotionally vulnerable and intimate (Weeks & Fife; 2014; Weeks & Treat, 2001). This can occur after coercive sexual experiences (Nielson et al., 2022). Other fears in one or both partners that could leave a couple at risk for the development of desire disorders include fear of anger, rejection, abandonment, exposure, feelings, or dependency (Weeks & Treat, 2001).

Dyadic

Relational risk factors might overshadow the course of treatment, as research indicates that the extent to which people are satisfied with their relationship is related to their sexual satisfaction (Vowels & Mark, 2020). For example, women with FSIAD tend to report greater degrees of relationship distress and less relational cohesion (Gambescia & Weeks, 2020; Trudel et al., 1993). Men tend to report conflict and feelings of anger or resentment (Hall, 2020). For women, sexual satisfaction is related to factors such as the way sex was initiated, the level of arousal, and the behaviors present in that interaction. Basson's (2000, 2001) model of female sexual response appears to support this interaction, in that she believes that women's sexual response cycles are connected to the amount of trust and intimacy in her relationship. Other relational risk factors include contemptuous feelings, criticism, defensiveness, power struggles, rigid adherence to sexual scripts (i.e., who should initiate sex), sexual monotony, and toxic communication (Gambescia & Weeks, 2020; Gottman, 1994; Hall, 2020). Desire disorder assessment procedures are detailed in a handout on page 208.

Sociocultural and Family-of-Origin Messages

Many of the risk factors, such as negative beliefs surrounding sexuality, are learned within the social and familial contexts of each partner. Sociocultural influences and family-of-origin influences are separate domains in the Intersystem approach (Weeks, 1987; Weeks & Gambescia, 2002). For the purposes of this chapter, however, we have combined them as the empirical literature often combines them in support of this construct. For example, attachment has been demonstrated to be connected to sexual desire in later life (Cherkasskaya & Rosario, 2019; Van Lankveld et al., 2022). In addition, Korean husbands have been found to internalize messages from their family of origin and culture and perceive sex as burdensome, thus creating a context for the development of sexual disorders (Park et al., 2022). For these reasons, it is essential that the therapist explore intergenerational legacies and other socio-environmental/cultural messages regarding sexual intimacy and desire.

TREATMENT OF DESIRE DISORDERS: THE THREE R's

Reduce Response Anxiety

When individuals notice and are distressed by the fact that they are not feeling desire for sex with their partner, they experience anxiety. As anxiety increases, the likelihood that they will experience that desire decreases, thereby increasing anxiety, and so on (Pascoal et al., 2020). One critical component to the treatment of HSDD and FSIAD is lowering the response anxiety (Weeks et al., 2020). It is important to treat this component first, as it can be both a cause and an effect of these desire disorders. There are several techniques to help reduce response anxiety. Response anxiety refers to not feeling the desire that a person thinks they should be feeling (Weeks & Gambescia, 2002). The therapist educates the couple about response anxiety by explaining the concept. The partners are then asked to observe what happens to their anxiety levels when they force themselves to feel desire for their partner. Cognitive techniques such as thought-stopping and thought-substitution are useful in treating response anxiety (Alvarez & Garcia-Marquez, 2011; Rowland & Kolba, 2018). Another technique is to confront irrational ideas that foster response anxiety, such as believing that the only way to have sex is via intercourse (Gambescia et al., 2021). In this case, the definition of sex is broadened to include behaviors that are less likely to cause response anxiety (e.g., noncoital sexual touching). Part of broadening this definition is to educate the client on ways to separate sex, intimacy, affection, and sensuality (Weeks et al., 2009; Weeks & Gambescia, 2002).

Paradoxical interventions can also be used if the therapist is familiar with such techniques (Weeks & L'Abate, 1982). One form is to intentionally prescribe a construct such as the use of humor. The therapist can ask clients to generate an image of a sexual activity they firmly believe is a must for the activity to count as sex – one that they would find entertaining. The more humorous the image, the less likely they are to feel anxious (Gambescia & Weeks, 2020; Weeks et al., 2009). This strategy may be one way to achieve distress reduction for HSDD, as identified by Hall (2020). Finally, the therapist can educate the couple on ways to create a sensual environment. Through trial and error, the couple alters their settings to allow themselves to positively anticipate and enjoy the sensual aspects of sexual intimacy, leading them to eventually become aroused by certain environmental factors (Weeks et al., 2009).

Reframing Responsibility

In couples who present with desire disorders, the symptom bearer is the partner who lacks desire, wants to have sexual desire, and feels the pressure to have sex to please their partner. In treatment, however, it is critical that the partner with the higher desire be an active part in the therapy (Gambescia & Weeks, 2020). Without this key component, the responsibility of the change may be placed on the symptomatic partner when, in fact, the other partner might have some invisible responsibility to the emergence and maintenance of the problem. The couple must be educated to view the desire disorder as a relational problem, not just the responsibility of the symptom bearer. Reframing is one technique the therapist can use to create the conceptual understanding of low desire as a couple issue (Weeks et al., 2009; Weeks & Gambescia, 2002). In reframing, the therapist works with each member of the system to help them identify what their role/involvement is in the problem. The therapist asks focused questions that become increasingly directed. In this way, the therapist can gain more information and present it back to the couple system. As couples begin to hear their own responses, they get a different picture of what is happening in the system. Once the couple can reframe their own perceptions and behaviors, the label of symptom bearer is dropped, and desire disorder is viewed as a relational problem by both partners (Gambescia & Weeks, 2020; Weeks & Gambescia, 2015; Weeks et al., 2009).

Recognizing the Intersection of Affective, Cognitive, and Behavioral Aspects of Desire

Psychological interventions are effective in reducing the severity of the symptoms and sexual satisfaction of women with hypoactive sexual desire disorder (Fruhauf et al., 2013). Throughout the course of sex therapy, the therapist continues to work with the couple to improve their sexual compatibility. This includes helping the couple to be more closely aligned with one another in their emotional, cognitive, and behavioral elements of their sexual relationship (Apt et al., 1996; Kolivand et al., 2021; Offman & Matheson, 2005). In a couple presenting with desire disorders, the therapist will need to continually assess the presence and influence of affect, behavior, and cognitions experienced by each partner throughout the course of treatment, especially since the etiology of desire disorders are often a mixture of psychological and biological factors (Brotto, 2017; Gambescia & Weeks, 2020; Schwartz & Southern, 2018; Weeks et al., 2009). For instance, the lower desire partner appears to have a lack of motivation for sex and a lack of affect. This lack of motivation causes a response anxiety which becomes part of the cycle. The higher desire partner is often more emotional, frustrated, and pessimistic (Gambescia & Weeks, 2020; Weeks et al., 2009). In these instances, the therapist should normalize these feelings and continue to direct the couple to explore, understand, and reassess their feelings over time.

We often warn clients that things may get worse before they get better; this helps to keep them in the treatment process when they feel discouraged and pessimistic. The therapist can then intervene by normalizing feelings for the couple as they learn to understand and support one another. In terms of addressing the cognitive components, the therapist should be aware that the partner with the desire disorder is thinking negative thoughts about sexuality (Kolivand et al., 2021). These thoughts, no matter how aware the client may be of them, can exert a powerful influence over affect and behavior.

TREATMENT PLANNING

Treatment plans can be as focused as addressing only the presenting problem or as broad as addressing one's relational, vocational, behavioral, emotional, and cognitive functioning. In the Intersystem approach, our goals are to examine the problem in context (Weeks et al., 2009; Weeks & Gambescia, 2015). In this way, the therapist connects the client's sexual desire problem to a larger concept in the relationship. Treatment should be collaborative where the therapist presents an idea and seeks the couple's agreement before proceeding.

Elements of the Treatment Plan

There are several elements to the treatment plan for desire disorders. The first is the focal point of the lack of desire. Because this is the problem that brought the couple into therapy, the treatment plan should reflect this issue. Second, treatment should generally improve the couple's overall level of sexual functioning, which include sexual satisfaction, sexual depression, sexual anxiety, and sexual compatibility (Gambescia & Weeks, 2020; Hall, 2020; Offman & Matheson, 2005; Weeks et al., 2009; Weeks & Gambescia, 2002). Certainly, impaired desire may be associated with other elements of the sexual relationship, specifically those that diminish the sexual experience. Discussing the wide variety of elements in the couple's life that can impact desire communicates to the client that the global quality of one's sexual life can be improved. The final element of the treatment plan is to improve the overall quality of the couple's relationship. If couples can effectively work together to solve their sexual problem, it will relate to greater improvements in the couple's relationship. We generally advocate for developing a treatment plan that attends to all areas of the Intersystem approach: individual biology, individual psychology, dyadic issues, family-of-origin issues, and sociocultural issues (Weeks & Gambescia, 2002). For an example of the structure of a treatment plan reflecting all five domains of the Intersystems approach, see Gambescia et al. (2021).

Setting Treatment Priorities

Once the goals for treatment are established, the therapist identifies which of those objectives takes precedence over the others. This is an important step, as some of the therapy goals may overlap or be addressed concurrently. A triage tree is presented in Gambescia et al. (2021) which highlights the importance of working with desire disorders prior to other sexual dysfunctions. As stated earlier, the therapist begins with the desire disorder prior to treating other sexual difficulties in either partner. If treating the desire disorder is ineffective because of the problems within the relationship, the therapist must address the relational issues that take precedence (Gambescia et al., 2021; Weeks & Gambescia, 2002). Further, if the partners cannot work together in conjoint sessions, the format can be changed to concurrent individual sessions on a short-term basis, bringing the couple back together later to continue to work on the relational issues and the desire problems. As the couple works together constructively, both the desire disorders and relational issues are addressed (Gambescia & Weeks, 2020; Weeks & Gambescia, 2002). The simplest problems are tackled first, moving gradually to the more difficult or complex. To triage problems in this way helps the couple to experience positive gains and increases hopefulness (Gambescia et al., 2021). The therapist and couple can begin to work on any other sexual difficulties once the presenting problem has been resolved to the couple's satisfaction. Finally, when the couple believes they have essentially eliminated their relational and sexual problems, the therapist can offer to assist with optimizing/enhancing their sexual and couple relationship.

Homework and Incremental Change

Homework is an important component of the treatment of sexual difficulties (Gambescia et al., 2021). It increases the chances of success, lowers anxiety, and creates a safe environment in which the couple can try out new behaviors (Jensen et al., 2020). Homework is intended as a way for the couple to take responsibility for creating positive changes in their relationship and to relearn how to function sexually. It also has been shown to help couples gain changes in their relationship more quickly than couples who do not do homework (Hawrilenko et al., 2016). Homework will gradually desensitize the couple, reduce anxiety, and promote enjoyment of sexual activity; therefore, many elements of homework must be structured for the couple and assigned in graduated increments. Throughout each step, the therapist encourages the couple to proceed slowly, engaging only in activities that have been assigned.

There are several structural elements of homework. The therapist and clients discuss who will be responsible for initiating the completion of the homework assignment. The therapist generally prescribes the client that initiates the homework to promote mental preparation for the activity. Scheduling is another element of homework. The therapist asks that the couple schedule the homework for two reasons. First, without the schedule, it is unlikely that the couple will complete the assignments. Second, when the couple schedules time to do the homework, they are intentionally setting aside time to do something meaningful with one another. Whenever the couple fails to complete the homework, the therapist must help them process and understand the reasons for noncompliance. Otherwise, the noncompliance may continue and sabotage the entire process. Finally, therapists should consider using text messaging to communicate with their client in between sessions to reinforce homework completion, as it leads to increased compliance (Alfonsson et al., 2019).

In the earlier stages of treatment, the duration of each homework exercise should be short and tailored to the needs of each couple; as the course of therapy continues, the therapist can extend the duration of each exercise. Initially, sensual touching is often assigned for a period of 5 to 10 minutes. As the couple can endure this activity, the therapist can extend the time frame to 20 to 30 minutes. The decision about duration of an assignment should be underwritten by the couple's comfort level. The frequency of homework assignments is also an important consideration. The therapist must keep in mind that this couple likely has not had positive sexual experience with one another for months or perhaps even longer. Nonetheless, the couple will need to have repeated assignments to become comfortable with sensual and sexual touch (De Villers, 2014). Typically, homework frequency is at least three times per week, but this prescription is adapted to each couple and adjusted as needed (Gambescia et al., 2021; Weeks et al., 2009). Finally, location is another aspect of the homework that must be addressed. Many couples connect sexual activity with the bedroom; it is likely that couples with desire disorders might have negative connotations of the bedroom because of the association with problematic sexual activity. The therapist should explore with the couple various locations that would work best for them in terms of reducing their anxiety and increasing compliance with treatment (Gambescia et al., 2021).

Promoting Compliance for Homework

There are a few ways in which the therapist can promote compliance for homework (Muise et al., 2017; Weeks & Fife, 2014). The therapist must respect the element of choice. Directing people to do something specific often removes the element of choice and creates psychological resistance. Therapists will fare better if they collaborate with the client in making decisions about homework. This collaboration can take the form of structuring the basics of the assignment for the couple and having the couple fill in the gaps. Couples need to have a vested interest in the process. Another important element of homework is what to call it. Clients might have negative connotations of the word "homework" (Kazantzis & L'Abate, 2007). In such instances, the therapist and/or couple can decide what to call these activities based on personal preference. The second way that therapists can promote compliance through homework is using depersonalization. This means that the therapist assigns homework by explaining to the couple that this work is "standard," "typical," or "needed" at this stage in the therapy. This relieves the therapist of being in a position of ordering the clients to a certain activity, also reducing the likelihood of resistance. Finally, the therapist can use implicit rather than explicit directions to describe the homework. In this way, the therapist might say "You might try . . ." and allow the client room to feel whatever might occur. See Weeks et al. (2016) for more detailed information.

Treating Comorbid Sexual Dysfunctions

It is not unusual for an individual to have more than one sexual problem; thus, it is possible that the impaired desire might be a part of another sexual difficulty such as physical discomfort during sex or trouble with orgasm (Gambescia & Weeks, 2020; Hall, 2020; Weeks & Gambescia, 2002). Sometimes the nonsymptomatic partner also has sexual difficulties, such as erectile dysfunction or premature ejaculation (Hall, 2020). Sexual difficulties in the partner can make intercourse less desirable, thereby increasing the possibility of continued desire problems. The role of the therapist is to educate the couple in how other sexual problems might contribute to the development and maintenance of the desire problem. Further, the couple is encouraged to make a commitment to working on all elements of the dysfunction, not just the desire problem.

Promoting Sexual Intimacy

In this treatment model, sexual intimacy is promoted in four stages. First, the therapist helps the couple to share their ideas about what it means to be intimate. In this stage, the partners discuss their views of intimacy, identify discrepancies in their definitions, and work toward a common definition. Next, the therapist helps the couple to understand that intimacy and sex are not distinct entities. The partners adopt attitudes and thoughts that will foster intimacy within their sexual relationship. Third, the therapist works with the couple to redefine sexuality by broadening their definition of sexuality to include more than intercourse, moving away from goal-orientated sex and helping the couple to focus on being in the moment with one another (Brotto, 2017; Gambescia & Weeks, 2020; Weeks & Gambescia, 2015). Finally, the couple needs to become aware of and identify the barriers that inhibit and prevent them from gaining greater intimacy.

Relapse Prevention

The therapist should help the couple to understand that sexual desire is maintained through active sexual contact with one another. Thus, the therapist assists the couple in relapse prevention by including strategies in the repertoire that involve sensual touching and caressing. Also, the couple will need help in solving conflicts and anger not related to sexuality, as this can inhibit desire. One of the signs that a couple is relapsing is their noncompletion of the homework assignments. Therefore, the couple is reminded to plan regular times/sexual dates. Another strategy for preventing relapse is to generate an agreement for the couple on what is expected from the initiation to the completion of the sexual activity.

Paradoxical strategies can also prevent relapses (Gambescia & Weeks, 2020; Weeks & Gambescia, 2002). One strategy is to ask the couple to identify the ways that they might sabotage their sexual relationship (Gambescia & Weeks, 2020; Weeks et al., 2009). The therapist also encourages the couple to seek more treatment if they have a continual dry spell in their sexual intimacy. Therapists can also ask the couple to predict the factors that might cause inhibited desire. Asking the couple to think about the ways that this therapy will be undone will increase the likelihood that these problems will not occur.

IMPLEMENTATION

Keeping couples engaged in the treatment process is critical to achieve a successful outcome. Brotto (2017) advocates for working within a biopsychosocial approach, including combining medical and psychological treatments, to reduce treatment dropout and improve outcomes. Therapists need to ensure that the couple has access to the medical professionals who can address any physiological etiology.

A great deal of the work done with desire disorder couples addresses the relational problems that contribute to and maintain the sexual difficulties. It is essential that the therapist be qualified and knowledgeable about couples and sex therapy techniques and know the circumstances under which the techniques will be most effective. The implementation of techniques should be tailored to the specific problems of each couple rather than utilizing a "one size fits all" method. Moreover, we suggest that when a technique is implemented during treatment, the couple should be aware of why it is being used and what the outcome is expected to be (Weeks et al., 2009). Clients are more likely to be compliant when they have an idea about how the technique fits into the scope of the treatment plan and when they are aware of any potential problems in implementing this technique. Again, couples must be active members of their treatment.

Process

The focus of treatment should be on the emotional processes that occur within the session. It is important for the partners to share their anticipations and beliefs about treatment and for the therapist to help them to come up with realistic expectations for the course of their therapy. In this way, the couple will learn to communicate about feelings (McKay et al., 2018). In treating desire disorder cases, the first process that should be addressed is that of the expectation of the couple.

STAGES OF TREATMENT AND RISK FACTORS

Intimacy-Based Approach to Treatment

Weeks and Fife (2014) were the first to advocate for an intimacy-based approach to couple/sex therapy. Their theory was that underlying fears of intimacy can create any number of dysfunctions in the individual/couple. By removing these fears and fostering intimacy, these dysfunctions can be eliminated. Sternberg (1986) provides a model of love in adult relationships that is clinically useful and includes intimacy as a central element. This model is primarily composed of three elements: commitment, intimacy, and passion. Commitment refers to the cognitive component of love. It is the decision one makes to commit exclusively to another person. There are many ways that a couple can express commitment to each other, such as through marriage, cohabitation, and so on. Intimacy in Sternberg's model refers to the extent of closeness people feel toward their partner. It is characterized by showing emotional support, demonstrating vulnerability, regarding the other in a positive light, being honest and empathetic with each other, and so forth. Passion signifies the aspect of Sternberg's model that relates to the physical attraction one feels for their partner. It is this passion that Sternberg believes motivates people to come together physically. Sternberg's model has been found to be psychometrically accurate (Askarpour & Mohammadipour, 2016).

Considering Sternberg's triangle model for describing love, we emphasize that passion, intimacy, and commitment are all related in cases of desire disorders. We believe that passion does occur within the context of an intimate and committed relationship. In this way, our treatment approach includes not only revitalizing the passion through sex therapy behavioral techniques, but also addressing the intimacy and/or commitment needs within the relationship.

Defining the Relationship in Terms of Sternberg (1986)

The therapist may provide a brief overview of the Sternberg model and demonstrate how each side of the triangle is interconnected to other parts. The therapist asks the couple about their fit to this model. One question is to ask whether both partners desire all three components as described in the triangle. This question elicits each partners' level of agreement and sets the stage for a conversation about how love and intimacy are present in the relationship. The therapist then asks whether each component of this triangle is needed in the couple's relationship. To what extent is each person committed? Desire intimacy? Desire passion? It is important to assess the discrepancies in the responses. For example, one partner may want passion and intimacy but is not certain they want to commit to the relationship. This would indicate another issue in the relationship that would need to be resolved prior to engagement in sexual skill building. It is also at this phase that the therapist assesses for any underlying intimacy fears (see section later in this chapter). Intimacy fears can be disguised as commitment fears and can occur in one or both partners. It is imperative that the therapist distinguish whether fears of commitment are truly the result of fear of intimacy.

Once the partners can establish whether they want or need certain aspects of the Sternberg model, the therapist can ask whether each partner wants the same level of intensity for each of the three components. Partners may agree they want commitment, intimacy, and passion in their relationship but disagree on the degree to which they want it. In some couples, one partner wants to be closer than another. The partner who does not want to be as close may engage in strategies to distance, of which one strategy may be removing themself from sexual encounters. The result of this distancing can leave the partner who wants greater closeness and intimacy feeling hurt and angry, thereby reducing this partner's desire.

As relationships progress, partners may determine that they need to balance the time they spend together with time spent on their own. Therefore, it is important that the therapist ask the couple about the amount of togetherness and individuation each partner wants in the relationship. Typically, it is easier for couples to talk about ways to spend more time together rather than ways where they can spend more time apart. Partners may avoid talking to one another about needs for individual time for fear of hurting one another's feelings. They instead find ways to take this time, whether it be working late, losing oneself in the computer all evening, and so on. Couples should be encouraged to discuss how they will balance their individual and togetherness needs within their relationship.

Couples are typically able to understand Sternberg's (1986) model from a cognitive standpoint, yet they may have difficulty being able to conceptualize how to express these three aspects of love in a real-world way. It is important for the therapist to understand what prevents the partners from being able to freely express themselves. These difficulties may be related to socialization and upbringing. Men, for example, are not typically socialized in the same way as women regarding emotional expression (Gaia, 2013; Montemurro & Riehman-Murphy, 2019). As a result, they may be unable to demonstrate intimacy in ways that would be recognized by their partners. It is also possible that partners have come from families that were detached from one another or cold. In such cases, it may behoove the therapist to employ a focused genogram depicting the way love was expressed in each partner's family of origin (DeMaria et al., 1999). This technique is detailed later in this chapter.

Couples also come into a relationship with expectations of themselves, each other, and what it means to be in a loving relationship. Some of these expectations might be mismatched, and partners are left feeling disappointed and sad upon the realization that these expectations will not come to fruition. There are also those expectations that are unrealistic from the start, such as believing that if your partner loved you, they would know automatically what you want (Hertlein et al., 2007). In cases where expectations are not met, one partner may misattribute this to their partner not caring about them enough and, as a result, withhold sex or desire (Thomas & Fletcher, 2003). The therapist should help the couple to develop realistic perceptions of themselves, what each can offer, and a realistic perception of love and all that it involves.

Creating Greater Intimacy

Once the couple has appropriately defined their relationship and has come to an agreement about what is meant by developing/maintaining intimacy in their relationship, it is time to combine it with action. The therapist instructs each member of the couple to make a list of actions they can do that will develop intimacy in the aforementioned areas (Weeks et al., 2009). It is important that the actions they choose be of value to their partner because if the partner does not view it as being valuable, the couple will not become closer. Partners are expected to check their list at the end of each day to determine how successful they were in performing the tasks on the list and to consider reasons that they may not have been successful.

We also suggest the "three A's" exercise. In this exercise, the A's stand for affection, appreciation, and affirmation. In this activity, we encourage the couple to show how much they like and value one another (affection), to show how much they appreciate one another (appreciation), and to make an expression of affirming the relationship, such as "I love you" (affirmation) (Hertlein et al., 2007; Weeks et al., 2009).

Couples also need to talk to one another on a process rather than content level. This means that the couple should become accustomed to talking about the emotional process during their relationship rather than strictly focusing on the content, or who said/did what when. Bernal and Barker (1979) identify levels that help the couple to assess where they fall in the continuum of cognitive to affective. These levels are:

1. *Objects Level*: The couple communicates in a factual, detached manner.
2. *Individual Level*: Communication is characterized by each partner discussing how other people are responsible for his or her actions.
3. *Transactional Level*: Partners in the couple can step back and look at their pattern of interaction.
4. *Relational Level*: The couple can make inferences about the reasons for their behavior and established patterns. The couple has developed awareness about why they make decisions to behave in a certain way and are able to express this rationale to their partner.
5. *Contextual Level*: The couple can connect present behavior with past experiences and history. The couple can explore their family-of-origin patterns and connect it to their present behavior, thereby providing further insight into their individual behavior and the way it affects the couple.

Couples often communicate only at the first two levels, which is not intimacy building. Levels 3-5 help the couple communicate about the way they relate and communicate. It is an important aspect of learning how to meta-communicate about their relationship. Couples will need to be coached on these levels in the session and then given homework to practice these skills at home.

The therapist should ask the couple to set aside time weekly for such conversations as well as opportunities to bond with one another. We recommend to our couples that they integrate all the levels of communication in their ways of talking with each other:

1. They must assume they are fully committed to each other.
2. They should assume that the other had good intentions and good will.
3. They should each assume that understanding each other can be achieved even when communication becomes difficult and frustrating.

In terms of communication and promoting intimacy, Gottman (1994) found that couples should try to maintain a 5:1 ratio of positive to negative exchanges, as couples who report their marriages are "working" maintain this ratio. Other strategies for working toward more effective communication include using "I" statements, validating one another, reflective listening, and learning to edit what you say (Weeks & Treat, 2001).

Working With Underlying Fears of Intimacy

Fears of intimacy and closeness, whether conscious or unconscious, are often exhibited through one's behavior (Weeks & Treat, 2001). It is important to address this issue in the treatment of desire disorders, as some partners may fear intimacy to the point where their sexual desire for one another becomes compromised. The therapist may share several of the underlying fears of intimacy described earlier. The couple is then given the opportunity to probe each one of these fears. They are usually deeply held fears which are not immediately recognized. In some cases, the therapist may help the partners identify their fears using a genogram that focuses on elements of one's upbringing that influence intimate behavior. The therapist educates the couple about the many reasons why individuals might fear intimacy so that they understand the origin of these fears and can connect these fears with the current problems. For example, a woman experiencing anorgasmia might equate having an orgasm with her partner as losing control, being controlled, or becoming dependent. Several of the common factors related to fear of intimacy include a fear of abandonment or rejection, fear of losing control, fear of being dependent on the other partner, fear of anger or conflict, fear of feelings, and fear of exposure.

In low-desire cases, a few of the factors related to fear of intimacy are more frequently seen (Gambescia et al., 2021; Weeks & Treat, 2001). For example, the fear of becoming dependent may manifest in relationships through a power imbalance that is so severe that one partner is perceived as a parent and the other a child. This issue has the potential to make sex feel almost incestuous. The fear of losing oneself is another common presentation. It relates to low desire and how this low desire is one aspect of the relationship that is in their control; the fear that their partner wants to potentially control them by telling them what to do and what to feel has the effect of reducing sexual desire for their partner. Another way to view this issue is that the low-desire person may submit to having sex (loss of control) but may unconsciously reject feeling any desire in order regain a sense of self-control. In addition, when a partner fears anger and/or conflict, they may be viewing anger as solely negative or potentially destructive to the relationship. They may attempt to avoid experiencing this emotion by avoiding all emotional contact instead of learning that anger (if expressed) need not destroy the partner or the relationship. The therapist can address this by helping the couple to understand their attitudes toward anger and identify what other emotions the anger might be protecting (Weeks & Treat, 2001).

There are several guidelines for treating intimacy fears (Gambescia et al., 2021). First, it is important to identify the fear. Next, the therapist uses cognitive therapy to help neutralize the negative thoughts associated with the fear and replace them with appropriate and adaptive cognitions. The therapist and clients then work to disrupt the pattern of avoidance that results from the fear. It is important to validate the fearful partner's emotions without agreeing with them, as agreeing would lead to continued avoidance of the feared stimuli and, consequently, the behavior. When the therapist is confident the couple can directly tackle the fear, the suggestion should be made that the fear is threatening to the present relationship and serves little or no purpose. It is essential that the therapist and couple explore the ways in which each person in the relationship contributes to the problem, rather than placing the blame solely on the person with the fear (Weeks et al., 2009).

Self-Monitor for Passive-Aggressive Behavior

Passive-aggressive behavior can also undermine treatment (Weeks & Fife, 2014). Passive-aggressive behavior tends to suppress desire. Forgetting, procrastination, and reporting that a request was misunderstood are all indications of passive-aggressive behavior. The therapist can educate about the advantages of expressing anger directly rather than in ways that are hidden and destructive. Another example is self-righteousness in a partner. This form of communication places the other partner in an inherently weaker position. In addition, self-monitoring for victimization is appropriate in circumstances where the low-desire partner accepts the role of the wounded party. In such cases, their partner is viewed as smarter, more assertive, and more verbal as support for their belief that they cannot defend themselves. Another aspect to self-monitor is the extent to which the partners rely on intellectualization and reasoning. Clients who use this as a shield for anger may not value emotions and instead depend on rationality to prevail (Weeks et al., 2009).

Use of Focused (Sex and Anger) Genograms

In sex therapy, tracking patterns of sexual interest and behavior is a key part of assessment and treatment. One way to do this is through the use of focused genograms. There are two that apply to the treatment of desire disorders: a sex focused genogram and an anger genogram. At first blush, anger does not seem to have a lot to do with sexual behavior, but withholding sex or desire is a common way anger is expressed (DeMaria et al., 1999).

DeMaria et al. (1999) identified the use of the genogram for tracking the patterns and expression of both sex and anger to increase the couple's awareness of how they are experienced. The following questions can be used to identify and explore intergenerational sources of sexual learning and history:

1. How did your parents explain the topic of sex?
2. What did you learn about sex from each of your parents?
3. What were your parents' expectations regarding sex and sexuality?

4. Was one parent more open about sex than the other?
5. What did intimacy look like for your parents? For example, did they kiss in front of you?
6. Were there any family "secrets" surrounding sex?
7. Was there a family member you felt more comfortable talking to about sex?
8. Did you ever walk in on your parents having sex? If so, how did they respond to it?
9. What role did your family play in forming your sexual values?

Additionally, the following questions can be used to identify and explore intergenerational sources of anger:

1. How did your parents deal with anger and conflict?
2. Did you see your parents work through anger/conflict?
3. When members of your family (name each one) got angry, how did other members respond?
4. What did you learn about anger from each of your parents?
5. When your parents became angry with you, how did you feel and what did you do?
6. How did members of your family respond when you got angry? For example, who listened to you? Who failed to listen to you?
7. Who was allowed/not allowed to be angry in your family?
8. What is your best/worst memory about anger in your family?
9. Was anyone ever hurt because of someone's anger? Who?

The therapist should educate the couple that appropriate expression of sex and anger can benefit their relationship. In fact, the couple can learn that expressing both sex and anger respectfully might bring them closer to one another. Moreover, it can reaffirm their expectations of one another and clarify their boundaries in the relationship.

Bibliotherapy

The therapist can recommend several books to clients which may be helpful to addressing fear of anger and conflict in a relationship. Harriet Lerner's *The Dance of Anger* (1989) focuses on the benefits of expressing anger, particularly for women, but this book can also be helpful for men. Alberti and Emmons's *Your Perfect Right* (1995) is written from a behavioral perspective and centers on communication, anger, and assertiveness. A helpful book that the therapist can recommend for addressing sexual expression is Lori Brotto's *Better Sex through Mindfulness: How Women can Cultivate Desire* (2018). The focus of this book is to explore the benefits of mindfulness when it comes to sexual difficulties, such as lack of desire.

Guidelines for Arguing Constructively

In clients with low sexual desire, there may be a tendency to circumvent conflict through avoiding anger or sex. The anger becomes underlying resentment which suppresses desire (Weeks & Gambescia [2015] first identified by Weeks [1987] in *Integrating Sex and Marital Therapy*). This results in a cycle of frustration, failed attempts to solve the problem, and ineffective processing of the issue. Once the couple understands the benefits of appropriate expression of anger or sex in their relationship, guidelines for arguing constructively can be provided. These guidelines emphasize the process of identifying the underlying feelings that is being protected (i.e., hurt, fear, etc.) through description of the problem as well as one's feelings about the problem. After the couple can identify their emotions related to an issue, the next guideline is to advise the couple on ways to make a clear complaint without blaming. Blameful statements will often produce anger and defensiveness in the other partner and perpetuate a cycle of blaming (Becker et al., 2008). Therefore, couples should be helped to use "I" statements to identify the reasons for their anger; thus, they are able to offer the complaint in a productive, non-accusatory manner. Using "I" statements helps each partner express their feelings without putting the cause of those feelings onto the other person (McKay et al., 2018). In desire disorders, some clients are angry or resentful toward their partners and express anger through avoidance of sex and inhibited desire. The therapist can assess how these clients might be feeling in certain situations and encourage them to overtly address hidden feelings of anger.

Another guideline is to instruct the couple to employ time-out procedures when appropriate. Once a time-out is called, the discussion should immediately end until it is revisited. Several specific rules apply when couples take a time-out. First, the time-out should last at least 20 minutes. Gottman's (1994) research indicates that individuals' physiology takes at least that long to return to its baseline. Further, the partner that initiates the time-out is responsible for beginning the discussion again.

The final guideline is to encourage an atmosphere of compromise and negotiation as opposed to winning or losing the argument. Once the couple has adopted the attitude of compromise, adaptive behaviors can be interjected into their pattern. Old destructive patterns are consistently monitored and identified as blocks to stopping effective communication as new behaviors are integrated. Couples are also given a list of behaviors to avoid as they are correlated with relationship discord. These behaviors include complaining, mind reading, defensiveness, demonstrating contempt, stonewalling, and criticism.

Steps in Conflict Resolution

As the couple is helped to learn to argue constructively, the therapist reinforces the guideline that everyone is responsible for their own actions and feelings. Principles of active listening are instituted. Active listening enables the partners to discuss problems without criticism, mind reading, blaming, defensiveness, or other toxic emotions. The partner with the issue is responsible for holding a discussion regarding the topic that needs attention. The other partner reflects both the initial complaint and feelings without responding defensively to the issue. Once the feelings and behaviors are understood, a response can be made. Then the initial speaker becomes the active listener. Next, the person with the issue should be responsible for posing a solution. The idea is for the couple to consider a wide range of possible solutions and choose one that appears as the most workable. Discussion should then focus on establishing a plan of implementation as well as periods of time where they return to the situation and evaluate its effectiveness. One excellent resource is *Messages: The Communication Skills Book* by McKay et al. (2018), which allows couples to practice effective communication in several different topic areas.

Sensate Focus, Mindful Touch, and Mindfulness Techniques

Because desire disorders are the couple's problem, the treatment requires that the partners be ready to work together effectively toward the common goal of pleasurable intimacy. When the therapist determines that the couple is sufficiently committed to treatment and to the relationship, sensate focus techniques are implemented. Sensate focus exercises consist of a series of graduated physical exercises to be performed at home. They are designed to reduce anxiety and promote relaxation during physical intimacy. The term sensate implies that the couple will learn to enjoy the sights, sounds, smells, and so on, related to physical touch. Moreover, the term sensual does not necessarily imply sexual. The physical prescriptions are nondemanding of intercourse and tailored to the needs of each couple. Thus, judicious timing and careful evaluation of each incremental step is essential.

There are several objectives in sensate focus exercises (Gambescia et al., 2021). The environment should be conducive to supporting sensate focus techniques, including an environment of collaboration and readiness for the techniques. During the exercises, the couple creates an intimate environment by making their physical surroundings comfortable and pleasant. Any source of distraction is eliminated (e.g., turning off phones, television, etc.) with a reliance on mindfulness techniques and a focus on the present. Low-desire partners are instructed to recognize any negative or antisexual thoughts that occur and to make a note of them later. They are asked to quickly return to the exercise mentally by staying in the moment, without judgment, focusing only on the pleasurable sensations and keeping those sensations present (Weeks et al., 2009).

Incorporating mindfulness in treatment has been demonstrated to be an effective component of working with desire disorders (Brotto et al., 2016; Kocsis & Newbury-Helps, 2016; Rashedi et al., 2022; Rullo et al., 2021). Programs involving mindfulness and teaching resiliency can be delivered online; they incorporate couples activities such as communication and sensate focus exercises, which result in improvements in desire (Rullo et al., 2021). Later, the negative cognitions are addressed in session and the partners learn techniques of thought-stopping and thought-substitution.

In desire disorder cases, the sensate focus exercises are instrumental in the assessment process as well as treatment. The sensate focus and mindfulness techniques, described for those experiencing sexual dysfunction, are also followed by clients with desire disorders with the caveat that transition to intercourse only occurs when the HSDD or FSIAD partner begins to feel some sexual desire. Educate the couple that at times it is natural to feel more desire than at other times. When they are ready to have intercourse, the couple is reminded to focus on the sensations, positive thoughts, and fantasies that were instrumental in reactivating the desire.

CONCLUSION

Treating desire disorders can be complicated as it might involve a series of contradictions. First, this disorder is the couple's problem, not just the individual's problem. Next, although the couple often believes that the partner with HSDD or FSIAD lacks interest or feelings about sexual intimacy, it may be a way of indirectly expressing strong emotions related to the individual's values, beliefs, and fears. Additionally, the individual experiencing low desire may develop this problem in response to conflict within the couple's relationship. Often, partners with this problem want to feel desire for their partner, yet the more they try to force themselves to feel desire, the more difficult it becomes to do so. The role of the therapist is to first perform an assessment of the couple's situation and to identify their fit for treatment. The Intersystem model can guide the therapist to decode and address the many problem areas in couples presenting with this complex dilemma. The therapist works with the couple to identify and reduce risk factors arising from sexual ignorance and faulty beliefs about sex and intimacy that existed prior to the present relationship. Each partner's individual risk factors are also addressed. Finally, the focal point becomes the couple's relationship. The therapist uses a variety of cognitive and behavioral techniques to help the couple communicate effectively and enhance physical and emotional intimacy.

Desire Disorder Assessment Handout

There are several phases in the assessment of desire disorders: the telephone evaluation, the preliminary assessment, the preliminary Intersystem assessment, and a cognitive assessment. Each of these phases is described below. These assessment procedures are more fully outlined in *A Clinician's Guide to Systemic Sex Therapy* (Gambescia et al., 2021).

The Telephone Evaluation

During this conversation, the therapist should ask how the client was referred and answer questions on the phone. The therapist should use the phone call to

- become familiar with the problem,
- identify ways to combine individual and couple therapy,
- develop a treatment plan, and
- find a way to get both partners into session.

The Preliminary Assessment

In the preliminary assessment phase, the therapist begins to gather data and generate a hypothesis to later be tested. This process is facilitated by

- noting initial impressions and reactions of the couple,
- taking an adequate history of the problem,
- recording recent significant changes in the client's life, and
- establishing goals by identifying the changes that each partner would like to occur in the relationship.

The Preliminary Intersystem Assessment

As part of the preliminary Intersystem assessment, the therapist employs rapid assessment techniques. The following questions can be taken home by the couple.

1. How often do you have sex?
2. How often do you feel like having sex?
3. Do you believe your desire level is too low?
4. When did you first notice yourself losing desire for sex?
5. What was happening at that time?
6. Did you lose desire rapidly or slowly?
7. What was your level of sexual desire earlier in your relationship?
8. What medications are you taking now?
9. Any changes in your health?
10. On a scale of 1 to 10, how much desire do you feel in general? Prior to sex? During sex?

Cognitive Assessment

Assess each partner's negative emotions about the self, about the partner, about the relationship, from the family-of-origin, and so on. The cognitive assessment helps to determine which of the thoughts can be changed though cognitive therapy techniques, and to assess other problems in the relationship that need to change through couple therapy.

Favorable Conditions and Contraindications For Therapy With Clients That Have Low Sexual Desire

The Intersystem treatment for desire disorders is favorable when:

- partners have positive sex beliefs and *want to* experience desire again.
- both partners are relatively free from psychiatric problems that can impede treatment.
- response anxiety is present in the presenting partner, or the pressure to feel desire in the absence of sexual desire is present.
- the client wants to feel desire rather than having no interest or motivation to work on feeling desire.
- there is treatable discord in other areas of the relationship, such as ineffective communication, unresolved anger, and expectations.
- desire disorders can be related to other sexual difficulties in either partner, such as erectile dysfunction, inhibited female orgasm, or vaginismus.

The Intersystem treatment for desire disorders is *not* appropriate when:

- couples are unable to break the cycle of negative sexual cognitions and obsessive thoughts that interfere with building sexual desire.
- clients with desire disorders keep a secret from their partner such as sexual abuse, physical abuse, or emotional abuse.
- negative sexual attitudes based on religious beliefs, internalized negative sex messages from the family-of-origin, and the resulting sexual guilt are present.
- situational life stressors such as divorce, severe work stress, or death of a loved one affect one partner.
- anxiety is present where there is a real or imagined loss of health, or when the individual or couple do not appreciate the normal physiological changes of aging and maintain the same expectations as they did when they were younger.
- difficulties in negotiating issues of power, control, inclusion, and autonomy are present.
- the couple's sexual script has not been successfully negotiated, or the partners may have different preferences or ease of arousal.
- the desire disorder partner does not wish for or care about sexual desire or has sexual aversion.
- the problem is viewed as solely belonging to the partner who lacks desire and the other partner is unwilling to participate in the therapy.
- there is a great deal of untreatable discord.
- couples are unable to work together cooperatively.
- one or both partners are not committed to the relationship.
- significant psychopathology is present in either partner, which makes couple/sex therapy problematic.
- one or both parties have a lack of commitment to treatment or the relationship, such as during an affair or active addiction.

Sensate Focus Objectives

- Partners learn to be focused on themselves rather than wondering if they are pleasing their partner.
- These activities provide an opportunity for both to communicate their likes and dislikes, wishes and desires, and so forth.
- The goal is to experience sensual pleasure from each individual activity without the pressure of having to complete the sex act with vaginal intercourse.
- Once couples begin to experience sexual intimacy in a positive manner, positive anticipation of future intimacy occurs and desire becomes enhanced.

Sensate Focus and Mindful Touch Techniques

- Ask that the couple not engage in intercourse until asked to do so at a later point, because forcing the goal of intercourse might increase anxiety and reduce relaxation.
- Discuss the rationale for sensate focus activities, explaining that it is a form of systematic desensitization.
- Begin with an assignment that is carefully selected ahead of time by the therapist and the couple (e.g., foot rubs, massages, back rubs, and other forms of loving touch). Partners are encouraged to experience as much pleasure as they can and to communicate about what feels good.
- Remind the couple not to exceed the prescription.
- Advise the partners to communicate with each other if something does not feel right and to do something else.
- Routinely check the completion of assignments. In other words, what worked? What did not work? This technique might involve many graduated steps until the couple is comfortable with sensual touch and ready to progress to genital stimulation.
- Gradually move to the phase of touching breasts and genitals. Follow this phase again with questions and activities.
- Gradually transition to intercourse.
- Educate the couple that at times, it is natural to feel more desire than at other times.

RESOURCES

Abdo, C. H. N. (2013). Treatment of premature ejaculation with cognitive therapy. In E. Jannini, C. McMahon, & M. Waldinger (Eds.), *Premature ejaculation: From etiology to diagnosis and treatment* (pp. 213-220). Springer-Verlag.

Alberti, R. E., & Emmons, M. L. (1995). *Your perfect right* (25th ed.). Impact.

Alfonsson, S., Englund, J., & Parling, T. (2019). Tailored text message prompts to increase therapy homework adherence: A single-case randomised controlled study. *Behaviour Change, 36*(3), 180-191. https://doi.org/10.1017/bec.2019.10

Alvarez, M., & Garcia-Marquez, L. (2011). Cognitive and contextual variables in sexual partner and relationship perception *Archives of Sexual Behavior, 40*(2), 407-417.

American Psychiatric Association. (2013). *Diagnostic and statistical manual of mental disorders* (5th ed.). https://doi.org/10.1176/appi.books.9780890425596

Apt, C., Hurlbert, D. F., Sarmiento, G. R., & Hurlbert, M. K. (1996). The role of fellatio in marital sexuality: An examination of sexual compatibility and sexual desire. *Sexual and Marital Therapy, 11,* 383-392. https://doi.org/10.1080/02674659608404452

Askarpour, A., & Mohammadipour, M. (2016). Psychometric properties of Sternberg love scale. *Journal of Fundamental and Applied Sciences, 8*(4), 2036-2047. https://doi.org/10.4314/jfas.v8i2s.164

Basson, R. (2000). The female sexual response: A different model. *Journal of Sex and Marital Therapy, 26*, 51-65. https://doi.org.10.1080/009262300278641

Basson, R. (2001). Are the complexities of women's sexual function reflected in the new consensus definitions of dysfunction? *Journal of Sex and Marital Therapy, 27*, 105-112. https://doi.org/10.1080/00926230152051725

Becker, J. A., Ellevold, B., & Stamp, G. (2008). The creation of defensiveness in social interaction II: A model of defensive communication among romantic couples. *Communication Monographs, 75*(1), 86-110.

Bernal, G., & Barker, J. (1979). Toward a metacommunication framework of couples intervention. *Family Process, 18*, 293-302. https://doi.org/10.1111/j.1545-5300.1979.00293.x

Bhasin, Enzlin, P., Coviello, A., & Basson, R. (2007). Sexual dysfunction 3: Sexual dysfunction in men and women with endocrine disorders. *The Lancet (British Edition), 369*(9561), 597.

Branson, D. C., Weigand, D. A., & Keller, J. E. (2014). Vicarious trauma and decreased sexual desire: A hidden hazard of helping others. *Psychological Trauma, 6*(4), 398-403. https://doi.org/10.1037/a0033113

Briken, P., Matthiesen, S., Pietras, L., Wiessner, C., Klein, V., Reed, G. M., & Dekker, A. (2020). Estimating the prevalence of sexual dysfunction using the new ICD-11 guidelines. *Deutsches Ärzteblatt International, 117*(39), 653-658. https://doi.org/10.3238/arztebl.2020.0653

Brotto, L. A. (2017). Evidence-based treatments for low sexual desire in women. *Frontiers in Neuroendocrinology, 45*, 11-17. https://doi.org/10.1016/j.yfrne.2017.02.001

Brotto, L. A. (2018). *Better sex through mindfulness: How women can cultivate desire.* Greystone Books.

Brotto, L., & Basson, R. (2014). Group mindfulness-based therapy significantly improves sexual desire in women. *Behaviour Research and Therapy, 57*, 43-54. https://doi.org/10.1016/j.brat.2014.04.001

Brotto, L., Chivers, M. L., Millman, R. D., & Albert, A. (2016). Mindfulness-based sex therapy improves genital-subjective arousal concordance in women with sexual desire/arousal difficulties. *Archives of Sexual Behavior, 45*(8), 1907-1921. https://doi.org/10.1007/s10508-015-0689-8

Chadwick, S. B., Burke, S. M., Goldey, K. L., & van Anders, S. M. (2017). Multifaceted sexual desire and hormonal associations: Accounting for social location, relationship status, and desire target. *Archives of Sexual Behavior, 46*(8), 2445-2463. https://doi.org/10.1007/s10508-017-0959-8

Cherkasskaya, E., & Rosario, M. (2019). Relational and bodily experiences theory: Attachment and sociocultural influences in a parsimonious model of sexual desire in women. *Archives of Sexual Behavior, 48*(6), 1719-1722. https://doi.org/10.1007/s10508-019-01492-1

Costa, R. M., Oliveira, G., Pestana, J., Costa, D., & Oliveira, R. F. (2018). Do psychosocial factors moderate the relation between testosterone and female sexual desire? The role of interoception, alexithymia, defense mechanisms, and relationship status. *Adaptive Human Behavior and Physiology, 5*(1), 13-30. https://doi.org/10.1007/s40750-018-0102-7

DeMaria, R., Weeks, G., & Hof, L. (1999). *Focused genograms: Intergenerational assessment of individuals, couples, and families*. Brunner/Mazel.

De Villers, L. (2014). Getting in touch with touch: A use of caressing exercises to enrich sensual connection and evoke ecstatic experience in couples. *Sexual and Relationship Therapy, 29*(1), 87-97. https://doi.org/10.1080/14681994.2013.870336

Foster, A. B., & Scherrer, K. S. (2014). Asexual-identified clients in clinical settings: Implications for culturally competent practice. *Psychology of Sexual Orientation and Gender Diversity*, *1*(4), 422-430. https://doi.org/10.1037/sgd0000058

Frühauf, S., Gerger, H., Schmidt, H. M., Munder, T., & Barth, J. (2013). Efficacy of psychological interventions for sexual dysfunction: A systematic review and meta-analysis. *Archives of Sexual Behavior*, *42*(6), 915-933. https://doi.org/10.1007/s10508-012-0062-0

Gaia, A. C. (2013). The role of gender stereotypes in the social acceptability of the expression of intimacy. *The Social Science Journal, 50*(4), 591-602.

Gambescia, N., & Weeks, G. (2020). Systemic treatment of sexual interest/arousal problems in women. In K. M. Hertlein, N. Gambescia, & G. Weeks's (Eds.), *Systemic sex therapy* (3rd ed., pp. 107-129). Routledge.

Gambescia, N., Weeks, G. R., & Hertlein, K. M. (2021). *A clinician's guide to systemic sex therapy* (3rd ed.). Routledge.

Goldstein, I., Kim, N. N., Clayton, A. H., DeRogatis, L. R., Giraldi, A., Parish, . . . Worsley, R. (2017). Hypoactive Sexual Desire Disorder: International Society for the Study of Women's Sexual Health (ISSWSH) expert consensus panel review. *Mayo Clinic Proceedings*, *92*(1), 114-128. https://doi.org/10.1016/j.mayocp.2016.09.018

Gottman, J. (1994). *What predicts divorce: The relationship between marital processes and marital outcomes*. Lawrence Erlbaum.

Hall, K. (2020). Male hypoactive sexual desire disorder. In K. M. Hertlein, N. Gambescia, & G. Weeks's (Eds.), *Systemic sex therapy* (3rd ed., pp. 41-59). Routledge.

Hawrilenko, M., Eubanks Fleming, C. J., Goldstein, A. S., & Cordova, J. V. (2016). Motivating action and maintaining change: The time-varying role of homework following a brief couples' intervention. *Journal of Marital and Family Therapy*, *42*(3), 396-408. https://doi.org/10.1111/jmft.12142

Hertlein, K. M., Gambescia, N., & Weeks, G. R. (Eds.). (2020). *Systemic sex therapy* (3rd ed.). Routledge.

Hertlein, K. M., Weeks, G. R., & Gambescia, N. (2007). The treatment of hypoactive sexual desire disorder: An Intersystem approach. In L. VandeCreek, F. L. Peterson, & J. Bley (Eds.), *Innovations in clinical practice: Focus on sexual health* (pp. 75-92). Sarasota, FL: Professional Resource Press.

Hertlein, K.M., Weeks, G.R., Gambescia, N. (Eds.). (2009). *Systemic sex therapy*, Routledge.

Jensen, A., Fee, C., Miles, A. L., Beckner, V. L., Owen, D., & Persons, J. B. (2020). Congruence of patient takeaways and homework assignment content predicts homework compliance in psychotherapy. *Behavior Therapy*, *51*(3), 424-433. https://doi.org/10.1016/j.beth.2019.07.005

Johnson, B. H., Palmer, L., & Foley, D. (2010). PIH5 diagnosis and treatment of women with hypoactive sexual desire disorder and depression/anxiety. *Value in Health*, *13*(3), A181-A181. https://doi.org/10.1016/S1098-3015(10)72882-5

Kalmbach, D. A., Kingsberg, S. A., & Ciesla, J. A. (2014). How changes in depression and anxiety symptoms correspond to variations in female sexual response in a nonclinical sample of young women: A daily diary study. *Journal of Sexual Medicine*, *11*(12), 2915-2927. https://doi.org/10.1111/jsm.12692

Kalmbach, D. A., & Pillai, V. (2014). Daily affect and female sexual function. *Journal of Sexual Medicine*, *11*(12), 2938-2954. https://doi.org/10.1111/jsm.12712

Kazantzis, N., & L'Abate, L. (2007). Introduction and historical overview. In N. Kazantzis & L. L'Abate (Eds.), *Handbook of homework assignments in psychotherapy: Research, practice, and prevention* (pp. 1-16). Springer.

Kocsis, A., & Newbury-Helps, J. (2016). Mindfulness in sex therapy and intimate relationships (MSIR): Clinical protocol and theory development. *Mindfulness*, *7*(3), 690-699. https://doi.org/10.1007/s12671-016-0506-z

Kolivand, M., Allahyari, P., Namdari, A., & Rahmani, K. (2021). The effect of cognitive-behavioral counseling on the sexual compatibility: A clinical trial study. *Current Psychology (New Brunswick, NJ)*. https://doi.org/10.1007/s12144-021-02289-z

Lara, L. A. da S., Duarte, A. A. F., Reis, R. M., Vieira, C. S., & de Sá Rosa-e-Silva, A. C. J. (2012). Endocrine disrupters: Potential risk factors affecting sexual function in both men and women. *Journal of Sexual Medicine*, *9*(3), 941-942. https://doi.org/10.1111/j.1743-6109.2011.02596.x

Lerner, H. (1989). *The dance of anger*. HarperCollins.

Lewis, R. W., Fugl Meyer, K. S., Corona, G., Hayes, R. D., Laumann, E. O., Moreira, E. D., Jr., . . . Segraves, T., (2010). Definitions/epidemiology/risk factors for sexual dysfunction. *The Journal of Sexual Medicine,* *7*(4pt2), 1598-1607. https://doi.org/10.1111/j.1743-6109.2010.01778.x

Malary, M., Khani, S., Pourasghar, M., Moosazadeh, M., & Hamzehgardeshi, Z. (2015). Biopsychosocial determinants of hypoactive sexual desire in women: A narrative review. *Materia Socio-Medica*, *27*(6), 383-389. https://doi.org/10.5455/msm.2015.27.383-389

Malmborg, A., Persson, E., Brynhildsen, J., & Hammar, M. (2016). Hormonal contraception and sexual desire: A questionnaire-based study of young Swedish women. *The European Journal of Contraception & Reproductive Health Care, 21*(2), 158-167. https://doi.org/10.3109/13625187.2015.1079609

McKay, M., Davis, M., & Fanning, P. (2018). *Messages: The communications skills book* (4th ed.). New Harbinger Publications.

Meana, M., & Steiner, E. (2014). Sex therapy in transition: Are we there yet? In Y. M. Binik & K. S. K. Hall (Eds.), *Principles and practice of sex therapy* (5th ed., pp. 541-557). Guilford Press.

Meston, S., & Stanton, A. (2017). Treatment of female sexual interest/arousal disorder. In W. IsHak (Ed.), *The textbook of clinical sexual medicine* (pp.165-168). Springer. https://doi.org/10.1007/978-3-319-52539-6_11

Montemurro, B., & Riehman-Murphy, C. (2019). Ready and waiting: Heterosexual men's decision-making narratives in initiation of sexual intimacy. *Men and Masculinities, 22*(5), 872-892.

Muise, A., Boudreau, G. K., & Rosen, N. O. (2017). Seeking connection versus avoiding disappointment: An experimental manipulation of approach and avoidance sexual goals and the implications for desire and satisfaction. *Journal of Sex Research, 54,* 296-307.

Neilson, E., Maitland, D. W. M., & George, W. H. (2022). Power-related emotions, alcohol intoxication, and nonconsensual sex intentions: The role of fear of intimacy. *Sexual Abuse: A Journal of Research and Treatment.* Advance online publication. https://doi.org/10.1177/10790632221096420

Offman, A., & Matheson, K. (2005). Sexual compatibility and sexual functioning in intimate relationships. *The Canadian Journal of Human Sexuality, 14*(1-2), 31-39.

O'Loughlin, J. I., & Brotto, L. A. (2020). Women's Sexual desire, trauma exposure, and posttraumatic stress disorder. *Journal of Traumatic Stress*, *33*(3), 238-247. https://doi.org/10.1002/jts.22485

Park, T-Y., Koh, E., & Park, Y. (2022). Sex is burdensome: Multiple case study on family therapy for Korean husbands with sexual disorders. *The American Journal of Family Therapy*, *50*(4), 348-367. https://doi.org/10.1080/01926187.2021.1922101

Pascoal, P. M., Raposo, C. F., & Roberto, M. S. (2020). A transdiagnostic approach to sexual distress and sexual pleasure: A preliminary mediation study with repetitive negative thinking. *International Journal of Environmental Research and Public Health*, *17*(21), 7864. https://doi.org/10.3390/ijerph17217864

Pulverman, C. S., & Creech, S. K. (2021). The impact of sexual trauma on the sexual health of women veterans: A comprehensive review. *Trauma, Violence, & Abuse*, *22*(4), 656-671. https://doi.org/10.1177/1524838019870912

Quinn-Nilas, C., Benson, L., Milhausen, R. R., Buchholz, A. C., & Goncalves, M. (2016). The relationship between body image and domains of sexual functioning among heterosexual, emerging adult women. *Sexual Medicine*, *4*(3), e182-e189. https://doi.org/10.1016/j.esxm.2016.02.004

Rashedi, S., Maasoumi, R., Vosoughi, N., & Haghani, S. (2022). The effect of mindfulness-based cognitive-behavioral sex therapy on improving sexual desire disorder, sexual distress, sexual self-disclosure and sexual function in women: A randomized controlled clinical trial. *Journal of Sex & Marital Therapy*, *48*(5), 475-488. https://doi.org/10.1080/0092623X.2021.2008075

Rowland, D. L., & Kolba, T. N. (2018). The burden of sexual problems: Perceived effects on men's and women's sexual partners. *The Journal of Sex Research*, *55*(2), 226-235. https://doi.org/10.1080/00224499.2017.1332153

Rullo, J. E., Sood, R., Fokken, S. C., Sood, A., Frohmader, K. S., Croghan, I. T., . . . Faubion, S. S. (2021). Couples' use of online stress management and resiliency training for sexual health concerns: A randomized controlled trial. *Sexual Medicine*, *9*(4), 100404-100404. https://doi.org/10.1016/j.esxm.2021.100404

Schwartz, M. F., & Southern, S. (2018). An integrative model for treatment of sexual desire disorders. *The Family Journal*, *26*(2), 223-237. https://doi.org/10.1177/1066480718775734

Seftel, A. D. (2018). Re: Testosterone replacement therapy: Improved sexual desire and erectile function in men with Type 2 Diabetes following a 30-week randomized placebo-controlled study. *The Journal of Urology*, *199*(3), 597-597. https://doi.org/10.1016/j.juro.2017.12.029

Shirazi, T. N., Self, H., Dawood, K., Rosenfield, K. A., Penke, L., Carré, J. M., . . . Puts, D. A. (2019). Hormonal predictors of women's sexual motivation. *Evolution and Human Behavior*, *40*(3), 336-344. https://doi.org/10.1016/j.evolhumbehav.2019.02.002

Steelman, S. M., & Hertlein, K. M. (2016). Underexplored identities: Attending to asexuality in therapeutic contexts. *Journal of Family Psychotherapy, 27*(2), 85-98. https://doi.org/10.1080/08975353.2016.1169014

Sternberg, R. (1986). A triangular theory of love. *Psychological Review, 93*, 119-135.

Strong, S., & Claiborn, C. (1982). *Change through interaction: Social psychological processes of counseling and psychotherapy*. Wiley.

Taylor, M. J., Rudkin, L., Bullemor-Day, P., Lubin, J., Chukwujekwu, C., Hawton, K., & Taylor, M. J. (2013). Strategies for managing sexual dysfunction induced by antidepressant medication. *Cochrane Database of Systematic Reviews, 2013*(5), CD003382–CD003382. https://doi.org/10.1002/14651858.CD003382.pub3

Thomas, G., & Fletcher, G. J. O. (2003). Mind-reading accuracy in intimate relationships: Assessing the roles of the relationship, the target, and the judge. *Journal of Personality and Social Psychology, 85*(6), 1079-1094.

Thornton, K., Chervenak, J., & Neal-Perry, G. (2015). Menopause and sexuality. *Endocrinology and Metabolism Clinics of North America, 44*(3), 649-661. https://doi.org/10.1016/j.ecl.2015.05.009

Trovão, J. N., & Serefoglu, E. C. (2018). Neurobiology of male sexual dysfunctions in psychiatric disorders: The cases of depression, anxiety, mania and schizophrenia. *International Journal of Impotence Research, 30*(6), 279-286. https://doi.org/10.1038/s41443-018-0077-8

Trudel, G., Ravart, M., & Matte, B. (1993). The use of the multiaxial diagnostic system for sexual dysfunctions in the assessment of hypoactive sexual desire. *Journal of Sex and Marital Therapy, 19*, 123-130.

Van Lankveld, J., Dewitte, M., Thewissen, V., Jacobs, N., & Verboon, P. (2022). Predicting sexual desire in daily life from an attachment perspective: An experience sampling study. *Journal of Sex & Marital Therapy, 47*(4), 311-324. https://doi.org/10.1080/0092623X.2020.1871141

Vowels, L., & Mark, K. P. (2020). Relationship and sexual satisfaction: A longitudinal actor-partner interdependence model approach. *Sexual and Relationship Therapy, 35*(1), 46-59. https://doi.org/10.1080/14681994.2018.1441991

Weeks, G. R. (1987). Systemic treatment of inhibited sexual desire. In G. Weeks & L. Hof (Eds.), *Integrating sex and marital therapy: A clinical guide* (pp. 183-201). Brunner/Mazel.

Weeks, G. R. (1994). The Intersystem model: An integrative approach to treatment. In G. Weeks & L. Hof (Eds.), *The marital- relationship casebook: Theory and application of the Intersystem model* (pp. 3-34). Brunner/Mazel.

Weeks, G. R. (2004). The emergence of a new paradigm in sex therapy: Integration. *Sexual and Relationship Therapy, 20*(1), 89-103.

Weeks, G. R., & Fife, S. (2014). *Couples in treatment: Techniques and approaches for effective practice.* Routledge.

Weeks, G. R., & Gambescia, N. (2002). *Hypoactive sexual desire: Integrating sex and couple therapy*. W.W. Norton.

Weeks, G. R., & Gambescia, N. (2015). Definition, etiology, and treatment of absent/low desire in women. In K. M. Hertlein, G. R. Weeks, & N. Gambescia (Eds.), *Systemic sex therapy* (pp. 125-151). Routledge/Taylor & Francis Group.

Weeks, Gambescia, N., & Hertlein, K. M. (2016). *A systemic guide to clinician sex therapy* (2nd ed.). Routledge.

Weeks, G.R., Gambescia, N., Hertlein, K.M.. (2020). *A clinician's guide to systemic sex therapy.* Taylor & Francis.

Weeks, G. R., Hertlein, K. M., & Gambescia, N. (2009). The treatment of hypoactive sexual desire disorder. In K. M. Hertlein, G. R. Weeks, & N. Gambescia's (Eds.), *Systemic sex therapy* (pp. 82-106). Routledge.

Weeks, G. R., & L'Abate, L. (1982). *Paradoxical psychotherapy: Theory and practice with individuals, couples, and families*. Brunner/Mazel.

Weeks, G. R., & Treat, S. (2001). *Couples in treatment: Techniques and approaches for effective practice* (rev. ed.). Brunner/Mazel.

13

Female Sexual Arousal and Orgasm: Pleasures and Problems

Belinda J. Chaffins

INTRODUCTION

A mere 70 years ago, the topic of healthy female sexual arousal and orgasm was hardly discussed in public, medical schools, or any branch of science. One exception was in psychiatry where an academic focus was on "female frigidity." Today, female sexual arousal and orgasm are incredibly important topics, as these aspects of female sexual health continue to evolve as significant areas of research and healthcare delivery in the first decades of the 21st century. This chapter gives an overview of the topic and references many clinically useful resources. It also reviews key areas of the topic, including how female sexual arousal and orgasm is represented in the *Diagnostic and Statistical Manual of Mental Disorders*. It includes an abbreviated summary of the most important historical contributions to our understanding of female sexuality, some brief notes regarding female anatomy and physiology, considerations regarding the clinical presentation of female sexual arousal/orgasm problems, and finally reviews treatment options across the spectrum of interdisciplinary perspectives. The chapter is written with a balanced view of healthy female sexual health and how to address challenges some women have in their endeavor to have a positive sexual image and rewarding sexual life. As this chapter begins, let us be reminded by one of the leading figures in the science of female sexuality, Beverly Whipple: "Be cautious diagnosing women with sexual disorders as there is much more we do not know about female sexuality than what we do know" (AASECT National Conference, Monterey, California 2014).

CURRENT THINKING ABOUT FEMALE SEXUAL PROBLEMS

Since the beginning of the "Sexual Revolution" of the 1960s and the invention of the birth control pill, women have been able to feel less anxiety about the possibility of pregnancy with intercourse. Has the pill contributed to women experiencing greater sexual satisfaction including arousal and orgasm? Prior to the 1960s, there was a paucity of empirical research on the subject of women's satisfaction beyond gender-biased psychiatric studies of the "problem of female frigidity." Change occurred when The National Health and Social Life Survey was started in 1957 for the purpose of securing accurate information on illness and disability. The survey included questions about the distribution and effects of illness and disability on sexuality. The survey also attempted to gain insight into how women feel about their own sexual experiences. The results indicated that 43% of American women between the ages of 18 and 59 reported having a sexual dysfunction (Michael et al., 1994).

Since the publication of the survey in 1957, many sex therapists expressed concerns regarding the results. One concern was that identification and definitions of female sexual dysfunctions have changed over time. The first *Diagnostic and Statistical Manual of Mental Disorders* (*DSM*; American Psychiatric Association) was published in 1952. With each new revision of the *DSM*, some female sexual dysfunctions were eliminated, others added and still others, redefined. The *DSM-III-R* (American Psychiatric Association, 1987) renamed Inhibited Sexual Desire to Hypoactive Sexual Desire Disorder. The latest edition, *DSM*-5, published in 2013, includes the diagnoses of Female Orgasmic Disorder and Female Sexual Interest/Arousal Disorder. Changes in understanding of women's sexuality through research and advances in technology and medicine have led to an awareness of how complex women's experiences of their own sexuality are continuing to be discovered.

The last revision of the *DSM* is not without flaws. Consider the woman who has never had an orgasm in her lifetime. According to the *DSM-5*, this occurs in about 10% of women. Further, consider the diagnosis of Female Sexual Interest/Arousal Disorder. Some women who report these "disorders" do not consider them a problem. For example, older women report less distress about low sexual desire than younger women. A common dilemma for many clinicians is treating couples with an issue of desire discrepancy. If her lower desire or lack of desire is not problematic for her, but her partner is distressed by it, who has the problem? How does a clinician treat the couple? It is important to understand, as a clinician, that sexual problems for an individual or couple are usually very complex. This is especially true for cases involving sexual dysfunction related to low or no sexual desire because of the multitude of variables influencing libido levels. Hence, a clinician needs to always keep in mind that sexual concerns for an individual or couple are almost never "just about sex." Therefore, taking a thorough biopsychosocial assessment is essential (as described in Chapter 2).

MAJOR EVENTS IN SEX RESEARCH AND THEORY REGARDING THE EVOLVING MODELS OF FEMALE SEXUAL RESPONSE

The field of sex therapy has been impacted by several noteworthy researchers over time. Each has made significant contributions by increasing the depth of knowledge and understanding of the human sexual experience, especially female responsiveness and what people actually do sexually. Professionals from many different areas of expertise including physicians, midwives, nurses, psychiatrists, psychologists, social workers, and zoologists have contributed to these advances. Sex research has also been influenced by social factors and innovations in technology and medicine. Over the years, the role of the clitoris has been brought to the forefront and then forgotten again, diminished, improperly illustrated, or omitted from textbooks. Women's genitalia including the words vagina, vulva, and clitoris have been absent from language in the media and education. However, proper naming of men's genitalia is more common and accepted, including the words penis, scrotum, and testicles.

A comprehensive list of sex researchers who have contributed to the understanding of female sexuality is well beyond the scope of this chapter. However, reading through the following brief summaries about notable researchers will help you appreciate the incredible body of science there is on women's sexuality as well as familiarize you with some of the key players.

Sigmund Freud

Including Freud as a contributor to the understanding of female sexuality is quite divisive, especially for women, as his contributions have to be weighed against the damage done by what are widely accepted as discredited misogynistic notions which are not based on science. Historically, Freud's work stated that the clitoris is "analogous to the male organ," however, an inferior sexual organ that does not serve a purpose (1931). Empirically, just the opposite is true as it is the only human organ solely dedicated to pleasure and serves an important basis for what is generally considered female sexual superiority over men. Freud believed that a woman should give up clitoral stimulation and switch to vaginal orgasms exclusively in order to become a "fully matured adult." Worst of all, his belief that women's reports of incest by their fathers were really representing their fantasies of having a penis (penis envy). Freud's theories about female and childhood sexuality have caused immeasurable suffering for women at the hands of some practitioners who utilize traditional psychoanalysis and psychoanalytically oriented psychotherapy. Many of today's therapists, especially older ones, have had the experience of treating women clients for sexual dysfunction and/or incest and who have a history of wasting much time and money being treated psychoanalytically. In addition, many of these women felt shame and guilt about their sexuality, in part due to having their incest memories literally ignored by their psychoanalytically trained therapist. In the field of sexual health, it is widely accepted that the women's movement of the 1970s introduced positive changes to start to repair the damage from Freud's views of female sexuality. Concurrently, the 1970s became a time of reexamination of the topic of child sexual abuse and the start of serious research on the topic after Freud's declarations, 80 years earlier, that memories and reports of childhood sexual abuse were mere fantasy.

At the same time, the effects of Freud's work also made some general positive impacts in society by bringing the topic of sexuality within accepted American public discourse and helping normalize sexuality as part of life. Freud is also credited for popularizing the idea of the "talking cure" and planting the seeds for the fields of counseling and therapy that we know today. Around the beginning of the 20th century, however, views of children's sexuality started changing due to the impacts of experts from many different disciplines. Prior to 1900, children's sexuality, especially masturbation, was viewed as pathological (Sauerteig, 2012) and a disease that required treatment (Peterson et al., 2020). Freud and other theorists debated this notion and Freud promoted the idea that sexuality is a normal part of childhood for both boys and girls. While Freud described the clitoris as an inferior sexual organ that does not serve a purpose, he also identified the clitoris as females' "leading genital zone" (Freud, 1931). As previously noted, he theorized that a woman's sexual life is divided between the clitoris and the vagina. The first was identified as masculine, analogous to the penis and the second as feminine. He postulated that females have an Electra complex and that she has to ("needs to/should") acknowledge males as superior. Furthermore, Freud believed women should give up masturbatory activity of the clitoris as it was viewed as inferior. He believed that if she didn't move toward the vagina as her primary source of sexuality, then she was considered "immature" or a lesbian. He did acknowledge that the clitoris continues to function throughout a woman's life in a way that was not understood at that time (Freud, 1931). In other words, Freud identified that the clitoris was likely a powerful part of a woman's sexuality and that he didn't understand its biological basis (true on both accounts)!

Marie Bonaparte

Marie Bonaparte, a descendant of the imperial Bonaparte lineage, was another controversial figure in the history of research of women's sexual health. She was profoundly interested in the study of medicine but forbade from pursuing it due to concerns it would lead to difficulty in securing her a prestigious marriage and improving the family's status (Moore, 2009). Bonaparte was a student of Freud's and associated with the expansion of psychoanalytic theory (Thompson, 2003). Additionally, in the 1920s, she was in therapy for 2 years with Sigmund Freud. She was conflicted by her intellectual pursuits, beliefs about her own "frigidity," and the social expectations of women in 1920s France. Bonaparte saw herself as "frigid" due to the teachings of Sigmund Freud, however, also recognized the importance of the clitoris in female sexual pleasure (Moore, 2009). She tried to conform to the social norms at the time, however, she also wanted to reduce the gender discrepancy of pleasure. Bonaparte knew she experienced desire but had difficulty experiencing orgasms through intercourse alone, which was not understood at the time. Bonaparte measured the distance between the underside of a woman's clitoral glans and the center of the urethral meatus of 200 women and published her research. She proposed that a shorter distance between the clitoral glans and urethral meatus resulted in a higher percentage of orgasms through intercourse alone. She believed this so strongly she had surgery to reposition the clitoris three times and all attempts were ineffective (Wallen & Lloyd, 2011). A total of five women had the surgical procedure and none found it helpful. Unfortunately, the notion that women who do not experience vaginal orgasms (or orgasms through intercourse only) are not mature, are less mentally healthy, or are inadequate in some way is still a myth perpetuated over 100 years after Freud first proposed this theory.

Alfred Kinsey

From the 1930s through the 1950s, Alfred Kinsey was a biologist and professor of entomology, zoology, and early sexologist (one who studies human sexuality empirically) at Indiana University. He conducted extensive research (based on 3- to 4-hour interviews) to find out what men and women actually do during their sexual behavior. His work, along with his colleagues Pomeroy, Martin, and Gebhard, created a new understanding, albeit with controversy, of what women do sexually with themselves as well as with others. Kinsey was one of the very first to use a scientific survey to gather information about human sexual behavior. Many experts before him had theories but had not actually developed scientific surveys to base their results. His groundbreaking book, *Sexual Behavior in the Human Female*, published in 1953, was a culmination of interviewing nearly 8,000 females who provided information regarding the types of sexual activity in which women engaged, from masturbation, nocturnal sex dreams, premarital coitus, extramarital coitus, same-sex contacts, and animal contacts. The findings were groundbreaking at the time. Kinsey also studied the physiologic, psychologic, hormonal, and neural factors that contribute to sexual responses. Results educated the American public that females were more similar to males than previously thought and different than the conventional mores of the time. His work disputed the idea that women are not sexual and also that vaginal orgasms were superior to clitoral orgasms as Freud had proposed. Results helped shed light on the incidence of same-sex arousal, sexual contact, and orgasm with other females. The female sample reported that by age 30, 25% experienced arousal, 17% reported sexual contact, and about 10% reported orgasm with another female (Kinsey et al., 1953). Kinsey also found that women's first erotic arousal and orgasm was achieved by masturbation, not contact with another male or female, with rates by about 27% for arousal and 40% for orgasm. Furthermore, and a fascinating finding, 2% of the women reported that no physical stimulation was needed at all to have orgasms. These women can experience orgasms by fantasy alone. This seems to indicate it is important for a woman to know her own body, where and what type of touch she finds pleasurable, and what type of thoughts or fantasies arouse her. She cannot expect her partner to know what she likes and "give" her an orgasm if she doesn't know her own body. Survey results showed 9% of the women in their late 40s had never experienced an orgasm. Kinsey's survey results are consistent with current statistics from the *DSM-5*. Additionally, he developed the Kinsey Scale to help people understand the broader spectrum of natural sexual expression through a range of sexual orientation between complete (100%) heterosexuality to complete (100%) same-sex interest, on a continuum from 0 (100% heterosexual) to 3 (equally attracted to men and women) to 6 (100% gay/lesbian).

Masters and Johnson

William Masters (an American gynecologist) and Virginia Johnson (a sexologist researcher) developed a model of sexual response in the 1960s based on the laboratory observation and physiologic measurement of over 10,000 orgasms. Their work was revolutionary in that they developed instruments to measure sexual responses (such as galvanic skin response) and used cameras to record changes to the vaginal linings of women during sexual arousal and orgasm (Masters & Johnson, 1966). Using this technology and method, they learned that the vaginal walls lubricate by forming small beads of moisture as a female becomes more aroused through sexual stimulation. This process of the formation of vaginal lubrication during sexual arousal is called transudation. This is just one of many scientific discoveries made at the Masters and Johnson Institute, which served as the basis for Tom Maier's book *The Masters of Sex* (2009) and the SHOWTIME series of the same name (2013-2016).

The Masters and Johnson model of sexual response includes four stages of what they described as the "sexual response cycle": Excitement, plateau, orgasm, and resolution. Their published work, *Human Sexual Response* (1966) was the culmination of 11 years of research in the world's first sex laboratory. They studied 312 men and 382 women, many of them married couples. However, they studied an estimated three times as many female sexual response cycles compared to men! This is an example of the complexity and underestimated capacity of women's sexual response.

The women in the study were mostly younger and well educated, with 84% of the women between ages 18 and 40 and many who had advanced levels of education. This was not surprising as much of their subject recruitment was from college campuses. Subjects were both married and single men and women in an attempt to determine differences in sexual response comparing the same married and single men and women. This research was discontinued as they quickly learned there was no difference in the anatomy and physiology of the human sexual response in regard to marital status. Interestingly, Masters and Johnson found many more similarities than differences in the physiologic sexual responses between men and women. One exception was they found women were much more able to have multiple orgasms and to be able to orgasm by fantasy alone.

The Masters and Johnson model was later criticized for being too simplistic, too phallocentric, and did not explain female arousal adequately even though they studied three times as many female sexual response cycles. Masters and Johnson acknowledged the female pattern of sexual responsiveness has "an infinite variety" compared to males (more evidence of female sexual complexity and power). However, they identified three patterns of women's sexual responsiveness in their book for brevity (which will not be described here also for brevity's sake). Masters and Johnson also studied the geriatric population, up to age 89, and concluded that increased age does not mean an end to gratifying sexual experiences for women!

Masters and Johnson identified the clitoris as having a dual role as both a receptor and transformer of sexual stimulation. Through their research, they determined clitoral and vaginal orgasms are not biologically different based upon their physiologic measures. They advocated for postmenopausal women to continue to behave as sexual beings understanding that there is no expiration date on female sexual pleasure. They suggested younger women can benefit from sex education to help increase women's sexual knowledge and acceptance. Excellent sexual health resources for women of any age include *For Yourself: The Fulfillment of Female Sexuality* (Barbach, 1975), *Reclaiming Your Sexual Self: How You Can Bring Desire Back Into Your Life* (Hall, 2004), *Come as You Are: The Surprising New Science That Will Transform Your Sex Life* (Nagoski, 2015), *Guide to Getting it On!* (Joannides, 2017), *The Gender Revolution & New Sexual Health* (Peterson et al., 2020), and *Read My Lips: A Complete Guide to the Vagina and Vulva* (Herbenick & Schick, 2011). The last book (*Read My Lips*) is dedicated to the sexual literacy and health of everybody and was written for "anyone who has a vulva, loves someone with a vulva, has come out of a vagina, or is just curious about these parts" (Herbenick & Schick, 2011, p. xiv).

Shere Hite

Shere Hite was an American and German researcher who wrote the *Hite Report: A Nationwide Study of Female Sexuality*, a culmination of 4 years of work and published in 1976. She analyzed over 3,000 questionnaires from women all over the United States. She wanted to find out women's experiences, in their own words. The questionnaire contained 58 items in five general areas: Orgasm, Sexual Activities, Relationships, Life Stages, and the final section titled "The Ending" that included a potpourri of items including questions about faking orgasms, fellatio, fantasizing during masturbation or with a partner during sex, sadomasochistic behaviors, and thoughts about the sexual revolution. Women described how they masturbate, what arousal feels like, what orgasm feels like, if they experienced more than one type of orgasm, and frequency of activities including intercourse, masturbation, and so forth. Most women in the study did not report orgasm through intercourse alone. Only about 30% of the sample reported orgasm regularly through intercourse, however, this statistic may be elevated for a few reasons. Hite cited that the women who had a "questionable orgasm" definition were also included; women don't want to appear frigid or feel pressure to say they had an orgasm and likely didn't; and some women had a different definition of intercourse, thinking all sexual activities were included in the definition. The rate of women who never experienced orgasm was 11.6% (Hite, 1976). Hite's work was very important at the time because it gave women the opportunity to provide information from their own experience rather than the usual male (patriarchal) perspective. She included items on lesbianism which helped normalize same-sex interest, activity, and relationships. Information regarding older women was included, normalizing menopausal women who were also interested in sex (with some expressing their satisfaction and experiences that had improved through the decades). One of the final chapters in her book examines the importance of a new female sexuality, acknowledging that women's sexuality was changing. During the 1970s, women were more independent, working outside the home and asserting their needs and interests. Sex was no longer just about intercourse and pleasing her male partner. More women learned it was normal to be interested in gaining pleasure for herself, either by herself or with a partner without the demand for orgasm. The "goal" can simply be the experience of pleasure and doesn't have to include intercourse or orgasm.

Helen Singer Kaplan

Helen Singer Kapan was an American psychiatrist who introduced the concept of desire into her model of normal sexual response in 1979. She proposed that desire leads to arousal, then plateau, orgasm, and resolution. Her seminal work was *The New Sex Therapy*, published in 1974. Kaplan was a sex therapist who developed the first clinic in the U.S. for sexual disorders at a medical school. She advocated that people should enjoy sex and that it was not dirty or harmful. She wrote that from her clinical experience, about 9% to 10% of the female population had never experienced orgasm and those women who do not orgasm during intercourse do not have a sexual disorder. She dispelled the idea that coital orgasm is superior compared to clitoral orgasm. She advocated that women can masturbate and take responsibility for their own sensations and arousal.

Kaplan also identified that women are capable of multiple orgasms throughout their lifetime. The women may not necessarily always want to have multiple orgasms with every sexual encounter, however, they are capable if interested. Additionally, Kaplan reported that female sexual responsiveness is much more variable compared to males. She proposed that for women who experience orgasmic dysfunction, treatment may include (a) Masturbation, (b) Use of a vibrator, (c) Resolution of fears of orgasm, (d) Distraction – to avoid "spectatoring" (allowing doubts and fear to interfere with your sexual pleasure and activity) by use of erotic fantasy, (e) Muscular Factors via awareness of contraction of vaginal and abdominal muscles to facilitate orgasm, and (f) Transfer orgasm to an interpersonal situation – after she has been able to learn how to consistently bring herself to orgasm.

Finally, Kaplan is the originator of the Sexual Tipping Point (STP) which was further developed by her colleague Michael Perelman. The STP model is described in detail in Chapter 9.

David Reed

David Reed was an American psychiatrist who proposed the Erotic Stimulus Pathway Model in 1989. This model of sexual responsiveness is often thought of as the "psychological stages" that accompany the physiological changes in the body during the sexual response cycle of Masters and Johnson (arousal, plateau, orgasm, and resolution). The Erotic Stimulus Pathway Model is comprised of (a) Seduction, (b) Sensation, (c) Surrender, and (d) Reflection (Stayton et al., 2005). The Surrender stage is about complete focusing on pleasure of the body and getting out of one's head. It may or may not involve or end with orgasm. The Reflection stage means contemplating questions such as *Did she enjoy the experience? Is this something she wants to do again? Does she want to be with this partner again?*

Beverly Whipple

In 1997, American sexologist Beverly Whipple proposed a more circular model of women's sexual arousal which is considered more nonlinear than previous theories. Whipple proposed that women's sexuality and sexual responses are complex and vastly different from men's response. Furthermore, she identified that women may not experience all of the phases of sexual response described in previous models. A woman may not experience sexual desire. However, she may experience arousal, orgasm, and satisfaction or a woman may experience desire, arousal, satisfaction, but not orgasm. Her work builds upon Reed's model (Seduction, Sensation, Surrender, and Reflection) by asserting that if a woman enjoys her sexual experience, it can lead to the seduction phase at the next experience in a circular fashion. More importantly, she expanded Reed's Erotic Stimulus Pathway Model to include nuanced features such as women's capacity to experience pleasure whether or not orgasm is present, and that this capacity is not a mandate to experience orgasm. While Whipple asserts that orgasm is not the be-all-end-all goal of sex, she is also the author (along with colleagues) of two ground-breaking books on the subject of orgasms: *The G-Spot* (with co-authors Alice Kahn Ladas and John Perry, 1982) and *The Science of Orgasm* (with co-authors Barry Komisaruk and Carlos Beyer-Flores, 2006).

Rosemary Basson

Rosemary Basson is a Canadian psychiatrist and sexologist who proposed a new circular model with no hierarchy and emphasizing the context of the relationship in which a woman is experiencing sex (Basson, 2000). She asserted that women experience orgasm very differently than proposed by Masters and Johnson. Basson's intimacy-based model proposed that women experience phases of sexual response in a manner that is not sequential as described by researchers and theorists in the past. She offered that women initiate or respond to sexual encounters for a variety of reasons including intimacy, commitment to her partner, and wanting to feel physically or emotionally close to or express that she cares for her partner. Like Whipple and others, she stressed that feeling "sexually satisfied" does not necessarily have to include orgasm. Another important reason Basson stressed women's variety of sexual responses is for the development of different treatment modalities relative to her assertion that intimacy needs are more important to women and that orgasmic response for women is highly variable compared to men. She indicated that women's sexual response may comprise of a single, multiple, or an extended orgasm. She may report a sense of well-being following the encounter, with or without an orgasm. She indicated that some women do not experience spontaneous desire and should be reassured they are normal. Basson also discussed the role of sexual guilt, interpersonal difficulties, nonsexual distractions, and "spectatoring" on a woman's arousal or lack thereof. She emphasizes the importance of normalizing a variety of women's experiences, especially if the woman feels satisfied and is not in distress regarding her experiences. This allows the questions: *Is anything really wrong? Does she really have a dysfunction or is this a factor of her partner's distress?*

Julia Heiman and Joseph LoPiccolo

American psychologists and sex researchers Julia Heiman and Joseph LoPiccolo developed an effective and widely acclaimed treatment program for women with difficulties concerning sexual arousal. Their program *Becoming Orgasmic* is a combined book/video set which was originally published in 1976 and updated in 1988, and is still commonly used in the field of sex therapy. Some of the best features of the *Becoming Orgasmic* program are that it is a "do-it-yourself" approach to resolving sexual difficulties and can be accomplished in the personal privacy of a woman's home and at her own pace of treatment (although doing the program in conjunction with consultation from a sex therapist is best). Either way, the program has been proven effective and is comprised of three stages of progression generally referred to as (a) Self-exploration, (b) Self-pleasuring, and (c) Self-sharing. A woman experiencing sexual dissatisfaction (with her ability to become aroused and/or climax) can go through the program solo or invite a partner to participate in the third stage of "self-sharing" (Heiman & LoPiccolo, 1988).

Michael Metz and Barry McCarthy

Michael Metz and Barry McCarthy are American psychologists and sex therapists that contributed much to the development of integrated sex and marital therapy. They proposed the *Good Enough Sex Model* in 2008 as a set of guidelines for maintaining sexual desire in long-term relationships. The Good Enough Sex (GES) model was originally developed for married couples in their 50s and beyond who experience erectile dysfunction and/or sexual avoidance behaviors (McCarthy & Farr, 2012). Four key factors in the GES model include: Sexual expression is foremost about giving and receiving pleasure-oriented touching; finding a comfortable level of intimacy for both; erotic scenarios and techniques; and lastly, develop positive, realistic sexual expectations (Metz & McCarthy, 2011). The GES model stresses that a person can be sexual for their lifetime, so couples do not have to throw away their active sex life just because she has gone through menopause or they are out of their childbearing years.

A VERY BRIEF NOTE ON THE ANATOMY AND PHYSIOLOGY OF FEMALE SEXUAL AROUSAL

Of course, an in-depth description of the anatomy and physiology of the vulva and internal reproductive system is far beyond the scope of this chapter. However, like the topic of research on female sexuality, there are some important notes that need to be highlighted. Female sexual interest/arousal difficulties are more difficult to observe and measure than male arousal problems, in part due to biology and in part due to our long history of repression of female sexual expression (and less awareness of the same). When a healthy male becomes aroused, he gets an erection. If he has some type of male arousal problem, it is often noticed via erectile dysfunction and it is much easier to evaluate. When a woman becomes aroused, her vaginal walls begin to lubricate and the clitoris swells. Due to these structures being almost entirely internal, it can be more difficult to observe and measure.

Women will naturally experience spontaneous or responsive sexual desire and arousal due to a combination of neural, endocrinological, and psychosocial influences. The solo function of the clitoris is pleasure, and it contains over 8000 nerve endings. The part of the clitoris that can be seen outside the body is a relatively small part of clitoral organ, which is somewhat of a wishbone shape. The visible parts of the clitoris are the tip or glans of the clitoris and the clitoral hood that covers it. The clitoris is comprised of three sections: The glans, the body, and the crura. The glans and body are a total of 2 to 4 cm long and the crura or base are each 5 to 9 cm long. Helen O'Connell used an MRI in the 1990s to investigate the characteristics of healthy normal clitoral anatomy (O'Connell et al., 1998; O'Connell & DeLancey, 2005). MRI imagery was consistent and complemented dissections performed on cadavers. The MRI results even necessitated updated changes in *Gray's Anatomy* textbooks and the one-dimensional teaching approach used with medical students regarding the clitoris.

Similarly, hormones have been recently discovered to play a role in arousal and orgasm for women. Nitric oxide is a naturally occurring chemical compound that is found in women's bodies and plays an important role for women's vaginal vasocongestion. Endocannabinoids are chemicals in the body that, when released, help to decrease symptoms of pain and increase the body's "feel-good self-medication." A recent study shows that masturbation to orgasm stimulates the release of endocannabinoids for women, which may contribute to rewarding and reinforcing these behaviors (Fuss et al., 2017).

CLINICAL PRESENTATIONS OF FEMALE SEXUAL AROUSAL PROBLEMS

Female sexual arousal involves what is happening in the body and how the woman feels about the physical sensations. Is she enjoying them? Is she repulsed? She may have a partner who she enjoys responding to or with whom she feels comfortable initiating sex. She may also have a history of sexual abuse which would likely decrease these behaviors and increase avoidance behaviors. The bottom line is this: *Does she see her body's sexual responsiveness (or lack of) as a problem?* This question circles back to Basson's question: *Does she really have a dysfunction or is this a factor of her partner's distress?* Very often, it is the latter.

Female Sexual Interest/Arousal Disorder is the current arousal disorder listed in the *DSM-5*. The criteria include absent/reduced experiencing of sexual arousal indicators, with at least three of the following five symptoms:

- absent/reduced interest in sexual activity, absent/reduced sexual erotic thoughts or fantasies
- absent/reduced initiation of sexual activity and typically unreceptive to a partner's attempts to initiate
- absent/reduced sexual excitement/pleasure during sexual activity in almost all or all sexual encounters
- absent/reduced sexual interest/arousal in response to any internal or external sexual erotic cues (e.g., written, verbal, or visual)
- absent/reduced genital or nongenital sensations during sexual activity in almost all or all sexual encounters

In addition, the identified symptoms have persisted for a minimum duration of approximately 6 months and the symptoms cause clinically significant distress in the individual. The sexual dysfunction is not better explained by a nonsexual mental disorder or as a consequence of severe relationship distress (e.g., partner violence or other significant stressors) and is not attributable to the effects of a substance/medication or another medical condition. The disorder may be lifelong or acquired, generalized, or situational in that it only occurs with certain types of stimulations, situations, or partners; and severity may vary from mild to severe.

The prevalence of this disorder is unknown and can vary in relation to age, culture, duration of symptoms, or distress. In a study in 1994, 19% of women who were premenopausal between the ages of 18 and 59 reported lubrication difficulties (Laumann et al., 1994). Lubrication is seen as a hallmark in women's arousal. In postmenopausal women, difficulties with lubrication tend to be higher, at 44% in one study (Rosen et al., 1993).

As females age through their 30s and 40s, they usually learn how to be orgasmic, however, many of them do not (approximately 10% according to the *DSM-5*). If a woman learns how to be orgasmic through masturbation and understands what type of touch she enjoys, it may be different with a partner. Results for sexologists found that women vary greatly in the manner in which they masturbate. One study found that approximately 73% of women masturbate their clitoral/vulva area with their hand while lying on their backs (Hite, 1976). Whether she is in a heterosexual or same sex relationship, it is in her best interest to take responsibility for her own orgasm and feel comfortable initiating different forms of self-pleasuring. She can assist her partner in learning what type of touch she finds pleasurable through communication and experimentation. This specific type of communication and learning is facilitated by sensate focus exercises (Peterson et al., 2020).

Sexual arousal and orgasm are normal functions for women and can be part of a woman's self-image. Women who have not experienced orgasm (or do not experience orgasm consistently) may not know what type of touch they like and haven't explored their bodies. In these cases, it is not unusual for some of these women to fake orgasm to get an encounter to end and avoid masturbation or sex play with a partner. A recent study of 1,008 women found that 19.2% had faked orgasm and still fake orgasm. Forty-one percent of these women who report they currently fake orgasm agreed that they would rather not talk about sex with their partner and think it should just come naturally to them (Herbenick et al., 2019). For heterosexual couples, she cannot expect her male partner to be the sexual expert, although this is still a common myth (Hite, 1976). Research does indicate, however, that as a woman ages, she is more likely to have experienced orgasm (Kinsey et al., 1953). Research also shows that women in relationships are more likely to have experienced orgasm (Kinsey et al., 1953).

Women's arousal and orgasmic response can be much more variable than described by Masters and Johnson. Orgasm for women is highly variable compared to men and Basson (2000) pointed out that women's sexual response may be comprised of a single, extended, or multiple orgasm. A woman may compare one orgasm as a "blip" and another as "mind-blowing." Women can report a variety of experiences after years of sexual experience and experimentation. She can learn to maintain tension or bring herself to a higher level of pleasure by a variety of methods such as tensing pelvic muscles, relaxing others, using rocking motions, a variety of positions, and breath work or holding her breath, focusing on physical sensations or use of fantasy.

COMMON BARRIERS AND CHALLENGES TO SEXUAL AROUSAL AND ORGASM

Medications

This is an area of growing concern as the vast majority of psychotropic medications have adverse side effects that can suppress sexual libido, arousal, and orgasm. Please refer to the excellent coverage of this topic in Chapter 5 ("Medications and Sexual Health" by Roa-Navarrete, Taft, and Pagano).

Illness and Disability

This important topic also has its own chapter concerning barriers and challenges to sexual expression faced by people of varied abilities due to illness or medical conditions which may suppress sexual libido, arousal, and orgasm. Please refer to the excellent coverage of this topic in Chapter 22 ("A Liberatory and Intersectional Approach to Sexual Health Care in Partnership With Disability Communities" by Dr. Julie Lynn Williams).

Alcohol

It is of paramount importance to note, foremost, that an individual has to be sober and not under the influences of any mood-altering substances in order to be able to give consent for sexual activity. The definition of sexual health involves consent, and the definition of consensual sex requires clear, explicit, and repeated verbal messages of permission-giving by an individual. When using alcohol or substances (e.g., cocaine, marijuana, or Ecstasy/Molly) an individual cannot do so because judgment is impaired. Alcohol consumption at lower levels (within recommended limits) tends to increase a woman's expectation of increased sexual arousal. However, alcohol at a higher level can lead to sexual dysfunction including reduced lubrication and orgasm (George et al., 2011).

Cocaine, Marijuana, and Other Substances

Cocaine is an illegal substance that has a reputation to be associated with increasing the intensity of orgasms. High doses seem to have the opposite effect. Marijuana seems to increase sexual desire and receptiveness but not result in improved orgasm ability or increased lubrication (Lynn et al., 2019). With the legalization of marijuana in many states and people using it to help relieve symptoms or treat medical conditions, some also use marijuana to help reduce symptoms of anxiety. CBD oil is also used by some to help reduce pain. Methamphetamines and heroin are examples of drugs that are definitely dangerous to one's health, impair judgment, and therefore, impair the ability to consent.

Opioids

Opioids have been prescribed for decades to treat cancer pain, pain from dental procedures, and other postsurgical pain. Increased awareness of long-term use or misuse of these drugs and risks has resulted in more careful prescribing by providers, usually meaning fewer pills per prescription and reduced dose or strength. However, for those women on long-term opioid medications, the results can include diminished libido (a common side effect) with some studies finding results of 69% (Reddy et al., 2010) and vaginal dryness (Grover et al., 2014).

Psychosocial Factors

A woman's arousal and orgasmic potential can be affected by many additional factors. Anxiety; unexpected stressors; and managing multiple responsibilities, roles, and deadlines can lead to difficulties relaxing and focusing on her own pleasure. Symptoms of depression, loss of a family member, or anticipatory grief such as a loved one having a terminal illness can impact mood and energy level. She may feel irritable and lack motivation and energy for intimacy. History of trauma including PTSD; military trauma; sexual, physical, and/or emotional abuse can lead to an aversion of sex and intimacy, especially with long-term or multiple types of trauma. Partner conflict as well as multiple sources of stress can contribute to decreased desire. In traditional heterosexual relationships, many tasks continue to fall upon women including child care, cooking, cleaning, and caregiving responsibilities of elderly family members, regardless of work outside the home. For gay and lesbian couples, a more equitable division of labor and child care responsibilities is the norm.

Negative sexual self-image can also be a concern for many women who are overly critical of their bodies, worrying one part is too small and another too large. Trends regarding what type of body is considered ideal has changed over the millennia. Worries about weight; fitness level; odor; underarm/pubic hair; and size and shape of breasts, buttocks, and vulva have been capitalized by marketers selling expensive weight loss products including diet plans, supplements, powders, pills and food, laser treatments, breast and butt implants, reductions, and lifts. Advertisements target women's insecurities about their body with the promise of feeling confident, sexy, desired, and loved. Women with poor body image may benefit from therapy that focuses on helping her appreciate her body; what her body is capable of; and understanding the range of "normal" in regard to shape, appearance, and size of various parts of her body. Additionally, when working with women who have body image issues, it is important to assess these issues carefully and secure appropriate treatment for those with clinical eating disorders.

CLINICAL TREATMENT OPTIONS FOR WOMEN'S SEXUAL AROUSAL AND ORGASM PROBLEMS

There are a growing number of treatment considerations for clinicians of which they should be knowledgeable when assisting women get to a goal of consistent sexual arousal and orgasm. The following list of treatment considerations are provided for review, including treatment strategies only available through the services of interdisciplinary colleagues. The list is in part based upon the International Society for the Study of Women's Sexual Health Process of Care for the Identification of Sexual Concerns and Problems in Women (Parish et al., 2019).

Hormones

Vaginal/Oral/Transdermal Patch Estrogens are treatment options for genitourinary syndrome of menopause, and women vary in their report of the impact of these treatments on libido and sexual functioning. Some women report a decrease in desire and arousability due to the impact of the exogenous estrogen on other hormones. Other women report a positive effect from the estrogen that may be partly psychological due to feminizing effects of estrogen on the skin, breasts, and vagina, and may also impact mood. Estrogen also stimulates nitric oxide production which is needed for vasocongestion. Progesterone is sometimes added to reduce risk of uterine cancer. Progesterone can also help reduce hot flashes or night sweats associated with menopause, and potentially improve sleep.

Testosterone Therapy is an option some women choose when reporting Hypoactive Sexual Desire Disorder (HSDD). Women may obtain a trial of systemic testosterone, off-label with close monitoring (Krakowsky & Grober, 2018) to evaluate the effects. A meta-analysis of postmenopausal women with low desire treated with testosterone (n = 3,035) demonstrated significant improvements in desire, orgasm, and sexually satisfying events with decreased personal distress. The FDA has not approved a testosterone transdermal patch for treatment of low sexual desire in women. No pharmaceutical formulations or doses have been developed for women at this time.

Medications

Flibanserin (Addyi) was approved, after multiple attempts, for treatment of HSDD by the FDA and with results that indicate limited improvement with this medication. First proposed as the "pink pill" and women's equivalent to Viagra, it is a very different medication. Addyi decreases the neurotransmitter serotonin and increases dopamine and norepinephrine. Addyi must be taken every day at bedtime and is only for premenopausal women. Alcohol is contraindicated with this medication due to risk of hypotension and syncope (Aftab et al., 2017). The most common adverse side effects are dizziness, somnolence, nausea, fatigue, insomnia, and dry mouth. In clinical trials, women reported one additional satisfying sexual event per month when taking the medication. The package insert also requires a Risk Evaluation and Mitigation Strategy (REMS) for the prescriber and the pharmacist. While this medication is only indicated for premenopausal women, it is postmenopausal women who are more likely to experience low desire. It appears more research is indicated, but if interested in obtaining the medication to help with low desire one can seek out an approved provider (who may be difficult to find outside large metropolitan areas). Critics propose that this is a lot of medication to take for only one additional pleasurable experience in one month's time.

Vyleesi (Bremelanotide) is an injection designed for women with low sexual desire. The FDA approved this drug in 2019 to inject in the abdomen or thigh about an hour before sexual activity. Like Addyi, this drug is approved only for premenopausal women with a diagnosis of HSDD. One side effect was nausea in 40% of users in a clinical study (Simon et al., 2019). As anyone would imagine, if a woman is feeling nauseous, she is very unlikely to pursue, continue, or be able to focus on enjoying a sexual experience. About 25% of the women treated with this medication reported an increase of 1.2 or more in their sexual desire score (with the range of 1.2 to 6.0, with higher scores indicating greater sexual desire) compared to 17% of those who took the placebo. No change was found in the number of satisfying events, and it does not enhance sexual performance. Other side effects include increased blood pressure and decreased effectiveness of naltrexone, a drug used to treat opioid dependency. As a result, women with uncontrolled hypertension or prescribed naltrexone are not good candidates for this medication.

Devices and Topical Aids

Mechanical devices such as vibrators are used to enhance vulvar, clitoral, and vaginal stimulation. Electric and battery-operated vibrators are very effective in enhancing women's pleasure and orgasm. It is possible to find any color, size, or shape of vibrator made from different materials and offering various levels of stimulation. Some are designed for clitoral or g-spot stimulation. A woman can purchase small one-use models that are inexpensive, offer varying intensities of vibration, and easily fit in a small purse. Eros, a clitoral therapy vacuum device, was approved by the FDA in 2000 for treatment of female sexual arousal disorder. The device stimulates blood flow to the clitoris and improves sensation, ability to achieve orgasm, sexual satisfaction, and lubrication. One drawback is the device is somewhat expensive, costing approximately $300 and cannot be returned for a refund if dissatisfied.

Lubricants can be used as desired with or without vibrators to reduce friction and enhance comfort during sexual activity. Lubricants come in a variety of forms including water-based, silicone-based, hybrid of water- and silicone-based, and oil-based. It is important to know the benefits and disadvantages of each type. Women are least likely to have an adverse reaction to water-based lubricants, however, it may need to be reapplied during extended sexual activity. Water-based lubricants are compatible with condoms and will not corrode latex. Water-based lubricants are usually preferred because they are more economical, have no taste, and do not interfere with oral sex. Glycerin may be an ingredient in water-based or other lubricants, which can be problematic for women who report frequent yeast infections. Silicone-based lubricants feel different and are not absorbed by the skin, so they last longer and do not need to be reapplied as often. A disadvantage to silicone-based lubricants is that they irritate some women if not rinsed off immediately after sex. Oil-based lubricants are incompatible with condoms, an important consideration when trying to prevent pregnancy or transmission of STIs. Also, oil-based lubricants should not be used in the shower and can stain the sheets! Petroleum-based lubricants such as baby oil or petroleum jelly may cause irritation for some women. For your clients who are new to anal play, give "go slow" messages. The anal walls are more delicate and thinner compared to vaginal walls. Anal play requires a lubricant that won't dry out easily and is thicker; a silicone-based lube is recommended. Some lubes offer additives to "spice it up." Some of these contain ingredients such as capsaicin, which is the active component in chili peppers. Other ingredients may be alcohol, herbal extracts, propylene glycol, or vitamins. For clients who report allergies or sensitivities to lubricants such as glycerin, encourage them to examine the ingredients, as many brands and options are available. Recent trends include more natural lubes with no parabens, artificial fragrances, or dyes, and some contain cannabis-related compounds. It is important to educate your client on the differences in order for them to make an informed choice.

Zestra is an oil-based product applied to the clitoris and vulva to enhance a woman's pleasure by providing a tingly and/or warming sensation. It can be used to enhance sensation during masturbation or foreplay. It is not a lubricant and should not be applied within the vagina. It contains borage seed oil, evening primrose oil, angelica extract, coleus forskohlii extract, theobromine, and vitamin C and E, and works by increasing smooth muscle vasodilation and increasing neurosensitivity. It should not be used with latex condoms, by women who have a yeast infection or an allergy to any of the ingredients, or is pregnant.

Physical and Other Exercises

There are far too many publications to cite that indicate regular physical exercise can help improve mood; reduce symptoms of depression and anxiety; improve sleep, core muscles, and body image; and lastly help improve a woman's sexual experience. Encourage your client to check with her doctor first to determine safety for exercise and which type of exercise(s) may be best for her.

Exercises to help a woman explore her body can help. Encourage your client to explore her body while naked and identify positives about every part of her body from the top of her head to her toes. This is an exercise that can be a lot harder for some women to do than it sounds. Many women have a disconnect of awareness and appreciation from the waist down. Another important part of this exercise is to encourage women to take a hand-held mirror to explore, identify, and appreciate her vulva, outer and inner labia, pubic hair, clitoris, vaginal opening, and so forth. Women are still taught not to touch or look at themselves. Once a woman takes the time to look, identify, and appreciate *all* of her body and what it does for her, she can feel much more confident, taking ownership of her entire body and pleasure.

Sensate Focus Exercises, developed by Masters and Johnson as previously noted, can help a couple learn a new way of communicating with one another and learn intimacy that is sensual rather than sexual. The purpose of sensate focus is not to experience erotic feelings or orgasm. The purpose is for a woman to tune into her own feelings and bodily sensations as well as learn to feel accepting of giving and receiving touch. Sensate focus is about touching for one's own interest, not about touching for sexual arousal. Additionally, the couple can learn that touching can be intimate, feel good, and be a way of communicating with a partner without the demand of intercourse. Sensate focus can be a useful treatment for women experiencing anxiety, arousal difficulties, or engaging in spectatoring during sexual activity.

Kegel exercises were developed by a gynecologist in the late 1940s and are a recommended treatment for women experiencing urine leakage, with expected improvement within a few weeks or months if done routinely. Kegel exercises help tone the pelvic floor muscles and may help improve orgasm.

Pelvic Floor physical therapy is for treatment of pelvic floor dysfunction that can be a result from childbirth, surgery, or aging. Physical therapists who specialize in this area can help women who report stress urinary incontinence, dyspareunia, vaginismus, vulvodynia, pelvic floor myofascial pain, or postpartum sexual dysfunction. Biofeedback may be used to help with relaxation or strengthening of pelvic muscles. Ice, heat, or electrical stimulation may be included. Vaginal dilators may be used to help women who have vaginismus or have had gynecological cancer treatment. Treatment is hands-on and may include both external and internal manual treatment such as massage or stretching. Patients are educated about their pelvic anatomy and how different elements of their anatomy work.

Medical Procedures

Labia rejuvenation surgery. Some women feel compelled to seek "rejuvenation" surgery, meaning some of their inner and/or outer labia is excised to provide an appearance that matches what they may have seen in pornography films. This type of surgery unfortunately is increasing with advertising. Women internalize that their inner labia are not sexually attractive and should not be visible outside the outer labia. Advertising for this surgery is intended to make women feel sexually unappealing and inadequate. This message (of not being good enough anatomically) is reinforced by what women see on reality TV, in which the stars schedule this surgery and sometimes girlfriends or sisters have the surgery at the same time to "bond" in recovery. What women are usually *not* told is that as some of the labia tissue is removed, delicate nerves that contribute to a woman's positive experience of sexual pleasure are also removed. Additionally, women are not informed that variation in the appearance of the vulva (including size, color, and shape) is very normal. There is little empirical evidence that this procedure increases women's sexual satisfaction, and recommendations to clients for their consideration of this option should be avoided.

Laser Intravaginal Devices. The fractional CO2 laser (DEKA SmartXide2 CO2 laser), marketed as the Mona Lisa Touch, is an example of such a device. The device is shaped like a long tube with tiny holes initially FDA-approved to treat vaginal warts. These laser devices were remarketed by the manufacturer as a tool to help women who reported vaginal dryness, atrophy, and pain with intercourse with the promise of lubricating more effectively and improved sexual experience. They are usually marketed as a series of three treatments, and the treatments are expensive. Providers usually recommend repeating the treatments over time as needed. The ACOG (American College of Obstetricians and Gynecologists, 2018) published a position statement warning physicians that the device was not cleared or approved by the FDA for the treatment of vulvovaginal atrophy and warned them of their ethical responsibility to provide accurate and current information to their patients. The FDA published a warning in 2018 that there was no research showing this was a proven treatment for vaginal dryness or laxity. In addition, the FDA warning included information that for some women, this treatment caused significant scarring and pain. Again, recommendations to clients for their consideration of this treatment option should be avoided.

Injection to G-Spot – The G-Shot. This "treatment" has been popularized by cable TV shows and advertised as helping improve women's pleasure and orgasm. The G-spot was identified in 1950 by Dr. Grafenberg, a gynecologist, as an erogenous zone approximately the size of half a centimeter on the anterior wall of the vagina. The injection involves fat transplantation or filler to temporarily increase the size of the area. The G-spot remains a controversial topic with much published data that a specific area does not exist. Some propose that more study is needed and that this is an area that is not well understood at this time. Research indicates women are not more likely to reach orgasm through intercourse alone after the G-shot treatment and risks include infection, bleeding, or scarring at the injection site. This is not a proven treatment and recommendations to clients for their consideration of this option should be avoided.

Injection – O-Shot. The O-Shot Involves the use of platelet-rich plasma (PRP) injected in the clitoris, labia, and G-spot to help improve their experience of orgasm. There is no scientifically proven evidence that this treatment can improve orgasm or overall sexual satisfaction.

Mental Health Therapy

Sex Therapy. The American Association of Sexuality Educators, Counselors and Therapists (AASECT) recommends the PLISSIT model for Sexuality Therapy. The model begins with Permission (P) giving which involves the therapist providing a comfortable climate for the client to discuss sexual concerns, often introducing the topic of sexuality and validating it as a legitimate health issue. Next, Limited Information (LI) consists of the practitioner addressing a specific sexual concern with attempts to correct myths and misinformation. Specific Suggestions (SS) constitutes the therapist compiling a sexual history of the client in order to define the issues and concerns, determine the course of how the issues have evolved over time, facilitate the client's understanding of the main issues, provide options for resolution, assist the client in formulating perceptions and ideas about sources of these concerns, and develop realistic and appropriate goals and solution plans. Intensive Therapy (IT) is indicated for cases that are complicated by other complex life issues or diagnosis such as depression, anxiety disorders, personality disorders, substance abuse, or interpersonal/intrapersonal conflict. Sexuality counselors are trained to identify situations that require intensive therapy and make appropriate referrals (Annon, 1976).

Case Vignette

Gina, a 26-year-old cisgender Caucasian female, has made an appointment reporting sexual health concerns. Gina has been married 3 years to her partner (Chris) and they have a 1½-year-old son. Gina was raised in South Carolina by a Pentecostal family and is the youngest of her 7 siblings. She had an aptitude for computers and was awarded a 4-year scholarship to a college in Arizona. Though reluctant to permit their daughter to go so far away for her education, her parents allowed it due to financial strain and wanting their daughter to have a better financial and educational future than they had. In college, when other young women in her sorority would talk about dating and sex, she felt uncomfortable due to lack of experience and her religious upbringing. When her girlfriends talked about experimentation, masturbation, and "earth-shattering" orgasms, asking her about the same, she would lie and say, "Oh yeah, it's awesome!" She stated that she feels as though her girlfriends knew a "great secret" about sex that she was never let in on. Due to her curiosity about women's issues, she signed up for courses and joined college clubs that increased her knowledge and discussed the women's equality movement, female leaders, researchers, and scientists. Shortly after graduation, she was hired by an innovative computer company and she stayed out West. She met her husband at her new job and she appreciated his gentle and kind nature, especially when it came to sex. Chris was raised Catholic, and Gina converted at his urging. Gina feels something is wrong with her due to feeling unfulfilled sexually. She was prescribed Prozac for a few years after being diagnosed with depression. She hesitantly disclosed that she has tried to masturbate a few times but stopped due to feeling conflicted. She also is not sure if she has ever had an orgasm. She has watched movies with her girlfriends or husband, feeling uncomfortable with sex scenes and inadequate about her own body. Gina is physically active and fit and has enjoyed swimming, bike riding, and hiking throughout her life. However, she saw her body as flawed because she didn't look like the women in the movies or other popular media, and her body changed after the birth of her son. Her husband usually wanted missionary position intercourse and she faked orgasms due to not wanting him to feel bad and also to get it over with. She said she doesn't want couple therapy because she fears hurting her husband's feelings and lying when he asks, "Did you come?" or "Was that good for you?" She wants to enjoy sex more "like my girlfriends have talked about," to be honest with her husband about sex and "not fake anymore," and to feel better about her body. What can be done to help her?

Treatment Recommendations for Case Vignette

As a general guideline, it is suggested that providers employ the PLISSIT model. Start by providing a comfortable climate for her to discuss her concerns, provide active listening, and validate her sexual concerns as important. Correct any myths or misinformation. Provide information that it is normal for most women not to have an orgasm with missionary position intercourse. Discuss the role of the clitoris and provide information or drawings of the structure. Normalize physical changes as well as possible fluctuations in desire and response after pregnancy. Compile a sexual history and work with her to determine realistic goals and solutions for treatment. Normalize that it can be difficult to discuss her concerns with her husband, though important to begin the process of improving her overall sense of sexual pleasure and satisfaction. Encourage her to talk to her prescriber about the possibility of a different antidepressant with decreased potential for sexual side effects such as Wellbutrin. Encourage her to use a hand mirror and explore her genitals, identify all the structures, and appreciate her own beauty and uniqueness. Encourage her to discuss her conflicted feelings regarding masturbating. If her concerns are due to religious teachings, process these with her. Suggest bibliotherapy such as *For Yourself* by Lonnie Barbach (1975). Encourage her to approach her husband, discuss her concerns, and have him accompany her to therapy. Provide instructions for sensate focus exercises and positive sexual self-image exercises. Enhance her sexual health through sexual literacy (Peterson et al., 2020). Employ the Becoming Orgasmic program (Heiman & LoPiccolo, 1988). Most importantly, develop a treatment plan that helps her work toward her treatment goals of accepting and appreciating her body, being more authentic with herself and her partner, and creating a more sexually fulfilling life.

CLOSING REMARKS

Clinical research toward the understanding of women's sexual health is still in its infancy after less than a century of study. There is still so much territory yet to be explored in women's sexuality. As innovators continue to develop new research, new techniques for treatment and continued advancements in science and imaging technology will help us to evolve and have a better understanding of the complexity of female sexual health and functioning. We cannot assume that our clients have adequate knowledge about sexual health.

It is up to us as clinicians to ask questions and provide a safe, welcoming environment for our clients to discuss their concerns. In my experience, many have found it a relief that a professional opened the door and let them know that their sexual health and pleasure are topics we feel comfortable talking about. As professionals, we must ask our clients if they have any concerns and address those concerns directly by never ignoring details of their personal story, promoting a positive sense of sexuality, and validating each client as a sexual being.

REFERENCES

Aftab, A., Chen, C., & McBride, J. (2017). Flibanserin and its discontents. *Archives of Women's Mental Health, 20,* 243-247.

American College of Obstetricians and Gynecologists. (2018). Fractional laser treatment of vulvovaginal atrophy and U.S. Food and Drug Administration clearance-[Position statement]. https://www.acog.org/clinical-information/policy-and-position-statements/position-statements/2018/fractional-laser-treatment-of-vulvovaginal-atrophy-and-us-food-and-drug-administration-clearance

American Psychiatric Association. (1987). *Diagnostic and statistical manual of mental disorders* (3rd ed., rev.).

American Psychiatric Association. (1994). *Diagnostic and statistical manual of mental disorders* (4th ed.).

American Psychiatric Association. (2000). *Diagnostic and statistical manual of mental disorders* (4th ed., text rev.).

American Psychiatric Association. (2013). *Diagnostic and statistical manual of mental disorders* (5th ed.). https://doi.org/10.1176/appi.books.9780890425596

Annon, J. S. (1976). *Behavioral treatment of sexual problems: Brief therapy*. Harper and Row.

Barbach, L. G. (1975). *For yourself: The fulfillment of female sexuality*. Doubleday.

Barbach, L. G. (1983). *For each other: Sharing sexual intimacy*. Doubleday.

Bartlik, B., & Goldberg, J. (2000). Female sexual arousal disorder. In S. R. Leiblum & R. C. Rosen (Eds.), *Principles and practices of sex therapy* (3rd ed., pp. 85-117). Guilford.

Basson, R. (2000). The female sexual response: A different model. *Journal of Sex & Marital Therapy, 26*(1), 51-65.

Basson, R. (2003). Women's difficulties with low sexual desire and sexual avoidance. In S. B. Levine, C. B. Risen, & S. E. Althof (Eds.), *Handbook of clinical sexuality for mental health professionals* (pp. 111-130). Routledge.

Brotto, L. A., & Luria, M. (2008). Menopause, aging, and sexual response in women. In D. Rowland & L. Incrocci (Eds.), *Handbook of sexual and gender identity disorders* (pp. 251-283). John Wiley & Sons.

Clayton, A. H., Kingsberg, S. A., & Goldstein, I. (2018). Evaluation and management of hypoactive sexual desire disorder. *Sexual Medicine, 6*(2), 59-74.

Freud, S. (1931). Female sexuality. In *The standard edition of the complete psychological works of Sigmund Freud, vol. 21, 1927-1931: The future of an illusion, civilization and its discontents, and other works* (pp. 221-244). Vintage.

Fuss, J., Bindila, L., Wiedemann, K., Auer, M. K., Briken, P., & Biedermann, S. V. (2017). Masturbation to orgasm stimulates the release of the endocannabinoid 2-arachidonolylglycerol in humans. *The Journal of Sexual Medicine, 14*(11), 1372-1379.

George, W. H., Davis, K. C., Heiman, J. R., Norris, J., Stoner, S. A., Schacht, R. L., . . . Kajumulo, K. F. (2011). Women's sexual arousal: Effects of high alcohol dosages and self-control instructions. *Hormones and Behavior, 59*(5), 730-738.

Grover, S., Mattoo, S. K., Pendharkar, S., & Kandappan, V. (2014). Sexual dysfunction in patients with alcohol and opioid dependence. *Indian Journal of Psychological Medicine, 36*(4), 355-365.

Hall, K. (2004). *Reclaiming your sexual self: How you can bring desire back into your life*. John Wiley & Sons.

Heiman, J. R. (2000). Orgasmic disorders in women. In S. R. Leiblum & R. C. Rosen (Eds.), *Principles and practices of sex therapy* (3rd ed., pp. 118-153). Guilford.

Heiman, J. R., & LoPiccolo, J. (1988). *Becoming orgasmic: A sexual and personal growth program for women* (Rev. ed.). Prentice Hall.

Herbenick, D., Eastman-Mueller, H., Fu, T. C., Dodge, B., Ponander, K., & Sanders, S. A. (2019). Women's sexual satisfaction, communication, and reasons for (no longer) faking orgasm: Findings from a U.S. probability sample. *Archives of Sexual Behavior, 48*(8), 2461-2472.

Herbenick, D., & Schick, V. (2011). *Read my lips: A complete guide to the vagina and vulva.* Rowman & Littlefield Publishers.

Hite, S. (1976). *The Hite Report: A nationwide study of female sexuality.* Seven Stories Press.

Joannides, P. (2017). *Guide to getting it on: Unzipped.* Goofy Foot Press.

Kaplan, H. S. (1974). *The new sex therapy: Active treatment of sexual dysfunctions*. Random House.

Kinsey, A., Pomeroy, W., Martin, C., & Gebhard, P. (1953). *Sexual behavior in the human female*. W. B. Saunders.

Kleinplatz, P. (2018). History of the treatment of female sexual dysfunction(s). *Annual Review of Clinical Psychology, 14,* 29-54. https://doi.org/10.1146/annurev-clinpsy-050817-084802

Komisaruk, B. R., Beer-Flores, C., & Whipple, B. (2006). *The science of orgasm.* Johns Hopkins University Press.

Kope, S. (2007). Female sexual arousal and orgasm: Pleasures and problems. In L. VandeCreek, F. Peterson, & J. Bley (Eds.), *Innovations in clinical practice: Focus on sexual health* (pp. 93-106). Professional Resource Press.

Krakowsky, Y., & Grober, E. D. (2018). A practical guide to female sexual dysfunction: An evidence-based review for physicians in Canada. *Canadian Urological Association Journal, 12*(6), 211-216.

Ladas, A. K., Whipple, B., & Perry J. D. (1982). *The G spot and other discoveries about human sexuality*. Bantam Doubleday Dell.

Laumann, E. O., Gagnon, J. H., Michael, R. T., & Michaels, S. (1994). *The social organization of sexuality: Sexual practices in the United States*. University of Chicago Press.

Leonhardt, N. D., Willoughby, B. J., Busby, D. M., Yorgason, J. B., & Holmes, E. K. (2018). The significance of the female orgasm: A nationally representative, dyadic study of newlyweds' orgasm experience. *The Journal of Sexual Medicine, 15*(8), 1140-1148.

Lynn, B. K., Lopez, J. D., Miller, C., Thompson, J., & Campian, E. C. (2019). The relationship between marijuana use prior to sex and sexual function in women. *Sexual Medicine, 7*(2), 192-197.

Masters, W. H., & Johnson, V. E. (1966). *Human sexual response*. Little, Brown and Company.

McCarthy, B. (2015). *Sex made simple*. PESI Publishing & Media.

McCarthy, B., & Farr, E. (2012). Strategies and techniques to maintain sexual desire. *Journal of Contemporary Psychotherapy, 42,* 227-233.

McCarthy, B., & McCarthy, E. (2012). *Sexual awareness: Your guide to healthy couple sexuality* (3rd ed.). Routledge.

Meston, C. M., Seal, B. N., & Hamilton, L. D. (2008). Problems with arousal and orgasm in women. In D. L. Rowland & L. Incrocci (Eds.), *Handbook of sexual and gender identity disorders* (pp. 188-219). John Wiley & Sons.

Metz, M., & McCarthy, B. (2011). *Enduring desire: Your guide to lifelong intimacy.* Routledge.

Michael, R. T., Gagnon, J. H., Laumann, E. O., & Kolata, G. (1994). *Sex in America: A definitive survey.* Little, Brown and Company.

Moore, A. (2009). Relocating Marie Bonaparte's clitoris. *Australian Feminist Studies, 24*(60), 149-165.

Nagoski, E. (2015). *Come as you are: The surprising new science that will transform your sex life.* Simon & Shuster.

O'Connell, H. E., & DeLancey J. O. L. (2005). Clitoral anatomy in nulliparous, healthy, premenopausal volunteers using unenhanced magnetic resonance imaging. *Journal of Urology, 173*(6), 2060-2063.

O'Connell, H. E., Huston, J. M., Anderson, C. R., & Plenter, R. J. (1998). Anatomical relationship between urethra and clitoris. *Journal of Urology, 159,* 1892-1897.

Parish, S. J., Hahn, S. R., Goldstein, S. W., Giraldi, A., Kingsberg, S. A., Larkin, L., . . . Faubion, S. S. (2019). The International Society for the Study of Women's Sexual Health Process of Care for the Identification of Sexual Concerns and Problems in Women. *Mayo Clinic Proceedings, 94*(5), 842-856. https://doi.org/10.1016/j.mayocp.2019.01.009

Perel, E. (2006). *Mating in captivity*. Harper Collins.

Peterson, F., Bley, J., & Frabotta, R. (2020). *The gender revolution & new sexual health: Celebrating unlimited diversity of the human sexuality hypercube.* Cognella Academic Publishing.

Pyke, R., & Clayton, A. H. (2017). What sexual behaviors relate to decreased sexual desire in women? A review and proposal for end points in treatment trails for hypoactive sexual desire disorder. *The Journal of Sexual Medicine, 5,* e73-e83.

Reddy, R. G., Aung, T., Karavitaki, N., & Wass, J. A. (2010). Opioid induced hypogonadism. *British Medical Journal, 341,* C4462. https://doi.org/10.1136/bmj.c4462

Rosen, R. C., Taylor, J. F., Leiblum, S. R., & Bachmann, G. A. (1993). Prevalence of sexual dysfunction in women: Results of a survey of 329 women in an outpatient gynecological clinic. *Journal of Sex and Marital Therapy, 19,* 171-188.

Sauerteig, L. D. (2012). Loss of innocence: Albert Moll, Sigmund Freud and the invention of childhood sexuality around 1900. *Medical History, 56*(2), 56-183.

Simon, J. A., Kingsberg, S. A., Portman, D., Williams, L. A., Krop, J., Jordan, R., . . . Clayton, A. H. (2019). Long-term safety and efficacy of bremelanotide for hypoactive sexual desire disorder. *Obstetrics & Gynecology, 134*(5), 909-917.

Stayton, W., Angelo, M., & Kaye, S. (2005, May). *Erotic stimulus pathways: The new sexual response cycle.* Presentation at the annual meeting of the American Association of Sexuality Educators, Counselors and Therapists. Portland, OR.

Thompson, N. (2003). Marie Bonaparte's theory of female sexuality: Fantasy and biology. *American Imago, 60*(3), 343-378.

van Lankveld, J. (2008). Problems with sexual interest and desire in women. In D. L. Rowland and L. Incrocci (Eds.), *Handbook of sexual and gender identity disorders* (pp. 154-186). John Wiley & Sons.

Wallen, K., & Lloyd, E. A. (2011). Female sexual arousal: Genital anatomy and orgasm in intercourse. *Hormones and Behavior, 59*(5), 780-792.

Weeks, G. R., & Gambescia, N. (2002). *Hypoactive sexual desire: Integrating sex and couple therapy*. W. W. Norton & Company.

Whipple, B., & Wise, N. (2014, June 7). *Women's sexual health: Where we have been and where we are going*. AASECT National Conference, Monterey, California.

Zoldbrod, A. P. (2005). *Sex smart: How your childhood shaped your sexual life and what to do about it.* PageFree Publishing.

14

Female Genital Pain

Jill W. Bley and Emma B. Schmidt

INTRODUCTION

Of all sexual problems, genital pain is possibly the most disturbing to the patient. It is also one of the most complex and difficult issues for the health care provider to treat. At times it is even difficult to make the differential diagnosis of vaginismus versus dyspareunia, as I will discuss below. So difficult, in fact, that some practitioners such as Bergeron et al. (2003) believe that there may not be any real need to differentiate the two because there is so much overlap of the symptoms and because they are both pain syndromes that happen to occur in the genitals (Reissing et al., 1999).

In 1834, Huguier described vaginismus in the scientific literature. Later, Sims called the symptom that had been described by Huguier "vaginismus" (Leiblum, 2000). Since that time vaginismus has been defined in the *Diagnostic and Statistical Manual of Mental Disorders* as recurrent or persistent involuntary spasm of the musculature of the outer third of the vagina that interferes with sexual intercourse (4th ed.; *DSM-IV*; American Psychiatric Association,1994). According to the medical literature there are two types of vaginismus: primary, which means that the woman has always had it; and secondary, which means that the woman used to be able to experience penetration but lost the ability (Katz & Tabisel, 2002).

Dyspareunia is described in the *DSM-IV* as recurrent or persistent genital pain associated with sexual intercourse in either a male or a female. Binik et al. (2000) pointed out some of the difficulties in this diagnosis. They reported that patients may describe their pain as dull/aching pain, burning/cutting pain, or sore/sharp pain. The pain may be at the vaginal opening, it may be experienced at different depths of the vagina, or it may be experienced only with thrusting. Katz and Tabisel (2002) described dyspareunia by dividing the presenting symptoms into onset, frequency, and location. They also described typical variations which may include primary, situational, deep (thrusting always hurts in missionary position, other positions are okay); secondary, situational, insertional (with current partner at beginning of penetration, goes away as soon as penis is halfway in and never happened with prior partners); primary, complete, superficial and deep (always had the pain with all partners, in all positions, throughout the sexual act); secondary, complete, superficial (initial penetration has been painful since gynecologic surgery regardless of lubrication or position).

A study that did not attempt to differentiate between vaginismus and dyspareunia conducted by Lauman et al. (1994) for the National Health and Sexual Life Survey reported that between 10% and 15% of women experienced sexual pain during the 6 months before taking the survey. Leiblum (2000) cited some studies on the prevalence of vaginismus that have indicated rates of from 12% to 17% with higher rates reported in Canada and Ireland. Katz and Tabisel (2002) concluded that we will never know the prevalence of these disorders because they are "private pains."

A study done by Andrew Goldstein and colleagues (2011) found that Dyspareunia affects 17% to 19% of women in the United States. In 2013, the *Diagnostic and Statistical Manual of Mental Disorders* was revised. The 5th edition combined vaginismus and dyspareunia into one diagnosis now referred to as Genito-Pelvic Pain/Penetration Disorder (GPPPD). Like previous research had suggested, the two diagnoses were tough to distinguish between and highly comorbid (*DSM-5*; American Psychiatric Association, 2013). The *DSM-IV* sexual disorders had subtypes which included lifelong versus acquired disorders, situational versus generalized disorders, and looked at combined factors versus psychological factors (*DSM-IV*; American Psychiatric Association, 1994). In the *DSM-5*, however, the subtypes only include generalized versus situational disorders and lifelong versus acquired disorders. Psychological and combined factors were not included due to both typically being present during a clinical presentation. In the *DSM-5*, one of the following has to be present to diagnose GPPPD:

- Persistent or recurrent difficulties with vaginal penetration during intercourse
- Marked vulvovaginal or pelvic pain during vaginal intercourse or attempts at penetration
- Marked fear or anxiety about vulvovaginal or pelvic pain in anticipation of, during, or as a result of vaginal penetration
- Marked tensing or tightening of the pelvic floor muscles during attempts at vaginal penetration

Similar to other sexual diagnosis criteria, the client has to have a duration of the symptoms for more than 6 months except in cases where there is a substance/medication-induced cause of the sexual dysfunction. This benchmark was noted in the *DSM-5* to not overdiagnose and to monitor the symptoms' persistence. Although the research is still limited in terms of the prevalence rate of genito-pelvic pain/penetration disorder, in North America around 15% of women report having continuous sexual pain (American Psychiatric Association, 2013). Irwin Goldstein et al. (2018) noted that dyspareunia alone in the United States was seen to be closer to 30%. That is 1 in 3 women. Their research also found that black women experienced pain to a higher degree on a daily basis than white women. For postmenopausal women, the prevalence went up to 45% for those who experienced GPPPD.

One study in 2015 by Marie-Andree Lahaie and colleagues looked at the relationship between dyspareunia/provoked vestibulodynia and vaginismus. Their goal was to see whether one would be able to distinguish between the two different sets of diagnoses in patients when tested. What they found was that genital pain among those with vaginismus and those with dyspareunia/provoked vestibulodynia did not have a significant differentiation. There was also a considerable amount of overlap when looking at muscle tension. The authors noted that their findings validated why physicians have had a tough time deciding between which diagnosis, vaginismus or dyspareunia/provoked vestibulodynia, would be the most appropriate.

Women with GPPPD tend to have a 50% comorbidity with other diagnoses. These comorbid diagnoses most associated with GPPPD are fibromyalgia, irritable bowel syndrome, female sexual interest and arousal syndrome, other pain disorders, and interstitial cystitis.

"The pelvic floor works as an emotional organ" (Dias-Amaral & Marques-Pinto, 2018, p. 789). This statement speaks to the psychological component that becomes intertwined into the somatic body. For instance, as we become anxious about an upcoming sexual encounter, we might subconsciously contract our pelvic floor muscles, indirectly causing pain to the vulvar area. One study observed women through electromyography. The results showed that there was a heightened state of tension in the pelvic floor during states of anxiety, more so than when they were experiencing sexual threats (Both et al., 2012). When it comes to anxiety, those with GPPPD tend to hold on to what are called negative schemas or negative messages about sex and apply those negative messages to future events. Research shows that those with healthier schemas are less likely to have GPPPD (Nobre & Pinto-Gouveia, 2009). Schemas that are often observed in women with GPPPD are anxiety about potential abandonment, avoidance of intimacy, loneliness, incompetence, feelings of rejection, and self-deprecation (Nobre & Pinto-Gouveia, 2008). The therapy modality that has been researched the most in GPPPD has been Cognitive Behavioral Therapy (CBT). Its efficacy is strong and shows improvement when addressing emotional dysregulation, cognitive distortions, and behaviors that are maladaptive regarding symptoms related to GPPPD. One piece that is notable in the research is that it still is unclear whether negative psychological schemas are a consequence or a cause of GPPPD (Dias-Amaral & Marques-Pinto, 2018).

What is clear is that the fear-avoidance cycle that happens to these women who experience pain is at a high level. For example, the woman experiences sexual pain, and the brain begins to translate that into a danger zone or catastrophizes what has happened. Hypervigilance begins to increase, and the body begins to experience the ideas of engaging sexually in a threatening way or as a fear state. Avoiding sexual activity, specifically penetration, becomes status quo. When she thinks about sex or sexual activity, her pelvic floor tightens up out of fear (pelvic floor hypertonicity) and it becomes difficult for her to be excited about sex, resulting in a lack of lubrication and leading back to experiencing sexual pain when engaged. The negative thoughts about sex only increase the body's tension, hypervigilance, and sensitivity to sexual pain. Studies are showing that high levels of stress, depression, and anxiety can be the contributors of dyspareunia and vaginismus and not necessarily always the opposite way around (genital pain causing anxiety and stress) (Basson, 2012).

Basson (2012) described "the vicious circle of female genital pain" as follows:

1. The woman experiences pain,
2. The woman and her partner catastrophize vocally or in private thoughts,
3. The woman begins to be hypervigilent about her body,
4. She experiences negative emotions (fear) and/or her partner is hostile or solicitous,
5. The woman avoids penetration,
6. Her pelvic floor muscles cause hypertonicity,
7. The woman experiences impairment of genital excitement with decreased lubrication, and
8. The vicious circle of pain repeats over and over.

Though the woman is the one experiencing GPPPD, the partner is impacted to a significant degree as well. What we find is that a woman will begin to not only avoid sex but also avoid her partner. Partners can become confused, frustrated, angry, and depressed by the experience and the cycle. When the couple does begin to engage in sexual activity, male partners can exhibit anxiety and sexual dysfunctions due to the fear of hurting the partner with GPPPD. Some partners with retrograde ejaculation might have been used to trying to have sex quickly as to avoid hurting their female counterpart for too long; others might experience erectile dysfunction due to anxiety and nervousness for fear of hurting their partner. Many partners fear that they are assaulting the woman, which can create a negative message around sex. These interactions can greatly decrease the relationship's satisfaction. The literature identifies that there is a higher likelihood for reduction in sexual pain when couples can work through the pain together instead of the woman working on it alone. However, if the partner is angry and expresses their frustration to the woman, this can intensify the negative pain cycle the woman experiences and can lead to more avoidance, negative messages, and pain (Rosen et al., 2014).

As the individual or couple begin to address GPPPD, it is important to have them set realistic goals about their treatment such as a reduction of pain versus the elimination of pain. It is recommended that the clinician begin treatment with psychoeducation and help the client break down myths around their body and around sex. The therapist can then guide the client through understanding the female body, its sexual functions, and teaching about the mind-body implications. Leading clients to see their situation through a biopsychosocial model can help them see all the ways that can impact and influence their GPPPD. After this has been established, the therapist can then begin to intertwine pain reduction behavioral techniques (Dias-Amaral & Marques-Pinto, 2018).

We will continue to break down Genito-Pelvic Pain/Penetration Disorder by taking a deeper look at vaginismus, dyspareunia, vulvodynia, and vestibulitis.

HISTORICAL APPROACHES TO THE TREATMENT OF SEXUAL PAIN

In their pioneering work *Human Sexual Response* (1966), Masters and Johnson mention dyspareunia only in the context of the aging female in a chapter with that title. They did not mention vaginismus at all. Eight years later, Kaplan wrote *The New Sex Therapy* (1974). She did not mention dyspareunia, but she did devote an entire chapter to vaginismus. She stressed the importance of treating the "phobic" element of the disorder and "in vivo deconditioning of the involuntary spasm of the muscles which guard the vaginal entry" (p. 418). She cited a "common method" recommended by Masters and Johnson, the gentle insertion of graduated catheters into the vagina. Kaplan stated that vaginismus is the most common cause of unconsummated marriage (1974).

In 1983, Kaplan wrote *The Evaluation of Sexual Disorders: Psychological and Medical Aspects.* She included a chapter written by Sherwin Kaufman, titled "The Gynecologic Evaluation of Female Dyspareunia and Unconsummated Marriage." Kaufman gave only one paragraph to the discussion of vaginismus. The rest of the chapter was devoted to dyspareunia. He categorized vaginal pain into pain on entry (vaginismus was included here), mid-vaginal pain, pain on deep thrusting, and pain on orgasm.

The first generation of sex therapists did not give much attention to these troubling problems, probably because the origin of the muscle spasms and pain is difficult to understand. There is often no obvious disruption of the sexual response cycle, for as Leiblum (2000) noted, some women with vaginismus can become sexually aroused, lubricate, and even have multiple orgasms with manual or oral stimulation. The spasms and/or pain also are almost never due to performance anxiety, per se. Therefore, the symptoms do not usually respond to sensate focus exercises or to traditional "talk" therapies.

Treatment of Vaginismus

As mentioned previously, Masters and Johnson advised that vaginismus should be treated using the gentle insertion of graduated sizes of catheters (1970). The use of catheters soon evolved into the use of graduated dilators developed for the specific purpose of helping a woman gradually desensitize to her fear of vaginal dilation and penetration. These dilators made it possible for clinicians to instruct a patient about how to use them, enabling her to practice relaxation techniques while using the dilators at home. This approach is called "in vivo desensitization." Schoen and Nathanson (1984) developed a 30-minute video (*Treating Vaginismus*) with sex therapist Joseph LoPiccolo that portrays therapy sessions during which LoPiccolo instructs a couple in the use of dilators. The film graphically shows the woman doing relaxation exercises and using the dilators. The dilators were sold and marketed to physicians. Hence, they were expensive, and many women could not afford the treatment.

Fuchs et al. (1978) described a method for treating vaginismus using hypnodesensitization therapy. This intervention is systematic desensitization during the hypnotic state either *in vitro* (where the patient imagines the stimuli) or *in vivo* (where the patient confronts the real stimuli).

In her 1975 book *For Yourself: The Fulfillment of Female Sexuality,* Lonnie Barbach suggested to women that they could use common objects found in their home, such as candles as dildos, for learning how to have orgasm. She paved the way for practitioners to begin to think "outside the box" for ways that the average woman with limited income could be treated for vaginismus. Many sex therapists began to suggest that women use implements and/or vegetables they might have in their home. They could start with very thin implements and graduate to larger things, such as carrots and cucumbers, that they could easily and cheaply obtain on their own. They could follow the self-help directions for learning to relax the muscles of the vagina as they insert objects that gradually increased in size. Since the medical dilators could only be ordered through a physician at a high cost, Barbach's ideas were (and continue to be) extremely useful to therapists who wanted to help those who could not afford the more costly dilators.

Another important part of the treatment of vaginismus is teaching the woman to learn to relax the musculature of the vaginal area. The therapist must instruct the woman in learning how to do these relaxation exercises. The exercises are described in the video *Treating Vaginismus* (Schoen & Nathanson, 1984) and the books *Women Discover Orgasm: A Therapist's guide to a New_Treatment Approach* (Barbach, 1980) and *Becoming Orgasmic: a Sexual and Personal Growth Program for Women* (Heiman & LoPiccolo, 1988). Heiman and LoPiccolo believed that some women with this problem seem to become more tense when they try to do muscle relaxation exercises. They recommended that women do exercises they called "body awareness." After she learns to relax her body, the therapist asks her to focus her attention to her vaginal muscles (primarily the pubococcygeal muscles) and to learn to isolate those muscles. She then learns to tense and relax them. Those exercises are called Kegel Exercises and were developed by Arnold Kegel (1948). They are described in the Heiman and LoPiccolo book and the Barbach book (both cited above), and a brief set of instructions is included in the Patient Handouts section in the back of this book.

Once the woman has mastered the use of the dilators, she is encouraged to use her fingers. The next step is to allow her partner to be present as she uses her fingers and shows him how she gently inserts her finger. Then she allows her partner to insert his finger as she guides him. Finally, when she feels that she is ready, she allows insertion of the penis with her controlling the insertion. The key to the treatment is to make sure that the woman feels that she is in control of the whole process. Therefore, it is important to solicit the cooperation of her sexual partner.

As many researchers have noted, treatment of vaginismus does not always produce positive results using the *in vivo* or *in vitro* desensitization techniques. There are times when the clinician has to learn more about what is causing the problem. Sometimes the origin can be traced to sex-negative messages that the young girl received from her parents, her church, or her friends. When these are the etiological factors, the clinician needs to help the woman relearn positive information about sexuality. The therapist needs to "normalize" behaviors such as masturbation, premarital sex, consensual sexual explorations, and so forth.

A recent study monitored 472 women from 2010 to 2019, all of whom were diagnosed with vaginismus (Zulfikaroglu, 2020). The research looked at a multifaceted approach utilizing dilation exercises, cognitive and behavioral therapy, hypnotherapy, and postcounseling. At the end of the treatment, all 472 women were able to engage in successful intercourse. This type of approach speaks to not only the effect of dilators, but dilators partnered with other approaches to help the woman understand the origin of her vaginismus.

Sometimes, sexual abuse is the cause. Other times genital trauma, such as intrusive and/or insensitive medical procedures, are the cause. More recently, clinicians are learning that it may be a reaction to vulvodynia (see the later section on dyspareunia) which is a very painful condition (Leiblum, 2000). When trauma is found to be the cause, approaches known to ameliorate the effects of trauma need to be used. As Bessel van der Kolk (2002) has pointed out, Eye Movement Desensitization and Reprocessing (EMDR) can be a very effective integrative psychotherapy tool.

Perhaps one of the most important reasons that some cases of vaginismus are difficult to treat is that the spasm-based definition of vaginismus may not be an adequate diagnostic marker. In 1999, Reissing and colleagues suggested that vaginismus should be considered a type of genital pain and that it should be described in terms of its quality, intensity, location, and time course. Later, in 2004, Reissing et al. found that clinicians were unable to differentiate between vaginismus and dyspareunia resulting from vulvar vestibulitis syndrome. They suggested that the diagnosis needs to be changed to include a multidimensional reconceptualization of vaginismus so that the clinician must consider whether or not the woman presents with pain and fear of pain, pelvic floor dysfunction, and behavioral avoidance. In 2018, Irwin Goldstein and colleagues continued to make the point that "research has failed to prove the presence of muscle spasm as a valid or reliable diagnostic criteria" (p. 252). They go on to say that muscle spasms alone do not make sense of the other emotional somatic pieces that arise such as pain, fear of penetration, and anxiety. Researchers still believe that it is challenging to differentiate between vaginismus and dyspareunia (I. Goldstein et al., 2018).

After the more traditional forms of treatment have not been successful to treat vaginismus, botulinum toxin, or what some people know as the brand name Botox, can be used to loosen the pelvic floor muscles. This allows for physicians, including pelvic floor physical therapists, to begin stretching the muscles back to their intended form. The Botox method is incredibly effective but is seen as a last resort effort, as loosening the pelvic floor can create other challenges such as prolapses if the muscles become too loose. This method is also not indicated if a woman is wanting to try to get pregnant in the future due to the loosening of the pelvic floor muscles (Pacik & Geletta, 2017).

Botox injections are administered on the inner walls of the vagina in the bulbospongiosus usually under local or general anesthesia. As the muscles relax, a dilator is inserted and left there while the patient is coming out of anesthesia. This allows for the patient to understand that penetration is possible. For some, the largest dilator can be inserted after the procedure. Dilators range from 2.5 inches in circumference to 6.25 inches in circumference. Some recommend keeping a dilator in throughout that night postprocedure to continue to encourage the muscle stretching as the botulinum toxin improves. In some cases, those with severe vaginismus were able to advance to the largest dilator the day after the procedure. Psychotherapy is recommended for patients pre- and postprocedure as many women experience a fear of penetration and oftentimes are inexperienced sexually (Pacik & Geletta, 2017). One reason botulinum toxin has been unsuccessful in some patients is due to a lack of dilation after receiving the procedure. Pacik and Geletta outline a protocol used for successful dilation with botulinum toxin. During the first month the patient should dilate 2 hours a day. This can be challenging for many clients as life can get in the way and doing dilation at all, let alone 2 hours a day for 30 days, is difficult. The goal is to advance comfortably to the second largest and largest size dilators. During the second month the patient is to use dilation for 1 hour per day while using the largest dilator. After that, the patient should reduce dilation to 15 to 30 minutes a day over the third month. The authors note that those who regressed in their progress were women who stopped doing the dilation exercises for the length of the 3 months. Because the botulinum toxin only lasts 2 to 4 months, it is important to not let dilation slip during that period. Due to fear of intercourse prior to botulinum toxin injections, addressing anxiety and fear is a critical part of the treatment. Though physically a woman might be able to have penetration, the fear of penetration, not actual pain, might contribute to her and her partner not engaging in sex a year postprocedure (Pacik & Geletta, 2017).

Treatment Example of Vaginismus

A young 25-year-old woman who was planning to be married in 2 months was referred for sex therapy by her gynecologist. Her gynecologist had attempted to do an exam but was unable to insert anything, even a swab, into the young woman's vagina. She was very distressed and fearful that she would not be able to have intercourse with her husband on her wedding night. She stated that she had "saved herself for the man she marries." She believed that sex was sinful outside of marriage. Her sexual history indicated that she was raised in an orthodox Christian faith and attended a Christian academy. Her parents had severely punished any sexual behaviors of her or her siblings. When she was 16 years old, her mother saw her kiss a boyfriend and insisted that she never see the boy again, stating that the boy only wanted "one thing" from her and that he was not a "gentleman."

She had never had a gynecological exam because her mother did not think it was necessary and she was told by her mother never to use tampons because she would no longer be a virgin if she did. When she went to college, she resisted her parents' desire for her to attend a private school. That was her first "rebellious" act. After graduating from college, she started medical school where she met her fiancé. She realized that she needed to have a gynecological exam but put it off until her fiancé put pressure on her to do so. Her sexual experience was limited to kissing and petting, but the petting did not include touching the inside of her vulva. She said that her fiancé would be very cooperative and helpful. He had assured her that he wanted to marry her whether she was able to have intercourse on the wedding night. He expressed confidence that she could overcome this problem.

The therapist decided that it would be important to the success of the treatment to explore with her what her own religious beliefs about sexuality were. She said that she was definitely more liberal than her parents, but that she shared their belief that sex should only be shared with the person to whom you are married. She felt that her parents' punishments of sexual behavior were inappropriate, but she was raised to be fearful of incurring her parents' wrath, so she complied with their dictates about sex.

During the therapy session she was instructed in progressive muscle relaxation which she was able to do very well. She was given a handout that had information about how to do Kegel exercises (see p. 595 for the handout that describes Kegel/pelvic floor muscle exercises). Her assignment was to practice the muscle relaxation and Kegel exercises every day during the next week.

She reported success in learning how to relax and in isolating her vaginal muscles. The homework for the next week was to do the relaxation exercises, then tense and relax the vaginal muscles. When she felt very relaxed, she was to use a hand-held mirror to look at her vulva. At the next therapy session, she said that she was ashamed to admit but it had been very difficult for her to look at her vulva. She was surprised at herself because as a medical student she had looked at many vulvas of other women. She realized that she felt very "disconnected" from her own body and could view other people's bodies in a detached "clinical" manner, thereby, did not need to feel her real emotions about vulvas and vaginas.

She was asked to continue the relaxation exercises, but this time, after she felt relaxed and started focusing on Kegel exercises, she should try to insert a swab into the vagina as she released the tension in the vaginal muscles. At the next session, she was upset because she began to cry every time she tried to insert the swab. The therapist used EMDR and asked her to close her eyes and recall the experience of trying to insert the swab. She began to cry and explained that her thoughts had immediately gone to an experience during childhood when her mother had found her playing "doctor" with a friend and had held her hand under hot running water for a long time while yelling at her and telling her how dirty her mind and hands were.

After this very intense session she was able to do the assignment. She progressed to larger objects until she was able to insert a tampon. She was elated at this achievement. When it was time to move on to larger objects her progress slowed a bit, however, she kept trying and eventually was able to insert a cucumber with a circumference slightly bigger than her (now) husband's penis. Although she was not able to allow penetration on her wedding night, she was able to enjoy her first intercourse 5 weeks after the wedding. One week before her first intercourse she was able to have her first gynecological exam.

Discussion of Case

This case had a very successful outcome because of the confluence of five key factors, as follows: (a) The client was very motivated to overcome her problem, (b) she was receptive to changing her cognitions about sexuality, (c) she was able to resolve childhood memories of abuse related to sexuality, (d) her fiancé/husband was respectful of her needs and cooperative with treatment, and (e) the symptom was not complicated (i.e., there was no other pain syndrome).

As Leiblum (2000) pointed out, not all cases of vaginismus are successful. Many women who achieve their goal of being able to tolerate penetration may continue to avoid intercourse. When this is the case the therapist may continue to probe to learn more information about the etiology of the avoidance symptoms. If the partner has not been a part of the therapy, he should be included at this point. The therapy may need to be redirected toward an emphasis on desire issues. With some couples, the partner is willing to have intercourse only when the woman is willing. However, a partner with that much patience and understanding is not the usual case. Therefore, working toward an outcome that both partners can accept will mean that the therapist must be able to provide an "integrated" approach (see section on Team Treatment Approach, pp. 245-247) to further treatment. However, success is often difficult to achieve even when multiple dimensions of the problem are treated.

TREATMENT OF DYSPAREUNIA

As those of us who have treated women presenting with genital pain know, sometimes vaginismus is a secondary manifestation of the primary cause, which is the experience of pain with penetration. The pain may be felt as soon as there is the slightest penetration, it may be felt as penetration reaches part way into the vagina, or it may occur with deep penetration and/or thrusting. Kaufman (1983) states there are some medical conditions that can cause pain in mid-vagina which are easily diagnosed by a physician, such as trigonitis (inflammation which is confined to the mucous membrane of the openings of the ureters and the urethra of the bladder), cystitis (inflammation of the bladder, usually associated with urinary tract infections), and urethritis (inflammation of the urethra). Likewise, there are many medical conditions that can cause pain with deep penetration and/or thrusting, such as endometriosis and pathology of the ovaries. Kaufman also stated that pain on entry may be caused by dermatological conditions of the vulva, pathology of the glands near the vaginal opening (the Skene or Bartholin glands), or vaginismus.

As noted earlier in this chapter, there is so much overlap between the two diagnoses of dyspareunia and vaginismus that it is often difficult and perhaps impossible to make the distinction. Bergeron et al. (2003) proposed that the two diagnoses be dropped, not only because the differential diagnosis of the two is difficult, but because they feel it is not clear why painful genital sexual activity is even considered a sexual dysfunction. They point out that other pain syndromes may interfere with sexual activity, such as lower back pain. They also point to the fact that lower back pain is never referred to as work-related pain, even though it frequently is the cause of being unable to perform one's work. They assert that the International Association for the Study of Pain (IASP) has included vaginismus and dyspareunia in their classification of chronic pain.

Bergeron et al. (2002) believe that most dyspareunia is caused by vulvar vestibulitis syndrome (VVS) which is a subtype of vulvodynia (painful vulva). Vulvodynia is believed to make up 8% to 12% of the general population (Rosen, 2018). VVS is characterized as a sharp pain located within and limited to the vulvar vestibule (vaginal entry) and elicited upon pressing or touching the vestibule of the vagina or attempted vaginal entry (Bergeron, 2002). They stressed the need for a multimodal approach to the therapy which is a "biopsychosocial model" that includes the "organic, cognitive, affective, behavioral, and relationship factors." They believed that even though the source of the pain is a medical issue, the pain gives rise to many psychological and social problems as well.

Dyspareunia as a pain disorder is an umbrella for other specific pain conditions in the vulva. The more common types are vulvodynia, vulvar vestibulitis, and vestibulodynia. At times it can be difficult to diagnose specific sexual pain and its underlying causes due to their overlap in similarities. Harlow and Stewart (2003) note that it takes women, on average, seeing three different doctors before receiving the correct GPPPD diagnosis. This is due to the lack of sexual health education that medical professionals receive during their time in school. Medical doctors report receiving little to no attention in their education about sexual health and sexual medicine. Some will receive a day lecture in sexual health or sexual concerns, some do not receive any, while others specialize in sex medicine and take a few courses on how to help with sexual problems. This is why therapists hear clients say that their doctors tell them to just drink some wine when they experience sexual pain, or that their pain is in their head, because many doctors were not trained in how to treat sexual concerns. As therapists, we need to understand the medical side in order to help provide our clients with appropriate resources and referrals to doctors who have training in properly diagnosing sexual pain concerns. Ethically, we are not medical doctors and should not provide medical advice. This is also why it is important to conduct a thorough sexual history. The Vulvar Pain Assessment Questionnaire Inventory provides great benefit to narrow down what type of dyspareunia a client may be experiencing (Dargie et al., 2016).

Vulvodynia is chronic pain in the vulva. It derives from the words "vulva" and the name of the Greek Goddess of Pain, Odyne. This word originated in the 19th century as doctors noticed hypersensitivity in the nerves of the vulvar area, typically described as a burning sensation, sometimes known as the "burning vulvar syndrome." It can also be characterized by irritation, raw sensation, and stinging. Later, researchers began to note the association of inflammation to the vulva. Due to the significance inflammation had in some forms of vulvodynia, the term "vulvar vestibulitis syndrome" (VVS) was coined to represent this subset. VVS is known for the painful touch to the vestibule area. In 1999, vestibulitis was renamed vestibulodynia (pain located throughout the entire vestibule). This came about as research started to recognize that vestibule pain was not solely due to inflammation. Vulvodynia then got differentiated into two different classes, provoked or unprovoked and localized or generalized (I. Goldstein et al., 2018).

Provoked vestibulodynia or PVD is known as pain localized to the vestibule where generalized vulvodynia is referred to as unprovoked pain to the entire vulva (I Goldstein et al., 2018). PVD impacts about 20% of women and has a lifelong prevalence rate of 12%. PVD is the most common of the GPPPD diagnoses. PVD can be described as rawness, along with stinging and burning sensations around the vulvar vestibule, opening of the urethra, labia minora, and hymen areas. Ways in which the provoked distress gets activated is usually by touching the vestibule, using tampons, gynecological exams, and penetration. PVD is broken down into two categories: "lifelong," referring to always experiencing this pain upon first vaginal insertions; and "acquired," meaning the individual used to not experience pain during vaginal insertion and now she does. This, as you can imagine, greatly impacts one's sexual desire and arousal states. While experiencing PVD, women can begin to develop negative messages about their sexual being and sexual relationship (Dunkely & Brotto, 2016). As stated previously, anxiety, depression, and stress can impact one's PVD, so much so that people who have had major depression and anxiety disorders are 4 to 11 times more likely to also have PVD (Khandker et al., 2011).

In assessing for dyspareunia, the questions a clinician should focus on asking are in areas such as:

- sexual desire
- arousal
- frequency
- orgasm
- sexual distress

- sexual satisfaction
- characteristics of the pain, such as onset
- duration
- location
- intensity
- thoughts and feelings around the sexual pain
- the couple's interaction in relation to the sexual pain
- fear of the pain
- avoidant tactics and behaviors
- partner's response
- anxiety and depression

Giving attention to other comorbid mental health diagnoses that could contribute, it is important to inquire about attempts in the past for treatment of the pain, domestic violence, nonsexual physical intimacy, other types of sexual intimacy that the individual engages in that are not painful, and past or present sexual abuse (I. Goldstein et al., 2018).

Medications can be another contributing cause for dyspareunia. Comparing the onset of the pain to the time when medication first started can add a benefit to what to rule out. Approximately 90% of women take a prescription drug. Irwin Goldstein et al. (2018) note that contraceptives that have hormones in them are the second most common drug used by women of a reproductive age, and when a woman has used these types of medications there is a high association to also experiencing dyspareunia, specifically vestibulodynia. In premenopausal women, vestibulodynia is the most common cause of sexual pain. They highlight that when women take contraception orally, they are 9.3 times more likely to also develop vestibulodynia. In another study they found that around 20% of women who took anxiety and depression medication were likely to experience a lack of lubrication and of sexual desire, both of which can lead to dyspareunia.

In understanding how to treat vulvar pain disorders, doctors would recommend noninvasive approaches such as physical therapy and psychotherapy. Today, doctors are trying to get more accurate with the treatment approach needed by looking at the client's history and results from past physicals and tests. Overall, researchers agree that an integrative approach is the most helpful for successful outcomes. Treatment approaches that have been found successful are sex therapy (I Goldstein et al., 2018), cognitive behavioral therapy, mindfulness-based cognitive behavioral therapy (Brotto et al., 2019), pelvic floor physical therapy, lidocaine, capsaicin, botulinum toxin type A (Botox), corticosteroids, interferon, hormonal treatments, systemic medications, surgery, and laser therapy (I. Goldstein et al., 2018). In 2016, Andrew Goldstein and colleagues found that surgery actually showed successful results that were as high as 60% to 90% for pain free symptoms in women, outweighing that of a CBT approach. Though the success rates were high, it was noted that surgery could eliminate different nerve endings that produce pleasure. Therefore, it was recommended that clients try other modalities first, like CBT and pelvic floor therapy, before surgery.

In 2015, the American Congress of Obstetricians and Gynecologists (ACOG), International Society for the Study of Women's Sexual Health (ISSWSH), the International Society for the Study of Vulvovaginal Disease (ISSVD), the International Pelvic Pain Society (IPPS), and the National Vulvodynia Association (NVA) came together to create a new name category for vulvodynia and vulvar pain. The categories of vulvar pain are now broken down into two categories: vulvar pain caused by specific disorders and vulvodynia which needs to be present for at least 3 months.*

*For more information about the new criteria, see I. Goldstein et al. (2018) *Female Sexual Function and Dysfunction: Diagnosis and Treatment*, pp. 250-253.

New studies have been showing a greater benefit in using mindfulness approaches in combination with cognitive behavioral therapy. Rosemary Basson (2012) found that utilizing mindfulness with CBT approaches with provoked vulvodynia showed promising results when scanning the brain during the utilization of these therapies. Lori Brotto et al. (2019) looked at a comparison between Mindfulness-Based Cognitive Behavioral approaches to that of Cognitive Behavioral Therapy when in relation to what they describe as the most common form of dyspareunia, provoked vulvodynia. They noted the success rate that CBT has had in reducing chronic pain and increasing sexual and psychological health, and wanted to see how Mindfulness-Based Cognitive Behavioral Therapy (MCBT) would hold up in comparison. The results reported that MCBT showed a greater effectiveness than the CBT. However, both have high success rates. The study was aimed to show that MCBT is an effective approach in reducing sexual pain, which it successfully did.

Studies also show that relationship interactions also greatly impact the way a woman experiences her sexual pain and her treatment outcome. Researchers note that a person's attachment style (specifically avoidant vs. anxious attachment) play a significant role in their treatment process (Charbonneau-Lefebvre et al., 2020). Levine et al. (2011) recommend that partners be involved early in the treatment process since a partner's role can have an important impact on the treatment outcomes. Their support and investment can be powerful and add to the healing process for the woman. When a partner is involved in the treatment (e.g., they attend doctor's appointments, help with dilators, engage in discussions around the treatment), women express feeling less like the sexual pain is solely their problem and responsibility and tend to feel more like help with their sexual challenges is a team approach. This adds another layer of connection and intimacy for partners to experience.

Team Treatment Approach

Some clinicians and research teams (Bergeron et al., 2003; Katz & Tabisel, 2002; Reising et al., 1999, 2004) have advocated an approach to the treatment of vaginismus and dyspareunia that requires a team approach. An example of this method is outlined in a book titled *Private Pain: It's About Life, Not Just Sex. Understanding Vaginismus & Dyspareunia* by Katz and Tabisel, (2002). They call their treatment the "DiRoss Treatment Approach." They describe it as a "hands-on, hands-in, hand-in-hand" approach. They believe that vaginismus is too complex to be treated at home and that the insertion of dilators does not prepare the woman for "The Five Penetrations of Life," which are inserting a finger, inserting an applicator, inserting a tampon, having intercourse, and having a pelvic exam. Further, they maintain that relaxation exercises do not help because the symptom of vaginismus is a "fight-or-flight" reaction rather than just a response to stress. They also think that teaching a woman to strengthen the pelvic floor muscles is not helpful because "vaginismus is not about voluntary muscle control or about strengthening weak muscles, but rather about the involuntary muscle component of the pelvic floor, which is strong and tight because of its ongoing fight-or-flight activity" (p. 194). They say that the treatment team includes a physician or physical therapist and a psychotherapist working together at the same time with the woman. Katz and Tabisel believe that since vaginismus is a body-mind phenomenon, it has to be treated through both the mind and the body. This approach includes medical and psychological management and a strong emphasis on educating the woman about her body, myths and misconceptions about sexuality, and identifying and eradicating the negative coping mechanisms she has been using. The pelvic floor musculature and how it works is an important part of the education process.

Most of the clinicians who advocate this team approach acknowledge that it is impossible to have that kind of team available to all therapists. Therefore, they strongly urge mental health providers to work closely with a physician and/or physical therapist throughout the treatment process. The call for a multidisciplinary approach provides a breakthrough in the treatment of these very distressful pain conditions. However, most mental health professionals do not have ready access to other professionals or the facilities needed to accomplish this ideal approach to treatment. Therefore, every mental health practitioner who attempts to treat dyspareunia or vaginismus should be well informed regarding the medical management and the physical therapy techniques used to control the pain. They must also be willing and able to interface with those professionals and to make the effort to coordinate the treatment so that, when necessary, they are providing simultaneous treatments.

The assertion that most dyspareunia is caused by PVD may or may not be true. Perhaps the setting in which the woman presents for treatment may bias the perception of the etiology of this symptom. Speculatively, one might surmise from the literature that the cases presenting in the medical facilities where a multidisciplinary treatment team exists may have certain characteristics in common: patients may be very well educated, they may have access to the internet which can direct them to those facilities, and they probably have insurance plans that can pay for the multiple providers necessary to access those treatment teams.

Private practice practitioners generally do not report their case outcomes for publication. Further, their failed cases may often become the cases that are eventually treated in the academic/hospital settings. The reported statistics from those treatment centers do not take into account the cases that are successfully treated by the individual practitioner. Clearly, there is a need for more research on the epidemiology of genital pain. There is also a need for more research on the successes and failures of the treatment of genital pain by private practitioners.

CBT and Mindfulness-based approaches are being shown to have a great impact in reducing dyspareunia in women. CBT alone shows a 34% to 85% success rate in reducing pain (Bergeron et al., 2001). This approach is considered a more preferred route over oral or topical medications as they seem to have a lower efficacy rate (Bergeron et al., 2008). CBT is used for PVD to reduce fears of pain that are anticipated, decrease vulvar pain, and increase positive sexual interactions. CBT contributes to reducing stress which, as discussed earlier, has an impact on the pain sensitivity a woman experiences in her vulva. Combining CBT with dilator exercises and sensate focus allows for a client to progress their treatment goals. CBT should "center on challenging maladaptive pain-related cognitions, change-oriented psychoeducation, and behavioral interventions, such as specific pain-relevant coping and self-management skills" (Brotto et al., 2016, p. 1907).

Mindfulness has recently been studied alongside CBT and at times seen as a great option in treating dyspareunia, especially if clients aren't responding well with CBT (Veehof et al., 2011). Mindfulness has been defined as the "state of mental focus that emphasizes acceptance and awareness of the present moment without judgment or evaluation. This state of mind or style of thinking can be thought of as a personal trait or as a cognitive skill that can be exercised and improved upon over time" (Brotto et al., 2016, p. 1907). Mindfulness is known for its stress-reducing impacts on people, and also has shown to be impactful in pain reduction on a broader spectrum than just genital pain (Ludwig & Kabat-Zinn, 2008; Matousek & Dobin, 2010). Research has been showing that mindfulness has great benefits to not only stress reduction but increase in emotional wellbeing, positive sexual outcomes, and cognitive wellbeing. In a state of mindfulness, the genital pain can be detached from one's physical sensations. This provides a reframe for how women view and experience their pain. Being able to stay focused on the present allows for the woman to get out of catastrophizing that anticipatory pain, which indirectly doesn't allow for the sensation of sensitivity in the body to increase, creating somewhat of a roadblock for hypervigilance to creep in. Along with pain reduction, mindfulness has also shown to be beneficial in increasing sexual arousal and desire, lubrication, sexual self-esteem, and overall sexual satisfaction (Brotto et al., 2016).

As you can see, mindfulness-based approaches along with CBT are great modalities to work with in reducing dyspareunia. So much so, that more recent studies began testing out what is called Mindfulness-Based Cognitive Behavioral Therapy or MBCT. It is suggested that the combination of the two therapies would provide an even stronger approach in reducing dyspareunia. Though the research is limited the literature discusses the promising impact that MBCT will have for dyspareunia (Brotto et al., 2016).

TREATMENT EXAMPLES FOR DYSPAREUNIA

Case Example 1

A tall and rather thin woman, age 35, was referred for psychological treatment of dyspareunia by her gynecologist. The gynecologist had diagnosed the problem about 3 months prior and had been seeing the patient two times per month. The treatment consisted of (a) very explicit education about the physiology and anatomy of the female genitals and sexual response, (b) pelvic floor exercises, and (c) gradual insertion of dilators. When the physician attempted to insert her fingers into the patient's vagina, the patient recoiled in pain and became tearful. Since penetration and dilation with the dilators had been successful, the physician was convinced that there must be some psychological issues related to penetration with a finger.

Although the patient was very motivated to eliminate the pain she experienced, she was unable to complete a detailed sex history form (see Sexual Health Assessment Questionnaire, pp. 539-551) that the therapist requested of her. She brought the form back to her second session and explained to the therapist that she had great difficulty as she tried to answer the questions. One reason was because she did not have very many memories about her childhood and early adolescent years, therefore, could not answer some of the questions about those years that were on the form. The other was that she became very anxious, almost to the point of a panic attack, when she had tried to answer those questions about which she did have memory. She could not explain her reactions and felt very inadequate to have to admit that she could not do such a "simple" task.

The patient was asked to try to answer the questions while wearing an EMDR audio-scan (a device developed by NeuroTek). As they went through the questions together over the next three sessions, the patient began to recall events from her past that she had not been able to remember before. The memories of events were generated by the patient without being "led" by the therapist. The memories were usually just informational but a few were very painful. She had watched her mother on a number of occasions, who had an eating disorder, put her finger down her throat and vomit. This memory elicited much emotion. As she began to talk about this memory, she realized that her mother had done this to her.

When she was about 12 years old, her mother began to "badger" her about her weight. Her mother believed that she was too chubby and that boys would never like her if she didn't start paying more attention to her appearance. Whenever she was "caught" eating something that her mother thought was fattening, her mother would take her in the bathroom and insert her finger down her throat to make her vomit. This continued with her mother inducing her to vomit until she was able to leave home to go to college at age 17. The patient did not continue this behavior after she left home.

She said that she was a very compliant child until she went to college. Once away from her mother's control she became rebellious. She ate whatever she wanted and soon found that she could eat without gaining weight. She became sexually involved with most of the men she dated. She did not have any problems having sexual intercourse until she became engaged to "the man of my dreams." They met 3 years ago and had a very enjoyable sex life until he proposed to her. She stated that it happened "overnight." One day she was able to have intercourse and thoroughly enjoy it, the next day he proposed, and the next day she experienced horrible pain when they tried to make love. She sought help from her gynecologist when her fiancé told her that he did not want to get married until the problem was solved.

Regaining the memories of the abuse from her mother enabled the patient to deal with her anxiety related to penetration. She was able to verbalize the connection between the forced penetration of her throat with her fear that if she allowed anyone to have "control" of her in a committed relationship, that person could also force penetration of her body. She worked with the therapist to desensitize her fears and was able to allow her gynecologist to insert a finger and then to have a complete gynecological exam.

Her partner joined in the treatment. They were given homework exercises that enabled *in vivo* desensitization to being penetrated. She faithfully practiced the pelvic floor exercises and the breathing techniques that she learned in sessions with both her gynecologist and her therapist. Soon she was able to insert her own finger into her vagina with her partner present. Then she was able to guide her partner's finger into her vagina. When she was comfortable with digital penetration, she was able to insert a dildo that was about the size of her partner's penis. Then she guided her partner while he inserted the dildo. When she was comfortable with the dildo being inserted, she was able to allow vaginal containment of her partner's penis as she guided the penetration. Finally, she was able to let her partner guide the penetration.

During the last few sessions of the psychological treatment, the focus was on helping the couple learn to enjoy their sex life again and dealing with fears (that they both expressed) that the symptoms may return. They were given advice about how to deal with a situation if pain should recur (i.e., taking a break, focusing on the pelvic floor muscles, breathing with the tensing and releasing of the muscles, and allowing her to control the speed and timing of penetration).

Case Discussion

This was a successful case because this patient was motivated and trusting enough to allow her gynecologist to work with her on the medical/physical issues. She was also trusting of the therapist and willing to try EMDR even though she was very frightened of what she might feel if she tried to answer the questions on the sex history form. This case illustrates how abuse other than sexual abuse can be the etiological factor for a sexual dysfunction. It also demonstrates the major goals of therapeutic interventions as stated by Binik et al. (2000): (a) reducing or controlling the pain, (b) dealing with the negative consequences of having experienced the pain, and (c) reestablishing a pleasurable sex life.

This case was not difficult to treat because the referring gynecologist had already begun the treatment and elicited the trust and hope from the patient that helped to motivate her to work hard. There are times, however, when a patient comes to the office of a mental health practitioner only to appease her partner and never having sought treatment from any other caregiver. The reluctant patient is always a challenge. She is a particular challenge when the issue is something as personal and embarrassing as sexuality.

Case Example 2

Client was a 38-year-old sullen and reluctant woman who presented for therapy with her husband. He called to make the appointment and informed the therapist that he may have to come alone because he wasn't sure that his wife would come with him. She came but announced almost immediately that she was there only because she felt that her husband would be angry if she did not. He stated that they had been married for 5 years. This was her first marriage and his second. He had left his first marriage because his wife of 3 years had an affair. They had no children but he desperately wanted a child. They were unable to have intercourse very often because she had, as she described, excruciating pain whenever he tried to penetrate her.

She was very outspoken about being angry with him for forcing her to be humiliated by talking to someone about this problem. She considered it to be a problem mostly for him because she was happy with the sex that they could have. She was able to enjoy some forms of stimulation sometimes. However, there were certain times when she felt pain even at the slightest touch of her genital area. She believed that her husband was inconsiderate because he did not accept the fact that her pain was "natural."

When questioned about her belief that her pain was "natural," she said that her mother told her that all women have pain when they have intercourse and that you learn to "grin and bear it." Her mother's prediction of pain with intercourse was confirmed by two of her high school girl friends who told her that they had bled when they had intercourse and that it hurt. The couple was asked to fill out a sex history questionnaire and return the following week to individual sessions where the therapist would review the questionnaire with them. The woman returned with her questionnaire minimally filled out with "yes" and "no" responses to all questions even those that obviously required more. She said that she thought that this whole process was ridiculous and did not see what anyone could do to change "the way things are."

Her history revealed that she had had intercourse with only one other partner prior to her husband. The first intercourse had been painful as she knew it would be. She was in love with her partner and felt that the pain was worth it until she learned that she had genital warts. Her physician informed her that this was a sexually transmitted disease (STD) and since she had never had sex with anyone other than that partner, she knew that he had had sex with someone else while they were dating. She ended the relationship and vowed never to have sex again until she was married.

The therapist asked her to do a test at home by taking a cotton swab and touch the vulvar area with it. She reported that the touch with the cotton swab had felt painful. She was asked then to go to see a gynecologist who was known to have expertise in working with patients with sexual problems. The gynecological exam indicated that the patient probably had vulvodynia, perhaps VVS. When the patient heard this diagnosis she felt justified about her pain and angrier with her husband for seeming not to understand her pain.

She was encouraged to pay attention to the timing of the pain throughout an entire menstrual cycle. She learned that the pain was most severe during the time that she was ovulating. This presented a major obstacle to conception and increased his despair about ever having a child. At this point the couple and the therapist determined that they needed to work out a comprehensive treatment approach which would necessitate each of them being totally honest about what they wanted in the relationship. They learned that they both wanted a child, but she was afraid of the potential pain involved in conceiving and in giving birth. They both wanted to have a fulfilling sex life but she could not imagine sex not being painful. After two sessions during which the therapist educated both partners about the physiology and anatomy of sexuality, talked about the myths and facts about pain with first intercourse, and emphasized the pleasures of sexuality, the woman was able to express hope that she could cope with and minimize her expectations of pain.

They decided to work to learn to control the pain. She eventually was able to have intercourse occasionally without pain. They decided to consult their physician about using artificial insemination if they could not have intercourse during ovulation. After making that decision, she found that she was able to have intercourse and endure the pain during one of the days when she would be fertile in her cycle. At termination of the treatment, they were not pregnant yet, but they were happy with their sexual relationship.

Case Discussion

This case was very interesting in that it was never clear whether the woman had VVS. Since she was infected with an STD, one could hypothesize that her knowledge that sexual intercourse caused the STD created the pain and, therefore, the pain was psychosomatic. It is also possible that the STD was the physical etiology of the VVS. It was clear that she developed many fears about sexual penetration as a young woman and those fears were confirmed for her. The therapy helped this couple to learn what their priorities were and how to achieve them together. It helped them to master the pain together instead of struggling against it and each other.

PELVIC FLOOR PHYSICAL THERAPY

We wanted to give special attention to pelvic floor physical therapy as it can play a large role in the treatment of Genito-Pelvic Pain/Penetration Disorder. As Andrew Goldstein et al. (2011) recommends in their book *When Sex Hurts: A Woman's Guide to Banishing Sexual Pain*, pelvic floor physical therapy should be used in almost all GPPPDs because of its incredibly efficacy.

The pelvic floor is what many describe as a hammock or bowl shape of muscles in your pelvis, stretching from your pubic bone wrapping down and under ending at the tailbone. The pelvic floor contains three different layers of muscles called the pubococcygeus muscle or the PC muscles. On top of those muscles, the pelvic floor holds the urethra, bladder, rectum, and perineum. When you have a bowel movement or during urination, the PC muscles are what contract and release during that process. In fact, if you try to squeeze your urethra right now like you're trying to hold in your urination and then release that squeeze you can feel your pelvic floor muscles working. This is also called a Kegel exercise. Knowing how this muscle feels is important during treatment because it allows you to become more mindful of how strong or weak your pelvic floor is. It also allows you more body awareness and control. For example, if you start to feel anxious to have sex due to vulvar pain, you can notice if your pelvic floor feels tense or relaxed. Sometimes the pelvic floor muscles can be too tense or too loose, making it more challenging to do this exercise. Having pelvic floor muscles that are too strong are called hypertonia and having pelvic floor muscles that are too weak is called hypotonia. Hypertonia, tighter muscles, are the cause for most sexual pain disorders while hypotonia, loose muscles, are the cause for prolapse. A prolapse happens when the pelvic floor is too weak or loose and the organs that were once held up by the pelvic floor start to collapse. We hear about this most often in women after they have given birth as a result of having weaker pelvic floor muscles. This is also common after full hysterectomies (A. Goldstein et al., 2011).

Pelvic floor therapists thus evaluate the tone of the pelvic floor muscles to assess for the degree to which the muscles need help strengthening and/or loosening. This is done through checking the patient's mobility along with an internal examination of the muscles. Different parts of the pelvic floor muscles are pressed to identify any trigger points, knots, spasms, along with having the patient squeeze their pelvic floor to feel the strength of the muscles (A. Goldstein et al., 2011).

So why does someone experience pelvic floor muscle tension? For many, their pelvic floor muscle tension is completely unconscious until they gain the mindfulness component of noticing the tension versus relaxation in their body. Pelvic floor muscle tension can occur for a number of different reasons. Chronic yeast infections, trauma, stress, generalized vulvodynia, and lichen sclerosis, just to name a few, can cause the pelvic floor to go into a protective mechanism state by clinching these muscles. Some people hold stress and tension in their neck and shoulders, while others might hold in their stress in their pelvic floor. If the pelvic floor has experienced pain and discomfort such as with chronic yeast infections, that natural protective mechanism gets activated. The most popular way professionals tend to describe muscle tension in the pelvic floor is when they liken it to touching a hot stove. Once you've touched a hot stove there is a mind-body association to touching the stove. Touching a stove is hot and it hurts. Your body clenches up if you go to touch a hot stove again. You try and avoid touching a hot stove. This is what happens in the pelvic floor area. If there's been pain, the mind can start to translate that experience into a mind-body association. When the pelvic floor muscles begin to tighten, lactic acid increases in that region of the body, creating nerve compressions which lead to pain (A. Goldstein et al., 2011).

There are a number of treatment approaches that pelvic floor therapists utilize when working with GPPPDs. First is education. Providing clients with what is happening in their body, body awareness, and an understanding of their condition can be empowering. For many patients this helps them realize that their pain is real and there are solutions to help (A. Goldstein et al., 2011).

Biofeedback through pelvic floor surface electromyography (sEMG) is an additional intervention that is commonly used during pelvic floor therapy. The device used provides sensors that stick around the pelvic floor area to check the pelvic floor's muscle tone. It assists in allowing the patient to practice tightening and loosening their muscles while being able to visually see the muscles contracting on the sEMG screen. During this exercise, the patient wears a medical garment such as a robe or sheet while lying on the physical therapy table. The physical therapist provides exercises for the patient to do at home to work on the strength of the pelvic floor (A. Goldstein et al., 2011). In one study of women who had vulvodynia, half of the women who did the homework showed progress on the sEMG (Carroli & Mignini, 2009).

Myofascial is what Andrew Goldstein and colleagues (2011) describe as a covering over bones, muscles, organs, and nerves. Typically, the fascia moves with the organs but when it is in an unhealthy state the fascia sticks to the internal parts of the body which makes stability and flexibility challenging. During myofascial releases, the physical therapist massages and stretches out that targeted area providing more space for the fascia to breath and release the lactic acid that has built up.

Myofascial trigger point release are areas that create too much tension or knots within the muscle that need to be loosened. Similar to myofascial releases, physical therapists use methods to try and release the trigger points with their fingers, elbows, and knuckles. When the hypertonic is severe, a more aggressive intervention might be used such as botulinum toxin (Botox), which relaxes the muscles and allows for a deeper stretch to occur.

The most common approach with pelvic floor physical therapy is pelvic floor retraining. Pelvic floor retraining focuses on sEMG, Kegels, and using vibrators and dilators for stretching and relaxing the pelvic floor muscles. Other interventions include connective tissue manipulation, neural mobilization, joint mobilization, spinal core stabilization, electrical stimulation, and therapeutic ultrasounds. Finding a pelvic floor physical therapist can be difficult. Thankfully, this is a field that continues to grow. To find someone near you, you can contact the American Physical Therapy Association (Levine et al., 2011).

CONCLUSION

Genital pain is perhaps the most disconcerting type of sexual problem that mental health professionals must confront. It is difficult to access and evaluate. It is difficult to predict what type of therapy is most likely to work. Most patients come to the therapist with a history of failed previous treatments that leave them feeling hopeless and inadequate. Etiology includes negative sexual messages as a child and young adolescent, to sexual abuse, emotional abuse, medical traumas, relationship dysfunction, personal psychopathology, anger with the spouse, and so forth. It can lead to other sexual problems such as loss of desire, loss of ability to have orgasm, loss of ability to lubricate, and sexual avoidance, all of which further complicate the treatment.

It is the successes that sex therapists have with these cases that keep them hopeful, motivated to keep studying, and learning new theories and treatment techniques. Perhaps because there are so many causes of genital pain, there are many treatment approaches that bring at least some relief to many patients. Hopefully, sexologists will continue to do the research that will provide the answers needed for women who are desperately looking for resolution to their complaints of genital pain.

REFERENCES

American Psychiatric Association. (1994). *Diagnostic and statistical manual of mental Disorders* (4th ed.).

American Psychiatric Association. (2013). *Diagnostic and statistical manual of mental disorders* (5th ed.). http://doi. Org/10.1176/appi.books.9780890425596

Barbach, L. (1975). *For yourself: The fulfillment of female sexuality.* Doubleday.

Barbach, L. (1980). *Women discover orgasm: A therapist's guide to a new treatment approach.* Free Press.

Basson, R. (2012). The recurrent pain and sexual sequelae of provoked vestibulodynia: A perpetuating cycle. *The Journal of Sexual Medicine, 9*(8), 2077-2092.

Bergeron, S., Binik, Y. M., Khalifé, S., Pagidas, K., Glazer, H. I., Meana, M., & Amsel, R. (2001). A randomized comparison of group cognitive-behavioral therapy, surface electromyographic biofeedback, and vestibulectomy in the treatment of dyspareunia resulting from vulvar vestibulitis. *Pain, 91*(3), 297-306.

Bergeron, S., Brown, C., Lord, M., Oala, M., Binik, Y., & Khalifé, S. (2002). Physical therapy for vulvar vestibulitis syndrome: A retrospective study. *Journal of Sex and Marital Therapy, 28*(3), 183-192.

Bergeron, S., Khalifé, S., & Dupuis, M. J. (2008, February). *Provoked vestibulodynia: A randomized comparison of cognitive-behavioral therapy and medical management.* Annual Meeting of the International Society for the Study of Women's Sexual Health, San Diego, CA.

Bergeron, S., Meana, M., Binik, Y., & Khalifé, S. (2003). Painful genital sexual activity. In S. B. Levine, C. R. Risen, & S. E. Althof (Eds.), *Handbook of clinical sexuality for mental health professionals* (pp. 131-152). Brunner-Routledge.

Binik, Y. M., Bergeron, S., & Khalifé, S. (2000). Dyspareunia. In S. R. Leiblum & R. C. Rosen (Eds.), *Principles and practice of sex therapy* (3rd ed.). Guilford Press.

Both, S., van Lunsen, R., Weijenborg, P., & Laan, E. (2012). A new device for simultaneous measurement of pelvic floor muscle activity and vaginal blood flow: A test in a nonclinical sample. *The Journal of Sexual Medicine, 9*(11), 2888-2902. https://doi.org/10.1111/j.1743-6109.2012.02910.x

Brotto, L. A., Bergeron, S., Zdaniuk, B., Driscoll, M., Grabovac, A., Sadownik, L. A., . . . Basson, R. (2019). A comparison of mindfulness-based cognitive therapy vs. cognitive behavioral therapy for the treatment of provoked vestibulodynia in a hospital clinic setting. *The Journal of Sexual Medicine, 16*(6), 909-923. https://doi.org/10.1016/j.jsxm.2019.04.002

Brotto, L. A., Chivers, M. L., Millman, R. D., & Albert, A. (2016). Mindfulness-based sex therapy improves genital-subjective arousal concordance in women with sexual desire/arousal difficulties. *Archives of Sexual Behavior, 45*(8), 1907-1921. https://doi.org/10.1007/s10508-015-0689-8

Carroli, G., & Mignini, L. (2009). Episiotomy for vaginal birth. *Cochrane Database for Systemic Reviews, 1,* CD000081. https//doi.org/10.1002/14651858.CD000081.pub2

Charbonneau-Lefebvre, V., Rosen, N. O., Bosisio, M., Vaillancourt-Morel, M-P., & Bergeron, S. (2020). An attachment perspective on partner responses to genito-pelvic pain and their associations with relationship and sexual outcomes. *The Journal of Sex Research, 58*(2), 235-247. https://doi.org/10.1080/00224499.2020.1761936

Dargie, E., Holdon, R. R., & Pukall, C. F. (2016). The Vulvar Pain Assessment Questionnaire Inventory. *Pain, 157*(12), 1. https://doi:10.1097/j.pain.0000000000000682

Dias-Amaral, A., & Marques-Pinto, A. (2018). Female genito-pelvic pain/penetration disorder: Review of the related factors and overall approach. (Perturbação de dor Gênito-pélvica e da penetração: revisão dos fatores associados e abordagem geral). *Revista Brasileira de Ginecologia e Obstetricia: Revista da Federacao Brasileira das Sociedades de Ginecologia e Obstetricia, 40*(12), 787-793. https://doi.org/10.1055/s-0038-1675805

Dunkley, C., & Brotto, L. (2016). Psychological treatments for provoked vestibulodynia: Integration of mindfulness-based and cognitive behavioral therapies. *Journal of Clinical Psychology, 72*(7), 637-650. https://doi.org/10.1002/jclp.22286

Fuchs, D., Hoch, Z., Paldi, E., Abramovici, H., Brandes, J. M., Timor-Tritsch, I., & Kleinhaus, M. (1978). Hypnodesensitization therapy of vaginismus: In vitro and in vivo methods. In J. LoPiccolo & L. LoPiccolo (Eds.), *Handbook of sex therapy* (pp. 261-270). Plenum Press.

Ghizzani, A., & Sestini, P. (2017). Sexual pain in women: Exploring the manifestations of vaginismus versus vulvodynia. *Minerva Ginecologica, 69*(1), 1-5. https//doi.org/10.23736/S0026-4784.16.03966-6

Goldstein, A. T., Pukall, C. F., Brown, C., Bergeron, S., Stein, A., & Kellogg-Spadt, S. (2016). Vulvodynia: Assessment and treatment. *The Journal of Sexual Medicine, 13*(4), 572-590. https://doi.org/10.1016/j.jsxm.2016.01.020

Goldstein, A., Pukall, C. F., & Goldstein, I. (2011). *When sex hurts: A woman's guide to banishing sexual pain.* Da Capo Lifelong.

Goldstein, I., Clayton, A. Goldstein, A., Kim, N., & Kingsber, S. (2018). *Female sexual function and dysfunction: Diagnosis and treatment.* John Wiley & Sons.

Harlow, B. L., & Stewart, E. G. (2003). A population-based assessment of chronic unexplained vulvar pain: Have we underestimated the prevalence of vulvodynia? *Journal of the American Medical Women's Association, 58*(2), 82-88.

Heiman, J., & LoPiccolo, J. (1988). *Becoming orgasmic: A sexual & personal growth program for women.* Prentice Hall.

Kaplan, H. S. (1974). *The new sex therapy.* Brunner/Mazel.

Kaplan, H. S. (1983). *The evaluation of sexual disorders: Psychological and medical aspects.* Brunner/Mazel.

Katz, D., & Tabisel, R. L. (2002). *Private pain: It's about life not just sex. Understanding vaginismus & dyspareunia.* Kromar Printing Ltd.

Kaufman, S. (1983). The gynecological evaluation of dyspareunia & unconsummated marriage. In H. S. Kaplan (Ed.), *The evaluation of sexual disorders: Psychological and medical aspects.* Brunner/Mazel.

Kegel, A. (1948). Progressive exercise in the functional restoration of the perineal muscles. *American Journal of Obstetrics and Gynecology*, 56, 238-248.

Khandker, M., Brady, S. S., Vitonis, A. F., MacLehose, R. F., Stewart, E. G., & Harlow, B. L. (2011). The influence of depression and anxiety on risk of adult onset vulvodynia. *Journal of Women's Health, 20*(10), 1445-1451. https// https://doi.org/10.1089/jwh.2010.2661

Lahaie, M. A., Amsel, R., Khalifé, S., Boyer, S., Faaborg-Andersen, M., & Binik, Y. M. (2015). Can fear, pain, and muscle tension discriminate vaginismus from dyspareunia/provoked vestibulodynia? Implications for the new DSM-5 diagnosis of genito-pelvic pain/penetration disorder. *Archives of Sexual Behavior*, *44*(6), 1537-1550. https://doi.org/10.1007/s10508-014-0430-z

Lauman, E., Gagnon, J., Michael, R., & Michaels, S. (1994). *The social organization of sexuality: Sexuality practices in the United States.* University of Chicago Press.

Levine, S., Risen, C., & Althof, S. (2011). *Handbook of clinical sexuality for mental health professionals.* Routledge.

Lieblum, S. R. (2000). Vaginismus a most perplexing problem. In S. R. Lieblum & R. C. Rosen (Eds.), *Principles and practices of sex therapy* (3rd ed., pp. 181-202). Guilford Press.

Love, P., & Robinson, J. (1990). *The emotional incest syndrome: What to do when a parent's love rules your life.* Bantam Books.

Ludwig, D. S., & Kabat-Zinn, J. (2008). Mindfulness in medicine. *JAMA, 300*(11), 1350-1352.

Masters, W. H., & Johnson, V. E. (1966). *Human sexual response.* Little, Brown.

Masters, W. H., & Johnson, V. E. (1970). *Human sexual inadequacy*. Little, Brown.

Matousek, R. H., & Dobkin, P. L. (2010). Weathering storms: A cohort study of how participation in a mindfulness-based stress reduction program benefits women after breast cancer treatment. *Current oncology, 17*(4), 62-70. https://doi.org/10.3747/co.v17i4.572

Nobre, P. J., & Pinto-Gouveia, J. (2008). Cognitive and emotional predictors of female sexual dysfunctions: Preliminary findings. *Journal of Sex and Marital Therapy, 34*(4), 325-342. https://doi.org/10.1080/00926230802096358

Nobre, P. J., & Pinto-Gouveia, J. (2009). Cognitive schemas associated with negative sexual events: A comparison of men and women with and without sexual dysfunction. *Archives of Sexual Behavior, 38*(5), 842-851. https://doi.org/10.1007/s10508-008-9450-x

Pacik, P. T. (2009). Botox treatment for vaginismus. *Plastic Reconstructive Surgery, 124*(6), 455e-456e. https://doi.org/10.1097/PRS.0b013e3181bf7f11

Pacik, P. T., & Geletta, S. (2017). Vaginismus treatment: Clinical trials follow up 241 patients. *Sexual Medicine, 5*(2), e114-e123. https://doi.org/10.1016/j.esxm.2017.02.002

Pridal, C., & LoPiccolo, J. (2000). Multi-element treatment of desire disorders: Integration of cognitive, behavioral and systemic therapy. In S. Leiblum & R. Rosen (Eds.), *Principles and practice of sex therapy* (3rd ed., pp. 57-81). Guilford Press.

Reissing, E., Binik, Y., & Khalife, S. (1999). Does vaginismus exist? A critical review of the literature. *Journal of Nervous and Mental Disease, 187,* 261-274. https://doi.org/10.1097/00005053-199905000-00001

Reissing, E., Binik, Y., Khalife, S., Cohen, D., & Amsel, R. (2004). Vaginal spasm, pain, and behavior: An empirical investigation of the diagnosis of vaginismus. *Archives of Sexual Behavior, 33,* 5-17.

Rosen, N. O. (2018). Genito-pelvic pain from a couples' perspective. *Canadian Journal of Pain, 2*(1), A1. https//doi.org/10.1080/24740527.2018.1452499

Rosen, N. O., Bergeron, S., Sadikaj, G., Glowacka, M., Delisle, I., & Baxter, M.-L. (2014). Impact of male partner responses on sexual function in women with vulvodynia and their partners: A dyadic daily experience study. *Health Psychology, 33*(8), 823-831. https://doi.org/10.1037/a0034550

Schnarch, D. M. (1991). *Constructing the sexual crucible: An integration of sexual and marital therapy.* W. W. Norton.

Schoen, M. (Producer) & Nathanson, B. (Director). (1984). *Treating Vaginismus* [Film]. Focus International.

van der Kolk, B. A. (2002). Beyond the talking cure: Somatic experience and subcortical imprints in the treatment of trauma. In F. Shapiro (Ed.), *EMDR as an integrative psychotherapy approach: Experts of diverse orientations explore the paradigm prism* (pp. 57-85). American Psychological Association. https://doi.org/10.1037/10512-003

Veehof, M. M., Oskam, M. J., Schreurs, K. M., & Bohlmeijer, E. T. (2011). Acceptance-based interventions for the treatment of chronic pain: A systematic review and meta-analysis. *Pain, 152*(3), 533-542.

Weeks, G. R. (2005). The emergence of a new paradigm in sex therapy: Integration. *Sexual and Relationship Therapy, 20*(1), 89-103.

Zulfikaroglu, E. (2020). Patient's characteristics and outcome of therapy in vaginismus: A single-center report of nine-year experience. *Journal of Sexual and Relationship Therapy*. https://doi:10.1080/14681994.2020.1722991

15

Assessment and Treatment of Erection Dysfunction

Frederick L. Peterson, Jr. and Jonathan Reid Hester

Perhaps no other area of sexual health has changed so rapidly and dramatically over the last 3 decades as has the treatment of erection dysfunction (ED). In 1993, The National Institutes of Health (NIH) convened a Consensus Conference on Impotence, which was the very first NIH conference organized to address a sexual health topic (NIH Consensus Development Panel on Impotence, 1993). The pioneering sex researcher William Masters was the keynote speaker at the Consensus Conference. After his return to his training center in St. Louis (the Masters and Johnson Institute, as described in SHOWTIME's *The Masters of Sex* series), Doc Masters provided the clinical staff a seminar based on his keynote address at NIH (Peterson et al., 2020). As a Clinical Fellow at the Institute at that time, the first author of this chapter was impressed by several central messages, and "Doc" emphasized the following:

1. Human beings have natural cravings for both food and sex; and these biological needs are very similar except, fortunately, you won't die if you don't have sex (although there are some physiological effects of sexual abstinence).
2. There are so many factors that interfere with a man's sexual interest and ability to have erections, it is quite remarkable most men have as much sex as they do.
3. "Impotence" can ironically serve as a stimulus for a man to become a better lover, because through sex therapy, getting a man to have erections and resuming sex is the easy part. Achieving an emotionally meaningful and satisfying relationship is the challenge.
4. At that historic conference, the term "impotence" was declared obsolete in favor of the more neutral as well as precise term "erection dysfunction."

ED is defined as the persistent difficulty to achieve and/or maintain an erection of sufficient rigidity to permit satisfactory completion of the sexual intercourse (NIH Consensus Development Panel on Impotence, 1993). According to the *Diagnostic and Statistical Manual of Mental Disorders* (5th ed.; *DSM-5*; American Psychiatric Association, 2013), the erection problem must be a continuing concern for at least 6 months, occurs the vast majority of attempts to have sexual activity (75%-100% of the time), and causes distress to the individual man. There are other qualifying stipulations (such as the erection problem can't be caused by medications or drug use) but that is the primary definition of ED.

Interestingly, based upon this definition, there are many men who do not have erections on a regular basis and do not have ED. Many of these men do not have sexual intercourse on a regular basis (or even "never" as in "it has been years ago") and do not have ED. These men are not diagnosed with ED because they (and their partners very often) do not define it as a problem.

The goal of this contribution is to help mental health professionals develop a better understanding of how to respond to clients who complain of ED from the context of the multidisciplinary field of sex health. To meet this objective, the chapter authorship represents expertise from the fields of psychology and medicine. Erection function as well as dysfunction, a best practice assessment approach, and empirically based treatment options will be reviewed. Because there are few published research studies on homosexual men with ED, this contribution discusses the assessment and treatment of heterosexual men with ED, although many, if not most, of the interventions would likely be effective with men of any sexual orientation. Several clinical vignettes are included to illustrate key principles and practices used with real patients.

This contribution is intended to provide a basic level of understanding for the assessment and treatment of ED, because providing all information needed for high proficiency in treating ED is well beyond the scope of this contribution. Mental health professionals who wish to pursue advanced skills in sex therapy are encouraged to join the membership of the American Association of Sexuality Educators, Counselors and Therapists (AASECT), which is an accrediting body offering four levels of certification of practice. The advantages of pursuing AASECT certification and the process of developing a sexual health component to one's mental health practice are described elsewhere in this text (especially in Chapter 1).

INTRODUCTION TO ERECTION FUNCTION AND DYSFUNCTION

To better understand how the various physical and psychological factors affect erections, it is important to be aware of the many processes that take place before, during, and after sexual tumescence begins. Under typical circumstances, a desire for sexual activity is generally thought to precede physical arousal. This is often not the case for normal function in men, as erections frequently occur independent of psychological libido, such as morning erections with men who have normal endocrinology and neurology (Peterson et al., 2020; Peterson & Furest, 2007).

Desire is influenced by both physical and psychological factors. The physical factors include adequate testosterone levels, medications, and the absence of other disease states or impairments. Assuming these factors are in balance, the message has to get from the brain to the penis by way of the nervous system. When the neural message arrives, the arteries start to dilate and more blood flows into erectile tissue in the penis (primarily the corpora cavernosa). Erection is accomplished by the release of nitric oxide that, in turn, causes the production of a chemical (cGMP), and cGMP relaxes the smooth muscle in the corpora cavernosa so that the penis becomes tumescent and rigid. As the penis fills with blood, the venous system becomes compressed; this allows increased pressure to take place, giving the penis the rigidity needed for penetration. Normally, there is an enzyme (PDE5 inhibitor) that breaks down the cGMP, allowing the smooth muscle to contract and decrease the blood flow into the penis (which ends the erection). Once orgasm has occurred, the arteries constrict, the veins open-up, and the erection subsides. This description represents the current understanding of the multiple factors involved in erectile function.

One of the best prevalence studies on ED was conducted in 1992 by the National Health and Social Life Survey (NHSLS) and consisted of a national probability sample of 1,410 men aged 18 to 59. The NHSLS estimated a point prevalence of approximately 5% and a lifetime prevalence of approximately 10% (Laumann et al., 1999). The Massachusetts Male Aging Study (MMAS), a large longitudinal study following men aged 40 to 70, reported findings consistent with the NHSLS. The MMAS found 10% of that sample having "complete impotence" and approximately 35% reporting "moderate to complete erectile dysfunction" (Feldman et al., 1994). If considering any level of erectile functioning (even mild and temporary), then the prevalence increases to 52% (Feldman et al., 1994). These studies and others demonstrate a consistent association between aging and erectile dysfunction for men. In general, the incidence and severity of ED increase as men age and are also affected by men's health status (Laumann et al., 1999; Masters et al., 1995).

Traditional approaches to understanding ED emphasized a division between two types of ED based on causality: physical (often called "organic") or psychological. Physical causes include pharmacological (such as use of antihypertensives), endocrinologic (diabetes), or neurologic (spinal cord injury) factors; lifestyle choices (e.g., smoking); or penile disease or trauma. Psychological risk factors for ED include sexual trauma history, depression, anxiety, guilt, or having significant conflict with one's sexual partner.

An integrated systems perspective has evolved which views the division of causal factors into "physical or psychological" as artificial and not reflecting the true nature of the client's experience. Although identification of the contributing factors to ED is paramount, most cases of ED have a multicausal etiology ("mixed etiology"), and causal factors often have reciprocal influences upon one another. For example, a significant percentage of men who develop diabetes mellitus will experience some level of erectile dysfunction. A man who has a predisposition for developing diabetes and who also has clinical depression may engage in behaviors that facilitate the development of diabetes, such as not exercising, failing to follow a healthy diet, abusing alcohol to self-medicate, and becoming obese. Once the diabetes becomes severe enough to cause ED, he may become more depressed, develop marital discord, and experience heightened anxiety when his partner leaves him. In such cases, patient satisfaction and outcome may be improved with counseling even when the ED is secondary to a medical condition or mixed etiology (American Association of Clinical Endocrinologists [AACE], 1998; NIH Consensus Development Panel on Impotence, 1993).

Clinical Vignette: Young Married Man With Erection Dysfunction*

This clinical vignette involves a heterosexual couple in their 30s, Jill and Dave (pseudonyms). They were a handsome pair of DINKs (Dual-Income, No Kids). They sought sex therapy for Dave's erection dysfunction (ED), which was secondary to injuries sustained in a motor vehicle accident. They had previously worked with a sex therapist to address communication issues as a young married couple, build sexual literacy, and get assistance dealing with the ED. They described the therapy as beneficial but short-lived, as the couple relocated from California to a mid-sized city in the Midwest.

Dave reported a history of normal erectile function before his injury at age 26. Immediately after his accident, he was fortunate enough to receive care at an excellent medical center that included sexual health as part of his rehabilitation. The professionals initially worked with him on understanding the specific injuries he suffered as a result of pelvic bone splintering into his vascular system and the subsequent scar tissue that developed from surgical removal of the bone. The physician started Dave on a first-line treatment of a vacuum constriction device (VCD, also known as the penile pump), which he found satisfactory in terms of helping him get and maintain erections suitable for intercourse. Dave was referred for outpatient follow-up to a psychologist who had specialized competence in sex therapy. As mentioned, the couple worked with their first therapist regarding sexual health literacy in general and specifically about the issues and myths about erection dysfunction. Dave wanted to try other treatment options as the couple found the VCD somewhat cumbersome and an interference with the natural flow of their foreplay.

Dave was started on a 50 mg dose of sildenafil citrate (Viagra) but without effect. He reported some improvement when using 100 mg, the maximum dosage for a 24-hour period. He denied any

*Names and identifying characteristics in all case examples have been changed to protect privacy.

significant side effects that were not tolerable. He recalled moving from a satisfaction rating of about "20" for getting and keeping erections to about "60+" with the pharmacological aid of Viagra. The couple was able to have sexual intercourse on a more regular basis, but Dave still was not satisfied with the level of firmness or rigidity of his erections. When the couple started with their second sex therapist (the first author of this chapter), Jill's response to Dave's improved sexual function became a focus of therapy, especially her ambivalent affective response to having sexual relations with Dave. It was obvious that Jill dearly loved her husband and that she was willing to do about anything sexually to please him. At the same time, she was experiencing mild to moderate feelings of discomfort and, on occasion, disgust when engaged sexually with him.

Jill denied any sexual trauma history or any lapse in her memory of childhood. Jill slowly started to identify aspects of her socialization as a female, especially messages from her parents about sex, which contributed to her adverse visceral response to sex. She always thought that "sex and I are not a good match" and that her negative feelings about sex were part of her biology; that she simply did not like sex like other people did. Some individual counseling to supplement the couple's sex therapy helped her come to an understanding that it was her socialization that was contributing to her negative visceral response. She literally described an "epiphany experience" that this realization facilitated, and almost immediately she reported feeling empowered in minimizing and eventually eliminating her negative visceral response to her own sexuality as well as sexual intercourse with Dave.

Dave wanted to explore enhancing his sexual relations with Jill. The personal growth Jill experienced in terms of fulfilling more of her own sexual health potential opened up the possibilities for further developing their sexual life together. Jill reported less frequent negative feelings, and she started initiating sexual relations. Dave felt his sexual initiatives were more often welcomed by Jill, and he was more comfortable exploring other treatment options for his ED. After reviewing patient health education videos regarding second-line treatment options, Dave consulted with his urologist regarding injection therapy. Using the product Caverject, Dave found a double benefit over his use of Viagra. First, he reported an increase in the rigidity of his erections. Secondly, Dave reported increased consistency (reliability) of getting and keeping erections (from "60% of attempts to over 80+") as well as some increase in the lasting duration of erections.

THE ASSESSMENT PROCESS FOR ERECTION FUNCTION

The comprehensive assessment of ED is a complex process which requires multidisciplinary input and review. This integrated, multidisciplinary approach is reflected in what Fagan (2003) refers to as "the perspectives," evaluating client data from disease, behavior, and life story points of view. This section informs mental health professionals of their role in this process and what to consider from the perspective of other disciplines. Comprehensive assessment includes a review of presenting complaints and the couple's expectations (including desired outcomes), psychosexual history, substance uses, standardized measurement of the severity of ED, psychological assessment of personality factors if indicated (depression), and medical examination/measurement if there is indication of medical conditions/factors contributing to the presenting complaint. Determining if the patient is clinically depressed, has a sexual trauma history, experiences anxiety and/or guilt regarding sex, or reports partner conflict are also key factors in the assessment of ED.

Assessment of ED, unless it is solely of psychogenic etiology, usually requires multiple sessions. Single-session assessment of ED by mental health professionals usually is not effective unless it is an extended-time single session (2-4 hours) and/or a low-complexity case, such as performance anxiety as the sole causal factor. Moderate- to high-complexity cases usually require multiple sessions to allow detailed developmental histories to be taken from both individuals and conferring with other healthcare providers for medical evaluations.

It is recommended that the assessment process comprise two to three assessment sessions followed by a results-sharing conference. If multiple-session assessment is to occur, this structure is best communicated to a client prior to the first face-to-face meeting. Multiple-session assessment allows more time for an in-depth evaluation of the client's medical, social, and psychosexual history. Because there is an emphasis on the relationship as well as the dysfunction in sex therapy, both the identified client and his partner should be involved in the assessment, including individual assessment without the other present. A sexual development history should be completed with both the male client and his partner. With heterosexual couples, this individual time allows for his, her, and their view of the problem to be explored.

The psychosexual history and interview are important to include with every client (NIH Consensus Development Panel on Impotence, 1993). A family-of-origin review, how the client learned about sex, family rules about communicating about sex, masturbatory history, first sexual contacts (same and opposite sex as well as animal contacts), sexual functioning with principle sexual partners, extramarital affairs, frequency of naturally occurring erections, and previous experiences with ED and what has been tried to resolve it should be included in the psychosocial history. Although standardized self-report instruments (discussed below) also measure severity of the ED, comparing both partners' subjective estimates on specific behavioral elements of ED (i.e., percentage of time attempts at intercourse are unsuccessful, time before erection is lost) is recommended. The content and frequency of current sexual fantasies should be explored to determine the degree of confluence between fantasy life and behavioral sexual expression.

It is important to note that most complaints of not achieving or maintaining erections suitable for intercourse lend themselves to the diagnosis of ED, and it is a matter of assessing the level of severity. Clients do anxiously present with situational erectile difficulties that are transient in nature, such as not achieving an erection after heavy use of alcohol, a day of strenuous exercise resulting in fatigue, or being with a new sexual partner. At times, these clients do not meet the duration criteria for a diagnosis of ED, and spontaneous remission often occurs.

Standardized self-report measures have an important role in assessing the complaints of ED and moving from presenting complaints to a diagnosis. Highly recommended is the International Index of Erectile Functioning (IIEF), a 15-item, self-administered scale useful as one evaluation strategy in a comprehensive assessment of ED (see the IIEF, included in this text, on 553-556). The scale has been normed cross-culturally (10 languages), is psychometrically sound with high reliability and validity, and demonstrates sensitivity and specificity for detecting changes in erectile functioning (Rosen et al., 1997).

Assessment of Psychological Etiological Factors in Erection Dysfunction

The objective of this section is to describe the process of evaluating five psychological factors associated with ED. A patient may be in need of sex therapy when there is coexisting concern that the patient is clinically depressed, has a sexual trauma history, experiences anxiety and/or guilt regarding sex, or reports conflict with his partner. Findings from further evaluation of these risk factors may lead to an array of psychosexual interventions designed to achieve symptom relief and allow the patient to enjoy his optimal level of sexual health.

There are six questions useful to mental health professionals related to screening patients for psychological risk factors for ED (Department of Veterans Affairs, 1999; Peterson & Furest, 2007). The first two questions indicate further in-depth evaluation if answered in the affirmative. These questions are as follows:

1. Do you have natural-occurring erections in the morning, and can you get an erection by yourself (via masturbation)?
2. Have you ever been sexually molested or sexually assaulted, either as a child or as an adult?

The last four questions are answered on the following 4-point scale:

0 = no, not at all   1 = yes, seldom   2 = yes, quite a bit   3 = yes, frequently

An answer of "2" or "3" on any of the four questions below indicates further evaluation and possible treatment.

3. Do you feel depressed?
4. Do you feel nervous or anxious regarding sex?
5. Do you feel guilty regarding sex?
6. Do you have significant conflict with your partner regarding sex?

A client's report of regularly waking up in the mornings with an erection is usually, but not always, a sign that the patient has normal neurologic and vascular function. This information is often used to indicate that complaints of ED have a psychogenic basis. Be aware that self-reports are not always reliable; nocturnal penile tumescence and rigidity (NPTR) testing is still recommended by some authorities (Montague, 1998). Additionally, those who oppose NPTR testing argue that sleep erections may be different in their causal mechanisms from erections occurring in response to sexual stimulation (Montague, 1998). If the patient reports morning erections and reports that he is able to masturbate to satisfaction (able to get and maintain erection, and experience orgasm and ejaculation), then it is highly likely there is a psychogenic basis to his complaints of ED when he is with his partner.

If the patient has a sexual abuse history, a careful evaluation of the trauma nature and severity is in order. Sexual dysfunction may be a long-term sequela of sexual trauma. Male victims of adult-child sexual contact are three times more likely to experience erectile dysfunction as men, especially if the patient had a female perpetrator and/or the patient is engaging in sexual activity similar in nature to the original sexual abuse.

If it is found that sexual trauma is related to the complaints of ED, then intensive psychotherapy focusing upon trauma resolution is indicated. The process of trauma resolution may be short- or long-term, depending upon the complexity of the case. Factors that increase case complexity include younger age at onset of the abuse, longer duration of the abuse, greater number of perpetrators, and degree of force and violence used. Male survivors who experienced mild to moderate levels of severity of the latter three factors are likely to find ways to feel safe and overcome the ED, provided that they have an understanding partner willing to participate in the therapy process. Severe degrees of these factors indicate a poor prognosis for overcoming ED. However, it is to be understood that sexual trauma by itself may not be related to the presenting complaint of ED and may not require psychotherapy focused on resolution of trauma issues.

Because a patient's complaint of ED may be related to depression, standardized screening for depression is recommended, such as the Beck Depression Inventory (BDI; Beck et al., 1996). BDI scores of 1 to 10 indicate a normal range of affect, but a score of 30+ indicates a severe level of depression, which likely needs treatment to resolve. Care should be taken not to exacerbate complaints of ED by prescribing antidepressants, which may further suppress erectile response (Beck et al., 1996).

Commonly, anxiety or guilt may serve as psychogenic obstacles to erectile response. The patient's anxiety may be more specifically related to sex and is frequently referred to as "performance anxiety," concerning whether he will be able to get and maintain an erection when with his partner. Guilt related to sex is most often associated with strict religious training that typically has a specific view of sexuality as something a man does only for procreation and within the confines of marriage. Men who have been widowed sometimes have transient experience with ED when they start dating again. The same is true for some men who have extramarital affairs or during and after a divorce.

Anger and resentment between the couple may be expressed sexually by avoidance of sexual relations, sometimes perceived as punishment by one individual. These perceptions often manifest in the history, especially when interviewing each person individually. If significant relationship conflict does exist, it needs to be resolved at least to a point where the couple mutually desires and is ready for physical intimacy.

Assessment of Substance Use Etiological Factors in Erection Dysfunction

Sometimes referred to as a "lifestyle factor," substance use should always be a part of the assessment of ED. Patients should usually be referred for specialty treatment when they have an addiction to alcohol, tobacco, or illegal drugs, which have adverse effects on erectile functioning. Addictions to substances, whether legal (alcohol and tobacco) or illegal (amphetamines, cocaine, heroin, marijuana, morphine, or steroids) represent risk factors for ED. These six illicit drugs are listed because they have been found to have adverse effects on erectile response (Kolodny, 1985; Process of Care Panel of the University of Medicine and Dentistry, New Jersey, 1998; Wilson, 1988).

As tobacco use is a significant risk factor for ED (Shabsigh et al., 1991), all patients should be assessed for their use of tobacco products (not just cigarettes). All patients who are smoking should be referred to an intensive smoking cessation program if cessation efforts fail in the primary care or private practice setting (AACE, 1998; Agency for Health Care Policy and Research [AHCPR], 1996). Addressing clients' smoking status and assisting them to be tobacco free is within the professional role of psychologists (Wetter et al., 1998) and psychiatrists (American Psychiatric Association, 1996). This is true for all clients, not just those complaining of ED, as smoking is widely considered the number one preventable cause of premature disability and death in the United States (AHCPR, 1996).

Patients with addictions to alcohol and/or drugs should be referred for further assessment and treatment to a polysubstance abuse program (Masters et al., 1995; NIH Consensus Development Panel on Impotence, 1993). There are four questions useful to mental health professionals for screening patients for addictions as risk factors associated with ED. These questions are referred to as the "CAGE" assessment and are often used to differentiate between social drinking and alcoholism (Fagan, 2003; Peterson, 2000). The four CAGE questions are as follows:

C – Have you thought you should CUT down on your drug use?
A – Have you been ANNOYED recently about being criticized for your drug use?
G – Have you felt GUILTY about your drug use?
E – Do you need an EYE OPENER in the morning by using your drug to get going?

Assessment of Medical Etiological Factors in Erection Dysfunction

When assessing ED, it is important for mental health professionals to have at least some basic understanding of medical and laboratory aspects of the patient's condition. That way, they can work better with the medical provider in assessing and treating the patient. There are basically five etiologic categories to be evaluated in assessing a patient with ED: (a) hormonal, (b) vascular, (c) neurological, (d) anatomical, and (e) psychological. In almost all cases, there is more than one etiological category involved. For example, diabetes can affect the hormonal balance, vascular supply, and nerve supply to the penis. In addition, there is usually an overlying psychological component, most often depression.

Clients often ask mental health providers about the relationship between testosterone and libido. It is important to note that a history of decreased libido does not predict low testosterone (Govier et al., 1996) and that low testosterone is found to be a contributing factor for ED in as few as 3% to 6% of cases (Buvat & Lemaire, 1997; Heaton, 1998). Unfortunately, there is not a standardized laboratory panel that is widely accepted to evaluate ED. The NIH recommends a moderate work-up with measurement of testosterone in all patients, and serum prolactin, complete blood count, urinalysis, creatinine, fasting lipid profile, fasting blood sugar, and thyroid function testing in many patients (Department of Veterans Affairs, 1999; NIH Consensus Development Panel on Impotence, 1993).

Specialized medical testing is sometimes used in the diagnosis of ED. Mental health professionals should be aware that these diagnostic measures exist and are sometimes recommended by medical providers: nocturnal penile tumescence (NPT) testing, nocturnal penile tumescence and rigidity (NPTR) testing, test injections of vasodilators, cavernosometry, cavernosography, and duplex ultrasonography (especially Color Duplex Doppler Ultrasound [CDDU]). For detailed information, readers are referred to Broderick (1998) and Montague (1998). NPTR and other specialized testing are being used less often with the shift to primary care management of ED (Peterson, 2000; Rosen, 2003). Mental health professionals do not need to understand these procedures in detail but should be aware of them in order to engage in discussions of the results with medical specialists.

Regarding, obstructive sleep apnea (OSA), there is a high correlation between OSA and erectile dysfunction, with a recent meta-analysis finding a relative risk of 1.82 when evaluating presence of erectile dysfunction in patients with OSA (Liu et al., 2015). This is important when considering the need to address the underlying etiologies of an individual patient's dysfunction, as proper treatment of OSA will be a contributing factor to the improvement of ED. When treating ED in patients with OSA, CPAP alone was found to be superior to placebo (though inferior to PDE5 inhibitors) in improving erectile functioning and combination treatment of CPAP with PDE5 inhibitors may be superior to either modality alone (Z. Li et al., 2019; Melehan et al., 2018).

Ending the Assessment With A Results-Sharing Conference

Once all assessment information is collected, a results-sharing conference should conclude the assessment process. A results-sharing conference includes at least three elements. First, the therapist should share the results of standardized measures and summarize what they have learned about the client from all sources (interviews, psychological testing, medical and lab reports, and reports from previous therapists). Second, the therapist should share the conclusions drawn from this information. Here the client should be told the diagnosis, the type of ED (mixed, organic, psychogenic), any other disorders found (such as depression), and severity of the ED. Finally, recommendations should be shared which are likely to lead to resolution of ED. The results, conclusions, and recommendations may be shared with the couple in written form as a draft treatment plan (see therapist guide "Sharing the Treatment Plan for Sex Therapy" on pp. 579-583). The draft treatment plan outlines key elements of the assessment, desired treatment outcomes, specific treatment goals, recommended treatment strategies to assist the couple in achieving their goals (inclusive of appropriate patient education on sexual health), evaluative criteria (by which clients will know progress is being made and a treatment end point is defined), and their client rights and responsibilities, which include all obligatory information to be shared with clients via professional ethics.

TREATMENT STRATEGIES FOR ERECTION DYSFUNCTION

Treatment of ED should always be based upon a foundation of a comprehensive assessment and adequate patient education. Whether this patient education is integrated into the assessment process (sometimes as part of the results sharing) or as part of the treatment process (more common) varies according to healthcare setting and provider. Recommended components of patient education for couples seeking professional help for ED include the following: typical communication and relationship strains that couples experience when dealing with ED, anatomy and physiology of male and female sexual response, causes and types of ED, and all treatment options for ED whether or not that particular healthcare setting provides all treatment options. There are several considerations that guide the selection of treatment for ED. The first question the provider should ask is if there is sufficient severity and duration of the problem to require treatment. Most times the answer will be in the affirmative. Occasionally, couples will seek out your assistance about their concerns, yet they are within a normal range of functioning or may have a mild level of severity. Appropriate interventions may include helping the clients normalize their situation or perhaps engage in some therapy designed at enhancing their present level of sexual satisfaction as opposed to treating them for a sexual disorder.

Second, before any treatment is initiated, the clinician should ask if there are any reversible causes of ED that could account for the presenting complaints. If so, working with appropriate professional colleagues to make changes in those factors would be in order. Third, noninvasive (lower risk) treatment options are considered before more invasive (higher risk) options. Considering risk, the treatment options for ED are prioritized into first-, second-, and third-line therapies. Reversibility, cost, and ease of administration are also considerations. Selection of treatments should be made considering a combination of client preference, appropriateness of treatment for the etiologic base of ED, medical conditions that may rule out some options, and patient reimbursement factors such as out-of-pocket costs (Process of Care Panel, 1998).

Interventions With Reversible Causes

Specifically, consider four factors: prescription medication use, nonprescription drug use (including legal addictive drugs of alcohol and tobacco), hormonal replacement, and penile anatomical abnormalities. Very commonly, prescription medications have unintended adverse effects on erectile functioning (as well as sexual desire, ejaculation, and orgasm). In particular, antihypertensives, antidepressants, antiarrythmics, antiandrogens, and H2 blockers most often are suspect. The patient will need to work with the prescribing healthcare provider to explore if adjusting a dosage or substituting another medication may relieve the ED.

Before the physiological mechanisms for erections were well understood, testosterone, sometimes used indiscriminately, was one of the most widely prescribed drugs for ED. Today it is understood that testosterone does not have a direct effect on erectile response, although it does influence libido, which in turn may alter erection function. Although low testosterone level as a causal factor for ED has a low hit rate (3%-6%), it is reasonable to use supplemental testosterone if low libido is part of the presenting complaints (Department of Veterans Affairs, 1999; Heaton, 1998).

Anatomical abnormalities of the penis may adversely affect erectile ability and may be reversible, especially in younger men (under age 45) who have suffered penile trauma. Microsurgical revascularization of the penis is usually what is most helpful, particularly if the ED stems primarily from an arterial occlusion without veno-occlusive dysfunction (Process of Care Panel, 1998). Peyronie's disease, which causes devastating penile deformity and affects up to 2% of men, should not be considered a reversible cause of ED. Men with Peyronie's disease, which usually affects those between the ages of 40 and 60, should always be referred to a urologist (Levine, 1998).

For any clients who are smoking, referrals should be made to specialized smoking cessation programs employing the AHCPR guidelines, which incorporate behavioral, educational, and nicotine replacement therapies along with oral medications as treatment options. Clients using alcohol and/or drugs should be asked to abstain from use to evaluate whether the drug has an acute effect on their sexual performance. Those unable or unwilling to abstain should be referred for further assessment and treatment to a polysubstance abuse program (NIH Consensus Development Panel on Impotence, 1993; Peterson, 2000). Addictions to substances represent risk factors for ED whether they are illegal addictions or legal addictions such as to alcohol and tobacco. Questions sometimes arise with providers and patients as to the "staging of treatment" or which addiction should be treated first (and if treatment of ED should proceed if addictive behaviors continue). Generally, treatment for addiction to illegal drugs is prioritized over treatment for legal addictions. As is often the case, if a patient is addicted to alcohol and illicit drugs, treatment for these addictions should be prioritized over smoking cessation.

Clinical Vignette: Middle-Aged Male With Reversible Causes for ED

A 45-year-old, obese male veteran came into the primary care clinic and completed a screening tool which indicated an elevation of symptoms for depression. Being referred from the nurse, the man was confused about why he was scheduled for an appointment with a "shrink." The depression score was explained to him and he accepted the evaluation because he felt "stressed out." The patient went on to report that he had been laid off from his employer and had been out of work for 6 months. He was feeling overwhelmed by financial obligations and experiencing marital discord because of his unemployment as well as having problems "in the bedroom." He went on to explain that he had recently been diagnosed with moderately high blood pressure and started on a hypertensive medication, which interfered with erection function.

The patient was not interested in counseling for his depressed mood or marital issues to improve his relationship with his wife. But, while being evaluated for depression, he acknowledged that he smoked about two packs per day; he also reported that his wife smoked one pack per day. He was counseled regarding his cardiovascular risk for heart attack and invited to join the smoking cessation program. He talked it over with his wife and they decided to join the program together to improve their health as well as save a significant amount of money per month that they spent on cigarettes.

During nutrition counseling, which is part of the smoking cessation program, they learned to improve their diet, cutting out high-fat and high-cholesterol foods as well as increasing their physical activity to minimize weight gain. This couple decided to start "mall walking" and at first could not walk more than 20 minutes before getting fatigued. Slowly they built up to walking 90 minutes three to four times per week.

As a result of improved diet and increased exercise over a 6-month period, this patient lost 35 pounds! From the combination of losing this amount of weight and not smoking (nicotine is a vasoconstrictive agent), the patient's blood pressure fell to normal limits without medication and he was able to discontinue its use. His erection function resumed and the marital sex relationship improved. Exercise is one of the best antidotes for depression and, additionally, the couple reported increased marital satisfaction through shared support and goal attainment. In addition to all these benefits, the couple saved hundreds of dollars by not purchasing cigarettes every month while reducing their risk for heart attack!

Antidepressant-induced Sexual Dysfunction

A major adverse effect associated with the use of certain antidepressants is broadly classified as sexual dysfunction, with various manifestations: decreased libido, erectile dysfunction, and/or delayed/impaired ejaculation among them. While the physiology of this phenomenon is not fully understood, increased serotonergic tone appears to be a common factor behind the medications that are most frequently associated with these adverse effects (Segraves, 1989). In modern day, SSRIs and SNRIs are the most widely used antidepressants that can cause sexual dysfunction. There are other antidepressants, such as mirtazapine and Wellbutrin, that are less commonly associated with these symptoms (Serretti & Chiesa, 2009). However, the relationship between sexual dysfunction and antidepressant medications can be confounded in individual cases due to psychogenic ED's high comorbidity with psychiatric diagnoses commonly treated with these medications. Treatment of antidepressant-induced sexual dysfunction can be achieved with several different general strategies: reducing dosage (or fully tapering), transitioning to a different antidepressant, or adding an additional medication that may mediate the dysfunction (Taylor et al., 2013). The treatment decision will depend on the goals of the patient and should be made in close coordination with the prescribing clinician.

Clinical Vignette: Young Male Treated for Anxiety With Medication-Induced ED

A 28-year-old male with no significant past medical history presented to psychiatric intake for significant generalized anxiety that had been present at its current level for the past 3 years since joining the military as an engineer. He always appreciated that he was "high-strung" dating back to high school but reported a significant exacerbation since graduating college and joining the work force. He found himself excessively worried about expectations and deadlines at work, making it difficult to adequately concentrate and perform his duties at the required level. He also struggled with significant irritability once at home for the day, finding that it started to cause dysfunction in his relationships with his friends and family.

At intake, the patient was diagnosed with generalized anxiety disorder, referred to individual psychotherapy, and started on sertraline 50 mg daily. At the follow-up appointment, he reported that the medication had been well-tolerated and was further increased to 100 mg daily. At the next appointment, the patient had reported significant improvement in his aforementioned anxiety symptoms as self-reported on a commonly used measure for anxiety, the GAD-7. It showed improvements with symptom reduction from 16 to 7. However, he also reported that he was experiencing significant erectile dysfunction, limiting his ability to masturbate and fully engage in intimacy in his new relationship. After discussion of risks/benefits, including option of cross-titrating to alternative SSRI/SNRI, the patient elected to augment current treatment with bupropion ER tabs (150 mg daily).

At a follow-up appointment 4 weeks later, he reported a significant improvement in his ability to attain and maintain an erection, only appreciating a modest delay in time to ejaculation. He reported that the latter concern was not dysfunctional and he was satisfied with his current level of sexual functioning. His anxiety symptoms remained stable, and this medication combination was continued. The patient considered his concern with erectile function resolved.

First-Line Therapies: Sex Therapy, Vacuum Constriction Devices, and Oral Medications

Sex therapy, vacuum constriction devices (VCDs), and oral medications are all considered first-line therapies because of the relatively low risk for adverse events (considering medical contraindications). Sex therapy is indicated as the best treatment for most psychogenic-based cases of ED and is considered an important adjunct therapy with most organic and mixed etiology-based cases of ED (AACE, 1998; Masters et al., 1995; NIH Consensus Development Panel on Impotence, 1993). Sex therapy and VCD use do not involve any invasive procedures, while oral medications (such as sildenafil citrate [Viagra]) introduce substances into the body that may have adverse side effects in a minority of men (Padma-Nathan, 1998).

Undeniably, oral medications have become extremely popular, partly due to people preferring a "quick fix" external solution to ED over an "internally learned" behavioral strategy that takes more time and money, even though the latter goes beyond ED into benefiting other areas of sexual health and an overall relationship. Clearly this indicates a major shift in the treatment of ED, from the domain of urologists and mental health specialists to that of primary care clinicians (Padma-Nathan, 1998; Rosen, 2003). The implication is far-reaching, as family medicine and general internal medicine physicians are being asked to practice sexual healthcare, an area in which most physicians have not received comprehensive training. Hence, there are expanding opportunities for mental health professionals who have proficiency, if not a specialty, in sexual health and sex therapy (Althof, 1998).

Sex Therapy

Sex therapy is the treatment of choice for most psychogenic-based cases of ED and can be an important adjunct therapy with most other cases of ED. Sex therapy focuses upon the five most common psychological factors associated with ED: sexual trauma, depression, anxiety, guilt, and marital discord. If sexual trauma is related to the complaints of ED, then intensive psychotherapy focusing upon trauma resolution is needed to break the bond between past trauma and present sexual functioning. The process of trauma resolution may be short- or long-term, depending upon the history of the trauma and complexity of the case. Paramount is the process of the patient finding ways to feel psychologically safe. Unfortunately, many male survivors experiencing severe ED never form long-term relationships nor come into treatment. When they do, partner education and participation in the therapy process is critical to treatment outcome. However, it is important to again note that sexual trauma by itself may not be related to the presenting complaint of ED and may not require psychotherapy focused on resolution of trauma issues.

When sexual trauma is pertinent to complaints of ED, it may be an underlying cause of depressive symptoms. When abuse history is not present and the patient's complaint of ED is related to depression, brief psychotherapy should be the first strategy to bring relief. If psychotherapy does not reduce the depressive symptoms in the short term, psychotherapy and psychotropic medication may be combined for more intensive treatment. Again, care should be taken not to exacerbate complaints of ED by prescribing antidepressants, which may further suppress erectile response (AACE, 1998). When anxiety or guilt serve as psychogenic obstacles to erectile response, they can be effectively treated through relaxation training, cognitive therapy, and behavioral prescriptions, as described below (Kaplan, 1986; Masters et al., 1995).

Sex therapy represents the combination of psychotherapy and prescribed behavioral exercises which focus on relaxation and skill acquisition related to sensual touch. Between talk therapy sessions, sexually related behavioral assignments are completed within the couple's own value system in the privacy of their home. The most common of these behavioral prescriptions are referred to as "sensate focus" exercises; their effectiveness has been extensively studied (Masters et al., 1995).

Sensate focus is defined as graduated touching exercises assigned to couples in therapy to reduce anxiety and teach nonverbal communication skills (Masters et al., 1995). Sensate focus exercises create a "nondemand" touching encounter, force a couple to attend to sensual aspects of their bodies other than erogenous zones, and allow the patient to relax and "let Mother Nature take over" so he can once again enjoy erections with his partner. The series of touching exercises becomes increasingly sophisticated, progressively including the entire body, and may involve vaginal containment of the male.

Vacuum Constriction Devices

Invented in 1962, vacuum constriction devices (VCDs) have been a popular treatment choice for men with ED since the mid 1980s, when they received FDA approval and were legitimized as medical treatments by some prominent urologists. Historically, VCDs were one of the first "alternative" therapies developed (other than implants which are surgical alternatives offered by urologists, and sex therapy offered by mental health specialists). A VCD consists of a plastic cylinder that is placed over the flaccid penis, a pump that is used to create an erection through negative pressure (vacuum) in the cylinder, and a tension ring used to constrict venous blood flow out of the penis. Additionally, a patient education videotape is usually included with the device for proper instruction. Even better, the client is instructed in use by in vivo demonstration before leaving the clinic. There are no restrictions on how many times the client may use the VCD per day or per week.

There are relatively few contraindications to using a VCD. The most important one to consider is whether the patient and/or his partner have the mental and physical capability to safely use it. They must be able to physically load the constriction band (for trapping the blood in the penis) onto the device. They also must be able to remove the band when finished. They need to understand that there is a 30-minute time limit for the band to remain on the penis. Another consideration is the patient on anticoagulation therapy. He might experience more bruising or even bleeding into the tissues of the penis due to the trauma of the vacuum device and its band. Treatment outcome is good but contingent on appropriate patient education and motivation.

Because they are nonpharmacological, VCDs have no drug interactions, and side effects are minimal. Side effects include occasional penile numbing, pivoting at the penile base, mild bruising from the tension ring, pain with orgasm, and decreased penile tumescence and ejaculation. The most frequent complaint from men using VCDs is the unnatural interruption of the act of making love to achieve an erection via use of the device (Trapp, 1998). VCDs are referred to by many names, including vacuum tumescence device, external vacuum therapy, or, informally, "the pump." Manufacturers report high levels of patient satisfaction, but this may reflect initial patient response, not long-term satisfaction. Once only available by prescription, VCDs are now being sold over the internet.

Oral Medications

One of the most significant advances in the treatment of ED has been the development of oral medication to help with erections. Currently, there are four FDA-approved oral medications for erectile dysfunction. All of them have basically the same mechanism of action but differ in their side effect profiles and duration of activity in the body. These medications are not aphrodisiacs, work well for most (but not all) men (about 70% efficacy), and are not approved for use in females.

As mentioned previously, the FDA approval and marketing of these orally administered agents for the management of ED has not only provided a new aid to sexual health, but also has greatly changed the clinical practice of sexual health, particularly sexual medicine. A good example of this is the Department of Veterans Affairs (DVA), one of the largest healthcare systems in the world and one that primarily serves older men. Although ED has been a condition plaguing veterans long before establishment of the VA some 150 years ago, ED could be argued to be the most underdiagnosed medical condition in the VA, if not everywhere medicine is practiced. Not until the release of these medications and the subsequent consumer demand was there a sustained national focus within the VA on the topic of ED. The lead author of this chapter served as the contributing psychologist to the National VA Technical Advisory Group that developed practice guidelines for primary care management of erection dysfunction (DVA, 1999).

These drugs are classed as PDE5 inhibitors. Remember, erections are accomplished by the release of nitric oxide that, in turn, causes the production of a chemical (cGMP). This relaxes the smooth muscle in the corpora cavernosa so the penis becomes tumescent and rigid. Normally, there is an enzyme (PDE5) that breaks down the cGMP allowing the smooth muscle to contract and decrease the blood flow into the penis, thereby ending the erection. The new medications inhibit the PDE5 so that blood flow remains increased and the erection is improved. Eventually, the body metabolizes these drugs and the whole system returns to a resting state.

The four major PDE 5 inhibitors are Sildenafil (Viagra), Tadalafil (Cialis), Vardenafil (Levitra), and Avanafil (Stendra). The efficacy of each of these medications is similar with slight variations in side effect profiles (Hakky & Jain, 2015). A new innovation in this field is an oro-dispersable film (ODF) formulation of sildenafil, to overcome limitations in ability to swallow and the situational limitation of needing to take with water. This ODF form of sildenafil has been found to have a similar efficacy and side effect profile to the traditional tablet formulation (Cocci et al., 2017). These medications are most commonly used on an as needed (PRN) basis, with a lead time range of 15 to 60 minutes prior to sexual activity, varying among the individual medication. A recent meta-analysis found no clinically significant difference between daily vs. PRN use of tadalafil when it came to erectile functioning (Bansal et al., 2018).

Absorption of Levitra and Viagra may be decreased if taken with a fatty meal, rendering them less effective. Cialis does not appear to have this problem. Another difference is in the length of action in the body. Viagra lasts 4 to 6 hours, Levitra 5 to 12 hours, and Cialis up to 36 hours. This does not mean the erection lasts that long. All it means is that the length of time to initiate sexual activity varies with the medication. The medication does not give a man an erection; it gives him an enhanced ability to have and maintain an erection when he is sexually stimulated.

As with all medications, there are risks and possible side effects that the practitioner needs to be aware of. All of these medications can cause headaches, facial flushing, nasal stuffiness, and occasional indigestion. Viagra, in addition, may cause visual disturbances, specifically changes in blue/green colors. Recently, there has been concern raised about more serious visual problems and possible strokes associated with this medication. The exact mechanism of these reactions is not clear, and it is also controversial whether there is an actual cause-and-effect relationship. It is known that certain medications will react with these drugs in a potentially fatal way. The most common problems occur with nitrates and alpha blockers. Nitrates are used to dilate heart arteries and relieve angina. There have been several reported fatalities when these drugs were taken during the same 24 hours. This was especially true for Viagra. The time span will be different for Levitra and Cialis. Alpha blockers are drugs used to lower blood pressure and also to relax the prostate to allow men to void better, reducing the need for surgery. There have been many reported adverse reactions to this combination, including some mortalities.

Second-Line Therapies: Intracavernosal Injections and Intraurethral Suppository

Intracavernosal Injections

In 1982, surgeon Ronald Virag was performing a routine procedure when he noticed that the injection of a vasodilating drug (papaverine) into a pelvic artery produced an erection in the anesthetized patient. One year later, Dr. Giles Brindley dropped his pants and injected himself in front of an audience at the American Urological Association to demonstrate the immediate effectiveness of erectogenic drugs, producing an erection without aid of psychological or tactile stimulation. Soon after, vasoactive injections revolutionized the urologic diagnosis and treatment of ED by providing the first direct test of penile health and the first specific drug therapy for ED (Broderick, 1998).

Patients often refer to self-injection therapy as "the shot." For those who chose to withstand the "wince factor," an effective therapy was created that proved successful for 70% to 80% of men. As dozens of men have reported, the exchange of 5 minutes of discomfort for a sustained erection of

60 to 90 minutes is a good trade, especially for those men who have not had an erection – let alone intercourse – in several years. The two medications used for injections are prostaglandin E1-alprostadil sterile powder and alprostadil alfadex (AACE, 1998). Appropriate dosing usually occurs in the physician's office to ensure proper patient instruction and erectile response. In 10 to 20 minutes, a sustained erection is produced which usually does not subside with orgasm or ejaculation. Full and natural tumescence is enjoyed independent of sexual desire (Montague et al., 1996).

Besides the "wince factor," the disadvantages include being limited to three injections per week, developing scar tissue at injection sites, needing to have good dexterity, ability to learn the multiple steps involved in self-injection, and risk of overdose producing priapism in less than 1% (Process of Care Panel, 1998). When the patient injects too high a dose or has an atypical reaction, priapism can result, with the patient having to report to the nearest emergency room if the erection lasts longer than 4 hours. Intracorporal injection therapy may be unsuitable in patients with inadequate hand dexterity (due to arthritis), visual impairment (due to diabetic neuropathy), or difficulty gaining sufficient access to the penis, such as with obesity (DVA, 1999).

Intraurethral Suppository

Intraurethral suppository therapy uses the same drug used in self-injection (alprostadil) but employs a different route of administration. A small plastic dispensing applicator is lubricated and inserted into the urethral meatus (the urinary opening at the tip of the penis). This method of administration is generally more acceptable than injection (AACE, 1998). These dispensing devices come individually and sterilely wrapped with a premeasured dosage ranging from 250 to 1,000 micrograms. Once fully inserted (approximately 2 inches), a small suppository of the medication in semisolid pellet form is deposited into the penis for absorption. The dispenser is extracted from the urethra and thrown away. As with the injected vasodilator, a sustained erection will develop which may last approximately an hour (AACE, 1998).

Absorption into the spongy tissue of the penis is 80% complete within 10 minutes. Soon after, an erection occurs (10-20 minutes). Approximately 65% of men using this therapy in the physician's office achieved erections suitable for intercourse, while efficacy dropped to 50% of men being able to complete intercourse when using the therapy at home (Process of Care Panel, 1998). Although transient penile discomfort may occur with most men, 5% to 10% of patients will have substantial pain that will preclude any further use of this form of medication administration. Priapism may also occur with urethral suppository use of vasodilators, although this is rare. Some clinicians give patients medications (adrenergic agents such as ephedrine) in case the erection lasts more than 2 hours. If the erection is sustained more than 4 hours, aggressive and immediate treatment is necessary (AACE, 1998).

Third-Line Therapy: Surgery

Surgical revascularization of the penis or venous ligation for venous leakage is sometimes performed on younger males. But after a review of the high rate of failure for these procedures, NIH issued a statement suggesting these procedures be done only as part of research protocols (NIH Consensus Development Panel on Impotence, 1993). Of course, special cases involving destruction of or severe injury to the penile artery in men under 45 years of age after trauma or radiation therapy may indicate specific consideration of revascularization surgery as the treatment of choice (AACE, 1998) provided there is no other evidence of vascular disease.

Penile implants were introduced in 1972 with semirigid prostheses being inserted into the physical space where corpora tissue naturally lies. Implants are always the "last resort" intervention because they are the most invasive of all treatments and because the man will permanently lose any ability to have unassisted erections (as a result of scarring of the corpus cavernosum). This is why many urologists will not consider patients for penile prostheses if they have had any naturally occurring erections in the last 6 months.

Semirigid rod prostheses have been the more common model implanted. Treatment failures attributable to infection, erosion, or mechanical failure (especially in patients with diabetes) previously was as high as 36% (AACE, 1998). The technology has greatly advanced. There are now several subtypes of the two general categories of implants: semirigid and hydraulic prostheses. Semirigid prostheses come in two subtypes: more popular malleable rods or the mechanical type with articulating segments made out of high molecular weight polyethylene. Hydraulic prostheses come in one- to three-piece models (Mulcahy, 1998). However, they all consist of cylinders for the erection, a reservoir, and a pump.

As hydraulic implant designs improved, they have come to be seen as the "Cadillac model" with higher patient satisfaction ratings. A disadvantage of the multiple component hydraulic prostheses is that there are more parts to malfunction. The overall satisfaction rate is high, with 80% to 90% of men and their partners reporting that they are happy with the results of the implants. Complaints of implant recipients include some reports of diminished penile sensitivity and the implant resulting in an erection that is shorter than the natural erection (Mulcahy, 1998).

Clinician Vignette: Older Male With Repeated Rejections of Penile Implant

A previous co-author of this chapter (Dr. Furest; Peterson & Furest, 2007) had extensive experience with penile prostheses and taking care of their complications. He had several patients who had multiple procedures to correct their implants due to infection and erosion that required the implant to be removed. Although it is technically challenging, new prostheses can be inserted in many of these patients. The following case is an example of one such patient who was able to return to a higher level of sexual function and sexual health.

A 64-year-old male patient came for a consultation in the urology department because of ED. His history was remarkable in that he had undergone several penile implants that were removed because of infection. He was not a diabetic patient. His current urologist had told him that all he could do for him was to reinsert a malleable prosthesis due to the build-up of scar tissue in the penis.

On examination, some scarring was found, but it was believed that a channel could be made for a malleable implant. An inflatable prosthesis could just as well be inserted, and that was what the patient really wanted. He was educated about the risks of the procedure (as described earlier) and acknowledged that he understood the risks and benefits of the prosthesis. Additionally, he understood that the urologist might not be able to insert any implant. Having confidence the patient was fully informed, it was decided to proceed.

Dr. Furest, was able to insert an inflatable device, and this time the patient healed without infection. When the patient was last seen (at approximately 3 months follow-up), he was getting married to his long-time partner who had been with him through all of his previous trials and tribulations. She now had an ear-to-ear grin and gave Dr. Furest a hug while sharing her thanks for restoring her husband-to-be's self-esteem as well as his sexual function.

Alternative Medicine and Nutraceutical Approaches

While recognizing the lack of high-quality studies in the specific area, the following is an attempt to summarize what has been explicitly studied in treating erectile dysfunction. There has been no evidence to suggest efficacy of acupuncture in treating erectile dysfunction (Lee et al., 2009). There is a widespread market for "natural male enhancement" supplementations, and patients may seek out these options and should be cautioned against this given its unregulated status and potential inherent dangers. The FDA has an extensive list of warnings regarding "tainted" supplementations that often contain unlisted ingredients, sometimes including phosphodiesterase inhibitors (United States Food and Drug Administration, 2019). There is modest evidence to suggest that both ginseng supplementation and Prelox® (pycnogenol and L-arginine aspartate) are separately effective in treating erectile dysfunction (Borrelli et al., 2018). Similarly, a recent meta-analysis found effectiveness in treating mild to moderate ED with arginine supplementations (Rhim et al., 2019). L-citrulline has also been found to be effective in treating mild ED (Cormio et al., 2011).

ERECTION DYSFUNCTION IN THE FUTURE

The future treatment of ED may pose intriguing possibilities. The oral medications described in this contribution are only the start of a parade of sexual medicines that will be discovered and placed on the market over the next few decades. The entire media buzz that Viagra started nearly 25 years ago will be minor in comparison to the anticipation of sexual medicines that increase sexual desire. This is the brave new world that sexual science may eventually bring us to – libido in pill form. Such early attempts to do so, such as the "pink pill" Addyi (flibanserin) have demonstrated modest effects and considerable limitations in early studies (Miller & Flinn, 2019). What is unknown is what the relationship between pharmacological aids to sexual desire will affect erection function.

In the near future, molecular biology may be used to study ED in penile smooth muscle cells and make needle biopsy a routine procedure in the differential diagnosis of ED, determining whether etiology is organic, psychological, or mixed (Christ, 1998). With the potential of the human genome project identifying tens of thousands of genes which play a role in penile tumescence and rigidity (which could be transferred), the future of genetic therapy for ED may be promising. There is a serious dearth of research comparing the efficacy of different treatments in large-sample, randomized studies. The clinical management of ED will hopefully benefit from empirical investigation of the most effective treatment regime, combining several clinical interventions from across disciplines.

An interesting recent treatment modality that shows potential for future effective treatment of erectile dysfunction is Low-intensity Extracorporeal Shock Wave Therapy (Li-ESWT). This treatment is available for vasculogenic etiologies of erectile dysfunction and seeks to encourage new vascularization of penile tissues to allow patients to experience spontaneous erections. There is also evidence to suggest that Li-ESWT may also promote penile nerve regeneration and myelination (H. Li et al., 2016). Evidence has been mixed regarding this modality, but overall, there appears to be a favorable outcome with Li-ESWT when compared to placebo, especially when the premorbid erectile dysfunction is at least moderate to severe (Dong et al., 2019). Hopefully, the science of sexual medicine will continue to develop additional effective treatments and make it conceivable that erection dysfunction will eventually become 100% correctable, if not eventually eradicated.

REFERENCES

Agency for Health Care Policy and Research. (1996). *Clinical practice guidelines on smoking cessation* (Centers for Disease Control and Prevention Publication No. 18). U.S. Government Printing Office.

Althof, S. (1998). New roles for mental health professionals in the treatment of erectile dysfunction. *Journal of Sex Education and Therapy, 23*(3), 229-231.

American Association of Clinical Endocrinologists. (1998). AACE clinical practice guidelines for the evaluation and treatment of male sexual dysfunction. *Endocrine Practice, 4*(4), 220-235.

American Psychiatric Association. (1996). Practice guideline for the treatment of patients with nicotine dependence. *American Journal of Psychiatry, 153*(10S), S1-31.

American Psychiatric Association. (2013). *Diagnostic and statistical manual of mental disorders* (5th ed.). https://doi.org/10.1176/appi.books.9780890425596

Bansal, U. K., Jones, C., Fuller, T. W., Wessel, C., & Jackman, S. V. (2018). The efficacy of Tadalafil daily vs. on demand in the treatment of erectile dysfunction: A systematic review and meta-analysis. *Urology*, *112*, 6-11.

Beck, A., Steer, R., & Brown, G. (1996). *Beck Depression Inventory manual*. The Psychological Corporation.

Borrelli, F., Colalto, C., Delfino, D. V., Iriti, M., & Izzo, A. A. (2018). Herbal dietary supplements for erectile dysfunction: A systematic review and meta-analysis. *Drugs*, *78*(6), 643-673.

Broderick, G. (1998). Impotence and penile vascular testing: Who are these men and how do we evaluate the etiology and severity of their complaints? *Journal of Sex Education and Therapy, 23*(3), 197-206.

Buvat, J., & Lemaire, A. (1997). Endocrine screening in 10,022 men with erectile dysfunction: Clinical significance and cost-effective strategy. *Journal of Urology, 158*,1764-1767.

Christ, G. (1998). The control of corporal smooth muscle tone, the coordination of penile erection, and the etiology of erectile dysfunction: The devil is in the details. *Journal of Sex Education and Therapy, 23*(3), 187-193.

Cocci, A., Capece, M., Cito, G., Russo, G., Falcone, M., Timpano, M., . . . Natali, A. (2017). Effectiveness and safety of oro-dispersible Sildenafil in a new film formulation for the treatment of erectile dysfunction: Comparison between Sildenafil 100-mg film-coated tablet and 75-mg oro-dispersible film. *The Journal of Sexual Medicine*, *14*(12), 1606-1611.

Cormio, L., De Siati, M., Lorusso, F., Selvaggio, O., Mirabella, L., Sanguedolce, F., & Carrieri, G. (2011). Oral L-Citrulline supplementation improves erection hardness in men with mild erectile dysfunction. *Urology*, *77*(1), 119-122.

Department of Veterans Affairs. (1999). *The primary care management of erectile dysfunction.* The Pharmacy Benefits Management Strategic Healthcare Group and the Medical Advisory Panel, Publication No.99-0014. U.S. Government Printing Office.

Dong, L., Chang, D., Zhang, X., Li, J., Yang, F., Tan, K., . . . Yu, X. (2019). Effect of low-intensity extracorporeal shock wave on the treatment of erectile dysfunction: A systematic review and meta-analysis. *American Journal of Men's Health*, *13*(2). https://doi.org/10.1177/1557988319846749

Fagan, F. (2003). Psychogenic impotence in relatively young men. In S. Levine, C. Risen, & S. Althof (Eds.), *Handbook of clinical sexuality for mental health professionals* (pp. 217-235). Brunner-Rutledge.

Feldman, H. A., Goldstein, I., Hatzichristou, D. G., Krane, R. J., & McKinlay, J. B. (1994). Impotence and its medical and psychological correlates: Results of the Massachusetts Male Aging Study. *Journal of Urology, 151*, 54-61.

Govier, F. E., McClure, D. R., & Kramer-Levien, D. (1996). Endocrine screening for sexual dysfunction using free testosterone determination. *Journal of Urology, 156*, 405-409.

Hakky, T. S., & Jain, L. (2015). Current use of phosphodiesterase inhibitors in urology. *Turkish Journal of Urology*, *41*(2), 88-92.

Heaton, J. (1998). Androgens, andropause and erectile function. *Journal of Sex Education and Therapy, 23*(3), 232-235.

Kaplan, H. (1986). Psychosexual dysfunctions. In A. M. Cooper, A. J. Frances, & M. H. Sacks (Eds.), *Personality disorders and neurosis* (pp. 467-479). Lippincott.

Kolodny, R. (1985). The clinical management of sexual problems in substance abusers. In T. Bratter & G. Forrest (Eds.), *Current management of alcoholism and substance abuse* (pp. 594-622). Free Press.

Laumann, E., Paik, A., & Rosen, R. (1999). Sexual dysfunction in the United States: Prevalence and predictors. *Journal of the American Medical Association, 281*(6), 537-544.

Lee, M. S., Shin, B.-C., & Ernst, E. (2009). Acupuncture for treating erectile dysfunction: A systematic review. *BJU International*, *104*(3), 366-370.

Levine, L. (1998). Peyronie's disease: A brief review of a difficult sexual dysfunction problem. *Journal of Sex Education and Therapy, 23*(3), 226-228.

Li, H., Matheu, M., Sun, F., Wang, L., Sanford, M., Ning, H., . . . Lue, T. (2016). Low-energy shock wave therapy ameliorates erectile dysfunction in a pelvic neurovascular injuries rat model. *The Journal of Sexual Medicine*, *13*(1), 22-32.

Li, Z., Fang, Z., Xing, N., Zhu, S., & Fan, Y. (2019). The effect of CPAP and PDE5i on erectile function in men with obstructive sleep apnea and erectile dysfunction: A systematic review and meta-analysis. *Sleep Medicine Reviews*, *48*, 101217. https://doi.org/10.1016/j.smrv.2019.101217

Liu, L., Kang, R., Zhao, S., Zhang, T., Zhu, W., Li, E., . . . Zhao, Z. (2015). Sexual dysfunction in patients with obstructive sleep apnea: A systematic review and meta-analysis. *The Journal of Sexual Medicine*, *12*(10), 1992-2003.

Masters, W., Johnson, V., & Kolodny, R. (1995). *Human sexuality*. Harper.

Melehan, K., Hoyos, C., Hamilton, G., Wong, K., Yee, B., McLachlan, R., . . . Liu, P. (2018). Randomized trial of CPAP and Vardenafil on erectile and arterial function in men with obstructive sleep apnea and erectile dysfunction. *The Journal of Clinical Endocrinology and Metabolism, 103*(4), 1601-1611.

Miller, A., & Flinn, S. (2019, January 24). Keep passing on the pink pill: Don't get Addyi now. *National Women's Health Network.*

Montague, D. (1998). Erectile dysfunction: The rational utilization of diagnostic testing. *Journal of Sex Education and Therapy, 23*(3), 194-196.

Montague, D., Barada, J., Belker, A., Levine, L., Nadig, P., Roehrborn, C., . . . Bennett, A. (1996). Clinical guidelines panel on erection dysfunction: Summary report on the treatment of organic erectile dysfunction. *Journal of Urology, 56*, 2007-2011.

Mulcahy, J. (1998). Review of penile implants. *Journal of Sex Education and Therapy, 23*(3), 220-225.

NIH Consensus Development Panel on Impotence. (1993). NIH Consensus Conference on Impotence. *Journal of the American Medical Association, 270*(1), 83-90.

Padma-Nathan, H. (1998). The pharmacologic management of erection dysfunction: Sildenafil citrate (Viagra). *Journal of Sex Education and Therapy, 23*(3), 209-218.

Peterson, F. (2000). The assessment and treatment of erection dysfunction. In L. VandeCreek & T. L. Jackson (Eds.), *Innovations in clinical practice: A source book* (Vol. 18, pp. 57-71). Professional Resource Press.

Peterson, F. & Bley, J. (2005). The development of a sexual health component in your practice. In L. VandeCreek & J. B. Allen (Eds.), *Innovations in clinical practice: Focus on health and wellness* (pp. 159-168). Professional Resource Press.

Peterson, F., Bley, J., & Frabotta, R. (2020). *The gender revolution & new sexual health: Celebrating unlimited diversity of the sexuality hypercube.* Cognella Academic Press.

Peterson, F., & Furest, D. (2007). Assessment and treatment of erection dysfunction. In VandeCreek, L., Peterson, F., & Bley. J. (Eds.), *Innovations in clinical practice: Focus on sexual health.* (pp. 119-134). Professional Resource Press.

Process of Care Panel of the University of Medicine and Dentistry, New Jersey. (1998). *The process of care model for the evaluation and treatment of erectile dysfunction.* Unpublished manuscript used for continuing education, UMDNJ - Center for Continuing Education, Princeton, NJ.

Rhim, H., Kim, M., Park, Y., Choi, W., Park, H., Kim, H., . . . Paick, S. (2019). The potential role of Arginine supplements on erectile dysfunction: A systemic review and meta-analysis. *The Journal of Sexual Medicine, 16*(2), 223-234.

Rosen, R. (2003). Erectile dysfunction in middle-aged and older men. In S. Levine, C. Risen, & S. Althof (Eds.), *Handbook of clinical sexuality for mental health professionals* (pp. 237-256). Brunner-Rutledge.

Rosen, R., Riley, A., Wagner, G., Osterloh, I., Kirkpatrick, J., & Mishra, A. (1997). The international index of erectile function (IIEF): A multidimensional scale for assessment and erectile dysfunction. *Urology, 49*(6), 822-830.

Segraves, R. (1989). Effects of psychotropic drugs on human erection and ejaculation. *Archives of General Psychiatry, 46*(3), 275-284.

Serretti, A., & Chiesa, A. (2009). Treatment-emergent sexual dysfunction related to antidepressants: A meta-analysis. *Journal of Clinical Psychopharmacology, 29*(3), 259-266.

Shabsigh, R., Fishman, I., Schum, C., & Dunn, J. (1991). Cigarette smoking and other vascular risk factors in vasculogenic impotence. *Urology, 38*(3), 227-231.

Taylor, M. J., Rudkin, L., Bullemor-Day, P., Lubin, J., Chukwujekwu, C., & Hawton, K. (2013). Strategies for managing sexual dysfunction induced by antidepressant medication. *Cochrane Database of Systematic Reviews, 5.*

Trapp, J. (1998). External vacuum therapy: A historical review. *Journal of Sex Education and Therapy, 23*(3), 217-220.

United States Food and Drug Administration. (2019). *Alternatives for erectile dysfunction: A risky proposition.* https://www.fda.gov/consumers/consumer-updates/all-natural-alternatives-erectile-dysfunction-risky-proposition

Wetter, D., Fiore, M., Gritz, E., Lando, H., Stitzer, M., Hasselblad, V., & Baker, T. (1998). The Agency for Health Care Policy and Research smoking cessation clinical practice guideline: Findings and implications for psychologists. *American Psychologist, 53*(6), 657-669.

Wilson, J. (1988). Androgen abuse by athletes. *Endocrine Reviews, 9*, 181-199.

16

Clinical Management of Ejaculatory Problems

Dalton Bourke and Frederick L. Peterson, Jr.

INTRODUCTION

When men seek out a sex therapist for consultation regarding ejaculation problems, usually one of two things happens. Men who have complaints of ejaculation happening very quickly (typically younger men but not always) are told "*Congratulations – your rapid ejaculation is a sign of your biological competence and, if you are going to have a sexual dysfunction, you have the one type that is most successfully treated within a few meetings.*"

Alternatively, men who have complaints of too slow ejaculation or none at all (usually older men but not always) are told something different. Those men are often not greeted as enthusiastically and, after a thorough assessment, are told something along the lines of "*We have effective treatments for what you have that involve several months of individual and couple sex therapy.*"

Male ejaculatory dysfunction ranges in severity from very mild to extreme and spans a continuum from ejaculation before intercourse can begin to complete inability to ejaculate. Other problems include penile pain on ejaculation, "dry" ejaculation (no fluids emitted), and ejaculation without orgasm. The most common ejaculation dysfunctions for men and the focus of this contribution are premature ejaculation (PE; rapid or early ejaculation) and ejaculatory inhibition (EI; delayed or retarded ejaculation).

The ejaculatory dysfunctions may coexist with another sexual dysfunction. For example, orgasm pleasure may be diminished when the man attempts to suppress ejaculation, or PE may occur when the man who worries about erectile dysfunction overcompensates with overanxious excessive sexual arousal.

This chapter will focus on (a) the potential causes and effects of PE and EI, (b) specific assessment and treatment strategies and techniques, and (c) a case illustration. While female sexual ejaculation is an interesting and well-documented phenomenon, this chapter addresses male ejaculatory problems.

UNDERSTANDING THE NEUROPHYSIOLOGY OF MALE EJACULATION AND ORGASM

Knowledge about the neurophysiology of ejaculation can help you understand ejaculatory problems, as well as the rationale for the strategies to teach the man and couple, such as whole-body physical relaxation, conscious focus on pleasure, and pelvic muscle relaxation which will be discussed in this chapter.

The Anatomy and Physiology of Ejaculation

The process of ejaculation usually involves several events: erection, emission, ejaculation, and orgasm (although there are variations that can cause distress, such as ejaculation without erection). These processes are integrated by a complex set of interactions between the neurological, hormonal, and vascular systems. Erection refers to the processes in the brain, nervous system, and vascular system leading to penile rigidity. Emission refers to the collection and transport of fluids from several glands that form the semen in preparation for ejaculation. Sperm from the testicles travel through the vas deferens, which joins in the prostate gland with the tube exiting the bladder to form the urethra tube. Then the urethra runs through the chestnut-sized prostate, then out through the penis. With arousal, the neck or exit of the bladder closes (that is why it is difficult to urinate when the man has an erection), the testicles draw up against the body, and semen collects in the verumontanum, a balloon-like chamber inside the prostate gland. When the man is highly aroused, the verumontanum fills with semen, enlarging to three times its normal size, and this rapid distension is indicative of impeding orgasm. This pressure triggers the sensation of "ejaculatory inevitability" and the reflex of ejaculation. Technically, ejaculatory control is actually emission control, because once emission occurs the man will ejaculate within seconds.

Ejaculation is the process of pushing the seminal fluids out of the verumontanum through the urethra and the penis. Ejaculation occurs when a critical level of nerve input reaches the spinal cord and causes the reflexive ejaculatory response. The pelvic muscles (PMs) are directly involved in ejaculation by rhythmically contracting to force the semen out. Learning to identify and relax the PM is a core psychosexual skill and one method of training is through Kegel exercises. Immediately after ejaculation the male enters a refractory period during which further orgasm or ejaculation is physiologically impossible. As we age, the refractory period increases due to oxidative stress in corporal smooth muscle cells and can range from 10 to 20 minutes in younger men to between 12 to 24 hours in older men.

Orgasm refers to the subjective experience of pleasure associated with ejaculation. Orgasm is a natural, healthy extension of the pleasuring-arousal-intercourse process. Orgasm and ejaculation are experienced as one and the same, although physiologically they are two distinct processes. Orgasm is primarily an experience in the brain. Though emission, ejaculation, and orgasm are integrated events and seem simultaneous, technically, erection is not required for ejaculation, and ejaculation is not required for orgasm, because they are controlled by separate neurological mechanisms. On rare occasion, these events can be out of synchrony (especially with aging), usually caused by physical and/or emotional fatigue.

Ejaculatory Neurophysiology

How the nervous system (neurophysiology) brings about ejaculation is only partially understood. Although ejaculation is technically a biological reflex involving the verumontanum in the prostate, the brain interprets sensual information, which may either augment ("turn on") or inhibit ("turn off") his arousal. Signals from the brain to the lower spinal cord link with neurologic impulses from the verumontanum to signal the ejaculatory system, which results in emission and activation of the pelvic floor muscles resulting in 2 to 10 rhythmic contractions of ejaculation.

Neuroimaging studies have also demonstrated different patterns of brain activation and inhibitory control in response to erotic stimulation (Yang et al., 2018) and even macrostructural differences (Atalay et al., 2019) in patients with lifelong PE. Brain regions related to central inhibitory control of ejaculation include the posteromedial bed nucleus of the stria terminalis, posterodorsal medial amygdaloid nucleus, posterodorsal preoptic nucleus, and the parvicellular part of the subparafascicular thalamus (Wolters & Hellstrom, 2006). These regions produce a basal inhibitory tone on the spinal mechanism of ejaculation via dopaminergic and serotonergic systems, which are underlying pharmacological targets.

Knowledge of how the sexual body works can help the couple ground their sexual expectations on accurate knowledge. For example, for a young couple to expect 45 minutes of vigorous intercourse without ejaculation is physiologically unreasonable. Understanding physiologic features such as the role of the brain as an "interpreter," the role of conscious regulation of arousal and physiologic relaxation, and the role of the PM as the means of ejaculation, can aid management of ejaculation.

DESCRIPTIONS AND PREVALENCE OF PE AND EI

Description of PE

What defines ejaculation as "rapid?" For whom is the ejaculation "premature?" There is no universally accepted definition for PE (Rowland & Slob, 1997). We describe PE as when the man does not have voluntary, conscious control, or the ability to choose in most encounters when to ejaculate, and this experience creates distress in the intimate relationship. Many men see this as a very "high bar" to clear in order not to meet PE diagnostic criteria, as few have control over exactly when they ejaculate in a sexual encounter with a partner.

PE has been defined equivocally (see Metz et al., 1997) in terms such as the length of time or duration of intercourse (e.g., less than 2 minutes); the number of intravaginal thrusts (e.g., 8 or 15 thrusts); or the capacity for voluntary control (and voluntary control is the most common criterion used for defining PE). Multiple criteria have been suggested such as a combination or continuum of time and voluntary control. Other approaches (e.g., Grenier & Byers, 2004) add the perspective of the man's partner as well as the types and level of severity (Metz & Pryor, 2000).

According to the *Diagnostic and Statistical Manual of Mental Disorders* (5th ed.; *DSM-5*; American Psychiatric Association, 2013), PE is a dysfunction of the ejaculation-orgasm phase of the sexual response cycle characterized by (a) a persistent or recurrent pattern of ejaculation occurring during partnered sexual activity within approximately 1 minute following vaginal penetration and before the individual wishes it, (b) symptoms present for at least 6 months and must be experienced approximately 75% to 100% of occasions of sexual activity, (c) causes clinically significant distress, and (d) not better explained by another cause. The description of sexual problems is further aided by considering additional diagnostic parameters: (a) lifelong or acquired, (b) generalized or situational, and (c) mild (30-60 seconds of vaginal penetration), moderate (15-30 seconds of vaginal penetration), or severe (prior to or within 0-30 seconds of vaginal penetration).

However, a drawback of the *DSM-5* definition is that it uses similar criteria for lifelong PE and acquired PE, which can be clinically different, and does not separate men who complain of early ejaculations but actually have a normal Intravaginal Ejaculation Latency Time (IELT), as is the case in variable and subjective PE (Waldinger, 2007). In the *DSM-5*, the use of a 1-minute pattern of ejaculation for all subgroups of PE ignores the existence of Acquired PE (IELT <3 minutes) and Subjective PE (IELT <approximately 6 minutes), both of which have been shown to be clinically and psychologically important (Waldinger & Schweitzer, 2019).

The International Society of Sexual Medicine (ISSM) defines PE as ejaculation which always or nearly always happens previous to or within about 1 minute of vaginal penetration (lifelong PE); or a clinically significant and troublesome reduction in latency time, often to about 3 minutes or less (acquired premature ejaculation), and the inability to retard ejaculation on all or nearly all vaginal penetrations, and negative personal results, such as distress, bother, frustration, and/or the avoidance of sexual intimacy (Serefoglu et al., 2014). Likewise, the ISSM discusses lifelong and acquired PE but differentiate timing between the two and fails to mention subjective PE.

The International Classification of Diseases and Related Health Problems 10th edition (*ICD-10*; World Health Organization, 2004) and 11th edition (*ICD-11*; World Health Organization, 2019) have also developed well-known definitions for PE. The *ICD-11* has added a third subtype of PE, subjective PE. In one study by Janssen and Waldinger (2019), a mathematical formula was developed based on data from two large epidemiological studies that after 1.5 minutes, the IELT distribution of males with complaints of PE becomes mathematically identical to that of the general male population. Therefore, Subjective PE starts after an IELT of 1.5 minutes and may imply that the current IELT cut-off point in Lifelong PE should be 1.5 minutes instead of the approximate 1 minute, as has previously been stated by the ISSM and the *DSM-5*. Regardless of societies and definitions, when a patient presents with concerns regarding PE, treatment is warranted.

Prevalence of PE

As would be expected, authors of surveys among different populations using different definitions reach variable conclusions about the prevalence of PE (Saitz & Serefoglu, 2016). Perceptions of normal ejaculatory times vary in different cultures and there is a moderate genetic contribution related to dopamine and serotonin transporter gene polymorphisms. Internationally, 20% to 30% of men ages 18 to 70 years report concern with how rapidly they ejaculate. However, using the *DSM-5* criteria, only 1% to 3% of men would be diagnosed with PE (American Psychiatric Association, 2013).

Using criteria reminiscent of the *DSM-5* (Waldinger, 2008), two studies in Turkey and China found the prevalence rate of four subtypes of PE to be, respectively: lifelong PE 2.3% and 3.2%, acquired PE 3.9% and 4.5%, variable PE 8.5% and 11.4%, and subjective PE 5.1% and 6.4% (Gao et al., 2013; Serefoglu et al., 2011).

A common myth among men, couples, and professionals is that PE will naturally improve with age. This does occur for many adult men as they gain sexual experience. For some men, there is a sexual "mellowing" with age (e.g., between 40 and 60 years of age), but aging does not resolve lifelong PE for the majority of men. Homosexual orientation was also associated with 28% lower odds of PE compared with heterosexual orientation (Barbonetti et al., 2019).

Description of EI

Ejaculatory inhibition or delayed ejaculation (DE) is the "secret male sexual dysfunction" and is rarely recognized or addressed publicly or professionally. Yet EI can be a source of infertility (unlike PE), seriously block the reward of sexual pleasure, and significantly disrupt relationship intimacy. Often men with EI avoid or stop sexual activity altogether.

The now discarded traditional labels "retarded ejaculation" and "ejaculatory incompetence" were quite negative and added to the sense of stigma. In assessing EI, it is particularly important to carefully examine both objective (e.g., intensity of stimulation, time to ejaculation, masturbation pattern) and subjective (e.g., level of distress, focus of attention, arousal continuum) arousal. The etiology and pathophysiology is unclear and taking a dynamic approach considering psychosexual, psychosocial, and relationship issues as well as genetic, neurobiological, endocrine, anatomic, infectious, and drug-induced factors (Abdel-Hamid & Ali, 2018). It is equally important to approach EI as a couple's issue also effecting the partner, employing the biopsychosocial model of assessment, treatment, and relapse prevention.

According to the *DSM-5* (American Psychiatric Association, 2013), EI or delayed ejaculation is a dysfunction of the ejaculation/orgasm phase of the sexual response cycle characterized by (a) marked delay in ejaculation or marked infrequency or absence of ejaculation without the individual desiring delay approximately 75% to 100% of partnered sexual activity, (b) persisted for a minimum duration of 6 months, (c) causes clinically significant distress, and (d) not better explained by another cause. The description of sexual problems is further aided by considering additional diagnostic parameters: (a) lifelong or acquired, (b) generalized or situational, and (c) mild distress, moderate distress, or severe distress.

The Third International Consultation on Sexual Medicine defined DE as an IELT threshold beyond 20 to 25 minutes of sexual activity, chosen as it represents 2 standard deviations above the mean, with negative personal consequences such as bother or distress (Rowland et al., 2010). However, this definition has been criticized as most men seek help due to the negative impact on sex or sexual intimacy, and most men's IELT range is approximately 4 to 10 minutes, and any deviation from the approximate 4- to 10-minute IELT range should meet the diagnostic criterion (Abdel-Hamid & Ali, 2018).

Primary EI (or lifelong pattern) refers to the man who has never or rarely ejaculated during intercourse. Most of these men are able to ejaculate with manual, oral, or their own self-stimulation, although some men are totally unable to ejaculate during partner sex. The great majority of men are able to ejaculate during masturbation, but for those who cannot, a careful medical evaluation is necessary.

The much more common form of EI is the secondary, intermittent pattern (or acquired pattern) which increases with age. This is often misdiagnosed as an erection problem because the man eventually does lose his erection. However, the chief problem with EI is that he loses his erection because he "runs out of sexual energy." He is objectively aroused, but his subjective arousal is impaired. He is unable to establish an erotic flow that culminates in orgasm. For example, an older man might have developed a sexual response pattern where he was used to being the "giving" partner, stimulating the woman so she was ready for intercourse. Traditionally, intercourse thrusting alone might have been enough for him to become orgasmic. In truth, as men age, there are more similarities than differences between male and female sexual response, including the need for partner stimulation to enhance erotic flow and orgasmic response. Men who are unaware of these normal changes (see Metz & Miner, 1998) or who become self-conscious about sexual response are vulnerable to EI. In other words, men (like women) need additional erotic stimulation during intercourse in order to increase arousal and become orgasmic.

Prevalence of EI

The prevalence of EI is unclear due to the lack of precise definitions and is the least common male sexual complaint. While some partners enjoy the prolonged IELT, others may experience pain, question their own attractiveness, or suspect the partner's infidelity and can be a leading contributor to men seeking help.

Approximately 75% of men always ejaculate during sexual activity and less than 1% report problems that last more than 6 months (American Psychiatric Association, 2013). The prevalence rate of DE among the general population of sexually active men ranges from 1% for lifelong DE to 5% for acquired DE and increases in prevalence as one ages (Abdel-Hamid & Ali, 2018). Prevalence may also be higher in homosexual men (approximately 38%) (Simons & Carey, 2001).

The secondary (or acquired) pattern's estimated frequency varies from 7% to 15% of men over 50 (Perelman, 2004), with men in their 80s reporting twice as much difficulty as men younger than 59 years old (American Psychiatric Association, 2013).

CAUSES AND EFFECTS OF EJACULATORY PROBLEMS

The causes, effects, and complications of ejaculation problems cluster into ten types of classifications, subdivided into physiologic and psychologic etiologies. Assessing these types serves as the basis for an individualized, comprehensive treatment plan. To overlook a contributing or maintaining cause, or a detrimental effect, will sabotage treatment effectiveness and frustrate both the couple and the clinician. The five *physiologic* types include:

1. Physical system conditions (e.g., congenital sexual physiologic problems), which is rare;
2. Physical illness (e.g., respiratory illness, prostate infection), which occasionally occurs and is more common with aging;
3. Physical injury (e.g., abdominal surgery), which is infrequent;
4. Drug side-effects (e.g., some medications or recreational drugs), which is common;
5. Lifestyle issues (e.g., smoking, poor physical conditioning, obesity), which is also common.

The four *psychologic* types include:

1. Psychological system problems (e.g., Obsessive-Compulsive Disorder, Generalized Anxiety Disorder), which occur infrequently;
2. Psychological distress (e.g., reactive depression or anxiety, grieving), which is common;
3. Relationship distress (e.g., empathy deficits, unresolved conflicts), which is common;
4. Psychosexual skills deficits (e.g., unrealistic expectations, "performance anxiety," lack of knowledge about pacing one's arousal), which is very common.

The tenth type is *mixed*, which occurs with another sexual dysfunction (e.g., erectile dysfunction and low desire, or PE and the partner's dyspareunia), which occurs perhaps a third of the time (Loudon, 1998).

EJACULATORY PROBLEMS ARE MULTIDIMENSIONAL

It is not just the causes that are complicated; so are the multiple effects. These effects play a role in the vicious cycle, making the PE or EI chronic and severe. In addition, ejaculation problems are also multidimensional. The subtle intermingling of each partner's thoughts, feelings, and behaviors adds to the complexity. There is an inevitable interaction between the physical, psychological, relational, and psychosexual skills dimensions. For example, the couple with PE who erroneously expects perfect ejaculatory control every time (psychosexual cognition) typically creates unnecessary emotional (psychological distress) and interpersonal (relationship distress) anguish because of such impossible expectations. For another couple, PE may interfere with the partner's ability to get pregnant (relationship distress), and the partner may feel she is not attractive enough (psychological distress) and does not want to have sex with them (psychosexual cognition), which can negatively affect communication (relationship distress), and influence feelings about whether they should stay together (psychological distress). The integrative approach helps organize and guide treatment of each dimension.

THE IMPACT OF PE OR EI ON THE INTIMATE RELATIONSHIP

There are often hidden negative cognitions – "meanings" – about the sexual dysfunction that increases the distress. Men with PE or EI commonly think they are inadequate or a failure, and feel ashamed, anxious, and/or frustrated. The partner may think there is nothing she can do and feel frustration, loneliness, and abandonment. For example, female partners of PE patients versus female partners of non-PE patients were nearly twice as likely to report an increased prevalence of sexual distress, a reduced quality of sexual life, and an increased anxiety score (Verze et al., 2018). Emotions are mediated by the cognitions that determine the meaning of the sex issue for each partner. For example, with PE, if the man (or woman) thinks, "This is okay; let's enjoy the touch, find an alternate way for lovemaking that bonds us," the negative emotional effect would be minimal. On the other hand, if the man believes, "She is angry with me for ejaculating rapidly. I must stop this, or she'll go to a different man!" or if she believes, "He is utterly selfish and doesn't really love me," the impact of PE will be major. These negative attributions are unrealistic, erroneous, and "catastrophize" the problem, and the subsequent negative feelings block partner cooperation. Helping the couple to identify and correct these attributions is important for couple cooperation.

One way to conceptualize the distress of the sex problem is to view it as a negative behavior (Behavior; e.g., premature ejaculation) that is enmeshed with negative thoughts (Cognition; e.g., "I am a failure, an inadequate lover"), and negative feelings (Emotion; e.g., shame, frustration) of either or both partners. The more negative these dimensions, the more severe the distress from the sexual dysfunction and the more detailed clinical attention will be required. Three common clinical examples are given:

1. There seems to be a higher prevalence of vaginal penetration disorders in men with PE (Bronner et al., 2015).
   a. Behavior – PE and vaginal penetration disorders
   b. Cognition – Male: "my partner does not enjoy sex with me." Female: "I am abnormal because having sex hurts."
   c. Emotion – Rejection, shame, sadness
2. PE is associated with anxiety and depression (Mourikis et al., 2015).
   a. Behavior – PE
   b. Cognition – Male: "My partner doesn't understand how I feel." Female: "My partner doesn't find me attractive anymore."
   c. Emotion – Lonely, anxious, upset, disconnected
3. Pornographic representations or male and female sexual experiences and orgasm may give couples unrealistic ideas of sexual performance (Séguin et al., 2018).
   a. Behavior – Not performing as one wants or has seen previously
   b. Cognition – Either male or female: "My partner doesn't like sex." "I must not be doing it right."
   c. Emotion – Shame, embarrassment, inadequate

Therapy seeks to alter the harmful meaning and create sexual and relationship satisfaction. This involves facilitating functional sexual behaviors but also realistic, constructive cognitions as well as positive and intimate emotions.

ASSESSMENT OF EJACULATION PROBLEMS

The two essential features in assessment are determining (a) the causes and effects ("types") and (b) the severity. Identifying the types clarifies, organizes, and focuses the resources required for comprehensive treatment, while the severity determines the level of detail that your therapeutic effort will require.

The role of each suspected cause and effect of PE must be addressed, otherwise therapy may be insufficient and ineffective. For example, the case may simultaneously involve the following:

1. A physiologic PE associated with a prostate infection that needs medical treatment (antibiotic);
2. Condition is exacerbated or maintained by relationship conflict and warrants couples therapy addressing relationship dynamics;
3. Psychotherapy for depression; and
4. Paying attention to the details of the man's sexual response, because psychosexual skills help the couple recover from PE caused by other factors.

PE is often an "*interactive dance*" of multiple causes with multiple effects affecting multiple dimensions of the individuals and couple, and each must be addressed to ensure healthy function and satisfying intimacy.

However, some causes of PE are more closely associated with certain diagnoses and would indicate more frequent screening. Of the patients with PE, the most common to least common codiagnosis were depression (69.81%), chronic prostatitis (62.26%), erectile dysfunction (56.60%), anxiety (45.28%), diabetes mellitus (30.19%), abnormal FSH or LH (24.53%), hypoprolactinemia (16.98%), hyperthyroidism (15.09%), and high testosterone (7.55%) (Culha et al., 2020).

To assess the type of sexual dysfunction, a sexual dysfunction decision tree (American Psychiatric Association, 2013; Metz, 2007a) can be used to guide consideration of all possible features of the case. Initially, one needs to assess if the sexual dysfunction has been lifelong or an acquired pattern of onset, and if it is generalized to all sexual situations or situational.

1. If lifelong onset and generalized context, consider:
   a. physical system (congenital, genetic, circulatory, neurological, hormonal, or urologic system problems)
   b. psychological system (e.g., bipolar, obsessive/compulsive, depressive, posttraumatic stress, or anxiety disorders)
   c. cultural/religious factors (inhibitions related to sexual activity or attitudes toward sexuality)
2. If lifelong onset and generalized/situational context, consider:
   a. psychosexual skills (unable to manage desire, arousal, or relax and focus during arousal)
3. If acquired onset and generalized context, consider:
   a. physical illness (e.g., diabetes mellitus, multiple sclerosis, hypothyroidism, neuropathy, cardiac disease, sleep apnea, autoimmune disease, chronic renal failure, vascular pathology, hypogonadism, sexually transmitted disease, epilepsy)
   b. physical injury (pelvic injury or neurologic trauma)
   c. drug side effects (antihypertensive, psychotropic, or chemotherapy)
   d. physiological lifestyle (e.g., obesity, smoking, cardiovascular conditioning, marathon athletics, sleep deprivation)

4. If acquired onset and generalized/situational context, consider:
   a. psychological distress (e.g., death of a loved one, partner separation, workplace stress, financial problems, moving)
   b. relationship distress associated with sexual dysfunction (emotional conflict, infertility, infidelity)
   c. partner factors (co-occurring sexual dysfunction, health status)

With each sexual dysfunction type, consider treating the underlying cause leading to the specific sexual dysfunction. This can include various medical options, lifestyle changes, pharmacotherapy, psychosexual skills training, cognitive-behavioral sex therapy, relationship therapy, or a combination of treatment options addressing multiple causes of sexual dysfunction.

Determining Arousal Style

Assessing the man's predominant style of sexual arousal is crucial. Mosher's (1980) concept of three types includes (a) self-entrancement (focusing on his own body's physical sensations), (b) partner interaction (focusing on his partner's body or their sexual interaction), and (c) role enactment (fantasy role play). Those men with psychosexual skills PE almost invariably use partner interaction arousal strategies and also use "spectatoring" (detached observation of his performance), which diverts sensual body focus. In addition, he typically initiates and anxiously pursues sex with highly arousing activity. He starts with oral-genital sex or immediate intercourse rather than with relaxed kissing and light massage and gradually increasing pleasurable stimulation, and he ultimately fails to connect with or even dissociates from his physical sensations during sexual activity. Men with EI often have difficulty "blending" the three arousal styles in a progression that builds arousal that can culminate in orgasm. Men with psychosexual skills PE and EI find it difficult to describe sensual and sexual details of an arousal sequence with graduated excitement.

Determining the Severity of PE

Severity of PE can be assessed with the "Premature Ejaculation Severity Index" (PESI), a 10-item self-report questionnaire that is based on important features such as the onset, percentage of sexual events that are PE, the man and partner's emotional distress, chronicity, and presence of another sexual dysfunction (Metz & McCarthy, 2007a). Scores on the PESI above 60 (high or extreme) almost always require referral to a sex therapist.

Individuals with PE may also have decreased perception of orgasmic intensity which can reflect both healthy sexuality and a healthy relationship. One study (Limoncin et al., 2016) looked at a new tool termed the "orgasmometer." It consists of five multiple-choice items, structured and based on a validated tool for perception of pain intensity. Scores of 11 or above indicate clinically significant PE.

Determining the Severity of EI

The severity of EI is assessed with the "Ejaculation Inhibition Severity Index" (EISI; Metz & McCarthy, 2007a). Also included in the EISI is a crucial assessment question to determine under what circumstances the man is easily orgasmic. For example, the man who is orgasmic with his own idiosyncratic masturbation pattern, but never with his partner, poses a very different therapeutic challenge from the man who is readily orgasmic with partner by manual and/or oral stimulation, but not during intercourse.

Another important assessment dimension is whether he uses erotic fantasies during self- and partner-stimulation, and whether these serve as a bridge to arousal or whether the fantasy is totally controlling of his erotic response and interferes with couple sex. It is also crucial to assess whether he feels subjectively aroused or whether he is struggling to be orgasmic at low levels of subjective arousal. In terms of situational factors, assess what types of stimulation, fantasy, situation, and partner activities facilitate high arousal and orgasm, and what types of factors inhibit arousal and orgasm.

TREATMENT FOR PE

The Psychosexual Skills for Managing PE

Clinicians of different training have varying explanations to explain PE. Psychodynamic clinicians focus on unconscious hostile thoughts and fears toward women and pleasure (e.g., fear that the vagina may injure them). Behavioral clinicians focus on sensory cues and conditioned responses to learned experiences (e.g., history of sexual abuse, hasty and nervous lovemaking in the back seat of a car). Cognitive therapists examine the distortions in thinking (e.g., catastrophizing, overgeneralization, mind reading, etc.). Family/relationship therapists emphasize the dynamics of the relationship (e.g., power and control, emotional and sexual intimacy). Most psychotherapists/sex therapists take a blended approach and use ideas from several different theoretical schools. They offer men or couples an integrated psychological treatment format that focuses on empowering couples to create change, providing a safe and understanding environment to explore distress, and instill hope and realistic expectations.

Comprehensive treatment of PE requires progressing through four basic phases to learn 11 steps of psychosexual skills. The psychosexual skills are based on a number of traditional and newer cognitive and behavioral sex therapy techniques (Metz & McCarthy, 2003; Zilbergeld, 1999). Contrary to the wish for simple cures, no one psychosexual skill by itself is enough to overcome PE. Rather, a number of distinct skills need to be integrated within the context of couple sexuality. The following are among the blend of skills.

1. Developing couple openness and comfort so they can work together as an "intimate team"
2. Pursuing the principles of "pleasure before performance" and couple cooperation
3. Learning physical relaxation during lovemaking
4. Identifying and respecting the point of ejaculatory inevitability
5. Learning self-entrancement arousal and later blending this with partner interaction arousal
6. Learning to use the pelvic muscle as a "monitor" of the degree of relaxation and as an arousal/ejaculation management technique
7. Moderating arousal using cognitive pacing techniques
8. Managing arousal using behavioral pacing techniques
9. Learning the penile "acclimation" procedure during intercourse
10. Developing an individualized relapse prevention program

Overview of the Steps to Treat PE

Coping With Premature Ejaculation (Metz & McCarthy, 2003) describes in detail 11 sequenced steps for couples for effective treatment of severe PE. For milder cases, judicious selection of fewer steps can be effective. Each exercise in the steps requires 30 to 60 minutes, completed at home between therapy sessions.

In **<u>Phase 1 - Comfort and Relaxation</u>,** the series of exercises promotes positive valuing of sex and individual and couple comfort with sexuality, and teaches individual cognitive and behavioral skills for relaxation. **In Step 1, Increasing Couple Sexual Comfort,** the couple is safely guided to talk of their sexual feelings in a positive way and develop openness. **Step 2, Training Your Mind**

and Body for Relaxation, establishes the foundation for ejaculatory control and pleasure in physiological relaxation. Relaxation is facilitated by learning **Step 3, Pelvic Muscle (PM) Control.**

Cognitive strategies involve identifying and learning to consciously manage sexual arousal. In **Step 4, Cognitive Pacing With the Sexual Arousal Continuum,** the man develops awareness of his unique arousal continuum ("map"). This involves mapping out different activities or images according to the excitement level on a continuum of 0 to 100. This allows him to begin lovemaking with relaxed arousal, the point of **Step 5, Relaxed Self-Entrancement Arousal**. Rather than focusing attention on his partner's body, their interaction, and highly erotic features, he focuses exclusively on his own physical sensations. This exercise teaches him how to find his "calm erection" (especially helpful for the man whose PE may be overcompensation for fears of erectile dysfunction).

In **Phase 2 - Pleasure Toleration,** the couple functions as an "intimate team" to maintain physiological relaxation with increasingly more erotic stimulation. He learns to welcome more – not less – pleasure, the focus of **Step 6: Relaxed Couple Pleasuring**. **Step 7, Partner Genital Exploration**, increases the challenge for the couple to establish and enjoy calm, relaxed touch in an otherwise erotic situation.

In **Steps 8 and 9, Stop-Start Pacing**, the couple develops comfort and confidence in arousal and ejaculation management. Here the man is integrating self-entrancement arousal with partner-interaction arousal while progressively pacing his arousal, pausing and resting when close to ejaculation, then slowing down, then blending partner-interaction arousal into sensual self-entrancement arousal. This blending of cognitive and behavioral "pacing" is a powerful strategy.

In **Phase 3 - Pleasure Saturation**, the couple learns how to have extended intercourse. The essential skill is to integrate the cognitive and behavioral skills and to cooperate as an "intimate team" during intercourse. In **Steps 10 and 11, Intimate Intercourse**, the couple learns how to initiate and adapt to prolonged intercourse and to "personalize" the experience. In the exercise called Initiating and Acclimating to Intercourse, he relaxes the PM while his partner inserts his penis; then, with as little movement as possible to maintain his erection, they wait for his penis to "acclimate" to her vagina. Acclimation may take as long as 5 to 25 minutes, but once reached (and keeping the PM relaxed), they can enjoy more vigorous movement without ejaculation. When they are ready for ejaculation, he tenses the PM and increases movement. In the exercise called Progressive Intercourse, the couple cooperates to integrate these skills, are open to spontaneity, and focus on enhancing pleasure for the woman.

Phase 4 - Long-Term Satisfaction, melds the cognitive-behavioral psychosexual skills into the couple's sexual style. The essential skill is to integrate the couple's gains and ensure long-term satisfaction with an individualized relapse prevention plan. Without this, couples will likely relapse and regress.

Success rates for psychotherapy are high (approximately 98%), maintained for up to 5 years, and group psychotherapy may also be an effective avenue for couples and can play a significant role in the treatment of PE. Combination pharmacotherapy (discussed later in the chapter) and psychotherapy is the most promising intervention for lifelong and acquired PE and offers superior efficacy to drugs alone. This is because men and couples learn sexual skills and address the intrapsychic, interpersonal, and cognitive issues that precipitate and maintain the dysfunction (Althof, 2016).

Fangzhongshu

Another concept worth consideration is an ancient sexual technique based on Taoist thoughts called *Fangzhongshu*. Zhu et al. (2016) discuss the five main principles of *Fangzhongshu* which incorporate aspects of psychotherapy, behavioral therapy, and acupuncture. Idea transferring helps reduce mental anxiety and stress to control ejaculation; suppressing Yin and raising Qi helps raise the ejaculation threshold; interruptions in sex to help control ejaculation and depress excitability; a special posture to help improve sexual satisfaction for both men and women; and touching three peaks and foreplay suggesting using foreplay to stimulate sexual desire with a method of thrusting to improve stimulation threshold for ejaculation. While *Fangzhongshu* contains some outdated elements and has not been studied in scientific settings, it is one method to help promote reproductive health while also promoting and respecting traditional Chinese culture.

DIY At-home Video-based Sexual Health Education

You Can Last Longer: Solutions for Ejaculatory Control (Marini, 1992) is Volume 8 (DVD) of the Better Sex Video Series by the Sinclair Institute (formerly the Sinclair Institute of Intimacy). Fortunately, this video gives men (and couples) a DIY at-home behavioral approach to learn simple methods to achieve greater ejaculatory control. A Harvard psychiatrist (Dr. Polonsky) and certified sex therapist (Dr. Dunn) take the patient through the details of the program using real couples who demonstrate in explicit detail the step-by-step self-help techniques prescribed by sex therapists. These behavioral interventions, including the Stop/Start Technique and the Squeeze Technique, have been proven to be 90% effective. The DVD comes with a Spanish language feature. A clinical vignette of an actual case involving a 26-year-old man and his wife demonstrates how a couple can effectively use *You Can Last Longer – Solutions for Ejaculatory Control.*

Case Vignette of
Lifelong Generalized PE: John

John is a 26-year-old European-American male who is a U.S. Air Force Officer and is planning to be married to his long-term girlfriend. He was referred to MH Clinic by his primary care provider after disclosing his chief concern of premature (early) ejaculation (PE). He feels he is at a "dead end" given that nothing he has been advised to try has been helpful. He acknowledged that he experiences anticipatory anxiety regarding intimacy related to sexual relations with his fiancée and he worries regularly regarding the PE situation.

John was born and raised in Oregon in an intact family. He reported that he felt cared for by his family as he was growing up and denied abuse. He stated he had good grades and played sports in high school. He attended college and received a degree in aerospace engineering. He and his fiancée have been together for 3 years. They live together without any children.

Regarding symptom description, this patient reported a history of rapid (early) ejaculation since adolescence, which is not unusual. However, he stated he ejaculates within 60 seconds of vaginal containment with his fiancée. Upon further questioning, he estimated his duration of intromission before ejaculation is 15 to 20 seconds. He stated this occurs on every occasion of intercourse and causes considerable distress (although he denied specific concerns with general anxiety or depressed mood). Hence, he meets diagnostic criteria for premature (early) ejaculation.

Regarding exacerbating factors, John reports nothing makes symptoms worse or better, that it is always the same. He had tried several "DIY strategies" which all failed to bring relief. He had done some research, and has spoken of trying the "stop/start method," numbing sprays and numbing condoms, and Kegel exercises for men. He even tried the "squeeze technique" which he read about on the internet. Upon further questioning, it was evident John was very motivated to correct his problem of rapid ejaculation but he had attempted the incorrect application of information regarding both the "stop/start method" and the "squeeze technique." John said this situation has caused much distress in his personal relationship with his fiancée and wished to have this condition resolved before he gets married.

John reported that he is not taking any kind of medication, including psychotropic medications. He did state that he took general vitamins but denied any other OTC. He also denied any use of illicit substances or tobacco. He did admit to consuming two alcohol drinks (beer) per week. He also admitted to drinking caffeinated coffee to a moderate degree (1-2 cups per day). Anticipating discussion of potential treatment options with him, John was asked if he was open to using medications for his concern regarding rapid ejaculation, which he was.

Per screening measures, John was within the normal range for symptoms of anxiety and depressive symptoms. On the Beck Anxiety Inventory, he scored 6, which is in the normal range (mild range starts at 11 with range of scores 0-63). On the Beck Depression Inventory, he scored 7, which is also in the normal range (mild range starts at 11 with range of scores 0-63). Verbally, John stated he was upset by the distress the rapid ejaculation caused in his relationship but also reported that all other aspects of the relationship are positive and would like to have resolution.

At the initial evaluation, John was found to meet full diagnostic criteria for Premature (Early) Ejaculation (Life-long, Generalized, and Moderate). Safety concerns and several treatment options were reviewed with him at the end of the consultation. It was explained to the patient that he could use the treatment options separately or in combination. The three treatment options were:

1. An SSRI medication utilized to "slow him down." He stated he is open to using pharmacology to aid him in his goal so he was referred to Psychiatry Service for an evaluation.
2. An at-home DIY video-based therapy program called *You Can Last Longer: Solutions for Ejaculatory Control.* This program has a well-researched approach to delaying a man's ejaculation.
3. Follow-up consultation was recommended to offer guidance via sex therapy (if needed). Patient was offered to be re-evaluated for his situation in 6 to 8 weeks after he had time to obtain the video. He could review it with his fiancée, and they could jointly decide whether they wish to pursue this treatment option.

John stated that he wished to employ all three options and return in 6 weeks for a follow-up consultation. A referral was placed to Psychiatry Service for an appointment to be made for the medication evaluation. The appointment was made but the patient cancelled stating he had a schedule conflict. Six weeks later, John was contacted by phone because he had not rescheduled another appointment with Psychiatry.

He stated that he obtained a copy of the DIY video and viewed it with a positive response from both him and his fiancée. The couple engaged in the behavioral treatment at home and the patient reported moderate success "slowing down" during intercourse and decided not to use to medication option. John also reported that he and his fiancée had gotten married the previous week. They both felt higher levels of sexual satisfaction, optimism regarding further improvements, and significant overall relationship satisfaction.

This clinical vignette is an example of a one-time consultation that resulted in a positive patient outcome. The PLISSIT applies to this clinical example as the patient was provided Permission (P) to talk about and seek assistance, provide Limited Information (LI) regarding his diagnosis and treatment options, and Specific Suggestions (SS) regarding how to proceed toward John's therapeutic goal of resolving the relationship stress caused by the diagnosis. Fortunately, John was satisfied with the results of the behavioral DIY approach and decided he neither needed Intensive Treatment (IT) via the use of medication nor follow-up sex therapy.

Surgical Considerations

Surgery has also been attempted to help individuals with PE. These surgical approaches are mostly used in Asia and have failed to gain acceptance in the rest of the world. Current evidence on the three surgical approaches has been outlined by Anaissie et al. (2016) which include dorsal nerve neurectomy (DNN), hyaluronic acid (HA) gel glans penis augmentation, and circumcision. DNN and HA were found to be relatively safe and effective (IELT increase of 2.7 fold and 2.9 fold, respectively), but with large trials lacking and unclear long-term safety and efficacy, the ISSM has not endorsed these procedures until more data is available. While circumcision is the most widely used surgical option across the world, and the cause of PE thought to be due to a redundant or excessive prepuce, the preponderance of evidence has led to ambiguous outcomes regarding its efficacy and safety. Due to these outcomes, the ISSM has excluded the recommendation for circumcision to treat PE at this time.

TREATMENT FOR EI

As with treating PE, comprehensive treatment for EI includes biomedical, pharmacologic, psychological, relational, and psychosexual skills components. An individualized treatment plan is necessary. For example, EI with a partner may result from an excessive masturbatory pattern (e.g., a 45-year-old man masturbating daily to internet pornography and then being unable to ejaculate intravaginally with his partner) (Perelman, 2004). This also causes psychological distress and/or relationship tension, and these effects must be addressed. Further, to narrow the scope of treatment strategies, it is important to consider mental disorders, sexual orientation conflicts, unusual masturbation techniques, strong religious convictions, hostility, fears, relationship factors, fertility issues, or paraphilic inclinations/interests.

Motivation for Change

Assessing both the man and his partner regarding motivation for change is a crucial factor. The most common motivation for young men with primary EI during intercourse is the desire to become pregnant (whether the woman's desire for pregnancy or his own). Sometimes, although not for the majority, the symptom has the function of preventing pregnancy. A more common pattern is that the man does not understand the EI but over the years has adapted to it and does not view it as a major problem. As a young, single man he had a reputation as a "stud," especially among male peers. He viewed intercourse as primarily serving the woman, with him being orgasmic either with her stimulation or his own afterward. Often, his partner is more motivated to address the EI than he.

Because most sexual problems, including EI and PE, are best conceptualized and treated as a couple problem, it is crucial to assess the woman's motivation. In the best case scenario, she is motivated to be his intimate sexual friend and to enhance mutual pleasure. In the worst case scenario, she views the EI as a personal rejection of her sexual desirability and his ejaculation as a pass-fail test of the relationship. Some women use the EI as a form of blackmail, threatening to tell others and humiliate him. Often the EI is part of a complex relationship power struggle.

It is important to assess whether the EI represents a hidden sexual agenda (a variant arousal pattern, a sexual orientation conflict, a preference for masturbation more than couple sex, or a self-punitive reaction to a traumatic sexual secret). Even more important than understanding the cause(s) of EI is to assess his (and his partner's) motivation for change. Is the emphasis on sharing pleasure and intimacy, or is the focus on sexual performance (i.e., working to ejaculate)? The performance approach of forcing ejaculation to prove something to himself or his partner is likely to fail and ultimately to cause male inhibited sexual desire and avoidance. A healthy motivation is to positively anticipate couple sex; to feel that he deserves sexual pleasure, enjoys receiving erotic stimulation, gets into an erotic flow, uses orgasm triggers, and allows high arousal to naturally flow to orgasm. The woman is viewed as his intimate and erotic sexual friend, and her arousal enhances his (Metz & McCarthy, 2007a).

Tailoring the Psychosexual Skills for Treating EI

In a way, EI is the inverse problem to PE. Rather than helping the man and couple "pace arousal" in order to delay ejaculation, you help the man and couple "pace arousal" in order to promote arousal and ejaculation. This means learning skills to develop a relaxed, cooperative style that respects the man's physiological and psychological conditions for arousal and orgasm.

Psychological interventions may include: (a) cognitive behavioral therapy and sex education; (b) masturbatory retraining and adjustment of sexual fantasies; (c) psychotherapy targeting the areas of conflict and sensate focus exercises; (d) altering one's orientation from oneself to one's partner; (e) sexual anxiety reduction by teaching the individual mindfulness and breathing techniques, progressive relaxation, and increasing sensory tolerance; (f) couples' sex therapy and the use of interactional techniques; and (g) the sexual tipping point model, which emphasizes the utility of a biopsychosocial-cultural perspective combined with special attention to the patient's narrative (Abdel-Hamid & Ali, 2018).

The cognitive-behavioral skills that facilitate orgasm include:

1. Physiological relaxation to create the non-demand foundation for sexual receptivity and responsivity.
2. Using his cognitive arousal continuum to promote graduated arousal. This includes reserving thoughts and behaviors that are more arousing until the couple is "turned on" and moving toward orgasm.
3. Relaxing the pelvic muscles in order to reserve them until shortly before he wants to ejaculate. Then he tightens, relaxes, and tightens to activate ejaculation.
4. Avoiding prolonged intercourse. Intercourse is reserved for high levels of arousal in order to prevent "acclimation."
5. Using the mutual excitement of the relationship to heighten arousal and erotic flow through self-exploration and stimulation.
6. Identifying behaviors that enhance immersion in excitation and decrease inhibiting thoughts, and exploring sexual fantasies that may need realignment to match those occurring during coitus.
7. Integrating masturbatory retraining, negotiating a reduction in masturbatory ejaculation or no orgasm within 72 hours of partner sex, and progressive shaping of sexual experiences to be closer to partnered sex (transition from manual to oral to coital stimulation is typical).

Prognosis, assuming the patient will adhere and accept guidance, is hopeful. Most patients find improvements within the range of a few weeks to months and success rates are greater than 75% with 20% experiencing an intravaginal ejaculation within 6 weeks (Perelman, 2016).

Intermittent EI

Intermittent EI is more common and increases with aging. The man has a positive history of regular ejaculation, but then finds his subjective arousal waning, and it becomes increasingly difficult to reach orgasm. His confusion about what is happening sexually is compounded by the fact that because he does not ejaculate he eventually loses his erection. He is afraid he is developing erectile dysfunction. Sexual problems seldom remain static; unless successfully addressed, they become more severe and chronic.

The sooner the man and couple address intermittent EI the better. As with any couple sexual dysfunction, it is crucial to do a careful individual and couple assessment. There are two common causes: The first is that the man approaches sex in a habitual manner and no longer receives sufficient pleasure and arousal to develop an erotic flow which would naturally culminate in orgasm. The second is that he has become increasingly isolated from his partner and obsessed with orgasmic performance. The major therapeutic interventions are to increase intimate, interactive sexuality, specifically so that he becomes open and responsive to making sexual requests, and to transition to intercourse at higher levels of arousal and engage in multiple stimulation during intercourse.

SPECIAL CONSIDERATIONS

Infertility Issues

As discussed, infertility issues may be one of the main reasons why couples present to treatment. Approaches that can be employed to aid the couple in achieving pregnancy if psychotherapy was ineffective include collection of nocturnal emissions, prostatic massage or catheterization, penile vibratory stimulation, and rectal probe electroejaculation. If assisted ejaculation is unsuccessful, minor surgical procedures including percutaneous vasal sperm aspiration or epididymal sperm aspiration can be considered (Abdel-Hamid & Ali, 2018).

Relapse Prevention

To expect that the man will never have another experience where he ejaculates rapidly or does not reach orgasm is unrealistic and sets the couple up for failure and a return to sexual avoidance. The key to relapse prevention is to establish positive, realistic expectations, including that arousal, intercourse, and orgasm are inherently variable. Whether once every 10 times, once a month, or once a year, PE or EI will reoccur. The reality of the Good-Enough Couple Sex model (Metz & McCarthy, 2004) is that problems with desire, arousal, and orgasm are an occasional part of most couple's sexual experience. The key is to cooperate as an intimate team, accept an occasional episode of sexual dysfunction as normal and as a lapse (a single event which is not overly significant), and commit to not allow it to be a relapse (a pattern perpetuated by anticipatory anxiety, tense sexual performance, and avoidance).

There are cognitive, behavioral, and emotional components of an individualized relapse prevention program. Cognitive components include reinforcing a pleasure rather than performance orientation, seeing the partner as his intimate friend, remaining receptive to stimulation and arousal, feeling genuinely satisfied with good-enough couple sex, and not feeling pressure to strive for perfect intercourse performance.

The behavioral components of relapse prevention of PE, for example, include maintaining a regular rhythm of sexual experiences, blending self-entrancement arousal and partner interaction arousal, pacing with use of the "arousal continuum," not transitioning to intercourse until the PM is relaxed, cooperating as a couple to allow the penis to acclimate to the vagina, treating an episode of fast ejaculation simply as a lapse alerting the man and couple to take more care to manage progressive arousal, and returning to structured arousal exercises (especially the "Stop-Start" exercise) to reinforce the psychosexual skills.

The emotional components of relapse prevention include continuing to value each other as intimate friends and reinforce a sense of acceptance and cooperation. Especially important is setting aside quality couple time to share feelings of intimacy and sexuality. The couple can be given a handout with a number of strategies to individualize a relapse prevention plan (McCarthy, 2001), or use the Personalized Health Maintenance and Relapse Prevention Plan handout included this text (pp. 597-600).

Painful Ejaculation, "Dry Ejaculation," and Ejaculation Without Orgasm

When a man repeatedly experiences painful ejaculation (e.g., pain in the tip of the penis during ejaculation, post-ejaculation headache), "dry" ejaculation (orgasm without ejaculation called anejaculation or retrograde ejaculation), or ejaculation without orgasm, a medical evaluation is warranted. Each could be a symptom of a medical illness. For example, pain in the tip of the penis during ejaculation may be a symptom of a prostate infection, which can often be treated effectively with an antibiotic. The most common etiology for retrograde ejaculation is diabetes mellitus, which may need more long-term considerations and could benefit from anticholinergics or sympathomimetic medication. From the integrative, biopsychosocial perspective, it is always wise to consider possible physiological or medical sources for such sexual concerns, as well as possible psychological and relationship stresses that might manifest with such sexual symptoms.

Integrating Medications Into the Couple Sexual Style

Some topical agents have been made available and are often considered first-line pharmacologic treatment options. Topical agents for PE include mixtures of anesthetics creams and premature ejaculation sprays, severance secret cream, resiniferatoxin, and over-the-counter treatments including medicated condoms, sprays, and wipes (Butcher et al., 2020). Of note, Porst and Burri (2017) discuss Fortacin, a eutectic-like mixture of lidocaine 150 mg/mL and prilocaine 50 mg/mL, which is the first topical treatment officially approved in Europe and trials are ongoing in the United States.

Several antidepressant medications (e.g., selective serotonin reuptake inhibitors [SSRIs] such as paroxetine, sertraline, duloxetine) and tricyclics (e.g., clomipramine) are sometimes prescribed "off label" to slow ejaculation speed, and dapoxetine has been approved in Europe but not available in the United States. Serotonergic antidepressant medications are known to cause three different types of sexual side effects including erectile dysfunction, low sexual drive, and inability to reach orgasm. Other medications that have shown some benefit include tramadol and phosphodiesterase type 5 inhibitors (Jian et al., 2018), with the latter often being combined with SSRIs. Several pharmacologic agents are also under study for possible FDA approval for ameliorating PE, and it is likely that agents to facilitate ejaculation for men with EI will also appear in the future. Other medications can also induce PE (e.g., dopaminergic parkinsonian medications) and should be considered when evaluating individuals with PE.

An integrative approach to PE (and EI) emphasizes the use of all available resources, including ejaculation-inhibiting medications – especially when PE is of the physical (neurologic) system type. The medication must be integrated into the couple's sexual styles. As is evident from research and clinical experience with the pro-erection medications (e.g., sildenafil), these medications are rarely effective as stand-alone treatments. The drop-out rate is relatively high, perhaps 40% to 80% (McCarthy & Fucito, 2005). One 2-year prospective observational study by Park et al. (2017) with the SSRI dapoxetine found that at 1, 6, and 24 months, rates of discontinuation were 26.4%, 79.1%, and 90.1%, respectively. Reasons for discontinuation were cost (29.6%), disappointment at the need for continued use for each sexual encounter (25%), side effects (11.6%), and poor efficacy (9.8%), with those having acquired PE discontinuing much earlier than those with lifelong PE. These results are often due to a failure to integrate medication with the partner; failure of the medication to alleviate low sexual self-esteem; or disappointment that the drug was not the miracle cure as shown on the TV advertisements, with real side effects. Thus, integrating psychotherapy is often an important factor in long-term treatment.

There are currently no proven medications to treat EI. Anecdotally, some sympathomimetics such as over-the-counter decongestant/cold medications taken prior to sex may help on a very limited basis, but there is no controlled study to support this impression. Of interest is the recent single-case report of the successful oral administration of 60 mg of lisdexamfetamine dimesylate 2 hours prior to masturbation in a patient with neurogenic anejaculation (AE) (Lyons et al., 2017). Health food stores promote agents (e.g., Yohimbine) that claim to cure delayed ejaculation, but they lack controlled, reliable scientific evidence to support such claims. For patients who suffer from antidepressant-related delayed ejaculation (DE) or AE, shifting to or adding another antidepressant (e.g., bupropion, buspirone, mirtazapine, vilazidone, nefazidone) or adding cabergoline if they have hyperprolactinemia may be the most prudent option. For patients with idiopathic DE, symptomatic management with a drug or a combination of drugs aimed at more than 1 therapeutic target may be an option of choice.

Medication is likely to succeed best when used along with the psychosexual skills program and integrated into the couple's sexual style of intimacy, pleasuring, and eroticism (McCarthy & Fucito, 2005). If the man depends on the medication to establish 100% ejaculatory control or ejaculation every time, he sets himself and the relationship up for failure. Sex is an interpersonal experience. Striving for perfect sexual performance subverts sexual function and satisfaction rather than promoting "Good-Enough Couple Sex."

Good-Enough Couple Sex

An important characteristic of satisfied couples is a realistic appreciation of the value of sex in their relationship. The concept of Good-Enough Couple Sex (Metz & McCarthy, 2004; 2007b) challenges couples to set realistic expectations for intimacy as the ultimate focus, pleasure as important as function, mutual emotional acceptance, and at times sex experienced as mature playfulness. Good-Enough Couple Sex is not mediocre sex, but positive and genuine sex. The quality of Good-Enough Couple Sex in well-functioning, satisfied couples varies from day to day: "very good" quality approximately 20% to 25% of the time, "good" (at least for one partner) 40% to 60% of the time, "okay" although not remarkable 15% to 20% of the time, and "mediocre" or dysfunctional 1% to 15% of the time.

An indicator of Good-Enough Couple Sex is the occasional presence of playfulness because, for play to occur, other aspects of intimacy must be functioning well: trust, mutual acceptance, priority on pleasure, freedom to be yourself, and deep valuing of the relationship – a "special feeling." Playful experiences personalize the bedroom.

Sexuality is integrated into the couple's daily life, and their daily life is integrated into their sex life to create the couple's unique sexual experience. Living daily life provides the opportunity to feel sexual experiences in a subtly yet distinctively personalized and enriched way. One time, sex is for anxiety release through orgasm. Another time it is for physical pleasure or for escape and fun or for emotional healing. Another time it is for romance and intimacy. Or another time, sex is a spiritual experience such as having gentle sex for emotional comfort after a death in the family. Good-Enough Couple Sex "fits" the couple's genuine lifestyle and allows personalized and enriched experiences.

Sexual Concerns in Transmen

Sexuality is an important aspect of quality of life for not only cisgender but also transgender persons. Transgender individuals have unique struggles before, during, and after gender-affirming treatment that require an inquisitive and understanding clinician that can manage not only gender issues but also sexual health issues. These issues are often multifaceted. Aspects of gender affirming treatment include endocrine treatment (which can affect sex drive and function), gender-affirming surgery (improved body satisfaction, but can have postsurgical pain), and psychological difficulties (including societal aspects and body image). Transmen who undergo hormone and surgical options experience increases in sexual desire, arousal, activity, frequency, and almost all achieve orgasm (Kerckhof et al., 2019).

In transmen who received more treatment, the trend toward fewer sexual dysfunctions was seen likely due to physical changes, with chest surgery seeming important for sexual self-esteem; with 25% of those intending to undergo further treatment, they found that not being able to ejaculate was distressing. Transmen found difficulty with initiating and seeking sexual contact (32%), had fear of sexual contact (22%), had difficulty achieving orgasm (15%), and had pain during or after sex (12% and 7%, respectively). Fear of injury (16%) was only calculated for transmen who had genital surgery (Kerckhof et al., 2019). Phallic sensation was maintained for approximately 71.5% of people who underwent surgery, and 97% were fully satisfied with the cosmetic outcomes (Garaffa et al., 2010).

Transgender health care often ends after medical treatment, but some participants might be just beginning to explore their sexuality after their medical treatment and often experience fluidity in sexual orientation. Sex counseling and/or sex therapy treatment might help transgender persons to improve their sexual health, not only after but also before treatment, to explore wishes and hopes about future sexual functioning.

Referral to a Sex Therapy Specialist

Sex therapy is a clinical subspecialty which is offered by several groups of professionals including psychologists, marital therapists, psychiatrists, social workers, and pastoral counselors. For a sex therapy referral, contact the American Association of Sexuality Educators, Counselors and Therapists (AASECT) at www.aasect.org for a list of certified sex therapists in your area. The website has a map that you click on (for your state) and give a listing of all certified sex therapists. Another excellent resource is the Society for Sex Therapy and Research (SSTAR) at www.sstarnet.org. To develop your skills as a sex therapist it is essential that you establish a consultation relationship with an established, credentialed sex therapist who can teach and supervise your growth. Organizations like AASECT and SSTAR are excellent resources for finding colleagues and consultants.

REFERENCES

Abdel-Hamid, I. A., & Ali, O. I. (2018). Delayed ejaculation: Pathophysiology, diagnosis, and treatment. *The World Journal of Men's Health*, *36*(1), 22.

Althof, S. E. (2016, August 1). Psychosexual therapy for premature ejaculation. *Translational Andrology and Urology 5(4).* https://tau.amegroups.com/article/view/10700/11769

American Psychiatric Association. (2013). *Diagnostic and statistical manual of mental disorders* (5th ed.). https://doi.org/10.1176/appi.books.978089042559.

Anaissie, J., Yafi, F. A., & Hellstrom, W. J. G. (2016). Surgery is not indicated for the treatment of premature ejaculation. *Translational Andrology and Urology, 5*(4). https://tau.amegroups.com/article/view/9555/11780

Atalay, H. A., Sonkaya, A. R., Ozbir, S., Culha, M. G., Degirmentepe, B., Bayraktarli, R., & Canat, L. (2019). Are there differences in brain morphology in patients with lifelong premature ejaculation? *Journal of Sexual Medicine*, *16*(7), 992-998.

Barbonetti, A., D'Andrea, S., Cavallo, F., Martorella, A., Francavilla, S., & Francavilla, F. (2019). Erectile dysfunction and premature ejaculation in homosexual and heterosexual men: A systematic review and meta-analysis of comparative studies. *Journal of Sexual Medicine*, *16*(5), 624-632. https://doi.org/10.1016/j.jsxm.2019.02.014

Bronner, G., Kitrey, N. D., Uziel, N., Eli, I., Raviv, G., Ramon, J., & Elran, E. (2015). Correlation between premature ejaculation and female vaginal penetration difficulties. *International Journal of Impotence Research*, *27*(4), 152-156.

Butcher, M. J., Zubert, T., Christiansen, K., Carranza, A., Pawlicki, P., & Seibel, S. (2020). Topical agents for premature ejaculation: A review. *Sexual Medicine Reviews, 8*(1), 92-99. https://doi.org/10.1016/j.sxmr.2019.03.003

Culha, M. G., Tuken, M., Gonultas, S., Cakir, O. O., & Serefoglu, E. C. (2020). Frequency of etiological factors among patients with acquired premature ejaculation: Prospective, observational, single-center study. *International Journal of Impotence Research, 32*(3), 352-357.

Gao, J., Zhang, X., Su, P., Liu, J., Xia, L., Yang, J., . . . Liang, C. (2013). Prevalence and factors associated with the complaint of premature ejaculation and the four premature ejaculation syndromes: A large observational study in China. *The Journal of Sexual Medicine, 10*(7), 1874-1881. https://doi.org/10.1111/jsm.12180

Garaffa, G., Christopher, N. A., & Ralph, D. J. (2010). Total phallic reconstruction in female-to-male transsexuals. *European Urology, 57*(4), 715-722.

Grenier, G., & Byers, E. S. (2004). Premature or rapid ejaculation: Heterosexual couples' perceptions of men's ejaculatory behavior. *Archives of Sexual Behavior, 33*(3), 261-270.

Janssen, P. K. C., & Waldinger, M. D. (2019). Men with subjective premature ejaculation have a similar lognormal IELT distribution as men in the general male population and differ mathematically from males with lifelong premature ejaculation after an IELT of 1.5 minutes (Part 2). *International Journal of Impotence Research, 31*(5), 341-347.

Jian, Z., Wei, X., Ye, D., Li, H., & Wang, K. (2018). Pharmacotherapy of premature ejaculation: A systematic review and network meta-analysis. *International Urology and Nephrology, 50*(11), 1939-1948. https://doi.org/10.1007/s11255-018-1984-9

Kerckhof, M. E., Kreukels, B., Nieder, T. O., Becker-Hébly, I., van de Grift, T. C., Staphorsius, A. S., . . . Elaut, E. (2019). Prevalence of sexual dysfunctions in transgender persons: Results from the ENIGI follow-up study. *The Journal of Sexual Medicine, 16*(12), 2018-2029. https://doi.org/10.1016/j.jsxm.2019.09.003

Laumann, E. O., Paik, A., & Rosen, R. C. (1999). Sexual dysfunction in the United States: Prevalence and predictors. *Journal of the American Medical Association, 261,* 537-544.

Limoncin, E., Lotti, F., Rossi, M., Maseroli, E., Gravina, G. L., Ciocca, G., . . . Jannini, E. A. (2016). The impact of premature ejaculation on the subjective perception of orgasmic intensity: Validation and standardisation of the 'Orgasmometer.' *Andrology, 4*(5), 921-926. https://doi.org/10.1111/andr.12220

Loudon, J. B. (1998). Potential confusion between erectile dysfunction and premature ejaculation: An evaluation of men presenting with erectile difficulty at a sex therapy clinic. *Sexual and Marital Therapy, 13*(4), 397-401.

Lyons, M. D., Lentz, A. C., & Coward, R. M. (2017). Lisdexamfetamine dimesylate (Vyvanse) for the treatment of neurogenic anejaculation. *American Journal of Men's Health, 11*(3), 618-619.

Marini, F. (Director). (1992). *You can last longer: Solutions for ejaculatory control* [video]. Sinclair Institute.

McCarthy, B. W. (2001). Relapse prevention strategies and techniques with erectile dysfunction. *Journal of Sex and Marital Therapy, 27,* 1-8.

McCarthy, B. W., & Fucito, L. (2005). Integrating medication, realistic expectations, and therapeutic integration in the treatment of male sexual dysfunction. *Journal of Sex and Marital Therapy, 31,* 319-328.

Metz, M. E., & McCarthy, B. W. (2003). *Coping with premature ejaculation: Overcome PE, please your partner, and have great sex*. New Harbinger Publications.

Metz, M. E., & McCarthy, B.W. (2004). *Coping with erectile dysfunction: How to regain confidence and enjoy great sex.* New Harbinger Publications.

Metz, M. E., & McCarthy, B. W. (2007a). Ejaculatory problems. In L. VandeCreek, F. L. Peterson, & J. W. Bley (Eds.), *Innovations on clinical practice: Focus on Sexual health* (pp. 135-155). Professional Resource Press.

Metz, M. E., & McCarthy, B. W. (2007b). The "Good-Enough Sex" model for couple sexual satisfaction. *Sexual and Relationship Therapy, 22*(3), 351-362.

Metz, M. E., & Miner, M. (1998). Psychosexual and psychosocial aspects of male aging and sexual health. *Canadian Journal of Human Sexuality, 7*(3), 245-259.

Metz, M. E., & Pryor, J. L. (2000). Premature ejaculation: A psychophysiological approach for assessment and management. *Journal of Sex and Marital Therapy, 26*(4), 293-320.

Metz, M. E., Pryor, J., Abuzzahab, F., Nesvacil, L., & Koznar, J. (1997). Premature ejaculation: A psychophysiological review. *Journal of Sex and Marital Therapy, 23*(1), 3-23.

Mosher, D. L. (1980). Three psychological dimensions of depth of involvement in human sexual response. *Journal of Sex Research, 16*(1), 1-42.

Mourikis, I., Antoniou, M., Matsouka, E., Vousoura, E., Tzavara, C., Ekizoglou, C., . . . Zervas, I. M. (2015). Anxiety and depression among Greek men with primary erectile dysfunction and premature ejaculation. *Annals of General Psychiatry, 14*, 34. https://doi.org/10.1186/s12991-015-0074-y

Park, H. J., Park, N. C., Kim, T. N., Baek, S. R., Lee, K. M., & Choe, S. (2017). Discontinuation of Dapoxetine treatment in patients with premature ejaculation: A 2-year prospective observational study. *Sexual Medicine, 5*(2), e99-e105. https://doi.org/10.1016/j.esxm.2017.02.003

Perelman, M. A. (2004). Evaluation and treatment of the ejaculatory disorders. In T. Lui (Ed.), *Atlas of male sexual dysfunction*. Current Medicine.

Perelman, M. A. (2016). Psychosexual therapy for delayed ejaculation based on the sexual tipping point model. *Translational Andrology and Urology*, *5*(4), 563.

Porst, H., & Burri, A. (2017). Fortacin™ Spray for the treatment of premature ejaculation. *Urologia*, *84*(Suppl 2), 1-10. https://doi.org/10.5301/uj.5000275

Rowland, D. L., & Slob, A. K. (1997). Premature ejaculation: Psychophysiological considerations in theory, research and treatment. *The Annual Review of Sex Research, 8,* 201-209.

Rowland, D., McMahon, C. G., Abdo, C., Chen, J., Jannini, E., Waldinger, M. D., & Ahn, T. Y. (2010). Disorders of orgasm and ejaculation in men. *The Journal of Sexual Medicine*, *7*(4), 1668-1686.

Saitz, T. R., & Serefoglu, E. C. (2016). The epidemiology of premature ejaculation. *Translational Andrology and Urology*, *5*(4), 409-415. https://doi.org/10.21037/tau.2016.05.11

Séguin, L. J., Rodrigue, C., & Lavigne, J. (2018). Consuming ecstasy: Representations of male and female orgasm in mainstream pornography. *Journal of Sex Research*, *55*(3), 348-356.

Serefoglu, E. C., McMahon, C. G., Waldinger, M. D., Althof, S. E., Shindel, A., Adaikan, G., . . . Torres, L. O. (2014). An evidence-based unified definition of lifelong and acquired premature ejaculation: Report of the second international society for sexual medicine ad hoc committee for the definition of premature ejaculation. *Sexual Medicine*, *2*(2), 41-59. https://doi.org/10.1002/sm2.27

Serefoglu, E. C., Yaman, O., Cayan, S., Asci, R., Orhan, I., Usta, M. F., . . . Kadioglu, A. (2011). Prevalence of the complaint of ejaculating prematurely and the four premature ejaculation syndromes: Results from the Turkish Society of Andrology Sexual Health Survey. *The Journal of Sexual Medicine*, *8*(2), 540-548. https://doi.org/10.1111/j.1743-6109.2010.02095.x

Simons, J. S., & Carey, M. P. (2001). Prevalence of sexual dysfunctions: Results from a decade of research. *Archives of Sexual Behavior*, *30*(2), 177-219.

Verze, P., Arcaniolo, D., Imbimbo, C., Cai, T., Venturino, L., Spirito, L., . . . Mirone, V. (2018). General and sex profile of women with partner affected by premature ejaculation: Results of a large observational, non-interventional, cross-sectional, epidemiological study (IPER-F). *Andrology*, *6*(5), 714-719. https://doi.org/10.1111/andr.12545

Waldinger, M. D. (2007). Premature ejaculation: Different pathophysiologies and etiologies determine its treatment. *Journal of Sex & Marital Therapy*, *34*(1), 1-13.

Waldinger, M. D. (2008). Premature ejaculation: Advantages of a new classification for understanding etiology and prevalence rates. *Sexologies*, *17*(1), 30-35.

Waldinger, M. D., & Schweitzer, D. H. (2019). Differences between ICD-11, MMS and DSM-5 definition of premature ejaculation: A continuation of historical inadequacies and a source of serious misinterpretation by some European Regulatory Agencies (PART 2). *International Journal of Impotence Research, 31,* 310-318. https://doi.org/10.1038/s41443-018-0108-5

Wolters, J. P., & Hellstrom, W. J. (2006). Current concepts in ejaculatory dysfunction. *Reviews in Urology*, *8*(Suppl 4), S18-S25.

World Health Organization. (2004). *International statistical classification of diseases and related health problems* (10th rev., 2nd ed.).

World Health Organization. (2019). *International statistical classification of diseases and related health problems* (11th ed.). https://icd.who.int/

Yang, X., Gao, M., Zhang, L., Liu, L., Liu, P., Sun, J., . . . Qin, W. (2018). Central neural correlates during inhibitory control in lifelong premature ejaculation patients. *Frontiers in Human Neuroscience, 12,* Article 206. https://doi.org/10.3389/fnhum.2018.00206

Zhu, Y., Chen, Q., Gu, Y., Yue, J., & Zeng, Q. (2016). Ancient Chinese fangzhongshu (sexual skills and methods) therapy for premature ejaculation. *The World Journal of Men's Health*, *34*(3), 173-178. https://doi.org/10.5534/wjmh.2016.34.3.173

Zilbergeld, B. (1999). *The new male sexuality.* Bantam.

17

Innovative Methods in Treating Patients With Sexual Trauma

Jill W. Bley

INTRODUCTION

This chapter addresses the devastating damage sexual abuse does to a person's sexual, emotional, psychological, and spiritual self. The content draws from the many years I have been treating victims of sexual abuse, going back to 1972, when I was part of a small group of women who started a rape crisis center in Cincinnati, Ohio.

During my 4-decade career as a clinical psychologist, I have treated hundreds of sexual abuse survivors. I have treated adults with no memory of any sexual abuse in their childhood or adolescence, but who are having extreme difficulty trying to be a sexual partner with someone they love. Try as they may, they find themselves crying during sex, getting violently angry at their partner, or avoiding sex at all costs – all for no apparent reason. When these clients began to remember what happened to them – that they were sexually abused during their childhood or adolescence and "repressed" or "denied" the memories – they are shocked but relieved that they have finally figured out why they have reacted so strongly to sex.

Many survivors are baffled by their reactions because they remember a time in their lives when they loved sex and had no negative reactions. What the clinician hears from them and their partners is how radically sex changed after the relationship entered into a commitment stage such as engagement, commitment ceremony, or marriage. For these people sex is not a problem until they feel that it is "obligatory." Feeling obligated to have sex brings to the surface not the visual memories of the abuse, but the emotional, psychological memories of the abuse. It is an unconscious reminder of having sexual touch forced on them as a hostage to their abuser. They are suffering from all the symptoms of sexual abuse but with none of the visual memories of the abuse.

Unfortunately, most people do not "believe" an emotional memory or a touch memory unless it is combined with the visual memory (as sex is all about emotional and touch experiences and memories). Our bodies have a huge number of touch receptors from the top of our heads to the tip of our toes, so it makes sense that if you are sexually abused you would store lots and lots of "touch" memories as compared to the visual memories. During abuse, victims may close their eyes, might be in a dark room, or the abuser might say things and/or do things to them that make them terrified to remember the visual experience.

I have also provided therapy to many people whose memories include the visual memories of their abuse. They come for treatment because no matter how hard they try to put those memories aside they are plagued by "triggers," especially sexual triggers. A "trigger" is anything in the here-and-now that causes them to have an unwanted memory (visual, touch, smell, auditory, emotional, or psychological) that they have been trying to avoid.

Before beginning the part of this chapter that will address the psychological aftermath of sexual abuse and treatment issues, I will cover some of the history of attitudes toward sexual abuse as demonstrated by the laws governing rape. I will briefly look at a case brought by prosecutors in California against a Stanford athlete who brutally raped a woman. This case clearly demonstrates not only some of the emotional and psychological symptoms following a rape, but some of the "blame the victim" attitudes that persist, even today, in our judicial system. An amazing letter follows, in an unprecedented response to this Stanford case survivor, written by none other than a sitting Vice-President of the United States. Then I will review some of the statistics related to sexual assaults.

The chapter continues with a brief review of how a diagnosis developed to describe a clinical condition that has become well known in mainstream American culture: Posttraumatic Stress Disorder (PTSD). Not only is PTSD described, but effective evidence-based treatments are explained to inform survivors, and anyone interested in understanding the harm done to survivors, of the hope of recovery. Finally, the chapter concludes with commentary regarding the promotion of a consent culture (as opposed to the tradition of a rape culture).

HISTORY OF LAWS GOVERNING RAPE

It has taken a very long time for humans to recognize how prevalent sexual abuse has been in almost every society on earth. It has taken even longer for us to acknowledge how severe the damage to the victim is or to acknowledge that sexual abuse is a crime and abusers should be punished. In 1975, Susan Brownmiller wrote *Against Our Will, Men, Women & Rape*. In it, she outlined the history of rape laws beginning with the Code of Hammurabi who was the sixth King of Babylon. This ancient code of law dates back to about 1754 BC. It describes the type of offense and the penalty that must be imposed. If a married woman was raped, the law required that she share the blame equally with the rapist. No matter what the circumstances of the crime, it was labeled "adultery" and both were bound and thrown into the river.

The ancient Hebrews were influenced by Hammurabi's Code but they were more specific regarding who the victim was and where the offense occurred. They also substituted drowning with stoning to death (Brownmiller, 1975). The Hebrew elders decided that if a woman was raped in the city limits, both victim and attacker were stoned to death, reasoning that someone would surely have heard her cries for help if it was really a rape. Therefore, since no one heard her cry for help, she must have been complicit. If the attack happened in the fields, where it was assumed no one might hear her screams for help, and she was a married woman, the attacker had to make restitution to her spouse and the spouse could decide her fate, which was usually to put her out. If the female in the field was not married, the rapist had to pay her father the bride price of 50 silver shekels and the attacker had to marry her. If the victim was betrothed to someone, then the rapist was stoned to death and the victim was not punished. However, she often experienced the same fate as the married woman who was raped in the fields. Notice that all of these laws assume that the woman is "owned" by a man and that men are never raped.

Brownmiller continued to trace the rape laws from Biblical times up until 1975 and ended with English law, upon which American law is based. Prestigious men of the Bar, such as English jurists Hale and Blackstone and American jurist Wigmore, warned against the female victim and worried about her motivations and reputation. These jurists were cited and quoted frequently in Case Comments and Law Journal articles whenever a case was being made for preserving rape laws that require corroboration and nonconsent (Bley, 1980) .

Preservation within the law of a need to establish nonconsent in order to prove rape sets this crime apart from other forcible assaults, as can be seen from this quote from a 1969 decision by the United States Court of Appeals for the District of Columbia:

> A man who handles a lady vigorously and with some force (against her will) is plainly guilty of an assault – of an indecent assault. But he does not have an intent to commit rape if his actions are taken in the hope or expectation of thereby awakening desire, and with the further intention of desisting if his approach does not arouse desire or lead to acquiescence but rather encounters continued resistance.
>
> When a defendant intends to use the kind of 'force' that is enough in his mind to test the existence or persistence of complainant's true intentions, but not enough to achieve sexual intercourse if she 'really' rejects him, there is no intention to commit rape. (*United States v. Bryant*, 1969)

Because of the laws requiring corroboration and proof of nonconsent, it has been rationalized that the rules of evidence should permit introduction of the sex history of the victim.

> Whether character evidence is presented as general reputation, personal opinion, or specific acts, it is admissible because the complainant's past conduct is considered relevant in an evidentiary sense to the issue of consent to a particular act committed. The underlying presumption of relevance is that an unchaste complainant is more likely to have consented to a sex act than to have been coerced. Theoretically, this presumption leads to an inference that the complainant has falsified his or her accusation of forcible assault. (Northwestern University School of Law, *Journal of Criminal Law & Criminology,* 1973)

In the 1970s and '80s, due to the influence of the Feminist Movement, there was a nationwide campaign aimed at changing each state's rape laws so as to keep information concerning the victim's sex life from being introduced as evidence in rape cases (Bley, 1980). At this point in time, 2023, all of the states have changed their laws making the process of reporting and prosecuting somewhat easier on the victim. The problem is that many victims are so traumatized by the crime that they do not want to report, let alone go through a trial and have to deal with the attacker in court. However, even with the changes in the law concerning the evidence that may and may not be admitted, the courts, at times, still render opinions and judgments that cause many women to continue to believe that they are better off "just forgetting" about it than to try to report and prosecute.

Part of the reason for their reluctance is that even though the laws have changed, the attitudes of many people in this country have not changed. In fact, more recently, a congressman and United States Senate candidate said, "If it's a *legitimate rape*, the female body has ways to try to shut that whole thing down" (Todd Akin, August 20, 2012). He was echoing a position that a physician, John Willke, stated when he started the Right to Life Movement in Greater Cincinnati and the state of Ohio. Dr. Willke said that he believed that the stress of rape caused the female body to inhibit conception. He stated, "Rape can radically upset (a woman's) possibility of ovulation, fertilization, implantation and even nurturing a pregnancy." He did concede that pregnancy following rape was "possible" but rare (*Cincinnati Enquirer*, 2012).

David Grimes, an obstetrician and gynecologist, who was also chief of the abortion surveillance branch at the Center for Disease Control, criticized Willke: "To suggest this doesn't happen is cruel, cruel, cruel. Rape is an ugly and common occurrence" (*Cincinnati Enquirer*, 2012). Another candidate for the U.S. Senate Richard Mourdock said, "When life begins with that horrible situation of rape that is something that *God intended to happen*" (October 23, 2012). Rick Santorum, who was a Senator and a Presidential candidate said, "The right approach is to accept this horribly created, in the sense of rape, but nevertheless . . . a gift of human life, and *accept what God is giving to you.*" On February 3, 2012, when he was a Congressman and a Presidential candidate, Ron Paul said, "If it's an *honest rape*, that individual should go immediately to the emergency room. I would give them a shot of estrogen." Paul Ryan, along with 214 other congressmen and congresswomen, voted to prohibit federal funding of abortions except in the instances of "an act of ***forcible rape***, or if a minor, an act of incest" (H.R. 3, 112th Congress, January 20, 2011). And then the most egregious statement of all was made by the Gubernatorial candidate Clayton Williams (TX) on March 25, 1990, when speaking about rape, *"If it's inevitable, just relax and enjoy it."* Note: these statements were all made by men who never have to face the soul-wrenching experience of dealing with a pregnancy caused by a devastating attack on one's body and forceful penetration of her genitals.

These attitudes have set the stage for the judiciary to ignore the severity of the crime of rape and the consequences to the victim, and focus the concern on the consequences to the perpetrator. We have seen this judicial attitude time and time again in this country and around the world. The effects of these attitudes are poignantly stated in a letter written by a woman who was the victim of a vicious rapist (charged with three counts of sexual assault), read aloud to her attacker after he was convicted of the charges and then given an incredibly light sentence by the judge. The perpetrator was also a Stanford student and an athlete. What follows are a few excerpts from that letter.*

> **WARNING: This rape account is graphic, even in this brief form. It may be a trigger if you are a victim. Even if you are not a victim, you may have a strong emotional reaction to her words. It makes me cry every time I read it. If you would like to read this letter in its entirety you can find it in *The Gender Revolution & New Sexual Health* by F. Peterson et al. (2020) or in a book written by the victim, *Know My Name*, by Chanel Miller (2019).**

> *You don't know me, but you've been inside me, and that's why we're here today.*

> *On January 17th, 2015, it was a quiet Saturday night at home. My dad made some dinner and I sat at the table with my younger sister who was visiting for the weekend. I was working full time and it was approaching my bedtime. I planned to stay at home by myself, watch some TV and read, while she went to a party with her friends. Then, I decided it was my only night with her, I had nothing better to do, so why not, there's a dumb party ten minutes from my house, I would go, dance like a fool, and embarrass my younger sister. On the way there, I joked that undergrad guys would have braces. My sister teased me for wearing a beige cardigan to a frat party like a librarian. I called myself "big mama," because I knew I'd be the oldest one there. I made silly faces, let my guard down, and drank liquor too fast not factoring in that my tolerance had significantly lowered since college.*

> *The next thing I remember I was in a gurney in a hallway. I had dried blood and bandages on the backs of my hands and elbow. I thought maybe I had fallen and was in an admin office on campus. I was very calm and wondering where my sister was. A deputy explained I had been assaulted. I still remained calm, assured he was speaking to the wrong person. I knew no one at this party. When I was finally allowed to use the restroom, I pulled down the hospital pants they had given me, went to pull down my underwear, and felt nothing. I still remember the feeling of my hands touching my skin and grabbing nothing. I looked down and there was nothing. The thin piece of fabric, the only thing between my vagina and anything else, was missing and everything inside me was silenced. I still don't have words for that feeling. In order to keep breathing, I thought maybe the policemen used scissors to cut them off for evidence.*

*"Stanford Victim Letter," https://www.sccgov.org/sites/da/newsroom/newsreleases/Documents/B-Turner%20VIS.pdf. Copyright in the public domain.

Then, I felt pine needles scratching the back of my neck and started pulling them out my hair. I thought maybe, the pine needles had fallen from a tree onto my head. My brain was talking my gut into not collapsing. Because my gut was saying, help me, help me.

I shuffled from room to room with a blanket wrapped around me, pine needles trailing behind me, I left a little pile in every room I sat in. I was asked to sign papers that said "Rape Victim" and I thought something has really happened. My clothes were confiscated and I stood naked while the nurses held a ruler to various abrasions on my body and photographed them. The three of us worked to comb the pine needles out of my hair, six hands to fill one paper bag. To calm me down, they said it's just the flora and fauna, flora and fauna. I had multiple swabs inserted into my vagina and anus, needles for shots, pills, had a Nikon pointed right into my spread legs. I had long, pointed beaks inside me and had my vagina smeared with cold, blue paint to check for abrasions.

After a few hours of this, they let me shower. I stood there examining my body beneath the stream of water and decided, I don't want my body anymore. I was terrified of it, I didn't know what had been in it, if it had been contaminated, who had touched it. I wanted to take off my body like a jacket and leave it at the hospital with everything else.

I tried to push it out of my mind, but it was so heavy I didn't talk, I didn't eat, I didn't sleep, I didn't interact with anyone. After work, I would drive to a secluded place to scream. I didn't talk, I didn't eat, I didn't sleep, I didn't interact with anyone, and I became isolated from the ones I loved most. For over a week after the incident, I didn't get any calls or updates about that night or what happened to me. The only symbol that proved that it hadn't just been a bad dream, was the sweatshirt from the hospital in my drawer.

I was not only told that I was assaulted, I was told that because I couldn't remember, I technically could not prove it was unwanted. And that distorted me, damaged me, almost broke me. It is the saddest type of confusion to be told I was assaulted and nearly raped, blatantly out in the open, but we don't know if it counts as assault yet. I had to fight for an entire year to make it clear that there was something wrong with this situation.

You are guilty. Twelve jurors convicted you guilty of three felony counts beyond reasonable doubt, that's twelve votes per count, thirty six yeses confirming guilt, that's one hundred percent, unanimous guilt. And I thought finally it is over, finally he will own up to what he did, truly apologize, we will both move on and get better. Then I read your statement.

My independence, natural joy, gentleness, and steady lifestyle I had been enjoying became distorted beyond recognition. I became closed off, angry, self deprecating, tired, irritable, empty. The isolation at times was unbearable. You cannot give me back the life I had before that night either. While you worry about your shattered reputation, I refrigerated spoons every night so when I woke up, and my eyes were puffy from crying, I would hold the spoons to my eyes to lessen the swelling so that I could see. I showed up an hour late to work every morning, excused myself to cry in the stairwells, I can tell you all the best places in that building to cry where no one can hear you. The pain became so bad that I had to explain the private details to my boss to let her know why I was leaving. I needed time because continuing day to day was not possible. I used my savings to go as far away as I could possibly be. I did not return to work full time as I knew I'd have to take weeks off in the future for the hearing and trial, that were constantly being rescheduled. My life was put on hold for over a year, my structure had collapsed.

I can't sleep alone at night without having a light on, like a five year old, because I have nightmares of being touched where I cannot wake up, I did this thing where I waited until the sun came up and I felt safe enough to sleep. For three months, I went to bed at six o'clock in the morning.

I used to pride myself on my independence, now I am afraid to go on walks in the evening, to attend social events with drinking among friends where I should be comfortable being. I have become a little barnacle always needing to be at someone's side, to have my boyfriend standing next to me, sleeping beside me, protecting me. It is embarrassing how feeble I feel, how timidly I move through life, always guarded, ready to defend myself, ready to be angry. Now to address the sentencing. When I read the probation officer's report, I was in disbelief, consumed by anger which eventually quieted down to profound sadness. My statements have been slimmed down to distortion and taken out of context. I fought hard during this trial and will not have the outcome minimized by a probation officer who attempted to evaluate my current state and my wishes in a fifteen minute conversation, the majority of which was spent answering questions I had about the legal system. The context is also important. Brock [the defendant] had yet to issue a statement, and I had not read his remarks.

The probation officer factored in that the defendant is youthful and has no prior convictions. In my opinion, he is old enough to know what he did was wrong. When you are eighteen in this country you can go to war. When you are nineteen, you are old enough to pay the consequences for attempting to rape someone. He is young, but he is old enough to know better. He is a lifetime sex registrant. That doesn't expire. Just like what he did to me doesn't expire, doesn't just go away after a set number of years. It stays with me, it's part of my identity, it has forever changed the way I carry myself, the way I live the rest of my life.

The judge in this case gave the defendant a sentence of 6 months in jail. Later the voters in the state of California recalled the judge.

After reading the powerful statement written by this courageous victim, when it went viral on the internet, Vice President Joe Biden, who was the sitting Vice President at the time, wrote an open letter to her. Vice President Biden was very concerned about the issue of violence toward women. In 1994 he wrote the Violence Against Women Act. He has been a strong advocate to spread awareness about campus sexual assault. Here is the letter* he wrote to her:

An Open Letter to a Courageous Young Woman

I do not know your name—but your words are forever seared on my soul. Words that should be required reading for men and women of all ages. Words that I wish with all of my heart you never had to write. I am in awe of your courage for speaking out—for so clearly naming the wrongs that were done to you and so passionately asserting your equal claim to human dignity. And I am filled with furious anger—both that this happened to you and that our culture is still so broken that you were ever put in the position of defending your own worth. It must have been wrenching—to relive what he did to you all over again. But you did it anyway, in the hope that your strength might prevent this crime from happening to someone else. Your bravery is breathtaking. You are a warrior—with a solid steel spine. I do not know your name—but I know that a lot of people failed you that terrible January night and in the months that followed. Anyone at that party who saw that you were incapacitated yet looked the other way and did not offer assistance. Anyone who dismissed what happened to you as

*Joseph Biden, "An Open Letter to a Courageous Young Woman." Copyright in the public domain.

"just another crazy night." Anyone who asked "what did you expect would happen when you drank that much?" or thought you must have brought it on yourself.

You were failed by a culture on our college campuses where one in five women is sexually assaulted—year after year after year. A culture that promotes passivity. That encourages young men and women on campuses to simply turn a blind eye. The statistics on college sexual assault haven't gone down in the past two decades. It's obscene, and it's a failure that lies at all our feet. And you were failed by anyone who dared to question this one clear and simple truth: Sex without consent is rape. Period. It is a crime. I do not know your name—but thanks to you, I know that heroes ride bicycles.

Those two men who saw what was happening to you—who took it upon themselves to step in—they did what they instinctually knew to be right. They did not say "It's none of my business." They did not worry about the social or safety implications of intervening, or about what their peers might think. Those two men epitomize what it means to be a responsible bystander. To do otherwise—to see an assault about to take place and do nothing to intervene—makes you part of the problem. Like I tell college students all over this country—it's on us. All of us. We all have a responsibility to stop the scourge of violence against women once and for all. I do not know your name—but I see your unconquerable spirit. I see the limitless potential of an incredibly talented young woman—full of possibility. I see the shoulders on which our dreams for the future rest. I see you. You will never be defined by what the defendant's father callously termed "20 minutes of action." His son will be.

I join your global chorus of supporters, because we can never say enough to survivors: I believe you. It is not your fault. What you endured is never, never, never, NEVER a woman's fault. And while the justice system has spoken in your particular case, the nation is not satisfied. And that is why we will continue to speak out. We will speak to change the culture on our college campuses—a culture that continues to ask the wrong questions: What were you wearing? Why were you there? What did you say? How much did you drink? Instead of asking: Why did he think he had license to rape? We will speak out against those who seek to engage in plausible deniability. Those who know that this is happening, but don't want to get involved. Who believe that this ugly crime is "complicated." We will speak of you—you who remain anonymous not only to protect your identity, but because you so eloquently represent "every woman." We will make lighthouses of ourselves, as you did—and shine. Your story has already changed lives. You have helped change the culture. You have shaken untold thousands out of the torpor and indifference towards sexual violence that allows this problem to continue. Your words will help people you have never met and never will. You have given them the strength they need to fight. And so, I believe, you will save lives.

I do not know your name—but I will never forget you. The millions who have been touched by your story will never forget you. And if everyone who shared your letter on social media, or who had a private conversation in their own homes with their daughters and sons, draws upon the passion, the outrage, and the commitment they feel right now the next time there is a choice between intervening and walking away—then I believe you will have helped to change the world for the better.

At the time of the Stanford rape, 2015, it was reported that there had been 30 known reported sex offenses on the Stanford campus that year. That means that there may have been two times that number since many sexual assaults go unreported. One study estimated that for every 1,000 college women, 35 incidents of rape occur each academic year; off-campus rape (66.3 %) is more common than on-campus rape (33.7%); less than 5% of completed or attempted rapes were reported to law enforcement; however, 66% did tell another person, usually a friend (Fisher et al., 2000).

In 2016 an online study of United States university students found that more than 50% of male athletes admitted to "sexually coercing a woman in a manner that meets the legal definition of rape" (Young et al., 2016). That is a mind-blowing statistic! One hypothesis that could be drawn from that data is that the "rape culture" in our country is strongest among men who play sports. Another hypothesis might be that athletes have learned that the universities in our country are more concerned about protecting their athletic programs than they are about protecting their students from sexual assault.

Of course, we all know that rape and other forms of sexual assault are not confined to college campuses. We have all been horrified by the accounts of sexual abuse perpetrated by members of the clergy, the Boy Scouts, some coaches, and doctors to athletes. The *#MeToo Movement* has put a national spotlight on just how frequent and insidious the incidence of sexual abuse is in this country. We have seen how many celebrities have been committing sexual abuse and assault for decades with no consequences; comedian Bill Cosby, movie producer Harvey Weinstein, financier Jeffery Epstein, even Presidents of the United States Bill Clinton and Donald Trump. The list goes on.

The news stories that caused Americans to be alarmed by the sexual abuse that has been perpetrated by some clergy and some leaders of the Boy Scouts has opened our eyes to the fact that victims of sexual abuse are not just female. Many, many victims are male. It took longer for us to see the overwhelming numbers of male victims in our country because we have, for centuries, been committed to believe all of the gender stereotyping that is so pervasive in our culture. Those stereotypes often favor male behavior over female behavior. But in the instance of sexual abuse, those stereotypes have caused most males who were sexually abused to report their abuse at even lower rates than females. In fact, most never told anyone, which meant that males rarely were able to get therapy for the abuse.

Stephen Braveman (2007a, 2007b), a sex therapist who practices in Monterey, California, wrote about his treatment of males. He listed these differences as they relate specifically to male victims:

Myths about Male Sexual Victimization

Myth #1 – Male socialization: Sometimes referred to as the "macho image." This means that males, even young boys, should not be victims or be vulnerable. Males should be able to protect themselves. In truth, boys are children and are weaker and more vulnerable than their perpetrators and cannot fight back. This is due to the perpetrator's power in terms of size, strength, and knowledge, position of authority or resources such as money, bribes, threats and whatever advantage taken to use the child for sexual purposes.

Myth #2 – Most sexual abuse of boys is perpetrated by homosexual males. Pedophiles who molest boys are not expressing a homosexual orientation any more than pedophiles that molest girls are practicing heterosexual behaviors. While many child molesters have gender and/or age preferences, those who seek out boys are, for the vast majority, not homosexual. They are pedophiles (adults sexually interested in children).

Myth # 3 – If a boy experiences sexual arousal or orgasm from abuse, this means he was a willing participant or enjoyed it. In reality, males can respond physically (have an erection) to stimulation even in traumatic or painful sexual situations. Therapists who work with sexual offenders know that one way a perpetrator can maintain secrecy is to label the victim's sexual response as an indication of his willingness to participate. Many survivors feel guilt and shame because they experienced physical arousal while being abused. Physical (as well as visual or auditory) stimulation is likely to happen in a sexual situation. It does not mean that the victim wanted the experience or fully understood what it meant at the time.

Myth # 4 – Boys are less traumatized by the abuse experience than girls. While some studies indicate males as less negatively affected, more studies find that long-term effects are quite damaging. Males are additionally damaged by society's refusal or reluctance to accept their victimization and the victim's belief that he must "tough it out" in silence.

Myth #5 – Boys abused by males are or will become homosexual. While there are different theories about how the sexual orientation develops, the human sexuality field does not see premature sexual experiences as playing a significant role in late adolescent or adult sexual orientation. It is unlikely that someone can make another person a homosexual or heterosexual. Sexual orientation is a complex issue and there is no single answer or theory to explain why someone identifies himself as homosexual, heterosexual, or bisexual. Premature sexual experiences on boys or girls, perpetrated by older males or females, is damaging in many areas, including sexual identity and orientation.

Many boys who have been abused by males erroneously believe that there is something about them to sexually attract a male, and this may mean the boy is homosexual or effeminate – again not true. Pedophiles who are attracted to boys will admit it is the lack of body hair and adult features that turns them on. It is the pedophile's inability to develop and maintain a healthy adult sexual relationship that is the problem, not the physical features of the sexually immature boy or the young adolescent male.

Myth #6 – The "Vampire Syndrome" (boys who are sexually abused, like the victims of count Dracula, go on to "bite" or sexually abuse others). This myth is especially dangerous because it can create a stigma for the child that he will become an offender. Boys might be treated as potential offenders rather than victims who need help. While it is true that most offenders have histories of sexual abuse, it is NOT true that most victims go on to become offenders.

Myth #7 – If the perpetrator is female, the boy or adolescent should be considered fortunate to be initiated into heterosexual activity. In reality, premature or coerced sex, whether by a mother, aunt, older sister, babysitter, or other female in a position of power over a boy, causes confusion at best, and rage, depression or other problems in more negative circumstances.

Belief in these myths is dangerous. If the survivor believes these myths, he may likely feel shame and anger and reinforce that it was his fault. It is never the fault of the child in a sexual situation. Perpetrators are quite skilled in making victims believe in these myths and that it is the fault of the victim. Remember, it is always the responsibility and fault of the offender.

Challenging these myths is difficult. Few can successfully accomplish such a task on their own. Joining forces as a team becomes an essential. However, male sexual abuse survivors typically have a very difficult time bonding with other men, especially if they were abused by a male. Therefore, it is important to introduce bonding exercises (Braverman, 2007a).

Given the overwhelming number of sexual assault victims in this country, it is likely that almost everyone who is reading this book has either been sexually assaulted, knows someone who has been sexually assaulted, is currently a friend or family member of someone who has been sexually assaulted but the friend or family member has not told you about their victimization, so you are unaware that you know someone who has been sexually assaulted. Therefore, it is important that you learn what the psychological, emotional, and behavioral aftermath of sexual assault looks like so that you can develop as much empathy and understanding for them as possible.

DEVELOPMENT OF THE DIAGNOSIS OF PTSD IN THE TREATMENT OF RAPE VICTIMS

Knowing about the laws that have governed sexual abuse until about 40 years ago will, hopefully, help the reader understand why it has taken so long for us to really investigate and learn how to provide effective treatment for survivors. Since victims were unlikely to come forward to report the crime, they were also not likely to talk about how the crime affected them. Therefore, there was very little discussion of the issue of sexual abuse in the psychological or psychiatric literature. Many mental health professionals relied on the beliefs that Sigmund Freud espoused about the topic. He did not do any controlled studies on the prevalence of sexual abuse in the population, nor on the credibility of those who spoke to him about it, or what type of symptoms were common among survivors.

But wait, that last statement is only half true. He did know something about the symptoms that many of his patients, who reported that they were sexually abused, were trying to cope with. He labeled those women "hysterical" because many of them had very similar symptoms. At first, he believed their accounts of sexual abuse and that the sexual abuse was the cause of the "hysterical" symptoms. His psychiatrist colleagues had heard similar stories from their patients but dismissed the stories as lies and fantasies. In April of 1896, Freud presented a paper titled, "The Etiology of Hysteria" to the Society for Psychiatry and Neurobiology in which he presented his belief that sexual abuse was the cause of hysterical symptoms (Freud, 1896). His colleagues gave his speech a very cold reception. After that experience Freud changed his mind and decided that his patient's stories of sexual abuse were, indeed, fantasies as opposed to actual accounts of childhood sexual abuse. In fact, he came to believe that these stories of abuse were actually related to a woman's unconscious desire for a penis.

Freud believed that the clitoris was the most inferior sexual organ which led girls to be very envious of their father's penis. It also caused them to be unable to develop into a strong, independent person with high moral standards. He believed that the ability to do so belonged only to men since they possessed a penis and, ergo, had no penis envy. However, he believed, as crazy as it may sound today, that if a woman were able to give birth to a penis (meaning a male baby), then their uterus would calm down and they would be less hysterical. In addition, these women were thought to be more willing to accept their inferior, dependent position in the world (Freud, 1927). By devising this theory about the consequences of not having a penis, he made it almost impossible for anyone who wanted to have a career in mental health to be able to help a woman who reported that she was a victim of sexual abuse. According to psychoanalytic theory (in original form) the treatment for such a woman would be for the diagnosis of hysteria. Her sexual abuse memories would be ignored.

The feminists of the 1970s did much to help liberate women from the horrors of Freud's sexist theories. The movement enabled many women to speak out about their sexual abuse. It also gave many researchers the opportunity to begin studying the effects of sexual abuse on the survivors. The effort to study the incidence of this abuse in the population led to recognizing how widespread it was in female populations (about 1 in 4) and in male populations, as well (about 1 in 6), before age 18 (Finkelhor et al., 1990). More recently, the FBI National Press Office released the 2015 Uniform Crime Reporting (UCR) Program on September 26, 2016. The report included a statement about an important change made by the FBI in how rape was defined. It stated:

> Prior to 2013, the FBI's UCR Program collected rape data in the Summary Reporting System under the category "forcible rape." In 2013, the program removed the term "forcible" from the title and revised the definition. The legacy UCR definition of rape is "The carnal knowledge of a female forcibly and against her will." The revised UCR definition of rape is

"Penetration, no matter how slight, of the vagina or anus with any body part or object, or oral penetration by a sex organ of another person, without the consent of the victim."

Of the 18,439 city, county, university and college, state, tribal, and federal agencies eligible to participate in the UCR Program, 16,643 submitted data in 2015. A high-level summary of the statistics submitted, as well as estimates for those agencies that did not report, found that in 2015 rape increased 6.3 percent, as compared to 2014.

It is reasonable to hypothesize that the increase noted in the reporting of rape may have been due to the very significant change in how rape was defined during the more recent reporting periods, (i.e., eliminating the word "forcible" and allowing that it happens to any person, not just females). However, no matter how hard reporting agencies work to learn what the prevalence of rape is, we probably never will know how many women and men are raped each year. What we do know is that those who do come forward asking mental health professionals for help are plagued with a variety of serious, debilitating symptoms.

When rape crisis centers began to open around the country in the early 1970s, there was not much known about the sequela of rape or how to help the victims. So, researchers began to study the victims. They learned that rape victims were likely to suffer from a number of behavioral, psychological, and physical symptoms and reactions that may last a very long time. They labeled the cluster of symptoms Rape Trauma Syndrome (RTS) (Burgess & Holmstrom, 1979). They observed that RTS progressed in stages. The Acute Stage begins right after the victim is able to grasp what has happened to her. It is a time of intense emotions with psychological, physical, and behavioral changes. In order to cope with the intensity of these emotions the victim will begin to appear to others as if she is okay – this is the Underground Stage. She tries very hard during this stage to go back to her pre-rape life. However, she is never able to go back to what her life was. She then enters the Reorganization Stage which is a time when she learns how to adjust to her new life as a survivor of rape (Burgess & Holmstrom, 1979).

At the same time that rape researchers were struggling to understand the sequela of rape, other researchers were trying to come to terms with the trauma they were observing in the men returning from the Vietnam War. They were seeing large numbers of Vietnam veterans in Veterans Hospitals who were presenting with symptoms similar but, in many cases, more severe than they had seen in veterans of previous wars, which was labeled "shell shock." The researchers were observing that men who had been discharged years prior were showing more severe symptoms than they had seen at the time they were discharged. Over time they came to realize that all of the veterans they were treating had symptoms that manifested in clusters that were labeled Intrusive Symptoms, Avoidant Symptoms, and Arousal Symptoms. The men with these symptoms all were describing traumatic war events that they were trying desperately to forget. But the horrible feelings were very easily "triggered" by something as benign as the sound of a helicopter overhead or the backfire of a car or truck.

In the mid-1970s, these clusters of symptoms were given a name, Posttraumatic Stress Disorder (PTSD). At first there was some controversy in the mental health field as to whether that diagnosis should be reserved for war trauma or if other traumas could cause such serious and often long-term symptoms. The end result of the discussions about PTSD was that a traumatic event was seen as a catastrophic stressor that was "outside the range of usual human experience" (*DSM-IV*; American Psychiatric Association, 1994). Therefore, PTSD is unique among mental health diagnoses because it is the only one that requires a "stressor criterion" (exposure to an event that is considered traumatic) in order to make the diagnosis.

You might wonder why placing a mental health diagnosis on a person is important. There are certainly many good reasons not to "label" anyone with such a diagnosis (e.g., sometimes the labels can cause a person to be rejected for life insurance, or a vindictive spouse may try to use it against their ex in a custody battle, etc.). However, clients and their families want to know the name of the disorder causing so much havoc in their lives. In addition, we as providers of mental health services need to know what we are treating in order to be effective and actually help our patients. People who have suffered with the symptoms of PTSD but misdiagnosed as having Bipolar Disorder, Borderline Personality Disorder, Dependent Personality Disorder, and so forth, were usually treated with drugs and/or (especially in the case of a personality disorder) dismissed due to the fact that many practitioners believe that a person with a personality disorder cannot be helped.

Fortunately, some evidence-based treatments have been developed that are effective in the treatment of PTSD. Many researchers have been studying the effects of trauma on the mind and body for a number of years. The research indicates that treatments that include asking the survivor to Recall, Revisit, and Resolve the memory of the event (3 R's) are the most effective modalities for treatment.

RECALL – The therapist asks the survivor to remember the details of the traumatic event and tell the story. As the person remembers and relates the details of the traumatic event, the therapist notes what pieces of the story elicit the most emotion. The therapist keeps in mind that there will probably be parts of the story that the survivor may not remember at this time.

REVISIT – The therapist asks the survivor to try to recall the event while applying a "desensitization" technique. There are various techniques that a therapist might use to help the survivor achieve the most vivid revisiting of the trauma possible. Those that this author has used are ***Progressive Relaxation***, which allows the survivor to be calmer and more relaxed before beginning to revisit the memory (Bernstein & Borkovec, 1973); ***Hypnosis***, which enables the survivor to go into a deep state of trance and also enhances their ability to relax and provides heightened focus on the memories of the event (Hammond, 1990); and ***Eye Movement Desensitization Reprocessing (EMDR)***, another evidence-based therapy which allows the desensitization to the memory to happen within a shorter period of time without the intense and prolonged anxiety that may accompany the other methods of desensitization (Shapiro, 2002). ***Cognitive Processing Therapy*** is a treatment modality that has been used extensively which focuses on "stuck points." Often survivors have some inaccurate beliefs and self-statements, especially about trust, self-esteem, and guilt. The treatment helps the survivor process and change these distorted perceptions. During the process of revisiting, the therapist makes sure that the aspects of the traumatic event that have elicited the most emotion receive a sufficient amount of attention and focus to facilitate trauma resolution.

RESOLVE – During this phase of the treatment the therapist pays attention to what beliefs about the event and the self may need to be corrected. For example, common self-beliefs that are problematic are: "It is my fault that I was raped because I was wearing a short skirt," "No one will ever want to marry me because I am not a virgin anymore," or "If I weren't so stupid this would never have happened to me."

The work is successful when the survivor reports that she is no longer plagued by unwanted, intrusive memories, dreams, emotions, reactions, or beliefs about the self that are related to the traumatic event. There is, of course, a caveat to this statement of "cure." As the survivor goes through life, there may be times when they will need to return to therapy or otherwise to deal with something new in their life that may be bringing up some parts of the trauma.

Eye Movement Desensitization Reprocessing (EMDR)

- In 1989, Francine Shapiro published the results of a study* she had conducted using a new technique that she had discovered and developed. In that study she called the technique EMD.
- She discovered that during a single session of EMD during which the generation of rhythmic, multisaccadic eye movements while the subjects concentrated on a traumatic memory successfully desensitized the subjects' traumatic memories and dramatically altered their cognitive assessments of the situation, effects that were maintained through the 3-month follow-up check. This therapeutic benefit was accompanied by behavioral shifts which included the alleviation of the subjects' primary presenting complaints related to rape, molestation, and combat.
- She believed that the movement of the eyes in an awake state enabled the brain to replicate the process that occurs in the brain during REM (dream) sleep. There are data that suggest that if a person is deprived of REM sleep for 1 week they will develop symptoms similar to psychosis. If allowed to sleep normally and REM activity resumes, the person will return to normal functioning. Therefore, she concluded that REM sleep is the main function of the brain that keeps us "sane."
- In this 1989 article she described the EMD procedure:

  Clients are requested to follow with their eyes the therapist's finger, which is moved very rapidly from side to side 10 to 20 times as a means of eliciting from them rhythmic, bilateral saccadic eye movements, while they simultaneously visualize the traumatic event and internally repeat the associated irrational cognition or negative self-statement. Preliminary testing suggested that the procedure had the capacity to:

  1. desensitize a highly traumatic memory within a short period of time (one session) without intense and prolonged anxiety;
  2. produce a cognitive restructuring of the verbalized self-statement or assessment, along with a redefined visual representation; and
  3. cause congruent and substantial behavioral shifts (Shapiro, 1989).

*Note: Further research has indicated that the "curative" function that REM sleep provides is a result of the fact that both hemispheres of the brain are activated during REM which is the reason that the eyes move back and forth. Therefore, providing a rhythmic bilateral auditory stimulation to the ears or a pulsing tactile sensation to shoulders, hands, and so forth, provides the same result as eye movement (Siegel, 2002; Van der Kolk, 2002).

Cognitive Processing Therapy (CPT)

In 1988 Patricia Resick began developing a treatment modality she called Cognitive Processing Therapy (CPT). She then worked with Candice Monson and Katherine Chard to further develop the treatment model (Resick et al., 2017). It is a trauma-focused psychotherapy that is considered to be a very effective treatment for PTSD. CPT is based on cognitive therapy theory.

CPT theory looks at how humans organize information into categories or schemas so that one can make sense of the world they live in and understand new information, thereby being able to predict and control, to some extent, their experiences.

The theory posits that traumatic events disrupt the organization of information, especially information related to trust, safety, self-esteem, and so forth. PTSD causes "stuck points" which are inaccurate self-beliefs and self-statements. This distorted information inhibits the victim's ability to recover from the traumatic experience. CPT can be provided to individuals and to groups.

CPT treatment typically consists of 12 structured sessions that include:

- educating the client about PTSD symptoms,
- informing the client about the usual thoughts and feelings related to PTSD,
- giving lessons to develop skills that help clients to challenge their thoughts, and
- helping clients to recognize the changes in their beliefs after they were traumatized.

Clients are asked to write an account of their traumatic event and to practice the cognitive techniques that they are learning.

DEVELOPMENT OF THE DIAGNOSIS OF DISSOCIATIVE IDENTITY DISORDER

Now we need to consider the victims of prolonged sexual trauma. As noted previously, when rape crisis centers were starting around the U.S. in the 1970s, we barely knew anything about the incidence of incest and other forms of prolonged sexual abuse. In the 1980s that issue entered the social conscience. We began to hear more and more patient stories of prolonged abuse, especially during childhood, and again thanks to the Feminist Movement we believed them. We also had a lot of data about the psychological aftermath of the abuse. The symptomatology of prolonged sexual abuse or any other kind of prolonged abuse is much more complex. There are some major differences in the presentation (symptoms) and treatment of a single event of sexual abuse and the sexual abuse perpetrated by one (or more) perpetrator who has control over a person for a number of years.

Most parents of young children want to protect their children from harm. Due to society's heightened awareness of the prevalence of sexual abuse, children are routinely told to be careful around strangers (Stranger Danger). They stress to their children that they should not take gifts from strangers, get into a car with strangers, leave school with a stranger who tells them that their parent sent them to pick them up, that no one can touch their "private parts," and so forth. All of this is excellent advice and if heeded, may prevent harm. The part that most parents do not talk to their children about is what to do if Uncle Frank or their best friend's Dad or the babysitter harms them.

Unfortunately, the most likely person to sexually abuse a child or adolescent is someone known to the child or adolescent. Ninety six percent (96%) of perpetrators are known to their victim (National Center for Victims of Crime, 2008). Only 4% were strangers. Often the person who perpetrates has continued and prolonged access to the child. When this happens the resulting trauma sequela is severe and complex. A seminal book about prolonged trauma was *Trauma and Recovery: The Aftermath of Violence – from Domestic Abuse to Political Terror* (Herman, 1992, 1997, 2015). In this very important book Judith Herman explained what she called "complex PTSD." She believed that when a person is exposed to prolonged trauma, especially when it is perpetrated by another human who has control over them, the symptoms of PTSD were not enough to describe the very intense and extreme symptoms survivors experience. So, in her earlier work she described those symptoms and suggested some methods of treatment.

Symptoms of Complex Posttraumatic Stress Disorder (PTSD)

1 History of subjection to totalitarian control including childhood physical or sexual abuse
2. Alterations in affect regulation
   - persistent dysphoria
   - chronic suicidal preoccupation
   - self-injury
   - explosive or extremely inhibited anger (may alternate)
   - compulsive or extremely inhibited sexuality (may alternate)
3. Alterations in consciousness, including
   - amnesia or hypermnesia for traumatic events
   - transient dissociative episodes
   - depersonalization/derealization
   - reliving experiences, either in the form of intrusive PTSD symptoms or in the form of ruminative preoccupation
4. Alterations in self-perception, including
   - sense of helplessness or paralysis of initiative
   - shame, guilt, and self-blame
   - sense of defilement or stigma
   - sense of complete difference from others (may include sense of specialness, utter aloneness, belief no other person can understand, or nonhuman identity)
5. Alterations in perception of perpetrator, including
   - preoccupation with relationship with perpetrator (includes preoccupation with revenge)
   - unrealistic attribution of total power to perpetrator (caution: victim's assessment of power realities may be more realistic than clinician's)
6. Alterations in relations with others, including
   - isolation and withdrawal
   - disruption in intimate relationships
   - repeated search for rescuer (may alternate with isolation and withdrawal)
   - persistent distrust
   - repeated failures of self-protection
7. Alterations in systems of meaning
   - loss of sustaining faith
   - sense of hopelessness and despair

The first edition of Herman's *Trauma and Recovery* was printed in 1992. Symptom number 3 points out the fact that loss of memory of abuse is a symptom that can be complete amnesia for the trauma (as mentioned at the beginning of this chapter). During the 1980s and 1990s, therapists were reporting that they were seeing more and more examples of loss of traumatic memories among their patients. The therapists were becoming more aware of the symptoms of sexual abuse and were more inclined to try to help patients with amnesia retrieve those traumatic memories. This change in awareness and treatment caused a sensational controversy among clinicians and researchers that received a lot of attention in the press. Were therapists planting memories that were not real in the minds of vulnerable patients and causing them to believe that a relative or family friend abused them? It became known as the "false memory" controversy. The controversy was so intense that some therapists were frightened to suggest to a patient that their symptoms may be the result of trauma, even though therapists knew that a number of the patients they treated, who had symptoms of trauma, had repressed the memory of the trauma.

The controversy ended when a graduate student of an ardent denier of repressed memory, Elizabeth Loftus (1994), did her dissertation on the topic of repressed memory. The graduate student, Linda Williams, decided to do a real-life study of the aftermath of trauma. She went to a hospital emergency room and was able to get the names and contact information for 129 women who presented in the ER with substantiated sexual abuse trauma in 1973 to 1975. She contacted the victims about 17 years after they had been seen in the hospital ER. She asked them about the abuse. Eighty of the women she spoke with reported that they recalled the abuse. Sixteen percent (16%) of those who recalled the abuse had forgotten it at some time in the past. Those with a history of forgetting the abuse were younger than the other victims at the time of the abuse and were less likely to have received support from their mothers (Williams, 1995). There have been other studies that support the fact that abuse survivors do repress memories or parts of memories of abuse (Briere & Conte, 1993; Van der Kolk, 1994).

Judith Herman and others continued to research and publish their findings about the complexity of the symptoms of prolonged sexual abuse and the treatment methods used to alleviate those symptoms. When the 1994 version of the *Diagnostic and Statistical Manual of Mental Disorders* (*DSM-IV*) was published, the diagnosis of Dissociative Identity Disorder (DID) was included. This diagnosis has replaced the concept of a Complex PTSD (which was never a diagnosis that was accepted for publication in the DSM).

Prolonged sexual abuse (e.g., incest, sexual slavery, domestic abuse - which often includes sexual abuse) causes in the victim a disruption of identity that can produce more than one personality. In the past, mental health providers believed that dissociative identity disorder was very rare. Now we know that it is much more common and can easily be misdiagnosed if the therapist doesn't identify the cause of the symptoms they are seeing.

The diagnosis of DID means that during the abusive events the victim has been able to develop a way to survive the overwhelming emotions and physical pain by psychologically removing herself from the reality of the trauma. She is able to preserve her psyche by blocking it out. Many victims describe their experience during the abuse from a perspective that is outside of their body. For example, "When I remember him getting in my bed and starting to touch my vagina, I am seeing me laying on the bed and him on top of me. I'm not in my body when I remember it."

Part of the treatment during the revisiting stage is to help the victim return to her body so that she can associate her visual memory of the abuse with her emotional and tactile memory of it. It is a scary process for the victim. Therefore, sufficient safety skills are required. The payoff for being able to actually revisit and relive the trauma is that the memory no longer has the same intense hold on her psyche. In the case of disruption of identity that is severe enough to create separate parts (personalities or ego states), the process of association is critical to being able to help the victim "integrate" the dissociated parts back into her psyche in order to form a whole person.

The reader might wonder why the author has taken time and space to talk about the diagnosis of PTSD, Complex PTSD, and Dissociative Identity Disorder (DID). The answer is because it is very important that the reader understand that the person who has been diagnosed with these syndromes is not inherently a "sick" person. They have, through no fault of their own nor due to their genetic makeup, developed the symptoms, problems, and issues. Essentially, survivors experience normal reactions to extraordinarily abnormal personal events. Many years of therapy have been wasted and many patients have suffered needlessly even after going to therapy because they did not receive the correct diagnosis which then resulted in receiving ineffective treatments.

Understanding that traumatic events produce a predictable set of symptoms has revolutionized the clinical practice of most mental health professionals. Once there was an understanding that the symptoms were the result of exposure to a traumatic event, many researchers began to develop treatment techniques that could help the person "resolve" the traumatic memory of the event. As discussed previously, that research has led to many treatment options that address the emotional, psychological, and physical symptoms.

Another reason is to help the reader understand how sexual abuse affects the victim. As the letter written by the Stanford University student illustrates, the damage to the victim is life changing. When another person penetrates the boundaries of someone's body against the will of that person, they set in motion a life-long struggle on the part of the victim to find peace and healing. The symptoms are intense, deeply rooted, long-lasting, and severe. The symptoms are manifested in every area of the victim's life and in every part of her mind, body, soul, and spirit. As one researcher put it, "The body keeps the score" and "The body does not lie" (Van der Kolk, 1994).

RAPE CULTURE VS. A CONSENT CULTURE

The attitudes and beliefs about rape in most cultures of the world have been based in large part on the attitudes and beliefs about the role of women in the culture. For most of recorded history, the roles assigned to women have been dichotomized as "Madonna" or "Whore." Women who accepted the role of wife and mother were "Madonnas," while women who did not accept these designated roles were perceived to be dangerous to the culture. The "wife" and "mother" titles were respected but also were believed to be inferior to the roles designated to men. Any woman who was perceived as being antagonistic to her role might get labeled as a "shrew," or worse, a "whore."

In order to maintain these cultural norms, most societies developed beliefs about female sexuality that could be labeled as a "rape culture." In fact, laws governing rape were based on these antiquated attitudes toward women (Brownmiller, 1975; Griffin, 1971) as seen in Brownmiller's book which was discussed at the beginning of this chapter under the section discussing the history of laws governing rape.

Rape has been defined in most cultures as having these three components: (a) Sexual intercourse, (b) forceful (some jurisdictions require that the victim prove that she resisted "to the utmost to the end"), and (c) against the will of the victim (Bley 1980). Given these criteria, the burden of proof is on the victim, who must be able to show that all three criteria were met (Brownmiller, 1975).

In a rape culture, the burden of proof is often overwhelming to the victim. She usually ends up wishing that she had never told anyone. The defense attorney can explore her sexual history to make sure that she isn't one of the "shrews" or "whores." She also has to show some evidence of force, such as photos of bruises or cuts (Bley, 1980). The problem is that if she took a self-defense course, she was probably told that if the rapist has a weapon, don't resist, lest he kills her.

Fortunately, the laws governing rape have changed in the last 60 years so that making a case is not as burdensome as it once was. However, many of the beliefs about female sexuality and a female's tendency to lie about rape when they want to punish someone continue to persist in our culture. These attitudes are particularly obvious in predominately male environments such as male locker rooms and fraternities and predominately male work environments.

What does a Consent Culture look like? We are beginning to see some evidence that a consent culture is possible. It would be a culture in which everyone knows that sexual touch can only happen when both parties are *clearly* saying "Yes." It is a culture in which women define their own roles and are free to pursue those roles without any harassment based on their gender. It is a culture where women feel free to come and go as they please, whenever they please, without fear of being labeled or of being raped. It would be a given that if there were a number of rapes (e.g., on a college campus), there would be a curfew for men on the campus and not for the women who are the potential victims, until the culprit is apprehended. It would be a culture in which males are taught to respect "No" even if her eyes say "Yes" (which is often the excuse to justify rape). It would be a culture where a woman could become intoxicated and not have to worry that someone will take sexual advantage of her condition.

What a wonderful world it would be if a *consent culture* became the norm!

REFERENCES

American College Health Association. (2016). *Addressing sexual and relationship violence on college and university campuses.* https://www.acha.org/documents/resources/guidelines/Addressing_Sexual_Violence.pdf

American Psychiatric Association. (1980). *Diagnostic and statistical manual of mental disorders* (3rd ed.).

American Psychiatric Association. (1994). *Diagnostic and statistical manual of mental disorders* (4th ed.).

American Psychiatric Association. (2000). *Diagnostic and statistical manual of mental disorders* (4th ed., text rev.).

American Psychiatric Association. (2013). *Diagnostic and statistical manual of mental disorders* (5th ed.). https://doi.Org/10.1176/appi.books.9780890425596

Bernstein, D., & Borkovec, T. (1973). *Progressive relaxation training: A manual for the helping professions.* Research Press.

Biden, J. W. (2016, June 9*). An open letter to a courageous young woman.* Buzzfeed.

Bley, J. W. (1980). *Effects of prior sex history and physical resistance evidence on verdicts of individuals and simulated juries in rape trials.* [Unpublished doctoral dissertation]. University of Cincinnati.

Braveman, S. (2007a). Innovative methods for treating patients with sexual trauma. In L. VandeCreek, Frederick Peterson, and Jill Bley (Eds.), *Innovations in clinical practice: Focus on sexual health* (pp. 197-206).

Braveman, S. (2007b). *Myths about male sexual abuse.* HAVOCA.org. Adapted from presentation at the 5th International Conference on Incest and Related Problems, Biel, Switzerland, August 14, 1991. https://www.havoca.org/survivors/sexuality/myths-about-male-sexual-abuse/?fbclid=IwAR24BA1cG3iNLal-LdA4bbN_wd3MDbnUvEY-8ozz8QsPRmjcidehBe1N6jo

Briere, J., & Conte, J. (1993). Self-reported amnesia for abuse in adults molested as children. *Journal of Traumatic Stress, 6,* 21-31.

Briere, J., & Elloitt, D. (2003). Prevalence and psychological sequelae of self-reported childhood physical and sexual abuse in general population. *Child Abuse & Neglect, 27,* 1205-1222. https://doi.org/10.1016/j.chiabu.2003.09.008

Brownmiller, S. (1975). *Against our will: Men, women & rape.* Simon and Schuster.

Burgess, A. W., & Holstrum, L. L. (1979). *Rape crisis and recovery.* R. J. Brady.

Burgess, A. W. & Holstrum, L. L. (1994). *Rape: Victims of crisis.* R. J. Brady.

Federal Bureau of Investigation National Press Office. (2016). *Uniform crime report.* https://ucr.fbi.gov/crime-in-the-u.s/2015/crime-in-the-u.s.-2015

Finkelhor, D., Hotaling, G., Lewis, I. A., & Smith, C. (1990). Sexual abuse in a national survey of adult men and women: Prevalence characteristics and risk factors. *Child Abuse and Neglect, 14*(1), 19-28. https://doi.org/10.1016/0145-2134(90)90077-7

Finkelhor, D., Ormrod, R., Turner, H., & Hamby, S. (2005). The victimization of children and youth: A comprehensive, national survey. *Child Maltreatment, 10*(1), 5-25. https://doi.org/10.1177/1077559504271287

Finkelhor, D., Turner, H., Ormrod, R., Hamby, S., & Kracke, K. (2009). *Children's exposure to violence: A comprehensive national survey* (NCJ 227744). U.S. Department of Justice, Office of Justice Programs. https://www.ncjrs.gov/pdffiles1/ojjdp/227744.pdf

Fisher, B., Cullen, F., & Turner, M. (2000). *The sexual victimization of college women.* National Institute of Justice, Bureau of Justice Statistics. https://www.ncjrs.gov/pdffiles1/nij/182369.pdf?hc_location=ufi

Freud, S. (1896, April 21). *The etiology of hysteria.* Paper presented to The Society for Psychiatry and Neurology.

Freud, S. (1927). The psychological consequences of the anatomical distinction between the sexes (James Strachey, Trans.). *The International Journal of Psychoanalysis, 8*(2), 133-142.

Griffin, S. (1971). *Rape: The all-American crime.* Know, Inc.

Hammond, C. (Ed). (1990). *Handbook of hypnotic suggestions and metaphors.* W.W. Norton.

Herman, J. (1992). *Trauma and recovery: The aftermath of violence - from domestic abuse to political terror.* Basic Books.

Herman, J. (1997). *Trauma and recovery: The aftermath of violence - from domestic abuse to political terror*. Basic Books.

Herman, J. (2015). *Trauma and recovery: The aftermath of violence - from domestic abuse to political terror.* Basic Books.

Krebs, C., Linquist, C., Warner, T., Fisher, B., & Martin, S. (2007). *The campus sexual assault (CSA) study*. National Institute of Justice. https://www.ncjrs.gov/pdffiles1/nij/grants/221153.pdf
Loftus, E., & Ketcham, K. (1994). *The myth of repressed memory: False memories and allegations of sexual abuse.* St. Martin's Press.
Martin, P. Y. (2016). The rape prone culture of academic contexts: Fraternities and athletics. *Gender & Society, 30*(1), 30-43. https://doi.org/10.1177/0891243215612708
McGovern, J., & Murray, P. (2016, January 13). *Consent communication: What does it mean for student athletes?* Paper presented at the NCAA National Conference, San Antonio, Texas.
Miller, C. (2019). *Know my name.* Viking Penguin Random House.
Mohler-Kuo, M., Dowdall, G., Koss, M., & Wechsler, H. (2004). Correlates of rape while intoxicated in a national sample of college women. *Journal of Studies on Alcoholism, 65*(1), 37-45. https://doi.org/10.15288/jsa.2004.65.37
National Center for Victims of Crime. (2008). *Child sexual abuse.* NCVC.org
National Sexual Violence Resource Center. (2011). *Child sexual abuse prevention - overview*. https://www.nsvrc.org/sites/default/files/2012-03/Publications_NSVRC_Overview_Child-sexual-abuse-prevention_0.pdf
Northwestern University School of Law. (1973). Complainant credibility in sexual offense cases: A survey of character testimony and psychiatric experts. (1973). *The Journal of Criminal Law and Criminology, 64*(1), 67-75. https://doi.org/10.2307/1142657
Peterson, F., Bley, J., & Frabotta, R. (2020). *The gender revolution & new sexual health: Celebrating unlimited diversity of the human sexuality hypercube.* Cognella.
Resick, P., Monson, C., & Chard, K. (2017). *Cognitive processing therapy for PTSD: A comprehensive manual.* The Guilford Press.
Saigh, P., Brenner, J. (Eds). (1999). *PTSD: A comprehensive text.* Allyn & Bacon.
Sanday, P. (1996). Rape Prone versus rape-free campus cultures. *Violence Against Women, 2*(2).
Shapiro, F. (1989). Efficacy of the eye movement desensitization procedure in the treatment of traumatic memories. *Journal of Traumatic Stress, 2,* 199-223.
Shapiro, F. (Ed). (2002). *EMDR as an integrative psychotherapy approach: Experts of diverse orientations explore the paradigm prism.* American Psychological Association.
Thomas, J. (2009). Report: Universities try to cover up rapes. *USA Today*, first published in the *Indianapolis Star.*
United States v. Bryant, 420 F.2d 1327 (D.C. Cir. 1969)
Van der Kolk, B. (1994). The body keeps the score: Memory and the evolving psychobiology of posttraumatic stress. *Harvard Review of Psychiatry, 1*(5), 253-265. https://doi.org/10.3109/10673229409017088
Williams, L. M., (1995). Recovered memories of abuse in women with documented child sexual victimization history. *Journal of Traumatic Stress, 8*(4).
Young, B., Desmarais, S., Baldwin, J., & Chandlar, R. (2016). Sexual coercion practices among undergraduate male recreational athletes, intercollegiate athletes and non-athletes. *Journal of Violence Against Women, 23*(7).

Section IV

Sex Therapy With Special Populations

18

Cultural Responsiveness in Sex Therapy: General Models and Considerations

Jennifer Cohen, Jouhaina Razzouk, and Frederick L. Peterson, Jr.

INTRODUCTION: CURRENT CULTURAL INFLUENCES AND MODELS OF MULTICULTURALISM

This chapter is about promoting effective cultural responsiveness that mental health providers are expected to practice within the contexts of counseling, therapy, and consultation. It first addresses the greater context of general cultural models and then highlights more specific models of cultural responsiveness for clinicians. The chapter is not intended to answer all questions of how to be culturally competent with all diverse client populations. Rather, the goal is to simply share the authors' experiences of what has worked well for them on their continuous journey toward further development on a spectrum of being culturally responsive to clients. The use of culturally respectful language is discussed related to addressing the sensitive topic of sexuality.

The nature and extent of clinical cultural responsiveness is, in large part, a reflection of the greater cultural understanding that we currently have about each other. At the time of writing this chapter, America was in the whirlwinds of change from the devastating loss of life resulting from the COVID-19 pandemic and the subsequent tanking of the national economy.

Simultaneously, there has been a majority-unifying repulsion to unrestrained police brutality exemplified by the killing of George Floyd (and the long list of others) and accompanied by vocal demands for social justice in the streets across this country. Not since the 1960s has there been such a shift in the American zeitgeist that has awoken the American consciousness to the immediate need for social, economic, and political change. A significant difference between then and now is the broader support for cultural sensitivity and cultural responsiveness, as well as demand for change from the White majority and other minority communities.

A predominant dimension of this national push for change has been the development of the Black Lives Matter movement, which stems from a long history of police killings of unarmed African Americans. Most, if not all, of these killings are unjustified. All killings of unarmed individuals are unjustified and reflect an institutionalized racism in America in general and specifically in law enforcement. The sheer number of killings and their social-media distribution has made mostly White Americans uncomfortable, angry, or perhaps for the first time since the Civil War, ready to support large-scale transformations for the Americans descended from those taken away from their homes.

Despite important advances in civil rights, our country still has a long road toward all Americans living in a "*more perfect union*" to which our U.S. Constitution aspires. Necessary to progressive reforms toward these ideals are recognizing and correcting our historical mistakes, from forcing fellow human beings into slavery and waging genocidal campaigns against native peoples to forced internment of Japanese Americans during WWII and economic exploitation of the poor and working classes. These unfortunate historical realities absolutely shape the worldviews of health care providers and facilitate the formation of their implicit biases, including those of mental health providers. Healing as a nation requires truthful acknowledgment of our past by educators and mental health providers, despite efforts to limit free speech and restrict discussion of race in classrooms within several states.

These worldviews are manifest in different models by which we are indoctrinated both as Americans as well as counselors, psychiatrists, psychologists, social workers, and therapists. Most people who are raised in America for any significant time are subtly indoctrinated to the "Great American Melting Pot" model, which was first touted as a blending of our cultural differences into one overarching and democratic "American identity." The trouble is it never worked that way. This model has been only theoretical without evidence of effective "democratization" of social acceptance of the racial and ethnic differences among Americans. This model is the reason why well-intentioned White Americans declare that they are "color blind" (an impossible task unless they are sightless).

While sometimes used in an effort to support the *ideal* of equality and sometimes used as a defense of one's own implicit biases, the phrase "I am color blind" has become out-of-favor and a sign of being out-of-touch with cultural sensitivity (as well as the research). People have slowly stopped using "I am color blind" much like the phrases "you people" and "where are you from?" (See the interesting story on pp. 324-325.) The declaration that "I am not racist, I am color blind" has been classified as a racial microaggression by some authors (Nadal et al., 2014).

Microaggressions are a topic often misunderstood, can be viewed as controversial, and not universally accepted as an evidence-based concept even by some mental health professionals. It is imperative that healthcare professionals, especially mental health providers, understand and accept:

1. the existence of "blind spots" within the framework of the Johari Window (see Figure 2 on p. 324)
2. the growing body of literature regarding implicit biases that influence our behavior in general as well as professional behavior as providers,
3. implicit biases reside within our blind spots and microaggressions are initiated from these biases, and
4. the adverse impact of microaggressions have nothing to do with the intent of statements or behaviors.

This is the reason the third author has been involved in teaching community-based zoom classes and university-based courses addressing the psychology of privilege with a special focus on the self-exploration of White privilege (Skillings & Peterson, 2022).

To illustrate the impact of microaggressions that people of color and minorities endure, Sue et al. (2007) introduced a taxonomy to delineate the different types of racial microaggressions. The taxonomy references eight different themes:

1. Alien in Own Land. This is when people make assumptions that a person of color was born outside the United States due to the likely assumption that all Americans are White.
2. The Ascription of Intelligence. This theme references the stereotype that some people are more intelligent or less intelligent than others depending on their race.
3. Color Blindness. This addresses the blending of racial realities to make all races a uniform one, as evidenced by the example of the melting pot as opposed to celebrating differences.

4. Criminality/Assumption of Criminal status. This refers to the stereotype that people that belong to certain races are generally more criminal than White people.
5. Denial of Individual Racism. This is when a person does not acknowledge their own biases and racism.
6. The Myth of Mediocrity. This is the faulty belief that a person's race is irrelevant in their lives and plays no role in success and denies the reality that a person of color's race does not serve as an obstacle in life.
7. Pathologizing Cultural Values/Communication Styles. This refers to the assumption that a White person's culture and mannerisms are the correct way to be and anything different from that is not considered normal.
8. Second-Class Citizen. This manifests when one person is given priority over another person because of their race.

Figure 1 is the cover of a theater program from a 1916 performance of *The Melting Pot: The Great American Dream*, written by Israel Zangwill. It told a story of a Russian Jewish immigrant family who arrived in America after their mother and sister were killed in the Russian pogroms (anti-Jewish violent riots). The plot was about coming to the United States to live a peaceful life free of prejudice and discrimination as Americans. For such a positive hope, the imagery is paradoxically foreboding of the racially conflicted history of Jews in America. The imagery in Figure 1 very well captures the spirit of the melting pot metaphor in which the cultural residuals of the "old country" are "melted away" to form new identities as Americans (Zangwill, 1909).

But the "Great American Melting Pot" is also the same model that provides a blind spot which hides implicit biases, deep sources of defensiveness, and a logical fallacy of those who argue that we now live in a "post-race society," and institutional racism does not exist (at least in the present). The election of an African American President is better support for the argument that our country is making progressive steps toward a "*more perfect union*" than the argument that we now live in a post-race society, where the color of a person's skin does not matter, or we have achieved "color-blindness." There is a whole body of scientific research which concludes, to a high level of empirical certainty, that "yes, the color of your skin makes a difference in 21st century America."

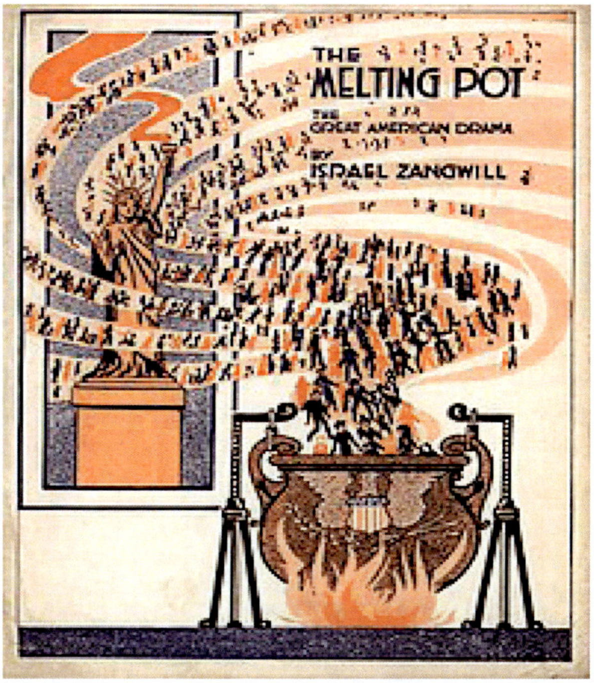

Figure 1. Cover of a 1916 theater program of *The Melting Pot: The Great American Dream*

The "Great American Melting Pot" supports the mythology of White supremacy because at the center of the model is an older, White male that visually represents what an "American" is supposed to look like. The model does not recognize the historical economic disenfranchising of women, the institutional racism reflected in financial red-lining practices, or the forced death-marches and relegation of native peoples to economically disadvantaged tribal lands. Perhaps just as devastating an effect of the "Great American Melting Pot" model is the perception that cultural differences are negative and somehow "un-American." The politicization of cultural differences, which is still very much present in our current political landscape, perpetuates prejudice and discrimination so that many Americans try to look "more American" in their language, appearance, and even by changing their family name.

More recently, different models have come into favor to replace the melting pot idea. One is the Salad Model which offers a visually colorful imagery of a salad with its many components. The green leafy vegetables (representing the land) are covered in red peppers and tomatoes, black olives and beans, brown mushrooms and nuts, white onions and sprouts, and so forth. You get the idea. The diverse collection of all these nutritious aspects of the salad are not yet complete without unifying the contents with a delicious dressing that "brings it all together" into a food that is incredibly joyful to eat because of both the unique tastes of the individual ingredients as well as the overall synergy of combined deliciousness. In short, this model feeds you cultural sustenance that is both emotionally satisfying and celebrates individual differences.

A third model that has also become popular and an effective replacement of the melting pot is the multicultural metaphor of quilting and the resulting product. Quilting has a long history among many cultural groups, including Afrolachians (African Americans who have inhabited Appalachia for generations and identify these mountains as home). African Americans and Appalachian Americans both share rich traditions of quilting to bring people together and to pass down oral family histories from generation to generation. Each panel is sown to represent some important aspect of the story of a family's struggle and/or celebration of birth, life, and moving forward.

It is no coincidence that in times of crisis, the practice of quilting has healing effects on a family, community, and national level. During the AIDS epidemic of the 1980s and 1990s, tens of thousands of Americans turned to quilting to support each other during times of loss and to memorialize their loved one. For years, a giant AIDS Quilt covered the National Mall every summer in Washington, D.C. until it became so big it had to be warehoused and archived. The use of a national quilt to represent the diverse humanity of all the Americans lost to AIDS is an example, on a societal level, of how diverse people can not only get along but also love one another. Our differences can add richness to our lives when we integrate them rather than dismiss them. The authors encourage you to use both the Salad and Quilt Models when thinking about multiculturalism. One feeds you and one comforts you with warmth. We need them both to survive.

The next section will introduce readers to three additional models that are very applicable to mental health providers who wish to become more culturally sensitive and responsive to their clients who look, sound, and perhaps act differently than the provider. These models of cultural competence development are: The Pyramid Model, the Mountain Model, and the Arranged-Marriage Model. Drawing from the research of multiculturalism, language to start discussions of cultural differences in sex therapy will be offered. It is clearly the task of the provider to address cultural aspects of sex therapy, to do so in a manner in which the client feels respected, and to make sure the client perceives that their cultural background is not only important but also a valued experience from which the provider can learn.

IMPLICIT BIASES: HOW THEY PREVENT PRACTITIONERS FROM MOVING FORWARD AND HOW TO OVERCOME THEM

While the current sociopolitical atmosphere in North America is charged with divisive rhetoric, laced by racist over- and undertones, the current zeitgeist of the field of clinical psychology continues to highlight the importance of clinicians being competent in multicultural therapy (MCT). This includes becoming aware of issues related to historical and current oppression, power dynamics, different worldviews, and social structures embedded within our value systems. It particularly highlights the importance of awareness of our own biases towards culture, race, ethnicity, sex, gender, religion, and so on. Moreover, literature in the psychology field reveals a push towards expanding the very definition of multicultural competence beyond general psychotherapy and counseling services that advocate for social justice for oppressed groups (Nadal et al., 2014; Skillings & Peterson, 2022; Vera & Speight, 2003).

In this chapter, we focus on culturally competent sex therapy. When the definition of sexuality is deconstructed, it proves to be beyond the physiological aspects of it as it carries in its very definition sociocultural, historical, and personal contexts (Lewis, 2004). The nature of sexuality as a concept has deepened to encompass the emotional, cognitive, and social facets (Barret, 1991). Hence, we as clinicians must extend ourselves to the unique experience of the individual while taking into consideration the sociocultural and historical experience with which our clients consciously and unconsciously present.

While it is encouraged to educate ourselves as clinicians about different cultures, it is important to be aware of our implicit biases that we bring into the therapeutic relationship. The Ohio State University's Kirwan Institute for the Study of Race and Ethnicity (2018) defines implicit bias as "the attitudes or stereotypes that affect our understanding, actions, and decisions in an unconscious manner." It often impacts our view of different cultural groups and manifests itself in stereotyping others. Implicit bias, as an occurring phenomenon in social and clinical settings, are the stereotypes or beliefs that we carry unconsciously about the world. While it organizes the world in reductionistic terms in our minds, it often ends up in likely unintentional prejudiced behaviors.

Examples of implicit biases that play a role in clinical settings are "Arab women are oppressed," "Black men are dangerous," and so forth. The question begs to be asked is: "How do clinicians work on their implicit biases if they are unaware of such biases?" Here are some suggestions to consider: Show curiosity about the unique experience and interpretation of a person's culture, exhibit a willingness to be educated or stand corrected, be open to feedback, and ask exploratory questions rather than presumptuous ones. More specifically, during a therapeutic interaction, ask oneself "What questions am I not asking this client that I may be asking someone else?" or "What questions am I asking this client that I would not be asking someone else?" Ask the client, "What would you like me to know about your culture that you would like me to be aware of?" Asking the client such questions reflects your openness and willingness to be educated. It also furnishes the client with a safe environment where they can give the clinician feedback if the clinician's implicit biases manifest themselves in interactions. Such difficult conversations prove to become very meaningful and can deepen the relationship between the clinician and the client. The safety that the clinician affords clients to have these difficult conversations becomes healing on its own as clients reflect a parallel process to their lives outside of clinical work in the wider social context.

A visualization of implicit biases can be demonstrated using the Johari Window (see Figure 2 on p. 324). It is a 2 x 2 matrix created by intersecting two perceptional dimensions: your self-perception and other people's perception of you. Cell one illustrates the public domain, which is information both the clinician and the client know. Cell two is information you know, but others do not know. They can be sexual orientation, cultural beliefs, and a diverse range of information you wish to keep to yourself. Cell three can represent our implicit biases, in which we, the clinicians, are unaware of our own biased beliefs, attitudes, and stereotypes. For example, we may subconsciously direct our attention to the female client when discussing household tasks in a couple's therapy. These biases can only be brought to conscious awareness through an open and safe dialogue with all parties. The same concept can be utilized to explain cell four; both the clinician and the client are not aware of how cultural experiences impact their interactions. This is probably particularly challenging in providing sex therapy given sexual practice can be such a taboo topic. We rarely discuss how we learned them, where we learned them, and what impact it has on our beliefs and values.

PERCEPTION Yours Others	**Things I Know About Myself**	**Things I Do Not Know About Myself**
Things Others Know About Me	Cell 1 Open/public domain	Cell 3 Blind spot/shadow domain
Things Others Do Not Know About Me	Cell 2 Private/undisclosed domain	Cell 4 The great unknown domain

Figure 2. Johari Window

In addition to some of the suggestions mentioned previously, here is another avenue to answer the question "How does a clinician work on their implicit bias, if they are unaware of such biases?" Pamela Hays (2008) developed the ADDRESSING model as a framework to help clinicians consider a broad range of diversity. They are Age, Developmental and acquired Disabilities, Religion, Ethnicity, Sexual orientation, Socioeconomic status, Indigenous group membership, Nationality, and Gender which all contribute to a multifaceted and complex understanding of a human being. Ask yourself what your beliefs are about these groups and how groups of people can bring up our deep-rooted biases and stereotypes. To combat these beliefs, it is important for clinicians to ask, "What does it feel like to be a minority woman immigrating to this country?" or "Tell me some of your experiences as a woman in relationships and sexual practices?" It is also okay to say, "I don't know, help me learn the right terms to call you," or "It is my mistake that I assumed this and can you correct me?" Sometimes, through trial-and-error, we begin to recognize how our cultures shape us and impact the way we see others and the world.

It is also important to note that in a world where multiple biases can intersect, such as race and sexual orientation, our biases are often hidden and not easily identifiable. You may have heard statements such as "I don't have biases; I just don't like Black gay men" or "You are beautiful for your race." These types of biases give prejudice and discrimination an opportunity to arise. It is even more problematic in a therapeutic relationship. As clinicians, we need to check our own prejudice as well as implicate biases.

One factor that may often be a double-edged sword is educating ourselves about other people's cultures. While it is an absolute must to remain committed to expanding our worldview and become more nuanced in our clinical work, it is just as important to understand that it carries with it the dangers of stereotyping. While well-intentioned, reading about general cultural issues may lead us to categorize the world in a way that does not feel accurate to the client. If one makes assumptions based on literature or experience, it inherently becomes a type of stereotyping although not fueled by prejudiced intentions. Every individual has a unique experience of their culture, and being aware of collective cultural experiences is not the same as assuming that such experiences are similar amongst all people belonging to that culture.

Consider this example: The question "Where are you from?" may be perceived as an invitation to discuss his or her cultural background to one immigrant, but to another immigrant, it was received as an attempt to make him further invisible and sidelined. This occurred in a real-life therapy session to a man who has been marginalized because of his Brown skin color. He explained that he perceived the question as being told "you do not look American enough," and it brought up traumatic experiences where he was told "Go back to where you came from." Because of established boundaries around safety and trust from the beginning of therapy, this client was able to share the impact of this seemingly mundane statement had on him. This example exhibits the need to be careful about what assumptions one's questions may mean to different people. In other words, not only is it important to empower clients, engage in social advocacy, and attend to the oppressive or racist social narrative, it is also important to introspect on ways we may be manifesting our own biases unconsciously even when we have the best of intentions.

This does not mean that one cannot ask someone else about where they come from, or questions that may be considered biased and/or insensitive. The authors do not intend to scare you, but to encourage you to be thoughtful with your questions and methods of approach. The example above was used as an illustration about how a seemingly benign question can trigger racial trauma and may even reflect implicit bias. If you place this same concept into the context of sex therapy, we hope one can understand how sensitive some of the questions may be to our clients. We believe the clinician must demonstrate a willingness to be open to feedback, reflect on their own biases, provide a safe environment, and have the clinical skill set necessary to unpack racial trauma and be able to process it.

It is nearly impossible to delineate all sociocultural and historical factors that make up sexuality for every individual. We must approach these factors with as much curiosity about them as we do the personal context. Just like we try to assume that we do not know much about the individual and allow them to tell us their story in assessment and treatment, similarly we must assume that how they have internalized their culture, history, religion, and ethnicity is unique to them. Surely, there is a common history, a collective unconscious, and a shared socio-political experience that we consider, but we must continue to be open to the client to educate us about how they have internalized and processed their circumstances. In 2015, a dress became a viral sensation over the internet when people argued about whether the dress was colored black and blue or white and gold. Most notable about this issue is that if people can perceive the same picture in significantly different colors, imagine how much more complex perceiving and interpreting similar cultural experiences can be.

Dr. William Hua (2019) listed the following steps that address implicit biases and minimize their impact on our work with clients.

1. Acknowledge our blind spots related to cultural issues; recognize the areas in which we are not experienced and rely on other sources to inform ourselves.
2. Consider taking the Implicit Association Test (Greenwald et al., 1998) which is geared towards assessing areas of potential biases such as age or skin tone.
3. Consider forming a consultation and accountability group aimed at highlighting each other's blind spots. Once trust and connection are established within the groups, peers are likely to challenge you in a way geared towards increasing your insight. This addresses the idea that we cannot address what we cannot see as is the case when we have a blind spot.
4. Consider utilizing the Cultural Formulation Interview (American Psychiatric Association, 2013) which offers clients the opportunity to describe their own presenting problem and the context in which that problem exists from their own cultural lens. This enhances the potential for a more collaborative relationship related to cultural issues.
5. Consider creating a culturagram (see Figure 3, p. 326) which helps to create a better visual for both the provider and the client about various aspects of an individual and family's culture (Congress, 1997).
6. Commit to continuous education by reading, attending workshops, and consulting about issues that relate to cultural bias.

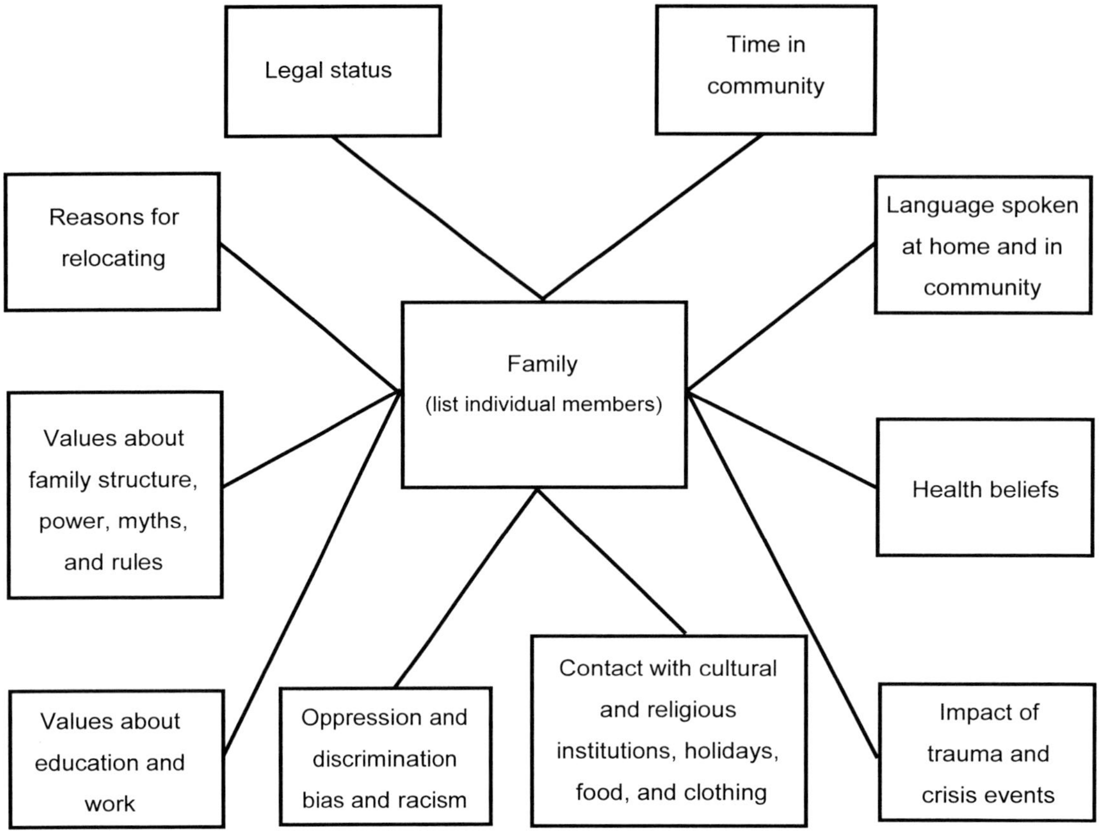

Figure 3. Culturagram

As we continue this journey of deconstructing implicit bias, please keep in mind that racial identities are cultural constructs. They are often used to establish systems of power and privileges. They are no longer accurate and do not represent today's ever-changing world of humankind. For example, when we ask, "Who are White Americans?" we tend to think of light skin-colored individuals from European nations. Well, many Americans of Spanish and Italian heritage may have disagreement about this assumption regarding skin color. Yet some Jewish Americans and Armenian Americans do not necessarily identify themselves as being in the mainstream category. There is much diversity within the White American community. That means we also have to challenge our implicit biases, attitudes, and stereotypes associated with White Americans. Ask the client "What would you like me to know about your racial and cultural identity?"

In addition, most White Americans in this country are descendants of Europeans. They often talk about their ancestors from Britain, Germany, Ireland, Italy, France, Poland, and so many other wonderful places. If you ask, they may invite you to their cultural traditions such as St. Patrick's Day and Oktoberfest. Americans also have small close-knit communities called Mennonites or Amish where they continue to carry on some of their original traditions, values, and beliefs. Our traditional definitions of racial/ethnic identities do not do justice to the rich cultural nuances in our current state of diversities.

Furthermore, Americans are seeing more interracial marriages as well as the integration of food, music, festivals, and cultural ideas from across the world. You can get Takoraisu, a delicious fusion of Japanese rice and Mexican tacos at some of the popular eateries in Los Angeles. Many Americans have attended Holi, a Hindu festival that celebrates the return of spring. Holi has become so popular that *USA Today* (Bleiberg, 2017) listed the ten best places to attend the holiday in the U.S. In this colorful world containing mixtures of culture, ethnicity, and other diversities, we need to construct new languages and ways of communicating our identity and experiences.

MULTICULTURAL TRAINING AND DEVELOPMENT USING MODELS

The American Psychological Association Council of Representatives adopted new multicultural guidelines for psychologists in August 2017 (American Psychological Association, 2017b). It includes ten guidelines and accompanying case studies to provide psychologists with a framework for providing multiculturally competent services. The goal is to address multiculturalism and diversity in education, training, research, clinical practice, and organizational change. According to its guidelines, mental health providers are ethically responsible in understanding the various cultural experiences that shape an individual client's life and presenting problems. In addition, there is research evidence that MCT is associated with positive treatment outcomes. Therefore, the authors want to illustrate three models that can help clinicians develop more culturally competent and responsive practices in assessment and treatment.

The Pyramid Model

The pyramid was selected as a metaphor of MCT for several reasons (see Figure 4). First, pyramids are familiar and readily recognizable. They are easy to conceptualize in terms of outside appearance as well as having interior contents. In addition, they represent one of the "wonders of the world" and reflect the different backgrounds among people inherent in MCT. Finally, pyramids represent strength and endurance, which are to be associated with ideals of strengthening the efficacy of clinical practices and increasing positive treatment outcomes.

The Pyramid Model synthesizes five factors to demonstrate the development of cultural competency for mental health professionals: (a) requisite life experiences, (b) awareness, (c) knowledge, (d) behavioral skills, and (e) intrinsic motivation (Peterson et al., 2007).

The first factor, requisite life experiences, serves as a solid foundation on which to sustain a pyramid over time. Requisite life experiences are similar to the roles that humanistic psychology gives to the importance of experience as described by Rogers (1961). It is the cultural soil from which each of us is nurtured and developed. Requisite life experience also involves having had experience with interpersonal relations sufficient to allow individuals to be predisposed to developing awareness of multicultural issues.

Then, there are three cornerstones of the pyramid that rest upon the foundation of requisite life experiences in this metaphor. They

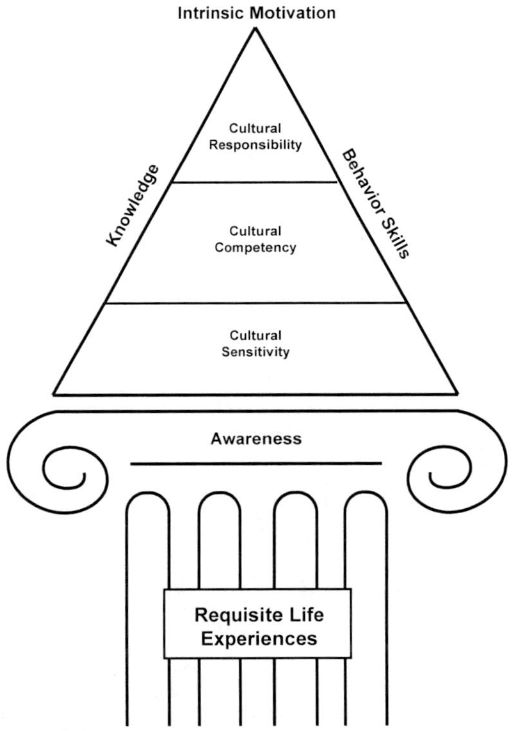

Figure 4. The Pyramid Model

are three components of cultural competency that have been discussed extensively in the literature: awareness, knowledge, and behavioral skills. The fifth factor is intrinsic motivation. It is the key factor that transforms the previously discussed three factors (representing a two-dimensional triangle) into a three-dimensional pyramid reflecting implementation. Motivation is at the apex of the pyramid and conceptually "activates" an individual to operationalize the knowledge, awareness/attitude, and behavioral skills. In other words, mental health professionals can know what to do and how to do it effectively but will not "activate" risk taking in the application of their knowledge and skills without the motivation to do so.

Having synthesized a five-factor metaphor of a three-dimensional pyramid, the pyramid directs and represents one's journey through three stages of self-development. The three stages of self-development are cultural sensitivity, cultural competency, and cultural responsibility (the latter we see as advanced proficiency of multicultural skill, also referred to as cultural responsiveness). Basic cultural sensitivity, the first stage and lower third of the pyramid, involves increasing awareness by acknowledging the value of cultural factors and deconstructing implicit biases associated with beliefs, attitudes, and stereotypes. This awareness serves as a foundation for further development of cultural knowledge and behavioral skill implementation.

Cultural competency, stage two and the midsection of the pyramid, involves continuing one's journey of cultural competency by putting knowledge into practice. With this second stage, basic competency can be achieved through personal growth in all three dimensions; expanded awareness, a shift in attitudes, and practicing culturally relevant behavioral skills in service delivery.

The final stage of development, represented by the top third of the pyramid, is cultural responsibility (responsiveness). It involves living life on a day-to-day basis by embracing an "integrated culturally relative identity." These individuals make multiculturalism a "natural" part of life by a long-term commitment to, and interaction with, pluralistic communities in multiple life domains (beyond their professional life). It is fundamentally based upon the premise that multiculturalism positively promotes acceptance and celebration of oneself as well as others. Hence, cultural responsibility is a concept and a lifestyle which can ultimately help facilitate the interaction of cultures in the Salad and Quilt Models.

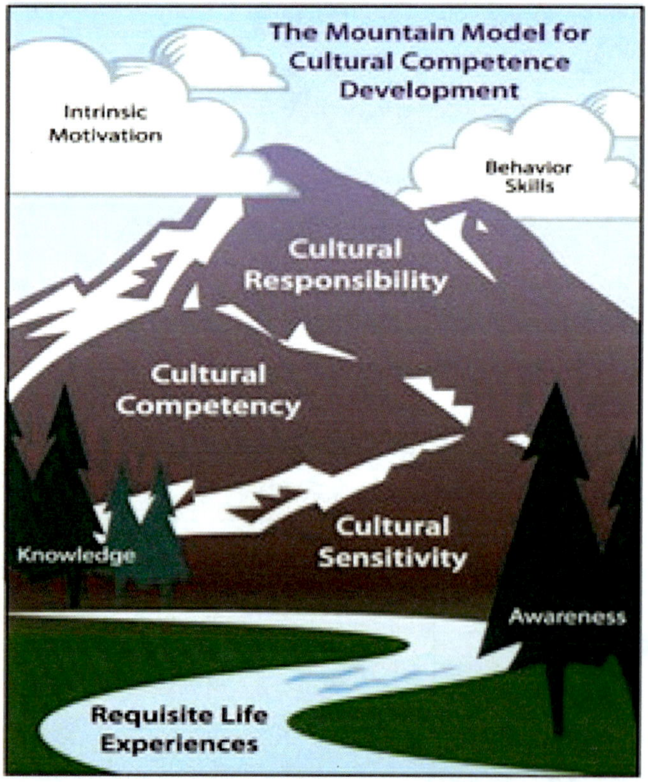

Figure 5. The Mountain Model

The Mountain Model

Another model that may be more relatable in the rural part of America is the Mountain Model (see Figure 5). In the Southern Ohio Appalachia country, where two of the authors have worked, the goal of training health care professionals is to promote transcultural encounters with clients that increase effective communication, enhance patient participation in self-care, and facilitate positive treatment outcomes (Cohen et al., 2013). The Mountain Model becomes a conceptual teaching tool to further advance the goals of transforming rural health care by integrating the extant literature of multiculturalism.

Like the Pyramid Model, the Mountain Model also consists of the five factors in cultural competency and three stages of self-development. Instead of having a pyramid that shapes and directs one's journey through cultural competence development, the Mountain Model spotlights the diversity and complexity of a journey to further illustrate the developmental nature of cultural competency. As we encounter culture experiences, whether in personal or clinical setting, our life experiences expand and even transform our surroundings like the flow of a river. Through the journey, we develop cultural awareness and cultural knowledge, especially by discovering our implicit biases. Our intrinsic motivation and behavior skills are dynamic like clouds because they too can be developed and nourish the journey of our cultural development. Cultural sensitivity, cultural competency, and cultural responsibility form a mountain that represents the curves and edges we can encounter in our interactions with one another. To help us gain competency in clinical assessment and treatment, there are four guiding principles in which the authors believe:

Principle 1. Every member of a health care team, clinical or administrative, has investment in and responsibility for individualized patient-centered care, which includes ensuring that services are delivered in a culturally contextualized and sensitive manner.

Principle 2. Implicit biases are outside a person's awareness and while individuals may be well-intended, their clinical behaviors may have unintentional consequences adverse to patient outcomes. Having an open and nonjudgmental conversation is crucial in overcoming implicit biases.

Principle 3. Race and racial identities are social construct. Consider Dr. Gregory H. Williams, the President of the University of Cincinnati and author of *Life on the Color Line: The True Story of a White Boy Who Discovered He Was Black* (1995). Dr. Williams makes the point that perception is what matters. De-categorizing, de-constructing, and de-mystifying these identities will only help us to build bridges toward a more collaborative clinical relationship with our clients.

Principle 4. Practicing cultural competency does not mean you have to know everything about every culture or even all about the individual culture of a specific patient population you serve. It does, however, mean knowing enough to deliver health care in a way that facilitates a culturally sensitive partnership with the patient (and family), which promotes effective cross-cultural interactions and results in improved health outcomes.

The Arranged-Marriage Model

Another model the authors want to introduce you to is the Arranged-Marriage Model. It was developed in response to the dual demand for a culturally sensitive health care system as well as the increasing need for a relationship-based approach to treatment. This model sometimes occurs in rural America simply because there are no other choices due to fact that more than 80% of psychiatrists and psychologists reside in urban areas, and this distribution has remained essentially unchanged for decades (Cohen et al., 2013). In addition to incorporating MCT in assessment and treatment, there are other circumstantial challenges that many patients face but are not properly addressed. A different approach to the current health care system needs a remodel, and therefore, a marriage between the cultural competency training and the relationship-based care model is the result.

Thus far, we know the value of developing cultural competency using the Pyramid Model and the Mountain Model as frameworks. We also know that cultural competency cannot easily be reduced to a technical skill in which clinicians use a "set of slogans" or "set of dos and don'ts" (Kleinman & Benson, 2006) that often lead to unexpected bad outcomes. Hence, it is beneficial for clinicians to educate themselves about their clients' racial and cultural backgrounds, because using general knowledge without understanding their clients' experiences may damage the therapeutic relationship. We believe this is where the relationship-based approach to assessment and treatment comes into play.

Traditionally, the medical practitioner has been the captain in managing their patient's health care. They are centered and surrounded by supportive staff along with patients. What the authors discovered is that many health care providers feel frustrated and demoralized when there is a lack of participation from their patients. We now know that the financial pressure in health care facilities is to have as many brief billable encounters with patients that can be fit into a workday. These systems do not work well for establishing positive and effective therapeutic relationships, especially when dealing with people from different cultural backgrounds. So, health care organizations are studying what matters most to patients and their families. High quality and safe care come from patients participating in decision-making at their chosen level (Joosten et al., 2008). A relationship-based health care approach was born out of the need for and recognition that patient involvement is crucial in management of various types of illnesses, such as sexual dysfunctions. The purpose is to promote a health care system that can increase effective communication and enhance an alliance-based, patient-centered relationship.

Considering just three relationships for the clinician that are presented in the model, there is the relationship with patients, the relationship with colleagues, and the relationship with self. To develop a trusting relationship with patients, the clinician needs to understand the client's unique life stories and how the client experiences an illness. Of course, it is impossible to accomplish this objective without exploring the client's cultural experiences. In addition, the treatment approach should incorporate all clinical disciplines to establish a team of providers in order to deliver a compassionate quality of care. The relationship-based care of this "Arranged-Marriage" model means team members can contribute and work interdependently to achieve a common purpose which is to improve the client's healthcare experience. With that said, the relationship with colleagues and among providers should be respectful and affirmative of each other's unique scope of practice. At last, all relationships begin with self-care. It means that the healthcare providers possess the knowledge and skills to manage their own stress, articulate personal needs and values, and balance the demands of the job with their physical and emotional health and well-being.

To dive into the Arranged-Marriage Model even further, this Model is particularly important in providing sexual health assessment and treatment. MCT traditionally focuses on increasing health equality and reducing disparities. The goal in sexual health assessment and treatment is to be culturally sensitive and responsive to your client's beliefs, values, and experiences, which in turn increases positive treatment outcomes. The challenge we know is that sex and sexual health is a taboo topic for many individuals and couples (especially ethnic minorities) to discuss with their medical providers. Therefore, developing a safe and trusting relationship is even more crucial before uncovering the discussion of such culturally sensitive topics. A relationship-based approach to health care essentially fosters an environment where clients can take charge of their medical and mental health needs from various experts. This empowerment will also likely increase the client's participation and the openly discussing of taboo topics such as sex. The Arranged-Marriage Model is a holistic approach to sexual health by focusing on understanding a patient's whole experiences, and not a narrow focus on symptoms.

The Arranged-Marriage Model emphasizes more than understanding an individual's cultural experiences; it helps to build a collaborative and fully engaging relationship between the clients and their providers. This approach will also allow mental health providers to move away from the medical practitioner-centered health care delivery system and toward a collaborative process that promotes the patient's ownership of the healing process. This is especially empowering in sexual health treatment where the etiology of sexual dissatisfaction and dysfunction could be a combination of biological, psychological, cultural, and circumstantial factors. In addition, training in the Arranged-Marriage Model frees trainees from being stuck in the mode of thinking that one-on-one psychotherapy for 50 minutes each week is the gold standard. It allows clinicians to incorporate family members, religious practices, and other components of their patients' lives into their service delivery model, as appropriate. Relationships among practitioners also provide the moral, ethical, and spiritual basis for support and self-care.

CULTURAL SENSITIVITY, CULTURAL COMPETENCY, AND CULTURAL RESPONSIBILITY

Historically, psychologists have been encouraged in clinical settings to remain apolitical and to steer away from issues of social justice (Brown, 1997). However, this traditional way of thinking and treating clients can become the reinforcement of racial disparities and inequality. In fact, Dobbins and Skillings (2004) had taken the idea one step further noting that "scientific racism" is still apparent and pervasive in professional fields. Psychology is no longer an isolated profession, and when utilizing various models discussed above, we can no longer act as a bystander of psychological issues resulting from social-cultural-political discord. To say that we are culturally sensitive and culturally competent, the authors believe that we need to follow up with actions. Becoming a culturally responsible clinician can be a controversial debate, but it is a crucial and important discussion in moving our profession forward. Today, psychologists are being asked to advance social justice issues within the context of MCT against all faces of oppression by becoming involved in public policy to increase awareness in social practices (Melton, 2018).

Ali and Lees (2013) believe that psychological practice has been dominated in recent decades by an emphasis on change at the individual level. While it can be effective in targeting psychological problems, it is not addressing racial inequalities, cultural issues, political injustice, and other isms that also impact today's psychological wellness. Thus, there is a need to incorporate interventions on a systemic or societal level to help our clients. Ali and Lees developed Anti-Oppression Advocacy (AOA), which is an approach that integrates social change and therapeutic change to support our clients' personal growth, sense of purpose, and environmental mastery. They argue that self-efficacy can be bolstered if health care systems can work to create positive change beyond the individual level. Through their research, they have found considerable psychological benefits, as well as symptom reduction, from such an approach to treatment.

Advocacy has been defined as "a process of informing and assisting decision makers," and that it requires developing active "citizen psychologists" who have at heart the interest of clients, health care systems, public health, and welfare issues, as well as professional psychology (Lating et al., 2009). With that said, becoming a culturally competent mental health provider also means having ethical obligations and responsibilities to advocate for our clients, and especially those with racial and cultural disadvantages. As many of us are experts in our fields and/or are community leaders, we should actively seek out opportunities to bring psychological and cultural issues into the awareness of health care systems at the organizational and national levels. Sullivan et al. (2007) suggested that a citizen psychologist should engage in grassroots advocacy, political giving, support of lobbying, and teaching advocacy. They consider these efforts as essential and standard to the professional identity and ongoing activities of mental health providers.

Dryjanska (2019) also believes that multicultural and social justice counseling go hand in hand, and they are at the core of our profession. As we mentioned earlier in the Mountain Model, while our cultural experiences expand, we the clinicians become more aware of cultural differences, as well as inequalities and privileges experienced by our clients from various groups. We then have the expertise in identifying mental health issues in social-cultural-political contexts, and we can engage ourselves in social initiates that would improve the current medical and mental health care delivery on a system level. Political actions can include strengthening the voice of psychology at the regulatory level, informing congress about psychology and its relevance to federal policy, advancing opportunities for education and training of psychologists, and advocating for increased support for federally funded psychological research and behavioral and mental health services (Dryjanska, 2019).

Allen and Dodd (2018) believe that avoiding political participation by our profession (intentional or unintentional) does not reduce the moral hazards inherent to political action itself. They specifically discussed current drug prohibition laws, the role that psychologists inevitably played in the political movement, and the negative consequences that impact society today. Psychologists' responsibilities have clearly expanded outside the realm of mere treatment provisions to include social justice advocacy and political action. Of course, we do so in consideration of the General Principles of the Ethics Code (American Psychological Association, 2017a) when we participate in these activities. The authors believe that the field of psychology at large should encourage open discussion and involvement in culturally sensitive, psychologically relevant political movements, such as Black Lives Matter.

Essentially, "multiculturalism is about social justice, cultural democracy, and equity" (Sue et al., 1998, p.197). MCT cannot be done if it does not address social justice and equality on an individual as well as organizational and societal levels. In the past, many psychologists have participated in advocacy efforts that resulted in policy and practice changes within the profession. For example, it was a group of gay and lesbian psychiatrists and psychologists that had advocated for the removal of homosexuality as a diagnostic disorder from the *DSM-III* (Peterson et al., 2020). Psychologists are capable of, and should, address the many psychological, cultural, societal, and political challenges facing our world.

Regarding sexual health and sexual wellness, many individuals who identify as a racial minority often do not seek interventions. One of the challenges is that many minorities feel distrust and anger towards a therapist typically coming from a different racial background. Without discussing these racial and cultural differences, we are really doing a disservice to the community of people who do care about current political movements and want to change the system. In addition, mental health providers are the experts in LGBTQI issues, gender inequality, health disparities, trauma, and violence. We now have ethical obligations and responsibilities in making changes in society.

The intergroup dialogues (IGDs) proposed by Nadal (2017) over the last 20 years are an "organizational and institutional approach to fighting oppression" (p. 936). IGDs are organized discussion groups that have been established across college campuses and federal agencies for building relationships across diverse groups. He suggests that such groups can be built in various work environments (such as hospitals and clinics) as a system approach in responding to health care disparity. This may be partially fitting in our proposed Arranged-Marriage Model in which dialogues about culture and racial identities are strongly encouraged among providers as well as between clinicians and patients.

A recent example of an IGD is the "dialogues on race" discussions conducted at the Wright-Patterson U.S. Air Force Base Medical Center during 2020. Discussion groups were designed to promote ideals of diversity and inclusiveness within military ranks. After a series of IGDs, one young African American female officer put a quote outside her door which said, "White privilege doesn't mean you haven't had a hard life, it just means your skin color is not a factor that made it harder." Soon after, a White doctor added another sign next to it, saying, "This is a great quote and now I get it. Thanks!" Only through these open and nonjudgmental dialogues, clinicians can begin to build trust with our clients, colleagues, and coworkers.

According to Goodman et al. (2018), clinicians can acquire advocacy skills through a variety of clinical work, such as working with clients outside the office and developing competencies in social engagements. Their research points out three core aspects of becoming an advocate: (a) internal grappling (through growing awareness and dialogue with peers and supervisors), (b) building the advocacy relationship (through empathy, integration of instrumental and emotional support, and learning to respect the client's goals), and (c) integrating advocate identity (through acquiring competencies, social justice commitment, and insight into oppression).

In addition to social advocacy, Mallinckrodt et al. (2014) endorsed the Scientist-Practitioner-Advocate Model as essential when it comes to training future mental health providers. The model incorporates social justice advocacy as part of a basic commitment to multicultural competence. Ratts and Ford (2010) have developed the Advocacy Competencies Self-Assessment Survey as a way to measure self-perceived advocacy competence. The American Psychological Association also features advocacy on its homepage (www.apa.org) and promotes advocacy as a way to "have a voice." All these trends show that current direction in the field of psychology confluents with the ideals of cultural responsibility in the Pyramid Model, Mountain Model, and Arranged-Marriage Model. There is a growing expectation that psychologists will also be advocates, and future trainees are becoming more equipped to take on such responsibilities.

DISCUSSION

As the United States becomes increasingly heterogeneous, a key skill for health care providers is to learn to work effectively with clients from various backgrounds. That means to provide culturally sensitive and responsive assessment and treatment. The authors presented the Melting Pot Model, the Salad Model, and the Quilt metaphor to illustrate the diversity represented in the American culture. We want to illuminate the idea that culture is not based on ethnicity alone. It is not black and white, or binary classifications. Culture is not about categories. It is not a set of rules or customs that people inherit from their ancestors. Culture is merely a social construct in which an individual experiences, evaluates, interacts, negotiates, and develops in the relationships and worlds around them. It is a process of continuous modification (Choi, 2002). Culture is multifaceted and encompasses many dimensions of an individual's life ranging from beliefs to everyday expressions.

In the context of multicultural training and development, the authors presented the Pyramid Model, the Mountain Model, and the Arranged-Marriage Model hoping to promote cultural competency development. The models depict the journey of moving along a continuum of cultural competency development – from cultural sensitivity, to cultural competency, and to cultural responsibility. The most essential learning is that humans are not concepts. Professional development is a continuous learning process as fascinating and complex, and parallel, to the incredible cultural diversity of the clients we serve.

The authors also believe that not addressing the topic of implicit biases and systematic racisms in today's culture and political climate would fail the goal of assisting mental health professionals to move toward a greater degree of cultural responsiveness in their practices. We proposed some of the recommendations from current clinical practices for helping clinicians overcome our own biases. We discussed ways of advocating for our clients, as well as making changes related to mental health (and health care in general) on individual, organizational, and societal levels.

Writing this chapter has been a particularly encouraging and empowering experience for the authors to explore our own beliefs and values in our collective multicultural practices. In a very real sense, the collaboration has been our own intergroup discussion (IGD) experience. We want to challenge you in taking on cultural responsibilities by participating in consulting work and advocating for your patients in the field of sexual health and assessment. Beyond the therapy room, we encourage you to engage in discussions about race, ethnicity, and gender with your family, friends, and colleagues.

One means of doing so was accomplished recently by an open-to-the-public self-study group experience on the topic of White privilege. One of the authors teamed-up with Dr. Judith Skillings to lead this personal exploration of what it means to have white skin privilege in 21st century America. Dr. Skillings is a psychologist deeply involved in discussions of race relations and how social as well as economic advantages are given to majority culture members with light skin (she was also referenced earlier in this chapter). For White mental health professionals (especially if they are male), examining the meaning, advantages and process by which White privilege is perpetuated is one of the most overlooked and underutilized methods of personal and professional growth.

Dr. Skillings counsels all therapists to continue to move towards greater levels of cultural competency throughout their professional career. "In the case of White therapists, they need to understand how White privilege mitigates for them in the culture at the expense of non-Whites. Without a basic grasp of this dynamic, the therapist is apt to be as inept as a male therapist who fails to take into account that a female client has probably noticed he is male. If the therapist is not conversant with the ways he has had different opportunities in life than the female client, that the world presents different threats to him than it does to the female client, his ability to be of service will be limited. The same is true for therapists who live with White privilege from cradle to grave who try to be of service to someone who must contend with an entirely different set of stressors on a daily basis, and often these stressors are presented to them by people who look much like the therapist" (J. Skillings. personal communication, May 7, 2020).

There is so much work to be done, but we do feel progress is being made in a positive direction in the field of psychology. It takes shifts in attitude and behavior. It takes the ability to undergo deep introspection into our own belief and value system that colors the lens through which we see the world. It entails our willingness to acknowledge that no matter how good our intentions are, old beliefs from a racist system may still be lingering in our collective and individual unconscious. It requires an understanding that racism and prejudice are not binary, and that good intentions do not always equal antiracism or antiprejudice. Indeed, it is imperative for providers to understand that intentions are secondary to the impact on the recipient.

Professional development is ideally based upon personal growth, which requires a certain level of internal strength to allow ourselves to be vulnerable enough to expose our belief systems to ourselves and to hold ourselves accountable before our clients, colleagues, and community. Despite the enormous responsibility that this chapter ascribes to clinicians, the authors hope that the reader not find this to be a daunting task but more a meaningful process that enriches the therapeutic process and strives toward a more just society. Instead of fearing (or tolerating) differences in other cultures, we can learn, grow, and celebrate differences in sex therapy.

RESOURCES

Ali, A., & Lees, K. E. (2013). The therapist as advocate: Anti-Oppression advocacy in psychological practice. *Journal of Clinical Psychology, 69*, 162-171. doi:10.1002/jclp.21955

Allen, L., & Dodd, C. (2018). Psychologists' responsibility to society: Public policy and the ethics of political action. *Journal of Theoretical and Philosophical Psychology, 38*, 42-53. 10.1037/teo0000077

American Psychiatric Association. (2013). Cultural formulation. *Diagnostic and statistical manual of mental disorders* (5th ed.; pp. 749-759).

American Psychological Association. (2017a). *Ethical principles of psychologists and code of conduct* (2002, amended effective June 1, 2010, and January 1, 2017). https://www.apa.org/ethics/code/ethics-code-2017.pdf

American Psychological Association. (2017b). *Multicultural guidelines: An ecological approach to context, identity, and intersectionality.* Retrieved from: http://www.apa.org/about/policy/multicultural-guidelines.pdf

Barrett, M. (1991). Sexual health education: Can a new vision avoid repetition of past errors. *SIECCAN Journal, 6*(4), 3-15.

Bleiberg, L. (2017, March 10). *10 great places to celebrate the Hindu festival of Holi.* Retrieved from https://www.usatoday.com/story/travel/destinations/10greatplaces/2017/03/10/holi/98946526/

Brown, L. S. (1997). Introducing critical psychology: Values, assumptions, and the status quo. In D. Fox & I. Prilleltensky (Eds.), *Critical psychology: An introduction* (pp. 51-67). Sage.

Choi, H. (2002). Understanding adolescent depression in ethnocultural context. *Advances in Nursing Science, 25*(2), 71-85.

Choi, Y., Tan, K. P., Yasui, M., & Pekelnicky, D. D. (2014). Race-ethnicity and culture in the family and youth outcomes: Test of a path model with Korean American youth and parents. *Race and social problems, 6*(1), 69-84. https://doi.org/10.1007/s12552-014-9111-8

Cohen, J., Peterson, F., Bottoms, J., Resch, W., Burgess, B., & Richards, M. (2013, March). *Healthcare in 21st century Appalachia: The arranged marriage of cultural competency training and relationship-based care approaches.* Southwestern Social Science Association Annual Conference, New Orleans, Louisiana.

Congress, E. (1994). The use of culturagrams to assess and empower culturally diverse families. *Families in Society, 75*, 531-540.

Congress, E. (1997). Using the culturagram to assess and empower culturally diverse families. In E. Congress, *Multicultural perspectives in working with families* (pp. 3-16). Springer Press.

Dobbins, J. E., & Skillings, J. H. (2004). White racism and mental health: Treating the individual racist. In A. Carter (Ed.), *Handbook of racial-cultural psychology and counseling: Training and practice* (pp. 427-446). John Wiley.

Dryjanska, L. (2019). Exploring advocacy in psychology in Italy: Exporting a term from the U.S. to a different cultural context. *Professional Psychology: Research and Practice, 50*(3), 184-194. https://doi.org/10.1037/pro0000227

Goodman, L. A., Wilson, J. M., Helms, J. E., Greenstein, N., & Medzhitova, J. (2018). Becoming an advocate: Processes and outcomes of a relationship-centered advocacy training model. *The Counseling Psychologist, 46*(2), 122-153. https://doi.org/10.1177/0011000018757168

Greenwald, A., McGhee, D., & Schwartz, J. (1998) Measuring individual differences in implicit cognition: The Implicit Association Test. *Journal of Personality and Social Psychology, 74*(6), 1464-1480. https://doi.org/10.1037/0022-3514.74.6.1464

Hays, P. A. (2008). *Addressing cultural complexities in practice: Assessment, diagnosis, and therapy* (2nd ed.). American Psychological Association.

Hua, W. (2019). Exposing our blind spots: How to tackle unconscious bias as a therapist. *Lyra Health.* Retrieved from https://www.lyrahealth.com/blog/unconscious-bias-therapists/

Joosten, E., Merillas, L., Weert, G. H., Sensky, T., van der Staak, C., & Jong, C. (2008). Systematic review of the effects of shared decision-making on patient satisfaction, treatment adherence and health Status. *Psychotherapy and psychosomatics, 77,* 219-226. https://doi.org/10.1159/000126073

Kirwan Institute for the Study of Race and Ethnicity. (2018). Implicit bias training for classroom teachers of English language learner students. Retrieved from https://kirwaninstitute.osu.edu/article/implicit-bias-training-classroom-teachers-english-language-learner-students

Kleinman, A., & Benson, P. (2006). Anthropology in the clinic: The problem of cultural competency and how to fix it. *PLoS medicine, 3*(10), e294. https://doi.org/10.1371/journal.pmed.0030294

Lating, J. M., Barnett, J. E., & Horowitz, M. (2009). Increasing advocacy awareness within professional psychology programs: The 2005 national council of schools and programs of professional psychology self-study. *Training and Education in Professional Psychology, 3*(2), 106-110. https://doi.org/10.1037/a0013662

Lewis, L. J. (2004). Examining sexual health discourses in a racial/ethnic context. *Archives of Sexual Behavior, 33*(3), 223-234.

Mallinckrodt, B., Miles, J. R., & Levy, J. J. (2014). The scientist-practitioner-advocate model: Addressing contemporary training needs for social justice advocacy. *Training and Education in Professional Psychology, 8*(4), 303-311. https://doi.org/10.1037/tep0000045

Melton, M. L. (2018). Ally, activist, advocate: Addressing role complexities for the multiculturally competent psychologist. *Professional Psychology: Research and Practice, 49*(1), 83-89. https://doi.org/10.1037/pro0000175

Nadal, K. L. (2017). "Let's get in formation": On becoming a psychologist–activist in the 21st century. *American Psychologist, 72*(9), 935-946. https://doi.org/10.1037/amp0000212

Nadal, K. L., Griffin, K., Wong, Y., Hamit, S., & Rasmus, M. (2014). The impact of racial microaggressions on mental health: Counseling implications for clients of color. *Journal of Counseling & Development, 92,* 57-92.

Peterson, F., Bley, J., & Frabolta, R., (2020). *The gender revolution & new sexual health: Celebrating unlimited diversity of the human sexuality hypercube.* Cognella Academic Publishing.

Peterson, F., Dobbins, J., Coleman, F., & Razzouk, J. (2007). Culturally competent sex therapy. In L. VandeCreek, F. Peterson, & J. Bley (Eds.), *Innovations in clinical practice: Focus on sexual health* (pp. 245-260). Professional Resource Press.

Ratts, M. J., & Ford, A. (2010). Advocacy competencies self-assessment (ACSA) survey: A tool for measuring advocacy competency. In M. J. Ratts, R. L. Toporek, & J. A. Lewis (Eds.), *ACA advocacy competencies: A social justice framework for counselors* (pp. 21-26). American Counseling Association.

Rogers, C. R. (1961). *On becoming a person.* Houghton Mifflin.

Skillings, J., & Peterson, F. (2022). *Workbook for the self-study exploration of White privilege.* [Unpublished manuscript in preparation for press].

Sue, D. W., Capodilupo, C. M., Torino, G. C., Bucceri, J. M., Holder, A. M. B., Nadal, K. L., & Esquilin, M. (2007). Racial microaggressions in everyday life: Implications for clinical practice. *American Psychologist, 62,* 271-286.

Sue, D. W., Carter, R. T., Casas, J. M., Fouad, N. A., Ivey, A. E., Jensen, M., . . . Vazquez-Nutall, E. (1998). *Multicultural aspects of counseling, Vol. 11. Multicultural counseling competencies: Individual and organizational development.* Sage Publications.

Sullivan, M. J., Newman, R., & Abrahamson, D. J. (2007). The State Leadership Conference: A history and appreciation. *Psychological Services, 4*(2), 123-134. https://doi.org/10.1037/1541-1559.4.2.123

Vera, E. M., & Speight, S. L. (2003). Multicultural competencies, social justice and counseling psychology: Expanding our roles. *The Counseling Psychologist, 31,* 253-272. http://dx.doi.org/10.1177/0011000003031003001

Williams, G. H. (1995). *Life on the color line: The true story of a White boy who discovered he was Black.* Dutton.

Zangwill, I. (1909). *The melting pot.* The MacMillan Company. Retrieved from https://www.gutenberg.org/files/23893/23893-h/23893-h.htm

19

Addressing Sexual Health Concerns of Lesbian, Gay, and Bisexual Clients

Kimberly Fuller

INTRODUCTION

Most clinical training programs incorporate some elements of cultural diversity throughout their training, and minimally introduce the topic of lesbian, gay, bisexual, transgender, and queer plus (LGBTQ+) identities. Codes of ethics for the American Psychological Association (APA), American Counseling Association (ACA), National Association of Social Workers (NASW), and the American Association for Marriage and Family Therapists (AAMFT) each have their own codes requiring clinicians to utilize cultural humility in their work with LGBTQ+ clients or require the thoughtful and intentional referral to an appropriate care provider. Many of these same codes of ethics outlaw conversion therapy as a method for treating sexual identity concerns. Treating LGB clients via sex therapy requires not only a basic foundational knowledge and acceptance of sexual minority identities – there is a necessity to understand the nuances differences within and across LGB relationships.

This chapter provides key knowledge about LGB health to guide providers in the best practices for treating these patients' needs. First, we briefly define LGB identities, both as sexual and romantic identities, and then discuss assessment, diagnosis, and treatment considerations for LGB individuals. Concepts of asexuality and consensual non-monogamy are introduced and explored as they apply to this broader topic. At the end of the chapter a clinical vignette is presented. This case describes the intersection of both sexual disorder work and sexual identity exploration. It does not address the intersectionality of transgender identities as this topic is addressed in detail in Chapter 20 within this text.

Although this chapter uses the language of lesbian, gay, and bisexual to encapsulate the larger community of sexual minority identities, the author acknowledges there are limitations in utilizing the term "LGB" to encapsulate such a broad categorization. This does not capture all the important identities that exist within the categorization of sexual minority identities. The amazing kaleidoscope of diverse sexual identities is addressed in Chapters 7 and 8 within this text as well as *The Gender Revolution & New Sexual Health* (Peterson et al., 2020).

UNDERSTANDING AND DEFINING SEXUAL ORIENTATION

Over the last decade, the language describing LGB identities has evolved to include greater specificity of identities and far greater nuanced differences amongst sexual identities. Concurrently, there has also been a resistance, particularly from younger generations, to utilizing labels to define sexual identities, as the language in existence seems too narrow to reflect the diversity of sexual identity (Adams et al., 2014; Coleman-Fountain, 2014). Sexual identities are most often defined by the gender(s) of their partner(s), which further limits the ways in which people are able to express their identities.

All sexual identities, including both sexual minorities and heterosexual people, can be described as either "allosexual" or "asexual." Someone who is allosexual has sexual desire, which may be specific to one gender (monosexual) or may desire people of multiple genders (plurisexual). Lesbian and gay people typically fall under the categorization of monosexual, while identities such as bisexual, pansexual, and queer would represent some ways people define their plurisexual identities. Someone who is asexual may have no sexual desire towards any person and may even feel repulsed by the idea of sex, regardless of the gender of their partner. Parallel language exists within romantic identities – alloromantic, monoromantic, pluriromantic, and aromantic.

Understanding Sexual Identity

The first attempts at understanding sexual identity was presented in Alfred Kinsey's 1948 book, *Sexual Behavior in the Human Male*, based on a comprehensive study of men's sexual histories (Kinsey et al., 1948). Kinsey measured sexual behavior of men by asking questions regarding their sexual experiences with other men. Those who shared same-gender attraction but did not act upon this attraction were not accounted for in this study. In his original model (The Kinsey Scale), sexual orientation was depicted on a six-point scale, ranging from exclusively heterosexual (0) to exclusively homosexual (6). Someone who identifies as a "3" would be considered equally interested in the same gender as in the "opposite" gender. However, this did not capture the true complexity of sexual orientation and implied that behavior was the only pivotal aspect of identity development.

There have been many alternative models of sexual identity developed over the last 100 years. One of the more comprehensive scales – The Orientation, Behavior, and Identity (OBI) Scale (Satterly & Dyson, 2010) expands the Kinsey Scale to three 6-point scales similar to Kinsey's scale, measuring sexual orientation, sexual behavior, and sexual identity. *Sexual orientation* is defined as sexual attraction or interest. Those whose sexual orientation falls between 0 and 6 might view themselves as attracted to both men and women, though not necessarily equally attracted to both or attracted to men and women in different ways (e.g., sexually or romantically). *Sexual behavior* includes all sex-related behaviors a person would consider engaging in with any gender they are attracted to, regardless of whether they have yet acted on behavioral desires. For example, a person who identifies between 1 and 5 on the sexual behavior scale may have had or would prefer to have sexual experiences with members of two or more genders, although they may be interested in some sexual behaviors more than others. The third scale, *sexual identity*, refers to how the person would actually identify themself and may include utilizing a label to define their identity (e.g., gay, straight, queer, pansexual, etc.). Labels, though, may be unimportant to the individual since sexuality can be more fluid, especially for women (Diamond, 2016). Unfortunately, this scale is still limited in its inclusion of attraction to nonbinary identities.

One of the most accessible methods to demonstrate the complexity of sexual and gender identities is the *Gender Unicorn* (Trans Student Educational Resources, 2015). Though not formally presented as a theoretical model, the Gender Unicorn depicts the differences between sex assigned at birth, gender, gender expression, sexual orientation, and romantic attraction. Most importantly, each of these dimensions are described as being on multiple spectrums, one representing feminine/women/female identities, a second representing masculine/men/male identities, and a third – most often described as Other, which can encapsulate nonbinary and gender nonconforming identities to allow the conceptualization of one's identity to be as broad as possible.

Asexuality

There is a wide gap in the literature on asexual identities, and much of what is written, especially in the sex therapy realm, does not appropriately distinguish between asexuality and hyposexual desire disorder or sexual aversion disorder. While researchers have attempted to explore causal origins of asexuality, including the link between sexual trauma and asexuality, and sexual aversion disorder (Parent & Ferriter, 2018), what exists has not been replicable across multiple studies. Further research is needed to determine whether sexual trauma is a true risk factor for asexuality and this correlation should be viewed with caution. While the low to no desire of one partner may be a challenge for a partner with a higher sex drive, being asexual does not often cause clinical distress, and is not diagnosable. Asexual people still thrive within relationships, but place value on other aspects of the relationship and may still have a deep emotional connection to their partner.

If an individual's asexuality is a presenting concern for any couple you may be working with, therapy should be focused on the discrepancy between both partner's desired levels of sexual frequency or type of sexual interests, without an emphasis on asexuality being the presenting problem. The partner's emphasis on sex and their underlying needs should be equally explored, and potential alternative mechanisms to meeting these needs should be a part of the broader contributing problems. While the low or absent desire may be presented as an issue, the other partner(s) should not be interpreted as devoid of any problematic contributing behaviors.

Romantic Identity – A Deeper View

Romanticism or *romantic identity* describes a person's emotional and romantic attraction to other people, which is distinct from sexual identity. Romantic identities are described similarly to sexual identities, using many of the same root words in their descriptions: hetero-romantic, homo-romantic, bi-romantic, pan-romantic, and a-romantic. Some people's sexual identity and romantic identities align, while for many others, they may experience extraordinarily different sexual and romantic attractions with their partners. For example, a person who is heterosexual may identify as hetero-romantic, feeling both sexually and emotionally attracted to people of the opposite/other gender. People who have differences between their sexual and romantic identities may be more or less inclined in one direction sexually (e.g., gay), but may find themselves more romantically inclined in another direction (e.g., hetero-romantic), and may choose their partners based upon both/either their sexual or romantic attraction. This may be one topic of discussion for sex therapists and their clients, especially if clients report varying levels of sexual interest based on a partner's identity. This can have an impact on sexual desire, which may appear as Hyposexual Desire Disorder, but may be better understood by more appropriately unpacking the individual's sexual and romantic identities.

Key Considerations in Sex Therapy

Although unpacking and defining LGB identities provides cultural insight into working with the LGB population, more often this is minimally emphasized in the work of a sex therapist and their clients. There are several other key considerations for working with this population.

Heteronormative View of Sexual Minorities, Oppression, and Discrimination

Most models of therapy were developed from a heteronormative perspective, and do not explicitly discuss how to apply these modalities differently for LGB people. LGB people often experience *heterosexism*, an automatic assumption that all people are heterosexual and where others speak and act in ways that assume a person is heterosexual. Heteronormativity "not only establishes a heterosexual/homosexual hierarchy, but also creates hierarchies among heterosexualities" (Seidman, p. 40) setting clear boundaries for how masculine and feminine men and women are supposed to present. An awareness of heteronormativity can begin at a young age and can affect if and when LGB adolescents choose to disclose their identities to family members and important others.

Coming Out and the Impact of Family's Rejection

Deeply rooted family or religious narratives can impact how a LGB person sees themselves and their relationships (Hossain & Ferreira, 2019). Heteronormativity, including family pressure or insistence to be straight, can lead to the development of internalized homophobia. Developing the feelings of internalized homophobia has been shown to sometimes prolong coming out (Weber-Gilmore et al., 2011), and has been shown to impact the quality of relationship development for LGB adults (Frost & Meyer, 2009).

Family rejection can also impact the physical and mental health of LGB adolescents (Newcomb et al., 2018). The family's unsupportive response towards their child's sexual identity has been linked to depression, anxiety, substance use, and obesity for youth. Although many clients appearing for sex therapy may be far past their initial coming out stage in life, there may still be residual effects from these responses present within their adulthood and causing problems in their romantic relationships and self-perception.

Homonormativity

Viewing life through a heteronormative lens may lead to the belief that all LGB persons desire the same life milestones and relationship goals as a heterosexual person in their similar socio-demographic. There are great discrepancies amongst LGB adults on whether they would like to achieve these milestones. Some believe that some LGB people want to achieve such goals only to blend into privileged, white, middle-class standards, a phenomenon known as *homonormativity.* This may be true for a subset of the population. For others, marriage and children are personal decisions made with their partner(s). For example, a 2013 poll found only 51% of LGBT adults in the USA were either currently parents or wished to have children someday through donor insemination, surrogacy, fostering, or adoption (Pew Research Center). As we ask LGB couples to share their relational milestones we must be aware of our own bias and values surrounding heteronormative life patterns. We must also be aware of how there may be parallel experiences between LGB and heterosexual couples. LGB people may find themselves in a situation where one partner would like to achieve these milestones, where the other may have no interest. This could be an essential component of your work with sex and relationship therapy.

Therapist Disclosure

Heteronormativity may make disclosing a sexual minority identity to a therapist extremely challenging, particularly when the burden falls on the client to disclose rather than the therapist to ask. The framing of questions is especially important. Since LGB people may not always engage in penetrative intercourse, thoughtful questioning about the type of sex can aid both the sex therapist's understanding of the client's experience and the client's reassurance that they are being understood. Heterosexism expands beyond the interactions of a therapist and their client to a broader societal level. The climate of heterosexism creates a culture that breeds oppression and discrimination, which can be found within our larger society, family systems, and even internally adopted and believed by the client herself. A study from 2020 found that during 2019 to 2020, at least 33% of people experiencing discrimination of some type was based on their LGBTQ+ identity (Center for American Progress, 2020).

Binegativity

Bisexual individuals are more likely to be criticized by both their partners for their sexual orientation, and these levels of criticism come from heterosexual as well as lesbian or gay partners. Bisexual individuals can experience a sense of invisibility and are more often perceived as either gay or straight, which is often dependent upon the optics of their partner's gender in any given situation. Some heterosexual people perceive bisexual people as actually being straight and temporarily "experimenting." These heterosexist biases view individuals who identify as bisexual as more promiscuous and sexual in nature, or even misinterpreted as being interested in open relationships or threesomes. Some gay and lesbian persons view bisexual people as indecisive and/or too scared or closeted to live their true life as gay or lesbian. Occasionally, individuals are unnecessarily concerned that their bisexual partner will be unfaithful to them with a person of another gender. Such discriminatory judgments fall under the umbrella term "binegativity," and despite evidence countering the above misconceptions, they persist. While these narratives are less common than 20 years ago, they still persist.

Consensual Non-monogamy

Approximately 3.5% to 5% of the general population currently practices *consensual non-monogamy* (CNM; Conley et al., 2012), and about 20% of adults have been in a non-monogamous relationship at some point in their life (Haupert et al., 2016). CNM is a broad term used to describe open relationships, polyamory, swinging, and other relationship agreements between a person and more than one partner (Conley et al., 2017). Researchers do not specifically know the number of LGB people who participate in CNM, but bisexual people and people engaging in CNM relationships are subjected to the same stigmatization and misperceptions surrounding fluidity of sexual partners, engaging in risky sexual behaviors, and the increased possibility of having STIs. Further nuances of CNM are discussed in detail in Chapter 21 within this text.

IMPLICATIONS FOR PRACTICE

There are several therapeutic elements to consider when working with LGB people.

Communication

At a baseline, all types of counselors in general, but especially sex therapists, should use affirming and inclusive language during the sexual history assessment. Questions about the client's experiences, partners, relationships, and sexual history should be framed in a way to gain access to the knowledge instead of making assumptions based on their sexual orientation. Sex therapists should also ascertain information regarding gender identity, as some LGB people may also present as more masculine or feminine and still identify with their sex assigned at birth. Their gender expression/presentation does not predicate a specific gender role in their sexual relationship, and assessments should not assume any specific sexual role based on gendered assumptions. Some LGB individuals may also engage in *kink* or other alternative sexual practices, which should be asked about during the sexual history in a neutral nonjudgmental manner.

Assessment

Once a counselor or therapist has established that someone identifies as a sexual minority, more specific questions should be considered during the intake.

Sexual Identity History

The client's sexual identity history should not only include a present assessment of the client's sexual identity, but also an exploration of the client's sexual identity development. During this segment of the sexual history, ask about when a person started to think about their sexual identity and how others have responded as they have disclosed. Experiences of rejection or discrimination by parents can affect relationship development for LGB individuals. It is important to note that any data gathered here may not be clinically relevant to sex therapy treatment. This information alone may help inform how you view the client but may not be one of the contributing factors to their presenting problem.

It can also be helpful to understand both attraction and sexual experiences with partners. Assess how a person has been able to explore their attractions, and any differences of experiences amongst partners, including distinction of experiences related to partner gender(s) and sexual identities.

Sexual Activity/Sexual Behavior

Counselors and sex therapists should recognize that broad definitions of sex go well beyond penile-vaginal intercourse. This is especially true for LGB individuals. Providers should explicitly ask about participating in kink or alternate sexual practices, consent in participating, and safety within the relationship. Counselors should also ask questions regarding non-monogamy of all clients and should be done so in a way that does not perpetuate the aforementioned stereotypes about bisexual individuals.

Due to the increased risk of trauma and interpersonal violence, a thorough trauma and safety history should be conducted. LGB individuals are also more likely to experience homelessness, especially due to parental rejection, which can lead to an increased need to participate in sex work (exchanging sex for pay or a place to stay). This can be especially true for trans women of color.

Sexual Dysfunction

Some LGB people will seek care for sexual dysfunctions unrelated to their sexual identity. The *International Classification of Diseases 11th Revision* (*ICD-11*) and the *Diagnostic and Statistical Manual of Mental Disorders - 5th Edition* (*DSM-5*) are useful resources for diagnosing sexual issues. While the specifiers for "situational vs. chronic" and "lifelong vs. acquired" are important to assess for all sexual dysfunctions across the general population, some of these criteria may be better explained by understanding an individual's sexual and romantic identity. Bisexual clients, for example, may notice fluctuations in sexual desire more related to partner gender, or even exacerbated in circumstances where their partner minimizes or rejects their bisexual identity. The mapping of key life events can be helpful as well. When mapping out a time line for the development of any sexual disorders, the patient should be asked explicitly about coming out (or being outed); family response to sexuality/level of "outness;" partner response to sexual identity; partner response to sexual behaviors; interpersonal violence; transmission of HIV or another STI; and acts of violence, harassment, discrimination, or micro-aggressions. Additionally, if someone reports low sexual desire, the sex therapist should explore further to determine if the client is presenting with Hyposexual Desire Disorder (HSDD) or may in fact be identifying as asexual.

SUMMARY

Counselors working with lesbian, gay, and bisexual clients have important cultural considerations in our work to be inclusive and affirming of our clients' lives and experiences. The background of your client should first be considered, even as far back to family of origin or other cultural groups the client was raised within. Elements of heteronormativity, homophobia/biphobia, and family/societal rejection can impact how clients view themselves and the relationships they have with their partners. Sex therapists must explore these topics in the overall biopsychosocial assessment.

Work should also be centered in the present. Experiences of heteronormativity, homophobia, and binegativity are still ongoing today. These may also be perpetuated within relationships. Individuals seeking treatment may also be seeking to understand more about their romantic and sexual identities, and a primary part of the clinical work may be centered on unpacking identities and their development. As clients may be learning more about their sexual identity, they may need help in deciding how and when to disclose to others. In these circumstances, validation is an essential function of effective sex therapy.

Clinical Vignette

Jessica was referred to a sex therapist due to a lack of sexual desire with her husband, struggling to become aroused during sex, and significant pain in her sexual experiences. The client and her husband have been married for 5 years and have been together for 7 years. The client's goal for therapy was to explore ways to build her connection to her husband and increase her sexual desire. She reported feeling no sexual desire and low to no romantic connection towards her husband. She also reported feeling extremely saddened about the detachment of their relationship.

Throughout the course of her sexual history, Jessica described significant messages from family and faith about their expectations of sex within the context of a relationship. Although sex was almost never discussed between Jessica and her parents, she was heavily involved in church settings throughout middle and high school where they believed that sex should be had only in the context of a marriage, and that relationships should only be between men and women.

As the therapist and Jessica began unpacking her early sexual and romantic experiences, Jessica disclosed early memories of liking women, but not being able to act on the experience out of fear and shame of her sexuality. The client describes moments of feeling relief that she liked men since it meant she had other options, and other times when the women she had feelings for were married or unavailable because it meant she couldn't explore those relationships further. She stated that she now wondered how exploring these feelings with women might have given her an alternative narrative to her sexuality.

Throughout their work together, the therapist and Jessica's explored feelings regarding women throughout her life. Jessica discussed high sexual attraction to women, including sexual fantasies with women. While she acknowledges lower romantic feelings, Jessica acknowledged that this may be due in part to her hesitance to allow exploration of these feelings, and not that the feelings weren't necessarily there. Jessica expressed that the more she talked about her feelings with women, the more anxious she felt, and the more she noticed her feelings towards her husband dissipating. It was clear that the more she was acknowledging about her own sexuality, the more this was affecting her desire and attraction to her husband.

Jessica discussed feeling like she never really had the opportunity to truly explore her relationships with women, and discussed a strong urge to do so, but feelings of internal shame. She mentioned sometimes making light of it with her best friend by making jokes about being gay, but this felt more like a protective front than her true feelings.

It was important for the therapist and Jessica to talk about these feelings as separate yet intertwined aspects of her sexuality. First, unpacking of feelings associated with her husband was necessary. Jessica's husband had mostly been receptive and understanding of her pain response earlier in their marriage, but as time went on, there were times when it was clear that she was in pain during intercourse and the sexual experience didn't stop. She also discussed a general dissipation of their connection. While she enjoyed spending quality time with him doing specific activities, she did not enjoy the intimate elements of their relationship, or feeling often emotionally connected with him, despite his own emotional vulnerability. Jessica acknowledged her own lack of desire to put an effort towards rebuilding this connection. Though saddened to admit it, she was no longer interested in a relationship with him.

At the same time, she felt compelled to explore relationships with women. This work required the client to reflect on her decision to engage in these relationships regardless of any changes that may occur in sexual desire, romantic connection, or sexual pain. Jessica was able to acknowledge that her decision to end her relationship with her husband wasn't dependent upon this new lens towards her own sexuality, or the potentiality of recognizing improvements within any of these areas.

At the time of this writing, Jessica decided to end her marriage. Jessica had also begun exploring romantic and sexual relationships with women. While her pain has not significantly dissipated with intercourse, she does not feel like this was impeding her sexual exploration. She had been finding ways to continue being sexual and recognized that she felt desirous and excited to have sex. She had also been able to build romantic and sexual relationships with women and reported feeling more fulfilled with the types of relationships she had established.

REFERENCES

Adams, J., Braun, V., & McCreanor, T. (2014). Aren't labels for pickle jars, not people? Negotiating identity and community in talk about 'being gay.' *American Journal of Men's Health, 8*(6), 457-469.

Center for American Progress. (2020). *The state of the LGBTQ community in 2020.* https://www.americanprogress.org/issues/lgbtq-rights/reports/2020/10/06/491052/state-lgbtq-community-2020/

Coleman-Fountain, E. (2014). Lesbian and gay youth and the question of labels. *Sexualities, 17*(7), 802-817.

Conley, T. D., Matsick, J. L., Moors, A. C., & Ziegler, A. (2017). Investigation of consensually nonmonogamous relationships: Theories, methods, and new directions. *Perspectives on Psychological Science*, *12*(2), 205-232.

Conley, T. D., Moors, A. C., Matsick, J. L. & Ziegler, A. (2012). The fewer the merrier? Assessing stigma surrounding consensually non-monogamous romantic relationships. *Analyses of Social Issues & Public Policy*, *13*, 1-30.

Diamond, L. M. (2016). Sexual fluidity in male and females. *Current Sexual Health Reports*, *8*(4), 249-256.

Frost, D. M., & Meyer, I. H. (2009). Internalized homophobia and relationship quality among lesbians, gay men, and bisexuals. *Journal of Counseling Psychology, 56*(1), 97-109. https://doi.org/10.1037/a0012844

Haupert, M. L., Gesselman, A. N., Moors, A. C., Fisher, H. E., & Garcia, J. R. (2016). Prevalence of experiences with consensual nonmonogamous relationships: Findings from two national samples of single Americans. *Journal of Sex & Marital Therapy, 43*, 424-440.

Hossain, F., & Ferreira, N. (2019). Impact of social context on the self-concept of gay and lesbian youth: A systematic review. *Global Psychiatry, 2*(1) 51-78. https://doi.org/10.2478/gp-2019-0006

Kinsey, A. C., Pomeroy, W. B., & Martin, C. E. (1948). *Sexual behavior in the human male.* W. B. Saunders Company.

Newcomb, M. E., Feinstein, B. A., Matson, M., Macapagal, K., & Mustanski, B. (2018). "I have no idea what's going on out there:" Parents' perspectives on promoting sexual health in lesbian, gay, bisexual, and transgender adolescents. *Sexuality Research and Social Policy, 15*(2), 111-122.

Parent, M. C., & Ferriter, K. P. (2018). The co-occurrence of asexuality and self-reported post-traumatic stress disorder diagnosis and sexual trauma within the past 12 months among U.S. college students. *Archives of Sexual Behavior, 47,* 1277-1282.

Peterson, F., Bley, J., & Frabotta, R. (2020). *The gender revolution & new sexual health: Celebrating unlimited diversity of the sexuality hypercube.* Cognella Academic Press.

Pew Research Center. (2013). *A survey of LGBT Americans: Attitudes, experiences and values in changing time.* https://www.pewresearch.org/social-trends/2013/06/13/a-survey-of-lgbt-americans/

Satterly, B. A., & Dyson, D. A. (2010). Social work practice with gay, lesbian, bisexual, and transgender persons. In J. Poulin (Ed.), *Collaborative social work: Strengths-based generalist practice* (3rd ed.,). Wadsworth.

Seidman, S. (2005). Polluted homosexual to the normal gay: Changing patterns of sexual regulation in America. In C. Ingraham (Ed.), *Thinking straight: New work in critical heterosexuality studies.* Routledge.

Trans Student Educational Resources. (2015). *The gender unicorn.* http://www.transstudent.org/gender

Weber-Gilmore, G., Rose, S., & Rubinstein, R. (2011). The impact of internalized homophobia on outness for lesbian, gay, and bisexual individuals. *The Professional Counselor: Research and Practice*, *1*(3), 163-175.

20

Addressing Health Concerns of Transgender Clients*

Jill W. Bley, Frederick L. Peterson, Jr., John Skicki, and W. Spencer Vicente

Many readers of this book likely have not directly had contact, lived, or worked closely with individuals who identify as transgender or gender nonconforming and, as such, lack adequate understanding of the daily life and ongoing stressors of these individuals. In this chapter we will review some of the literature related to transgendered individuals. This chapter will also explain how the diagnosis of gender dysphoria is made and the therapeutic best practices therapists should follow when treating these individuals. This chapter will also present the clinical case history of a transgender person who was the client of the first author of this chapter. After discussion of the case, we will relate the story of Gage and Devin, who were interviewed by the second author of this chapter at a "Drag" pageant in Dayton, Ohio.

LITERATURE REVIEW

Since initial publication and distribution of the World Professional Association for Transgender Health (WPATH) *Standards of Care for the Health Of Transsexual, Transgender, and Gender-Nonconforming People* (WPATH, 2012), literature focusing on further refining treatment and practices for care of transgender populations has grown substantially, with two broad focuses of treatment emerging: treatments focused on the transition process and challenges/hurdles that must be overcome to affirm ones gender throughout the lifespan; and treatments focused on evaluation and treatment of diagnoses/disorders among individuals who identify as transgender, with emphasis on a clear distinction between the two patient populations.

While the WPATH recommendations continue to be the gold standard of care for evaluation and treatment of this population during the transition process, further revisions, primarily with regard to multidisciplinary teams and interdisciplinary work and collaboration, have taken center stage in the updated recommendations by Wylie and colleagues (2014). Standards of practice for multidisciplinary teams recommend clear established practices of communication between providers, as well as clear terms of engagement with treatment, rules of confidentiality when communicating care between providers and patient, and clear plans for transfer of care across the lifespan (e.g., adolescence to adulthood, or older-adulthood). Paramount to this continued communication and transition across the lifespan are recommendations of ongoing access and/or engagement as desired with mental health

*Some of the information in this chapter was adapted from a chapter in *The Gender Revolution & New Sexual Health: Celebrating Unlimited Diversity of the Human Sexuality Hypercube* by Peterson, Bley, and Frabotta (2020), Cognella Academic Publishing. Copyright © 2020 by Peterson, Bley, and Frabotta. Adapted with permission.

treatment. However, beyond mental health involvement for diagnosis and ongoing evaluation and treatment of mood changes, clear communication of potential negative behaviors that could impact health and progression of transition should also be communicated between team members. These recommendations include diet compliance, smoking cessation (as these may affect the healing process), and exercise regularity or changes (as these may impact body image or the healing process and mobility postsurgery).

Mental health providers' key roles in this process include initial specialty evaluation and assessment for gender dysphoria diagnosis, as well as exploration of gender identity in the event that there is ongoing distress or confusion regarding the decision-making process for gender affirming procedures. In a slight departure from WPATH original guidelines, while diagnoses of concomitant mental health diagnoses is not grounds for halting gender affirming procedures, recommendations for temporary cessation of these services is advised when a mental health condition is present that may conceivably give rise to a misdiagnosis of gender dysphoria (e.g., complicating diagnoses such as PTSD or personality disorders), or in the event that co-occurring symptoms may reasonably hamper safe or efficacious transitioning.

Literature regarding complicating factors for gender affirming surgery has additionally focused on co-occurrences of learning disabilities and/or Autism Spectrum Disorder (ASD), with some literature suggesting higher prevalence rates of ASD among individuals also receiving treatment for gender dysphoria (Glidden et al., 2016). In these cases, recommendations outlined by WPATH and updates by Wylie and colleagues (2014) indicate that services, particularly mental health services, should be provided by an individual who is competent in the treatment of gender dysphoria and individuals with intellectual or developmental disabilities, in conjunction with close cooperation with an organization able to create an inclusive treatment plan for the individual. The treatment plan should be one that the individual is able to reasonably follow and consent to. As described in the literature and recommendations, no limits should be prescribed based on dual diagnoses of ASD and gender dysphoria (i.e., individuals with ASD are perfectly capable of making medical decisions in most cases). However, as discussed above, some limitations in cases involving intellectual disability may warrant additional evaluation for accommodations that will allow the individual to make medical and care-related decisions.

Following the initial evaluation and decisions regarding the transition process (e.g., hormone therapy, top and/or bottom surgery or other gender affirming surgeries), best practice recommendations include continuity of care throughout the process (pre- and postgender-affirming surgeries) as well as throughout the lifespan (from initial transition through older age), with additional emphasis on collaboration and transparency between mental health providers and other specialties including primary care, endocrinology, mental health, surgery, urology, and others that are involved throughout the lifespan. Interestingly, ongoing research in this area of study, with emphasis on psychotherapy techniques during the transition, have also examined best practices in both individual format and group format.

Of particular interest, in more recent research, are the therapeutic dynamics that predict more positive or negative outcomes and rapport for individual therapy. Mizock and Lundquist (2016) identify several key factors that may adversely impact rapport, specifically, the following "therapeutic missteps":

- Education burdening (patient is burdened with educating the therapist)
- Gender inflation (hyper-focusing on gender concerns to detriment of potential other concerns)
- Gender narrowing (applying restrictive notions of gender onto client)
- Gender avoidance (avoiding discussion of gender issues)

- Gender generalizing (making assumptions that all transgender clients are the same)
- Gender repairing (attempting to "fix" a patients gender)
- Gender pathologizing (treating gender identity as a disorder or pathology)
- Gate-keeping (focusing the psychotherapists role as restricting access to resources)

In contrast, additional compiled literature has generally focused on several "keys to success" that have been most strongly associated with positive clinical outcomes. Strongest factors associated with positive clinical outcomes include strong peer support and mentoring, consistent family support, positive self-image in new social gender role, consistent speech and language therapy, and (along with general positive self-image) facial feminization/masculinization. In each of these recommendations, a strong incentive is placed on continuing mental health care in order to bolster self-confidence, assist the individual in maintaining or altering current relationships, and seeking out available services in a timely manner.

Group therapy best-practices, as described in several more recent literature reviews, have focused on treatment emphasizing creating an affirmative atmosphere in the therapy setting. More specifically, studies focusing on dynamics cultivated by the therapist during session have emphasized the importance of providing an inviting space for patients to discuss, disagree, and converse regarding struggles, norms, and changes throughout the transition process. Additionally, integration of psychoeducation regarding potential difficulties or changes during the transition process (i.e., normalizing concerns such as mood changes, "coming out" to relatives/friends, etc.) as well as specific focus on cognitive coping strategies and affective regulation (e.g., relaxation exercises, breathing retraining, etc.) are associated with the positive establishment of rapport and improvements in coping during the transit.

GENDER DYSPHORIA AND BEST PRACTICES

The WPATH has published a manual that defines the *Standards of Care* (SOC) *for the Health of Transsexual, Transgender, and Gender-Nonconforming People* (2012). The original SOC were published in 1979, and were dubbed the "Benjamin standards of care," due to the fact that Harry Benjamin is the man who advocated for those standards in order to set guidelines for the treatment of people who experience gender nonconformity. WPATH states all who work with and are charged with the care of person's with gender dysphoria understand, "a disorder is a description of something with which a person might struggle, not a description of the person or the person's identity. Thus, transsexual, transgender, and gender-non-conforming individuals are not inherently disordered" (WPATH, 2012, pp. 5-6).

It is important to note here that some of the nomenclature used by WPATH when they published the manual outlining the standards of care in 2012, such as "transsexual" (which is no longer used unless the individual prefers it) or "genital surgery" (which is more appropriately referred to now as "gender affirming" surgery) is outdated and may be offensive to some individuals. However, where we are quoting from the manual, we cannot change the language of the quote without violating the copyright. Therefore, we will use the nomenclature that is currently accepted in this chapter when not quoting another source.*

For many years, even today, people living with gender dysphoria are misunderstood and often severely mistreated by others, including those who are responsible for protecting the rights of all peo-

*At the time of this text's publishing, Version 8 of the *Standards of Care for the Health of Transsexual, Transgender, and Gender-Nonconforming People* (2022) had not been released, but now is available. See Coleman et al. (2022) or visit the WPATH website: https://www.wpath.org/soc8

ple. Due to the treatment many people living with gender dysphoria experience in our culture, they are often reluctant to disclose their true selves or the pain they are going through even to their loved ones. Therefore, it is essential that transgendered individuals can trust they will find helpful, caring, and informed providers when they take the plunge to engage in psychotherapy.

Finding the help transgendered individuals need can be difficult since many health providers are not properly trained in rendering the care they need. They need knowledgeable professionals; a primary physician, a psychiatrist, a psychologist, a team of surgeons, nurses, and social workers who are competent in the unique needs of transgendered individuals.

Criteria for hormone therapy and surgeries are defined by WPATH (2012):

1. Persistent, well-documented gender dysphoria;
2. Capacity to make a fully informed decision and to give consent for treatment;
3. Age of majority in a given country (If younger, follow the SOC for children and adolescents);
4. If significant medical or mental concerns are present, they must be reasonably well controlled. (p. 34)

Since we (the first two authors) are clinical psychologists, we will describe the SOC that should be followed by a clinical psychologist when a person struggling with gender dysphoria comes for help. The first step is to conduct a thorough psychological and social assessment. The assessment is used to aid in understanding the person's diagnosis and their needs. The following are definitions of the three categories of gender dysphoria taken from the WPATH (2012, pp. 96-97) manual:

> Transsexual - Individual who seeks to change or who has changed their primary and/or secondary sex characteristics through feminizing or masculinizing medical interventions (hormones and/or surgery), typically accompanied by a permanent change in gender role. *(As noted previously, this term is outdated.)*
>
> Transgender - A person who crosses or transcends culturally defined categories of gender. The gender identity of transgender people differs to varying degrees from the sex they were assigned at birth (Bockting, 1999).
>
> Gender-nonconforming - an individual whose gender identity, role, or expression differs from what is normative for their assigned sex in a given culture and historical period.

The assessment is also used to determine if there are other psychological or emotional problems that need to be addressed, such as depression and/or anxiety.

The next step is to develop a treatment plan based on the results of the assessment and to begin the treatment. If the assessment indicates the person is suffering from concomitant problems (i.e., problems that have a high probability of resolving themselves as the person is transitioning), it may not be necessary to address those issues immediately. However, if the problem is related to something as debilitating as Posttraumatic Stress Disorder (PTSD), then it will be necessary to treat the PTSD first. PTSD is common among this population for a number of reasons.

Some reasons have to do with childhood abuse. Existing literature suggests that LGBTQ+ populations are disproportionally more likely to experience childhood trauma compared to their heterosexual counterparts, with the mental health symptoms/effects lasting into adulthood (Schnarrs et al., 2019). This research further indicated that variance in mental health disparities (i.e., higher likelihood of mental health diagnoses or poorer scores on mental health measures due to childhood trauma) within the LGBTQ+ community along trans vs. cisgender lines. This suggests that transgender individuals were more likely to experience significant mental health symptoms due to childhood trauma, most commonly as a result of physical abuse and neglect, even in comparison to other LGB samples. Potential explanations posited for this occurrence include that violence was perpetrated against the child and/or adolescent because the people in their family and/or society could not cope with allowing the person to be "different." Lastly, regarding adult trauma, members of the transgender community, particularly transgender Black or Native American women, are significantly more likely to be the victims of violence. They are also the targets of discriminatory practices in work settings, housing availability, and other social settings which can have a lasting impact on mental health and internalized beliefs. Further, transgender women are disproportionately incarcerated at higher rates than other minority groups, with transgender women of color also significantly more likely to be victimized while incarcerated. One study cited 47% of 3,878 respondents experienced victimization while incarcerated (Reisner, 2014; Sonoma, 2019). Another potential reason is due (in males, primarily) to the desire to "prove" their masculinity to themself and others by involving themselves in very dangerous occupations or sports.

Another common problem that the assessment may identify is addiction. Because of the lifelong struggle to come to terms with their gender dysphoria and/or because of the abuse they have had, many have tried to cope through the addictive use of alcohol, drugs, or sex. Therefore, the therapist must be skilled in treating addictions or be able to make a referral to a therapist who has those skills.

If the person is transgender or gender nonconforming, they have probably already been presenting publicly in a variety of ways, perhaps by cross-dressing, participating in drag shows, binding breasts or penis, enhancing breasts, enhancing buttocks, ridding the body of hair, and so forth. The therapist should help the person identify and deal with any behaviors that may be risky, such as anonymous sex and sexual encounters where safe-sex practices are not used.

If the person is transsexual, the treatment is more complex. In order to begin the process of transitioning toward genital surgery, hormone therapy must begin (unless hormones are not clinically indicated for the individual) (WPATH 2012), and if the person has not already done so, they need to acquire a wardrobe and begin presenting to their world as the gender they wish to be. There are a number of changes to the body which occur when hormone therapy begins, and the person needs to be prepared for the changes.

They may want to have electrolysis treatments, breast enhancement (after a minimum of 12 months of hormone therapy so that breast growth has been maximized), or mastectomy, which may include the creation of a male chest, shaving of the Adams apple, and perhaps some facial surgery. The person needs to be fully informed of the medical risks of both feminizing and masculinizing hormone therapies. Therapists should explore issues related to fertility and sexual functioning before hormone therapy begins, and encourage the person to discuss these issues with their intimate partner, if they are in an intimate relationship. The changes they will go through might have a negative effect on the relationship.

In order to proceed to the gender affirming surgery, the person must be able to provide the surgeon with two referrals from two health care providers. Usually, one letter must come from a medical provider and the other from a mental health provider. The reason these letters are required is because up to this point the transition is reversible. One can quit taking the hormones and return to life as it was, if that is their choice. Surgeries that remove the gonads and reconstruct the genitals are not reversible.

If the patient is only going to have surgery to remove the uterus, ovaries, or the testicles, the four criteria listed on page 348 must be met along with the following:

A. Twelve continuous months of hormone therapy as appropriate to the patient's gender goals (unless hormones are not clinically indicated for the individual).

B. If the person is going to have genital reconstruction surgery, the first 4 criteria must be met along with 2 continuous months of living in a gender role that is congruent with their gender identity.

Although it is not an explicit criterion, most recommend that the patient has regular scheduled visits with a mental health or other medical professional. Rationalization for this recommendation is based on previous literature indicating that hormone therapy and other procedures that are part of the masculinization or feminization process may result in fluctuations in mood and temperament. Therapy during this time is geared towards normalization of experiences and management of resulting changes in mood. Of course, the information that has been presented here is only an overview of the treatment process for gender dysphoria. There is much more that providers must know in order to deliver quality, professional, and ethical services for this population.

Now we are going to tell you the story of a gender dysphoria case, treated by one of the authors of this book. The names and identifying personal information have been changed or altered in order to protect the privacy of this remarkable person's journey. Her story is told in this book with her permission.

SUCCESS STORY – ALEX

When Alex came to my office for the first appointment he was rather shy. However, as our conversation progressed he began to relax and was able to provide information that was asked of him. He was clear he was very determined and confident about the process that laid ahead of him. He stated:

> I want surgery to feel complete. I wore the macho mask for years. I have never dressed as a woman but I do wear a bra for support. I don't know how I will handle some aspects of this, such as my business. I realize this will be a long and difficult road ahead of me, but I want to do it!

His determination was contagious. From that initial encounter until the end of the time that we met, I knew that he would make the journey to transition and would thrive afterward. He had already told me how many friends he had who were supporting him. In fact, two of those friends did the research to help him find the physician he had been seeing, who then referred him to me for the psychological part of his treatment journey. He had a very kind, gentle, warm, and welcoming aura. Miraculously, he had a wife who was very supportive of his transition. That didn't happen overnight, but his patience and kindness and strong need for the change won her over to the point that she even helped him get a wardrobe during the transitioning.

Developmental History and Evaluation

Alex was referred by his psychiatrist for a psychological evaluation and psychotherapy. At intake he said that he wanted treatment because he was told that in order to have a sex change operation, he had to see a psychiatrist and a psychologist to "make sure I wasn't crazy." He had already contacted three facilities that provided the genital reconstructive surgery (GRS) and knew what was going to be expected of him. He stated that he was married and that his wife knew about his desire to be a woman and that she was supportive of him doing so. He said that he married a girl he dated in high school. "I tried the gay routine in High School but that wasn't me. I had sex with several women while picturing myself as a woman." He and his wife had never had sex because neither one of them really wanted to. However, they were very affectionate toward one another.

He said that his mother was also aware of his intentions and that she was supportive. He had not told his father and had asked his mother not to tell him yet because he was sure that his father would be angry and verbally abusive toward him if he knew. His father had been verbally and physically abusive toward him during most of his childhood, but not toward his 5 siblings. His father ridiculed his "sissy" behavior and tried to "make a man" out of him by severely beating him for even small transgressions. He said that he was locked in closets many times by his father. His mother had no authority in the home and appeared helpless to protect him. On occasion he was able to stay with his grandparents who were "extremely good to me." He also reported that he was raped by a female babysitter.

His greatest solace during his childhood was to withdraw into music which he loved to listen to and to play. He said that he could play just about any instrument without taking lessons, just by listening to someone else play.

During the treatment he revealed that from a very young age, probably as early as 3 or 4, he had felt that he was more like his sisters than his brothers. He wanted to play with his sisters, get the same kind of toys for holiday gifts, and he desperately wanted to wear dresses. His first memory of a severe beating from his father was at about age 4 when his father found him wearing his sister's clothes. He recalled many times during preadolescence daydreaming about being a girl and drawing pictures of himself in girls' clothing. He was terrified of his father's anger about his desire to wear girls' clothes, so he contented himself to make drawings and hide the drawings.

By adolescence he had endured so much pain and humiliation about his "girly" behaviors that he was determined to make himself into the strong male that his father, siblings, and friends seemed to need him to be. He decided to join the military as soon as he was old enough because he kept hearing how the military could make you a man. At age 17 he enlisted in the navy and trained as a navy seal. He said that he became a "skilled warrior" and served his country well in Vietnam. Alex was often part of a team that went into enemy territory, sometimes to assassinate a target and other times on rescue missions. He received many honors for his valor. However, his military experiences caused him to have a serious emotional breakdown that required a brief hospitalization.

After the military, he married a woman with whom he had a friendship since he was in the fourth grade. He got a job as a police officer in a small town. He stated that he was a good "peace officer" but realized that his efforts to make everyone believe that he had finally become a man were making him more and more depressed and withdrawn. He quit his job and opened a small business making and selling musical instruments in a large city. He decided that he needed to be in a community where he might find support for and more acceptance of his desire to be a female.

He confided his concerns to some very close friends. They were understanding and empathic. He was amazed that someone understood him. He found a psychiatrist who was willing and able to treat his depression but was not knowledgeable about the treatment of his gender issues. She referred him for the psychological evaluation and treatment. His description of his history indicated a diagnosis of Gender Dysphoria, transsexual type who was sexually attracted to females. In fact, he stated that he thought that he was probably a lesbian and that "will work well for me and my wife, if she is a lesbian too." He thought that she might have those tendencies but had never "had the nerve to ask her."

The psychological testing indicated that he had no serious pathology; that he was depressed and anxious, that he had a mild to moderate level of Posttraumatic Stress Disorder (PTSD), and that he had many preferences that are typically viewed as feminine. He agreed to work in the therapy to resolve his childhood abuse issues and the traumatic aftermath of his navy seal experiences, which included having to kill people, including a woman, during a clandestine attack to rescue some prisoners.

He disclosed how killing people had made him feel intense guilt and shame. He worried during that time that he was becoming like his father. He tried to console himself by reminding himself that he was following orders and had chosen to be a part of the military, therefore, he was only doing his duty. He disclosed that after discharge he experienced terrifying, violent nightmares in which he was carrying out a military mission and everyone on the seal team, including himself, began to scream and yell and kill anyone they saw. All of their faces looked exactly like his father's face and then he would see his reflection in a puddle, or a mirror, or a pond (depending on the dream) and see that he too looked like his father. He would wake screaming and sobbing and needing his wife to hold and comfort him so that he could calm.

Treatment

After consultation with his psychiatrist and his physician, during which a collaborative treatment plan was developed, the treatment began. The first focus of the treatment was on resolving the childhood abuse issues. He was very motivated. He was willing to have two treatment sessions per week. Eye Movement Desensitization Reprocessing (EMDR; this treatment technique is discussed in Chapters 14 and 17) was the primary mode of treatment. He eventually was not only able to talk about his childhood without crying or feeling a lot of anger, but also was eager to go to his childhood home and tell his father his plans to become a woman.

The confrontation with his father went much better than he expected. He also reported that his siblings were somewhat okay with it too because his mother had talked with each one and asked them to support him. After resolving those family concerns, he was ready to work on the navy seal traumas. That work was a little more difficult for him to deal with than the childhood traumas because he felt much grief and sorrow that his attempts to be a "man" led him to kill people (this is a type of PTSD that has been called "moral stress syndrome").

The client's wife attended some of the therapy sessions. She was a very quiet, withdrawn woman who rarely made eye contact. She was very attached to her spouse and was supportive and encouraging toward him. She stated that she was eager to help him have the surgery he wanted because she knew he would be happier as a woman. She admitted that she had fears about the changes he was making, but she felt confident that the relationship could accommodate the changes and survive.

The only issues that she had with her spouse were that he didn't do as much around the house as she wanted him to do and that she would like to work part-time. She felt he did not make enough money since he started his new business and much of what he made was being saved to pay for his surgery. They both felt that the money issue would improve as soon as they saved enough for the surgery.

At this point in the treatment, I wrote a letter to the client's physician recommending him to begin hormone treatment. He was started on estrogen and an antiandrogenic medication. He also sought out and underwent electrolysis to remove facial hair and cosmetic surgeries to enhance his breasts and remove fatty tissue. As soon as the breast enhancement surgery was completed he began to dress as a woman and assume a female identity. The client emerged as a rather attractive middle-aged woman. Her spouse was complimentary of her and stated that she was a little jealous of her good looks. They used most of their therapy time talking about and figuring out how to deal with the reactions of their friends, families, and neighbors to the gender change.

After about 8 months living as a woman, the client selected a surgical facility and made plans to have the complete gender reassignment surgery. Those of us on the treatment team (her psychiatrist, her physician, and I) all wrote letters of recommendation to the surgeon and mental health professional at the surgery facility. Five months after first applying for the surgery she was admitted to the facility and the surgery was performed. The surgery and the recovery period went well. The client and her spouse remained in treatment for 6 months postsurgery. The general theme of the therapy during those final months was to help the couple adjust to their new relationship. The client's spouse expressed that she was finding herself to be more and more sexually attracted to her partner. At the final session they were experimenting with sexual touching. They were both enjoying it and feeling that the surgery had helped both of them learn to express their lesbian feelings.

Ten years after the treatment was completed, I telephoned Alex. She stated that she was still doing well as far as the gender issues were concerned. However, she was grieving the loss of her wife, who had died the previous summer of cancer and didn't feel that she could talk about it at that time. Later she wrote this to me:

> I will tell you that my wife and I had a GREAT (sic) life together. We were as one. We loved each other so very much. We hugged and kissed every day and told each other, "love you." We never liked being apart even for 1 day. We were together since fourth grade.
>
> Our great love and life never changed through the years. We always worked together and helped each other on everything. Our lives were always a success. My business was always good, and she retired from teaching after 30 years. Through sickness and health, we were always as one. I held her hand and hugged her until the end, telling her I loved her.
>
> Dr B. that is about all I can say. What the future holds is unknown for now. I will work in my shop and keep working at our county airport, where I have been an administrator for many years, and see what happens.
>
> My wife was a great quilter, and very popular, so I set up a large Memorial Quilt Library in her name at our county airport where her quilt club and friends meet. Hope this little information helps you. I just don't feel like talking right now . . . I miss her.

I was so touched by her love story. How tender, sweet, and rare is that!

Case Discussion

Of course, this case is not the usual way in which these cases unfold. I choose to tell about this client because it was a case that illustrates a motivated, relatively mentally healthy individual who was willing to accept and follow a treatment plan that conforms with the Standards of Care as outlined by the Harry Benjamin International Gender Dysphoria Association and WPATH. Another element of this case that made it a therapist's dream case was that she had a partner who was not only supportive, but who also benefited from the gender change. Plus, they were a couple who truly, dearly loved one another.

Many of the people who present with a desire to change their gender have been so frustrated by the lack of knowledge, understanding, and acceptance of their issues that they do not want to follow a treatment plan. They may perceive the plan as just another obstacle to getting what they so desperately need. Many others are very ambivalent about what they want to do because of their fears (real and imagined) of what will happen to them in their marriages, their jobs, their extended families, and their communities when people find out about their "secret."

With these cases the first task of therapy is to confront and deal with these issues. The person who is eager to "get it done" has to be able to see the value in taking the time necessary to ensure long-term emotional, psychological health before they have the surgery. The person who is ambivalent because of the perceived repercussions the gender change would have on their life needs to work to resolve those fears by considering all of the options and the consequences of those options.

Multiple forces converge on the therapist who is presented with the challenge and opportunity of working with a client who identifies as lesbian, gay, bisexual, or transgender and who is seeking help with a sexual health concern. Those forces include attitudes, knowledge, and values as they relate to sexual expression, gender expression, relationships, and social context.

The following section presents to the reader the story of two men and their journey toward sexual liberation and sexual health. Their story is included here as an example of the diversity of human sexuality. Their story makes clear how important it is for mental health professionals to educate themselves about the sexual hypercube which is described at length in *The Gender Revolution & New Sexual Health: Celebrating Unlimited Diversity of the Human Sexuality Hypercube* (Peterson et al., 2020). The human sexuality hypercube is also described in Chapter 8 of this book in a briefer form.

GAGE AND DEVIN'S JOURNEY

"I love you too" Devin says into his smart phone as he responds to another pageant contestant in between bites of food. It is the first night of a week-long pageant so Devin and Gage are really too busy to meet with me. But like Gage says, "We have to eat." So there we are, the three of us at the Siam Pad Thai restaurant trying to eat dinner, me trying to conduct an interview, and the two of them taking calls from people freaking out because of hotel room changes, substituting judges, and problems with videographing Divas during the first night's evening wear. Gage looks right at me with a wry smile and adds, "It isn't pageant week if something isn't f-up."

"Holy wow! This is amazing yum-yum. What is this called again?" I declared. "It's called Thai tea," Devin explains. It was sweet, cool, and delicious. And very needed for anyone like me who can't even eat food with #1 rating on the 1 to 4 spicy range. A video message comes in from another contestant who is just wanting to send his love and inform Devin that he has arrived in Dayton for the pageant. "This is a crazy business" Gage says with animation. One of their staff then calls talking about last-minute changes to the gifts and awards they get for the judges and staff. Gage explains they have seven judges, four officials, two contestant liaisons, and one all-purpose runner-utility man.

The reason all these people are needed and that the pageant lasts all week is that 70 individuals from across the country qualified to compete. Each of them participated in an evening wear competition, talent competition, and interview. Some came to compete in the Miss USofA Diva pageant, some for the Mister USofA MI (Male Illusionist) pageant, and the rest for the USofA MI Classic pageant. Gage explained that the "MI Classic" competition is for the more senior contestants that have been around awhile (33 years or older). "Like me," he says. Gage has been competing and transitioning for well over a decade. Having served as a mentor to many contestants, he humbly accepts an unofficial title of the "Godfather of Drag." "For the record," he adds, "all the contestants have to be assigned as a female at birth (perceived as baby girls), so they identify as either women or trans-men. They compete *with* each other as opposed to against each other. It's a Brotherhood."

Sitting within this whirlwind of food, conversation, and video calls, I wondered how these two remarkable individuals got to where they are. Among the many stories of fluid expressions of sex and gender (not only in this book but anywhere), there are only a few which cover such a wide spectrum of gender experience within one person as the story you are about to read. It begins with two young girls and ends with two men named Devin and Gage who are nationally known performers and national pageant producers in the world of male impersonators. Gage has been at his journey of transition a bit longer and sees himself as more at the masculine end of the traditional gender binary. Devin sees himself as more gender fluid and just being himself, Devin. They were gracious enough to share their stories in an effort to help promote understanding of people who are gender nonconforming, gender fluid, and otherwise considered transgender individuals.

This chapter continues with Gage's story (as he is older and been transitioning longer), then Devin's story, and how the two found each other, to live and love each other in one of the most unique sets of lives described in this book. To keep it easier to follow these stories (gender-wise) and use their preferred pronouns – all personal references used will be masculine, regardless of how Gage and Devin have been viewed by society in the past. In addition, this short chapter is a very brief description of a long and detailed history which is fascinating and beyond the scope of this chapter.

Gage's Story

Gage was born as a female in Jacksonville, Florida with a family that was full of military men – father, uncles, and grandfather. In other words, there was a lot of macho while Gage grew up as a girl and he always remembers wanting to join the military. During his childhood, he went back and forth in terms of gender-conforming. At times, he followed the socially sanctioned norms as a little girl and played typical activities as a girl. In eighth grade, though, there was a small rebellion. Gage decided to cut off all his hair to get negative attention. He liked the negative reactions of being thought of as a boy, but then later decided to grow it long again and conform to female expectations once the bullying got worse. As a teenager, he eventually felt compelled by social convention and dated boys.

Through typical sexual exploration, Gage eventually got pregnant and birthed a son at age 17. He and the father lived together as teenage parents for approximately 2 years but could not make it as a family. As a teenager, Gage was not ready for parenthood or marriage, and the parents never wed. Gage lost custody because he was living as a lesbian, had cut his hair short again, and was living with a Jamaican girlfriend in Virginia. The father was living in a small Jim Crow town in Florida. Gage even married a good friend of his (a man) in an attempt to avoid losing custody of his son (he was also planning to join the service and it was a problem being a single parent in the military). Although he loved his son, a court order eventually gave custody of the boy to the father when his son was about 5 years old. The marriage between Gage and his friend was for practical purposes and ended a year after they wed.

Gage continued to struggle with women's roles, and particularly his role, in a society that limits women's participation. Gage felt very similar to a popular song sung by Gwen Stefani (of No Doubt) which says, "Don't you think I know exactly where I stand, this world is forcing me to hold your hand . . . Cause I'm just a girl, I'd rather not be."

However, Gage was strong, brave, and wanted to break social expectations of women, so he joined the military. This was something that was still uncommon in the 1990s. He always knew something was "out of sync" with how he saw himself – already living as a lesbian but knowing there was more in terms of his growing identity as a male. He joined the U.S. Army (1996-1999) and was assigned to a detail of mortuary affairs. This was quite traumatic for Gage in terms of dealing with death, serving as a technician assistant during autopsies, and getting bodies back to their families for burial. Not only did Gage feel compelled to serve his country 4 years in the U.S. Army but, remarkably, he then joined the U.S. Navy!

This was even more uncommon; Gage was an aviation ordnanceman, and he demonstrated not only a deep commitment to country but also a sense of adventure and wanted to be in male-dominated environments. While Gage felt more comfortable in nonconventional situations, he was not happy as he still had sexist expectations placed on him as an active duty woman. The problem was that he was seen as a woman and he did not feel like a woman, did not want to be a woman, and wanted to correct the problem of wrong anatomy. Gage started to play with his gender during his Navy service, spending a year getting more masculine. He was the first of female Navy personnel to serve as a line coach on a firing range helping sailors to improve their firearm skills. However, the stresses of his job in the Army (which gave him PTSD) in combination with the stress of gender dysphoria resulted in a medical discharge for Gage. Although Gage loved military life and it never stressed him out, his job of dead bodies did. His 3 years of service in the US Navy ended in 2003.

Finished with the military? No way! Unbelievably, Gage could not let go of military life even after a medical discharge! What a guy! He could not resist the opportunity of joining the U.S. Army Reserve and serving as a military police (MP) officer. He started to bind his breasts down and doing all the required physical training (PT) to the male standards. After 2 more years of service, Gage finally ended his military career (in 2005) after figuring out what he wanted to do next.

After his final military year, Gage wanted to start gender-specific treatment. Although he felt like a man, he was still a bit unsure of social reaction to his commitment to fully transition until a key event occurred that propelled him further on his gender-transition journey. While he was surrounded by a very strong military family, Gage's experience of family support for sexual reassignment was patchy and less than enthusiastic. One day while Gage was at a family gathering, his man-among-men grandfather took him aside and in front of all to hear, told Gage that he loved him and whatever Gage wanted to do with his life, his grandfather would support him. It was this show of strength and love between them that helped Gage feel he had all he needed to move forward with his plan. He knew if his grandfather threw his support behind him, then many others would as well or at least try. And those who would not, Gage knew he would have to leave behind.

After leaving the military, Gage really started to ramp up his gender transition by exploring the world of drag kings, where women dress as males and usually impersonate famous male singers (like Elvis). New to the world of male illusionists, Gage met many new friends and found creative expression extremely rewarding. It was freedom to be himself and Gage thrived. Gage excelled at his performances and developed a highly celebrated performance impersonating country star Tim McGraw. He soon started to tour nationally winning many titles, appearing regularly on television, and being covered in numerous publications (visit his website for details: https://gunnergatlyn.wixsite.com/master-mi/gage-gatlyn).

Yet Gage still struggled with his gender and eventually came to the conclusion he was a transgender man. Gage began hormonal transition and he began to exhibit secondary male characteristics with his voice changing to a more masculine tone, increased facial hair, a more muscular body, and had a double mastectomy and a hysterectomy. Gage's goal was to successfully transition to male, and after completing the necessary legal paperwork, Gage had his social security card, driver's license designation, passport, and legal name all changed.

Enter Devin

In 2005, Gage met Devin Dame – another male illusionist at a drag king pageant. Gage became a mentor to Devin for performance and they become dear friends as well as co-performers. They were friends for about 3 years until eventually they found themselves in a romantic relationship. As their relationship progressed, they became lovers and began to live together. Gage's role as mentor transitioned to husband. Gage was then legally recognized as a man and then asked Devin to marry him. This was before same-sex partners were legally allowed to marry but it didn't matter because Gage was a man in what was seen as a heterosexual relationship. Gage and Devin became husband and wife and enjoyed a marriage as a heterosexual couple. So the transformation of Gage (as perceived by the world) included being a heterosexual mother, to a lesbian woman, and then transitioning to a man in a heterosexual relationship. So let's pause again for a moment to appreciate the sexual fluidity going on here. Using different terms, let's take stock of the transitions with this individual named Gage. At his first transition, he changed from a heterosexual wife and mother to lesbian woman and then transitioned to a heterosexual husband.

Let's introduce Devin's background, which includes being born in a small town of Woodsfield, Ohio but later was raised in Middletown, Ohio. He comes from a good family with positive support for him as a young girl. He was active in sports and describes his childhood in very positive terms. Devin knew early on in his childhood that he was attracted to other girls and identified early as being lesbian. He did share that he dated guys for a short while as a teenager but when he was age 18, came out to others as a lesbian. For the most part, Devin sees his family as supportive of his gender-nonconforming behavior, gender fluidity, and transitioning to male more recently.

As he always considered himself gender nonconforming, Devin always wanted to join the military. At age 20, he joined the U.S. Army and was first assigned to duty in heavy construction but later transferred to operations when our country was under attack on 9-11. He had to keep track of several hundred soldiers at all times, knowing exactly where they were and what they could do for the defense of our country. Devin was injured during his service in the Army and medically discharged in 2003. After separation from the service, Devin started working in the family business. His confidence was greatly increased when he underwent significant breast reduction surgery in 2012. Recently, Devin had a cancer scare and had a full double mastectomy, which is protective of his health but also consistent with his moving further forward toward masculinity.

In retrospect, Devin considers his drag king/male illusionist experience as a catalyst influence moving him more toward male identity, but he always saw himself as gender divergent. Devin has been with Gage for 8 years and they have been married the last 4. Devin was seen as the woman in the beginning of the relationship, but not anymore. As sexually fluid as this story reflects, it does not end here. Devin continues to transition to male, thus making Gage and Devin a homosexual couple as two gay men. Said differently, as Devin fully transitions hormonally to male status, the couple will have been on a journey that started as a lesbian couple, then changed to a heterosexual couple, and is now changing to a gay man couple.

Gage and Devin are now advocates and activists in gender and trans equality, run a transgender support group, and have become LGBTQ community leaders in the greater Dayton area as well as being known nationally. They lead a transgender support group in Dayton and have sponsored similar groups in other states. The mission of Gage and Devin's groups are to raise awareness, provide education, and act as an outlet for transgender, nonconforming gender-identity individuals, and their allies. Through their work, they also provide safe meeting places, social functions, newsletters, and referrals to LGBTQ-friendly professionals.

Their story is very unusual to say the least, but perfectly demonstrates the fluidity of sexual identity and diversity of human sexual expression. By physical appearances as male or female at birth, society tries to keep us in designated boxes with absolute binary labels. *It is a common function of the human brain – to generalize and oversimplify a very complex world.* As human beings, we do this to struggle to understand a very complex world but in the process confuse ourselves by missing many important nuances of gender variations, which are natural and frequently occurring. The resiliency of the human spirit and need to live authentically prove that there is an unlimited diversity to human sexual expression.

Today, society's traditional gender expectations can no longer keep an individual's inner identity from emerging. An individual's mind, heart, and soul need authentic expression for balance and happiness. Each of us, transgender and cisgender, can strive to become more authentic and comfortable with expressing our true selves. Gage and Devin are exceptional examples of this process.

Back to the Pageants

Three national pageants were produced by Gatlyn Dame Group in Dayton, Ohio during March 5-12, 2017. I went downtown to check out Gage and Devin's handiwork. It was about midnight Saturday evening at Club Masque and the place was packed. The stage was lit up with an amazing digital backdrop accompanied by equally dazzling light show and sound system. Several folks, including Devin and Gage, walked around wearing red and white college-style letterman jackets with "MI" on the front like they were wearing their school's initials. A skinny and handsome half-naked waiter came up to me and offered refreshment with a tray of shots. I passed on the alcohol but appreciated the tattoo displayed prominently across his chest: Live life with courage and conquer death. Right behind him strutted a 300-pound, seven-and-a-half-foot-tall drag queen (including her pumps and bouffant style wig). Of course, drags shows of both king and queen varieties bring out the best of us with fun, interestingly diverse crowds!

The divas and male illusionists were competing with each other for the crowns of Miss USofA Diva 2017, Mister USofA MI 2017, and Mister USofA MI Classic 2017. The coveted jewel crowns for the top competitors were prominently displayed upon the top of a red satin cloth above an elevated part of the bar. The contestants performed their hearts out for the judges and the audience was very appreciative of the diverse styles of performances, from the Beyoncé impersonator and way-big-boy cowboy to the duets and the dance ensemble composed of the male illusionist and several back-up singer/dancers. Apologies to country singer Luke Bryan, but I will never think of his song "Country Girl Shake it for Me" the same after the MI version was performed that Saturday night. To see lists of the participants and pictures of the crown winners, please check out www.MisterUSofAMI.org and www.MissUSofADIVA.org.

Regarding the son that Gage had many years ago, both Gage and Devin have a positive relationship with him. Several years back, a young man contacted Gage over social media asking, "Do I know you?" Gage responded, "You should, I'm your mother." That was when Gage's son was 14 years old. Over a period of reconnecting, the son came to live with Devin and Gage for about 3 years. During that time, he earned a degree from a community college and the two got to know each other again as son and parent. The young man then returned to Florida, is gainfully employed, and is happy living with his girlfriend.

Besides managing drag king/male illusionist pageants across the country, Devin and Gage stay busy being spokespersons for the LGBTQ communities, conducting LGBTQ-affirming groups, and educating medical students and other healthcare professionals. When they are not serving as advocates or running competitions, they enjoy their lives together in Dayton with their seven dogs, five cats, a turtle, and a bearded dragon!

Standards of ethical practice require knowledge and understanding of the particular issues which impact the lives of the LGBTQA (Lesbian, Gay, Bisexual, Transgender, Queer, Asexual) community (APA, 2015). Many issues addressed in sex therapy remain the same regardless of the orientation or gender identity of the client. However, there are some differences which exist including frequency of certain diagnoses, sexual identity issues, variety of sexual practices (Nichols, 2000), and the effects of oppression on sexual identity. As a caveat, the danger with considering the differences between sex therapy with heterosexual clients and sex therapy with LGBTQA clients is that it may implicitly communicate that heterosexual sexuality is normative and other forms of sexual and gender expression must be understood in relation to heterosexuality.

In contrast to this notion, this book attempts to elucidate those issues which are specific to LGBTQA persons with the assumption that the reader simply may be less familiar with them, not with the assumption that they are defined by points of departure from some heterosexual norm.

REFERENCES

American Psychological Association (APA). (2015). Guidelines for psychological practice with transgender and gender nonconforming people. *American Psychologist, 70,* 832-864.

Austin, A., & Craig, S. L. (2015). Transgender affirmative cognitive behavioral therapy: Clinical considerations and applications. *Professional Psychology: Research and Practice, 46*(1), 21.

Benjamin, H. (1966). *The transsexual phenomenon.* Julian Press.

Bockting, W. O. (1999). From construction to context: Gender through the eyes of the transgendered. *Siecus Report, 28*(1), 3-7.

Bockting, W. O., Knudson, G., & Goldberg, J. M. (2006). Counseling and mental healthcare for transgender adults and loved ones. *International Journal of Transgenderism, 9,* 35-82. http://dx.doi.org/10.1300/J485v09n03_03

Brown, L. S., & Pantalone, D. (2011). Lesbian, gay, bisexual, and transgender issues in trauma psychology: A topic comes out of the closet. *Traumatology, 17*(2), 1-3.

Carroll, L. (2017). Therapeutic issues with transgender elders. *Psychiatric Clinics, 40*(1), 127-140.

Chen, D., Edwards-Leeper, L., Stancin, T., & Tishelman, A. (2018). Advancing the practice of pediatric psychology with transgender youth: State of the science, ongoing controversies, and future directions. *Clinical Practice in Pediatric Psychology, 6*(1), 73.

Coleman, E., Radix, A. E., Bouman, W.P., Brown, G.R., de Vries, A. L. C., Deutsch, M. B. . . . Arcelus, J. (2022). Standards of care for the health of transgender and gender diverse people (Version 8). *International Journal of Transgender Health, 23*(S1), S1-S260. https://doi.org/10.1080/26895269.2022.2100644

Collazo, A., Austin, A., & Craig, S. L. (2013). Facilitating transition among transgender clients: Components of effective clinical practice. *Clinical Social Work Journal, 41,* 228-237. http://dx.doi.org/10.1007/s10615-013-0436-3

Cousino, M. K., Davis, A., Ng, H., & Stancin, T. (2014). An emerging opportunity for pediatric psychologists: Our role in a multidisciplinary clinic for youth with gender dysphoria. *Clinical Practice in Pediatric Psychology, 2,* 400-411.

de Vries, A. L. C., Cohen-Kettenis, P. T., & Delemarre-van de Waal, H. (2006). Clinical management of gender dysphoria in adolescents. *International Journal of Transgenderism, 9,* 83-94. http://dx.doi.org/10.1300/J485v09n03_04

Edwards-Leeper, L., Leibowitz, S., & Sangganjanavanich, V. F. (2016). Affirmative practice with transgender and gender nonconforming youth: Expanding the model. *Psychology of Sexual Orientation and Gender Diversity, 3*(2), 165.

Glidden, D., Bouman, W. P., Jones, B. A., & Arcelus, J. (2016). Gender dysphoria and autism spectrum disorder: A systematic review of the literature. *Sexual Medicine Reviews, 4*(1), 3-14. https://doi.org/10.1016/j.sxmr.2015.10.003

Heck, N. C. (2017). Group psychotherapy with transgender and gender nonconforming adults: Evidence-based practice applications. *Psychiatric Clinics, 40*(1), 157-175.

Heck, N. C., Croot, L. C., & Robohm, J. S. (2015). Piloting a psychotherapy group for transgender clients: Description and clinical considerations for practitioners. *Professional Psychology: Research and Practice, 46,* 30-36. http://dx.doi.org/10.1037/

Hendricks, M. L., & Testa, R. J. (2012). A conceptual framework for clinical work with transgender and gender nonconforming clients: An adaptation of the Minority Stress Model. *Professional Psychology: Research and Practice, 43*(5), 460.

Hope, D. A., Mocarski, R., Bautista, C. L., & Holt, N. R. (2016). Culturally competent evidence-based behavioral health services for the transgender community: Progress and challenges. *American Journal of Orthopsychiatry, 86*(4), 361.

Levine, S. B., Brown, G. R., Coleman, E., Cohen-Kettenis, P. T., Hage, J. J., Van Maasdam, J., . . . Schaefer, L. C. (1999). The standards of care for gender identity disorders. *Journal of Psychology & Human Sexuality, 11*(2), 1-34. https://doi.org/10.1300/J056v11n02_01

Mizock, L., & Lundquist, C. (2016). Missteps in psychotherapy with transgender clients: Promoting gender sensitivity in counseling and psychological practice. *Psychology of Sexual Orientation and Gender Diversity, 3*(2), 148.

Nichols, M. (2000). Therapy with sexual minorities. In S. Leiblum & R. Rosen (Eds), *The principles and practice of sex therapy* (3rd ed., pp.335-367). Guilford Press.

Peterson, F., Bley, J., Frabotta, R. (2020). *The gender revolution & new sexual health: Celebrating unlimited diversity of the Human Sexuality Hypercube.* Cognella Academic Publishing.

Reisner, S. L., Bailey, Z., & Sevelius, J. (2014). Racial/ethnic disparities in history of incarceration, experiences of victimization, and associated health indicators among transgender women in the U.S. *Women & health, 54*(8), 750-767. https://doi.org/10.1080/03630242.2014.932891

Schnarrs, P. W., Stone, A. L., Salcido, R., Jr, Baldwin, A., Georgiou, C., & Nemeroff, C. B. (2019). Differences in adverse childhood experiences (ACEs) and quality of physical and mental health between transgender and cisgender sexual minorities. *Journal of Psychiatric Research, 119,* 1-6. https://doi.org/10.1016/j.jpsychires.2019.09.001

Schulz, S. L. (2018). The informed consent model of transgender care: An alternative to the diagnosis of gender dysphoria. *Journal of humanistic psychology, 58*(1), 72-92.

Shulman, G. P., Holt, N. R., Hope, D. A., Mocarski, R., Eyer, J., & Woodruff, N. (2017). A review of contemporary assessment tools for use with transgender and gender nonconforming adults. *Psychology of sexual orientation and gender diversity, 4*(3), 304.

Sonoma, S. (2019, June 18). Black trans women want the media to show them living, not just dying. *Vox.* https://www.vox.com/first-person/2019/6/18/18679295/black-trans-women-murder-violence

Van Der Miesen, A. I., Hurley, H., & De Vries, A. L. (2016). Gender dysphoria and autism spectrum disorder: A narrative review. International Review of Psychiatry, 28(1), 70-80.

World Professional Association for Transgender Health. (2012). *Standards of care for the health of transsexual, transgender, and gender nonconforming people* [7th Version]. https://www.wpath.org/publications/soc

21

Consensual Non-Monogamous Relationships: The Paradox of Contemporary Relationships

Tori E. Stevens and Ronald Skip Carter

One of the major milestones in the human experience is the development of intimate and romantic relationships (Doyle & Molix, 2014). Historically in America, society set a standard that people should be sexually exclusive, having one sexual partner at a time in relationships. Ideally, the romantic notion was monogamy in a life-long relationship and if that was not achieved, then the practice of serial monogamy was acceptable. Before societal norms started to relax in the late 1960s, the expectation was to have as few sexual partners as possible. The belief has been to find the "one" love that satisfies all one's needs (psychologically, emotionally, spiritually, and sexually), get married, and spend eternal bliss with them. Both parties are expected to remain sexually monogamous, be exclusive throughout the entirety of the relationship, and try to keep the flame burning and the sex satisfying.

Barker and Landridge (2010) define mononormativity as the "dominant assumptions of the normalcy and naturalness of monogamy, analogous to such assumptions around heterosexuality inherent in the term heteronormativity" (p. 752). Ferrer (2018) describes the monogamous expectation as "Western mononormative culture" which generally refers to sexually exclusive, pair-bonding romantic relationships that evoke a sense of stability and security. In many ways, this mononormative expectation of one person checking every box (emotionally, spiritually, sexually, psychologically, and economically) potentially sets relationships up for failure. To date there are no psychological theories that address relational adjustment and development outside of a dyadic configuration (Conley et al., 2017). Most refer to any relationship that is not dyadic as triangulated, where the goal is to de-triangulate. The assumption is that triangles are unhealthy and should be avoided (Bowen, 1978). Some theories such as Emotion-Focused Couples Therapy (Greenberg & Goldman, 2008) assume bias in the name of their theory; the word couple meaning two. To avoid repeating this mistake in this body literature, the authors have opted to utilize the term "partners" rather than using terms that indicate the number of people in the relationship. Greenberg and Goldman do not explicitly state that Emotion-Focused Couples Therapy is only for dyads, but the assumption throughout the text is such. There is no mention of different relationship configurations. In fact, the only reference made to the possibility of more than one person in a relationship is when they discuss infidelity. Although most research and theories appear to assume relationships to be dyadic, and the only valid relationship orientation, that is not reality. While the monogamous relationship has been the societal expectation, some people are choosing an alternate relationship style. They decide to achieve relational and sexual satisfaction by engaging in consensually non-monogamous relationship configurations. These relationships are referred to as consensual non-monogamous (CNM) relationships. Cohen (2016a) defines CNM relationships as configurations in which there is a sexual agreement characterized by implicit or explicit rules for extra-dyadic sexual activities. When theory, research, training, and practice fail to address this valid relationship orientation, the needs of an entire population go unmet. Even worse, it invites stigma and bias to permeate the counseling profession and negatively impact people who dare to structure their relationships outside of the prescribed monogamous norm.

It is the authors intention to provide a more in-depth understanding of CNM. CNM relationship configurations look vastly different than the monogamous counterpart and can look quite different from each other. We hope that this chapter will start to shed some light on the various ways people construct their relationships and the various labels and terms associated with CNM. This chapter will provide a brief overview of what research shows regarding the stigma and bias CNM-identified people face, what research shows regarding the differences and similarities between monogamous and CNM relationships, and the motivation people have for engaging in CNM relationships. Additionally, this chapter will outline best practices and guidelines for working with CNM-identified people and provides a case example.

BRIEF HISTORY OF CNM AND DEFINITIONS

CNM is an umbrella term used to describe relationship structures in which sexual, romantic, and/or emotional exclusivity within a relationship is not expected. There are numerous CNM relationship labels and structures, each with its own particular emphasis and variations. These include such relationship structures as polyamory, swinging, open relationships, relationship anarchy, polygamy, and monogamish. It is important to note that this list is not exhaustive, and that language and labels change over time. The following relationship structure labels and definitions are a starting place to deepen understanding of CNM relationships but may not fit for some people who identify as consensually non-monogamous. The authors encourage a flexible of understanding of these relationship structures and labels.

Polyamory has been defined numerous ways within the literature. For example, it has been defined as a way of navigating relationships in which each person in the relationship has the option of pursing other romantic relationships at the same time, and most importantly, each partner in the relationship has given consent to this relationship agreement (Weitzman, 2006). Some scholars define polyamorous relationships as being non-hierarchal (Chapman, 2010), while others define it in terms of primary and secondary partners with most of their time and energy being spent with the primary partner (Weitzman, 1999). Additionally, Easton and Hardy (2009) note that some people use the term as more of an umbrella term that encompasses any relationship orientation that is extradyadic, and others use the term to indicate relationships characterized by committed love relationships in which emotional connections are present and the relationship is not solely based on sexual activity and engagement. One of the defining features of polyamory that sets it apart from other CNM relationship structures is the emphasis on relationships being more long-term and committal in nature (Sheff, 2005). For example, some partners in polyamorous relationships seek out singles or couples who join the partners in emotional and sexual relationships.

Open relationships are another form of CNM relationships that have multiple definitions and multiple ways of structuring. In open relationships, partners seek out others for dates or continuing sexual experiences. McCoy and colleagues (2015) define an open relationship as a relationship structure in which the two partners involved in a relationship can seek out additional relationships with other people, but those people do not usually interact with the other partner. Other scholars define open relationships as one in which a primary relationship is identified and that each partner may establish a secondary relationship with different partners; the main focus and commitment is to the partner in the identified primary relationship (Weitzman, 2006). This highlights the potential overlap in defining various relationship orientations. Sheff (2014) also discusses how the term open relationship can be used to describe all types of consensually non-monogamous relationships. Open relationships tend to have specific rules, expectations, and boundaries in place (Sheff, 2014).

One of the more widely known relationship orientations, and often the one most associated with CNM, is swinging. Williams and Prior (2015) define swinging as a relationship orientation that identifies the existence of a primary relationship and allows for sexual contact with other people. Swinging tends to emphasize having sexual relationships with people besides a primary partner within specific circumstances but does not include forming more intimate or emotional connections with anyone outside of the primary relationship (Chapman, 2010; Weitzman, 2006). Sexual encounters generally happen in a place where both partners are present, although that is not always the case. Swinging can be open or closed: open swinging is when a partner is participating in sexual behaviors in the same room as their primary partner, and closed swinging is when partners go to a different room or place separate from their primary partner.

Along with swinging, polygamy is also one of the more widely known CNM relationship orientations. Polygamy is characterized as a type of marriage consisting of three or more partners (Sheff, 2014). The most common form of multiple partner marriage is polygyny, a marriage of one husband and multiple wives, in which the wives are sexually exclusive with the husband and the husband engages in sex separately with each wife in the relationship (Sheff, 2014). This type of relationship orientation has been seen in mainstream media through reality television series Sister Wives and the HBO fictional series Big Love. Both shows depict one man with multiple wives. Williams and Prior (2015) note that polygamy can also consist of one woman with multiple husbands. However, this formation is seen with far less frequency.

Sex-advice columnist, podcaster, and author Dan Savage coined the term *monogamish* to signify committed relationships in which the partners are "mostly monogamous. However, there's a little allowance for the reality of desire for others and a variety of experiences and adventure and possibility" (Karpel, 2011). The boundaries, expectations, and agreements in these type of relationship structures can vary widely from one relationship to another. Partners practice varying degrees of consensual non-monogamous behaviors such as letting a significant other flirt, kiss, fondle, or explore others sexually. Partners create their own rules that govern their sexual behaviors and experiences. An example of rules can be "while being sexually active with other people, the couple will not engage in a particular sexual act, such as kissing. Kissing is only done by the couple, as they feel it is sacred between them." Monogamish people primarily want stable, long-lasting partner bonds with the potential for sexual experiences outside of the primary relationship.

Relationship anarchy is another way that some people define their relationship orientation, although this label is encountered far less frequently than the others. In fact, while studying and researching CNM, this term was only found a few times. Sheff (2014) notes one of the most prominent themes in this type of relationship orientation is the resistance to putting demands, expectations, and boundaries on the partners involved in the relationship. Another key philosophy in this type of relationship orientation is that the people involved do not place certain relationships above other relationships; there is a rejection of creating hierarchical relationship structures. Therefore, intimate relationships are no more important than friendships and are not subjected to a hierarchy of importance (Sheff, 2014).

TABLE 1. Other Key Terms Defined	
Relationship Orientation	This refers to the way in which people construct and engage in intimate relationships. This is related to how relationships can vary from monogamous to any form of non-monogamous configurations.
Hierarchical	These are relationships that are characterized as having some level of hierarchy within the relationship structure which delineates between primary, secondary, and tertiary relationships. Typically, primary relationships are considered more important than secondary and tertiary relationships.
Non-hierarchical	These relationships do not utilize terms such as primary or secondary partners. Relationships that are non-hierarchical do not consider any relationship to be more important than any other relationship.
Primary Relationship/ Partner	In relationships with a hierarchical structure this is often the closest relationship with the highest level of intimacy that may involve the most time, energy, and resources spent within that relationship and with that partner.
Secondary Relationship/ Partner	In relationships with a hierarchical structure this is often the second closest relationship and is characterized as requiring less time, energy, and resources as compared to the primary relationship. Secondary partners may or may not meet primary partners.
Tertiary Partner	In relationships with a hierarchical structure this is often the third closest relationship and is characterized as requiring less time, energy, and resources as compared to the primary relationship and secondary relationship. These partners may or may not meet primary or secondary partners.
Compersion	A feeling of pleasure and joy that comes from seeing a person you love experience joy and love with someone else.
Closed CNM Relationship	These are CNM relationships in which all partners of the relationship are exclusive with only the partners within the relationship. Individuals do not have permission to seek out other sexual and/or romantic relationships outside of the established relationship.

SUMMARY OF LITERATURE

A review of the literature on CNM shows the limited research that exists, although it is an area of research that continues to gain traction. Haritaworn et al. (2006) noted that the majority of the literature is in the form of self-help books and generally intended for people who are already familiar with CNM. People who identify as consensually non-monogamous are largely understudied (Rodrigues et al., 2016), with a lack of specific research concerning these relationships due to the societal stigma and potential consequences related to participating in CNM and nontraditional relationships. Due to this, obtaining accurate estimates of the prevalence of CNM has been difficult. McCoy et al. (2015) note that accurate estimates are unclear due to limited empirical research and the type of population that is being examined. Moors et al. (2015) used unpublished data in a study that indicated approximately 4% to 5% of the population engages in CNM. This is a similar percentage found in a study by J. D. Rubin et al. (2014). Haupert et al. (2017) found that more than one in five participants in their national study indicated they had engaged in a CNM relationship at some point in their lifetime. Given the difficulty with assessing how many people engage in CNM, it has also proven difficult to find a consensus on *who* is engaging in CNM relationships.

J. D. Rubin et al. (2014) found that men and women were equally likely to engage in consensual non-monogamy, White people and people of color were equally likely to engage in consensual non-monogamy, and heterosexually identified people and sexual minorities were equally likely to engage in CNM relationships. However, a more recent study analyzing a national sample found that men were more likely to engage in CNM than women and that sexual minorities were more likely than heterosexual-identified people to engage in CNM (Haupert et. al., 2017). Haupert and colleagues also found that age, education level, income status, religion, region, political affiliation, and race are not related to previous engagement in CNM relationships. Seguin et al. (2016) found some support for sexual orientation differences in relationship orientations. They found that a higher percentage of heterosexual-identified participants identified as monogamous, a higher percentage of homosexual-identified participants reported engaging in open relationships, and a higher percentage of bisexual-identified participants reported engaging in polyamorous relationships. The authors encourage utilizing a critical lens when examining what the research shows regarding the demographic make-up of those who engage in CNM relationships.

Sprott et al. (2017) describe how there is a bias against CNM behaviors in the foundational understanding of healthy relationships. Research also shows that there are misconceptions about CNM relationships and that some aspects of society perceive this behavior as deviant and immoral. Consensual non-monogamists are perceived as being deviant by mainstream society in part because this type of activity is in contradiction to our societal norm of monogamy (Serina et al., 2013). More broadly, mainstream culture views anything that is not classified as monogamy as if it were cheating (Mint, 2004). Conley et al. (2013) conducted a study that not only highlighted that the public views monogamy as superior to CNM but that there is also a halo effect surrounding monogamous relationships as well. Specifically, monogamous relationships were rated more favorably on arbitrary traits as well as specific relationship characteristics. Meaning, people were viewed as having better relationships and being a better person overall simply by being in monogamous relationships. Moors et al. (2017) found that people associate monogamy with higher quality relationships, more desired personality characteristics, greater intelligence, and a better quality of life compared to CNM.

Changing the societal understanding of what constitutes a healthy relationship would help destigmatize and could legitimize these relationships in the eyes of the public. Would changing the paradigm of relationships lead to the acceptance of CNM? Moors and Schechinger (2014) believe that researchers must place importance on examining assumptions underlying psychological frameworks that are pertinent to how romantic relationships are perceived. While further research is recommended to help people who participate in CNM to feel less stigmatized, there have been some studies that compare monogamous relationships to CNM relationships.

There is a perception that people who are in monogamous relationships are more satisfied with their relationships than people who engage in CNM relationships (Cohen, 2016b). Research is starting to debunk the myth that monogamous relationships are different, or better, than non-monogamous relationships. Relationships can be secure regardless of the relationship orientation (Moors & Schechinger, 2014). One study found no differences between male same-sex relationships with non-monogamous agreements and male same-sex relationships with monogamous agreements regarding relationship health, including self-reported relationship satisfaction, hostile conflict, feelings of constraint in the relationship, confidence in the relationship, and relationship instability (Whitton et al., 2015). Both participant samples reported confidence in their relationships, overall relationship satisfaction, and low levels of negative relationship experiences (e.g., destructive conflict, felt constraint, relationship instability, and individual depressive symptoms).

Conley et al. (2017) found no major differences between monogamous-identified people and CNM-identified people on ratings of satisfaction, commitment, and passion in their relationships. Additionally, they found that CNM-identified people reported less jealousy and greater trust in their partners compared to people in monogamous relationships. Other research has challenged the belief that CNM relationships are not as long-term and stable as their monogamous counterparts. A. M. Rubin and Adams (1986) conducted a follow-up study from their 1982 study comparing monogamous and non-monogamous couples. They found that 68% of the sexually open couples were still together and 82% of the sexually exclusive couples were still together. Participant happiness was also found to be stable from the first study to the follow-up study.

In addition to myths surrounding non-monogamous relationships, there are also myths surrounding the people who engage in non-monogamous relationships. One such myth is that people who engage in CNM are at greater risk for negative sexual health experiences and are viewed as more sexually risky (Hutzler et al., 2015). Contrary to this assumption, studies have shown that people involved in CNM relationships are more likely to engage in safe sex practices and engage in open communication about past and current sexual partners (Conley et al., 2012; Lehmiller, 2015). Moreover, operating under the belief that monogamy minimizes sexual risk can actually be detrimental to a person's sexual health (Moors et al., 2017). Other scholars found that people who engage in CNM relationships report higher sexual satisfaction than people in monogamous relationships, helping to dispel the myth that monogamous relationships result in greater sexual satisfaction (Conley et al., 2018). Conley et al. (2012) found that sexually unfaithful people, meaning people who are in committed monogamous relationships who are engaging in sex with other people without their partner's consent or knowledge, were less likely than people engaged in negotiated non-monogamous relationships to use condoms and other forms of safe sex such as using gloves for genital touching and sterilizing sex toys. They also found that sexually unfaithful individuals were significantly less likely than individuals engaged in negotiated non-monogamous relationships to have discussed their sexual history, including their history of Sexually Transmitted Infection testing. Lehmiller (2015) came to similar conclusions regarding safe sex practices of people engaged in CNM versus people engaged in monogamous relationships. Approximately one-quarter of the monogamous partners in the participant sample reported engaging in sex outside of their primary relationship and most of them indicated that their primary partner did not know about their infidelity. The non-monogamous participants in Lehmiller's (2015) sample did report more lifetime sexual partners than their monogamous counterparts, however safe sex practices were more present with the non-monogamous-identified people. These studies help to debunk the myth that people engaged in non-monogamous relationships are at greater risk for negative sexual health experiences and can ultimately give people a greater understanding of CNM relationships overall. Mogilski et al. (2017) conducted a study examining mate retention strategies in monogamous and CNM people. Compared to their monogamous counterparts, CNM-identified participants reported greater satisfaction with the communication and openness they experienced in their relationships. They suggested that the openness and communication in CNM relationships may be a form of mate retention that is unique to these types of relationships. They also conclude that monogamous partners and CNM primary partners are treated similarly in the respective relationships.

Research has focused on various experiences of people who identify as non-monogamous. Some qualitative studies have explored identity development, authentic ways of living, and the construction of CNM relationships (McLean, 2004; Robinson, 2013; Sheff, 2005). The question of how one comes to identify as non-monogamous or be involved in this type of relationship orientation has been examined, although it has been piecemeal and based on small sample sizes (Yarber & Sayad, 2010).

Barker (2005) suggests that people come to this identity one of two ways. Some people have always felt different in how they view relationship dynamics, meaning that they never identified with a dyadic relationship structure. Others, Barker (2005) said, have struggled with fidelity and then realized they could construct a relationship where they could be honest and open about multiple relationships at the same time. McLean (2004) conducted a qualitative study with CNM-identified people and found that the most notable and prevalent ground rules established in these types of relationship orientations is that of honesty and communication with the partners involved in the relationship. Other research has highlighted how engaging in CNM relationship orientations allows some people to be more authentic. Moors et al. (2015) found individuals lower in avoidance attachment style were more likely to be in a CNM relationship than in a monogamous relationship. They also found that men reported higher levels of avoidance but more positive attitudes toward CNM, and greater willingness to engage in CNM than women did. This finding suggests that gender role socialization and stereotyping might impact how people view various relationship orientations.

Some authors assert that there are many benefits for CNM relationships. One advantage (and motivation) for partners to practice CNM is to have the security of a stable relationship with a primary partner and also experience sexual satisfaction with others in an honest manner without deceit (Peterson et al., 2020). Cooney (2018) describes how partners in non-monogamous relationships create better communication styles, are better at setting boundaries and relationship negotiations, and managing jealousy. In addition, these relationships tend to be high in mutual respect.

However, CNM can have pitfalls and difficulties just like traditional relationships. In some cases, participating in CNM may cause cognitive dissonance and create internal conflict because of societal norms and pressure to only engage in monogamous relationships. The alternative, however, is to either live a monogamous life or to live in secrecy which can also potentially create psychological and/or relational distress. CNM relationships can cause concern among some people because they believe that the practice of CNM legitimizes alternative relationships which do not reflect traditional values. Doyle and Molix (2015) detail how social conservatives often argue that the legalization of alternative relationships such as same-sex marriage is wrong because it is a slippery slope that would lead to the legalization of other nontraditional marriages. Because CNM-associated behaviors go against the heterosexist social construct of one man and one woman, the idea of CNM is thought to be pathological. For some, consensual non-monogamy represents a line that must not be crossed (Rubel & Bogaert, 2015).

Those of traditional American values would pose the question: Why or how could anyone gleam happiness or satisfaction from letting one's significant other have sexual experiences with other people? Woods (2014) describes this phenomenon by explaining how those who participate in CNM derive a shared happiness called *compersion* which are overwhelmingly positive feelings that one gets from their partner's happiness during experiences with other people. An example of compersion is the feeling a parent gets when their child succeeds, such as winning a race or an award. These shared feelings can create a stronger bond and healthier relationship.

We have examined how the public views CNM, but what about mental health professionals? Are mental health clinicians understanding and accepting of varied relationship structures? What are the clinical implications if mental health professionals are not anymore accepting than the public? To date, there is limited research on the stigma and attitudes mental health professionals hold toward CNM. However, the research that has been conducted shows a clear pattern of stigma and negative attitudes toward non-monogamy held by therapists (Hymer & A. M. Rubin, 1982). It is worth noting that most of the research on mental health professionals' views on non-monogamy was conducted over 30 years ago. This represents a large gap in the research and should be explored and examined to gain a better understanding of how mental health professionals currently view and understand CNM relationship structures.

One of the first studies conducted on therapists' attitudes toward CNM found that over one third of the family therapists in the study believed that people engaged in sexually open marriages and swinging are neurotic and have personality disorders (Knapp, 1975). Knapp also found that one fifth of those therapists thought that people engaged in sexually open marriages or swinging were likely to have antisocial personality traits. Roman et al. (1978) also conducted research on psychotherapists' attitudes toward non-monogamy: 23% of their participants reported group sex was unacceptable and 13% reported extramarital sex was unacceptable, they used an alternative lifestyles measure that showed 11% of the participants believed group marriage was not okay and 35% said it was "possibly okay," and 16% of the participants thought swinging was unacceptable and 36% said it was possibly okay.

Research has also shown that people who have engaged in non-monogamous relationships and sought therapy experienced bias and little to no support from their therapists (Graham, 2014; Hymer & A. M. Rubin, 1982). Perel (2006) notes that non-monogamy, even if consensual, is viewed as suspect and that therapists often view it as a fear of commitment or a fear of intimacy. Even when therapists self-report being open and accepting of non-monogamous relationship orientations, they still hold problematic views and understandings that seep into their work (Finn et al., 2012). Finn et al. (2012) conducted a qualitative study with psychotherapists who reported using affirmative therapy with non-monogamous clients. While all the therapists professed their commitment to being open to working with the CNM population, they made several statements indicating they still held some biases toward this population.

Striving for multicultural competence is expected in the field of counseling (American Counseling Association, 2014; American Psychological Association, 2010; Association for Lesbian, Gay, Bisexual, and Transgender Issues in Counseling, 2012; D. W. Sue & Sue, 2003). D. W. Sue et al. (1992) developed cultural competence guidelines for counselors. They describe three dimensions of a culturally competent counselor. First, they assert that counselors must have an awareness of themselves to understand how that will impact their work with clients. Second, they assert that counselors must understand and have respect for culturally diverse clients without negative judgments toward clients. The third dimension of a culturally competent counselor addresses the skills and interventions utilized in therapeutic process, meaning interventions utilized should be appropriate and sensitive to the clients' culture and needs. Outside of the guidelines themselves, one of the most important pieces of becoming a culturally competent counselor is that this is an active process with no endpoint and that counselors must continually strive to increase their competency (D. W. Sue & Sue, 2008).

Current research has shown that therapist openness and acceptance of clients' identities is important. Fowers and Davidov (2006) suggested that therapists should possess an openness to strive for multicultural competency. They asserted that openness is a necessary component of cultural competence and it should inform training and practice. Cultural humility has been defined as engaging in a pattern of interpersonal connection that is focused on others rather than the self and in a way that shows respect for another's cultural background and experiences (Hook et al., 2013). Hook et al. (2013) found that cultural humility in therapists can lead to more positive outcomes in the therapy process.

In addition to multicultural competency guidelines, clinicians in the counseling field are also governed by codes of ethics. Even though these guidelines and codes do not specifically address varied relationship structures such as CNM, it does not mean that the established ethical and cultural competency guidelines are not applicable to clinicians working with CNM-identified people. One of the American Counseling Association's (2014) current ethical guidelines addresses counselors imposing their own values on clients. Section A.4.b. is concerned with personal values, and more specifically the personal values of counselors and how those are managed in work with clients. This guideline explicitly states that counselors are to avoid imposing their own values, attitudes, beliefs, and behaviors on their clients. It goes on to highlight that counselors should seek training and education in areas where there may be a risk of their values conflicting with their clients' values. Like sexual orientation, relationship orientation also represents a specific culture that has its own values, attitudes, beliefs, and behaviors. If therapists are guided by the ethics code of the American Counseling Association (2014) and they hold negative, stereotypical, and discriminatory attitudes and beliefs toward CNM, they are setting themselves up for ethical violations. The American Psychological Association's (2010) ethical code governs psychologists in their research and work with clients. The most notable guideline regarding relationship orientation is Principal E, which is concerned with respect for clients' rights and dignity. As with the ACA's (2014) ethical code, there is no specific mention of relationship orientation. However, Principle E does explicitly state that psychologists should be aware of and respect clients' cultures.

CNM is a valid and practiced way of constructing relationships (Barker & Landrige, 2010; Cohen, 2016a; Moors & Schechinger, 2014). As such mental health professionals should be, at the very least, minimally aware of CNM relationships and the guidelines that exist for working with this population. The question is not about "if" a clinician works with CNM-identified people but "when."

GUIDELINES FOR COUNSELORS

First and foremost, mental health clinicians should educate themselves on the topic of CNM. This is not to say that mental health clinicians must be experts in this area; quite the opposite. Having a basic understanding of what CNM is, how it may be expressed, and the potential challenges CNM-identified people face is likely to go a long way in regard to building a therapeutic alliance with clients who engage in CNM. Schechinger and colleagues (2018) found CNM-identified people were more likely to continue a counseling relationship with clinicians who did not rely solely on the client to educate them about CNM, but instead took steps to educate themselves outside of the therapeutic relationship.

Following this, clinicians should engage in their own process of reflection and be honest, at the very least, with themselves about the values they hold and how those impact their understanding of CNM. For example, during graduate school training one of the authors was talking about her research and clinical interest in CNM with a cohort mate in the same graduate program. This cohort mate mentioned she was working with a polyamorous-identified client, but that she did not believe that her client actually loved each partner equally and that she believed the client was just not being honest about which partner she liked more. On the surface, this belief may not seem overly harmful to the client. However, how might this belief have been impacting the way the clinician conceptualized the client? How might that belief be reflected in the interventions the clinician chose to utilize with that client? Holding the belief that the client must have loved one partner more than the other is dismissive of the client's actual experience. Understanding your own biases and beliefs surrounding CNM should go beyond just merely asking yourself if you agree or disagree with people constructing their own relationship configurations outside of the established monogamous expectation. As you were reading about the different ways to construct CNM relationships, did you have different reactions to certain relationship structures? Did you find yourself thinking that engaging in certain forms of CNM was appropriate, but other forms were not acceptable? It is a mental health clinician's ethical duty and responsibility to identify and understand their own values and beliefs related to CNM.

Mental health clinicians should work with and understand the labels and definitions that each unique client or partnered clients bring to therapy (Bairstow, 2017). As outlined previously in this chapter, there are many different labels that people assign to their relationship orientation and there are many ways to construct those relationships. The authors recommend using the labels and definitions given earlier as a starting point to understand how varied relationship configurations can be, but not as something that is set in stone.

Mental health clinicians need to consider and be aware of the client(s) level of outness regarding their relationship orientation and to whom and in what areas of their life they are out. Cooney (2018) describes how individuals are often scared of losing their jobs, not getting a promotion, losing family or friends who will not respect them anymore, or scared that their children will be taken away. There can be profoundly serious consequences for people when and if they come out about their CNM relationships. Understanding the outness of a client will give context to possible contributors to overall distress in a client's life, which will better inform the clinician regarding treatment. Additionally, outness can directly impact the level of social support clients do or do not have.

Mental health clinicians should not assume that clients who identify as CNM are coming to counseling because of their CNM identity and relationship. Just like people who are in monogamous relationships who seek therapy, their relationship may or may not be the impetus for counseling. Understanding a client's relationship can aid in conceptualization and help clinicians to know their clients holistically, but the relationship itself is not always part of the presenting issues. Clients will terminate the counseling relationship early if they feel like the counselor is holding judgment and pathologizing their relationship structure (Schechinger et al., 2018).

Additionally, counselors should not be afraid of or shy away from talking openly about a client's relationship structure and any potential difficulties clients are having related to their relationships. Clients are more likely to maintain counseling relationships when they have a counselor who is willing to discuss their CNM relationships and structures (Schechinger et al., 2018). Addressing concerns with clients regarding CNM can look different from client to client. This may include addressing the varying concerns each partner may have about CNM or their relationship, addressing any infidelity that may be present or that may have been present in the past, and understanding that opening a relationship and maintaining it is an ongoing process (Bairstow, 2017).

Lastly, the authors would like to caution counselors regarding jealousy in CNM relationships. Jealousy happens. Jealousy can be a part of any relationship, monogamous or non-monogamous. When partners in CNM relationships experience jealousy, it does not mean they are "doing CNM wrong" or that they should not be in a CNM relationship. The important part of experiencing jealousy in relationships is the way in which the partners and the counselor confront it and manage it. It should be processed in a way that helps partners understand why a partner is feeling jealous and how partners can work through the jealousy together.

CLINICAL VIGNETTE

The Story of Tim and Danielle

Tim sought our clinic because in his words he "wanted a therapist who understood his marriage lifestyle and not be judged because of it." At our first session Tim asked two questions: Did I understand what consensual non-monogamy was and did I know what compersion was? Tim told me he was seeing a therapist prior to finding our clinic and it did not go well. Tim said that he spent several sessions having to explain his lifestyle to the therapist. Tim shared that he felt judged by the therapist and noticed that the therapist seemed uncomfortable with him. Tim and Danielle had been married for 22 years and at the time he came to see me had two older adolescent daughters. Tim reported he loved Danielle very much and could not see his life without her and that he was also missing a stronger connection to her.

Once Tim felt that I was not going to judge him, he started explaining their story. Tim and Danielle made the decision to start playing with other couples about 4 to 5 years earlier. They would meet different couples, and at times individual males, for sex play. Eventually Danielle decided that she did not like swinging because of the lack of connection she made with the other males. Danielle felt cheap due to the lack of emotional connection and asked Tim about making their relationship polyamorous. Tim agreed to this change in their relationship boundaries but added that he wanted to seek out other couples rather than single individuals. So, they stopped swinging and started looking for a couple to start a relationship with.

Tim and Danielle met Dave and Jen at a meet-and-greet social event for swingers. The group meets twice a month on Friday nights at different locations for drinks and social conversation. Dave approached Danielle one Friday evening and they really hit it off. She explained that "sparks" kind of flew between them. The following Saturday evening the four made plans to go out and a quad was born. Tim recalled how there was great chemistry among the four of them and the four have been in a polyamorous relationship ever since. Dave and Jen have no children and live about 10 minutes from Tim and Danielle. Tim and Danielle never told their daughters that they are in a polyamorous relationship with Dave and Jen, but all six do activities as a group such as cookouts, pool parties, holidays, birthdays, and other special occasions.

Tim started struggling with situational depression caused by feelings of envy related to the strong connection Danielle had with Dave. Tim and Jen also engaged in sexual activity with one another; however, Tim explained that their chemistry was not anywhere close to Danielle and Dave's sexual chemistry. As time went on Tim wanted to find someone who he could experience a similar connection with. One Friday evening Tim met a couple named Joe and Brittany. Over the course of the evening Tim and Brittany seemed to experience a strong connection. The quad was not interested in adding another couple, so it was decided that Tim and Brittany would see each other individually. Over the next couple of months Tim and Brittany became really close. Tim and Brittany had the sexual chemistry and intimacy that Danielle and Dave had. Things went really well for everyone for about 8 months and then Brittany started canceling dates with Tim and their communication started becoming less and less. Eventually Brittany explained that she and Joe were having marital problems and Joe wanted to have a closed relationship while they sought therapy together. Eventually Brittany and Tim stopped seeing each other and communication was limited to a "text or two" per month. Tim sought comfort from the group as he grieved the loss of his relationship with Brittany. Over the next several months as Tim was trying to deal with the loss of his and Brittany's relationship, his depression continued to get worse. Then one day he ran into Brittany at a store while shopping, and they talked for about 30 minutes catching up with each other. Brittany said that her and Joe's marriage was getting better and that she missed Tim. However, Brittany and Joe were still in a closed relationship.

Sneaking around was not an option, so they said goodbye and went their own ways. Tim's depression began impacting his relationship with Danielle as well as the other relationships in the quad. After a group meeting, they suggested that Tim seek therapy which led him to the previous therapist, and then eventually to me.

Tim and I worked collaboratively to determine that our primary focus of counseling would be to help him decrease and manage his depression symptoms and to help him feel more secure with and connected to Danielle. We first focused on the more immediate goal of symptom reduction regarding his depression. After Tim began to report minimal to no depression symptoms for several weeks, we turned our therapeutic focus to his relationship with Danielle.

Danielle frequently reassured Tim that she loved him and was committed to the relationship; she told him she would never do anything to sabotage their relationship. Even with reassurance, Tim struggled to feel connected. We explored the differences in their relationship now as compared to when Tim felt more connected. Tim and Danielle were able to establish new boundaries within their relationship that helped Tim to feel more secure and connected in the relationship. Some examples of the changes they made were Danielle would not engage in sex with Dave on days that were dedicated to intimacy between Tim and Danielle, Danielle would stop engaging in specific sexual acts with Joe, and a few nights out of the week would be dedicated to Tim and Danielle's family only.

Additionally, we worked on changing Tim's cognitive distortions that contributed to him feeling insecure as a man and as a husband. We identified that the breakup with Brittany had triggered old thoughts and insecurities from when he was an adolescent. The breakup made him feel like he did in high school, that something was wrong with him and this caused people to reject him. Even though he understood the reasoning behind why Brittany ended their relationship, he still experienced negative thoughts and ruminating negative self-talk that contributed to significant insecurity. Once we understood his distortions, we improved his thoughts and stopped the ruminating negative self-talk. This, combined with the renegotiated boundaries and expectations in his relationship with Danielle, led to the remission of Tim's depression symptoms and increased his feelings of connection with Danielle.

CONCLUSION

Consensually non-monogamous relationships are valid. They are not inherently wrong or destined to fail. For many people there are numerous relational benefits to having a consensual non-monogamous relationship. That does not mean there are not pitfalls and difficulties, much like with monogamous relationships. There are several key factors to establishing and maintaining healthy CNM relationships that clinicians should consider and assess for when working with CNM-identified clients regarding their relational health and functioning.

The level of willingness of each partner engaged in a CNM relationship can impact the overall health and functioning of that relationship. Individual partners in a relationship may vary on their comfort level regarding CNM. It is not unheard of for partners to agree to a CNM relationship configuration despite not being completely comfortable with the idea. In fact, clinicians may find themselves working with partners struggling with this. Many factors can impact a person's willingness to engage in and be comfortable with CNM relationships. This would be beneficial to explore in the context of a therapeutic relationship. Hangen et al. (2020) proposed and developed the Triple-C model that addresses and assesses the foundational building blocks of a healthy relationship. They propose that mutual consent regarding relationship boundaries and expectations, level of comfort with the relationship structure, and the ability to engage in ongoing and open communication all impact the overall relational health of any intimate relationship, monogamous or non-monogamous. Exploring and understanding these components for all partners in a CNM relationship can provide clinicians with valuable information that will help them conceptualize and work with clients who might be experiencing relational distress.

As the Triple-C model (Hangen et al., 2020) highlights, communication is an extremely important factor in constructing and maintaining healthy CNM relationships. Communication impacts everything in a relationship from establishing relationship agreements to navigating conflict and tension as it happens. No relationship is without some experience of conflict or tension. This is a normative aspect of all relationships. Being able to identify tension and then subsequently being able to appropriately alleviate that tension requires communication within the relationship between all partners. This includes emotional honesty, even when it may be difficult for one, both, or all partners. Meaning, individuals should be willing to share their emotional experiences even when doing so may cause them distress, whether it is their own distress related to sharing their feelings or distress related to how their partner(s) may react to their feelings. Likewise, individuals should also be willing to hear their partner's emotional experiences without becoming defensive to the point that they stop hearing what their partner is communicating. This relational concept is called differentiation which comes from Family Systems theory developed by Murray Bowen (1978). For clinicians, when working with CNM-identified people, assessing partners' level of differentiation within the relationship structure can help to provide a blueprint for communication difficulties that can lead to increased tension in the relationship. Communication is one of the most important aspects of relational health for all relationships and it is no different for CNM relationships.

Another key factor that contributes to the overall relational health in CNM relationships is the ability to establish boundaries and expectations within the relational system and a willingness to revisit them and renegotiate them as needed. Boundaries and expectations for relationships should be clear and specific and all partners should have input regarding the agreements that are made. For example, rather than having an agreement that says, "we can have sex with other people outside of our primary relationship," there should be very specific agreements about what "sex with other people" means. Does this include all kinds of sexual activity? Is oral sex with another partner okay? How about kissing? Or, in the case example of Tim and Danielle, what about different sexual encounters with different people on the same day? There are many different things to consider when establishing boundaries and expectations for CNM relationships, too many to list here. The above is just one example of the specificity in agreements that is needed in CNM relationships to promote healthy relationship functioning. However, once initial agreements are made does not mean they cannot or should not be revisited. In fact, a hallmark of healthy CNM relationships is the willingness and ability to revisit and renegotiate agreements as needed in the relationship.

There are many reasons that relationship agreements may need to be renegotiated. Rather than attempt to list all the reasons that renegotiation may be needed, we would like to focus on the process of renegotiation. When there is a partner unwilling to explore how and why relationship agreements may not be working, this is cause for concern. As the context of people's lives change, so might their relational needs, wants, and desires. At the core, revisiting agreements is about open and honest communication when something is not working for one or more partners in a CNM relationship. Renegotiation should first address what is not working and why. It is important that each partner feel heard and understood regarding the difficulties they are experiencing with the current relationship agreements. Then, possible solutions can be identified and discussed. Renegotiation is not always easy. Just like in monogamous relationships, there may be aspects of the relationship that a partner feels cannot be renegotiated. The case vignette of Tim and Danielle is again a great example of how renegotiation can work and help to solidify the relationship. This may not always be the case. It is important to remember that a willingness to explore changing relationship agreements does not mean that those agreements will be or should be changed. For example, Danielle agreed to not engage in sexual activity with Dave on days in which physical intimacy was scheduled with Tim. However,

Danielle was under no obligation to agree to that change, and had she not agreed to it, a vastly different conversation would have been had. Renegotiation takes work and effort, and each partner should engage in their own self-reflection about what they want for the relationship and what they feel cannot be compromised.

In closing, this chapter is not meant to be a complete and exhaustive guide to working with CNM-identified people, but rather is meant as a starting point for learning about CNM relationship structures and a way to start developing a framework for how clinicians can approach their work with CNM-identified people. The authors encourage continued study in this area for clinicians who are interested in working with this population or who find themselves working with this population. Remember, with approximately 4% to 5% of the population engaging in CNM relationships the question is not "if" you see CNM-identified clients but "when." CNM relationships can be healthy and provide relationship satisfaction for those who engage in them. CNM relationships can also experience difficulty, tension, and conflict, just as is true for monogamous relationships. It is imperative that mental health clinicians engage in self-reflection regarding their views and beliefs on consensual non-monogamy in order to avoid inflicting harm upon clients.

REFERENCES

American Counseling Association. (2014). *ACA Code of Ethics.* https://www.counseling.org/docs/default-source/default-document-library/2014-code-of-ethics-finaladdress.pdf

American Psychological Association. (2010). *Ethical principles of psychologists and code of conduct.* https://www.apa.org/ethics/code

Association for Lesbian, Gay, Bisexual, and Transgender Issues in Counseling (ALGBTIC): A division of the American Counseling Association. (2012). *Competencies for counseling with lesbian, gay, bisexual, queer, questioning, intersex and ally individuals.* http://www.counseling.org/docs/ethics/algbtic-2012-07.pdf?sfvrsn=2

Bairstow, A. (2017). Couples exploring nonmonogamy: Guidelines for therapists. *Journal of Sex and Marital Therapy, 43*(4), 343-353. https://doi.org/10.1080/0092623X.2016.1164782)

Barker, M. (2005). This is my partner, and this is my...partner's partner: Constructing a polyamorous identity in a monogamous world. *Journal of Constructivistic Psychology, 18*(1), 75-88.

Barker, M., & Langdridge, D. (2010). Whatever happened to non-monogamies? Critical reflections on recent research and theory. *Sexualities, 13*(6), 748-772.

Bowen, M. (1978). *Family therapy in clinical practice.* Jason Aronson.

Chapman, M. (2010). *What does polyamory look like? Polydiverse patterns of loving and living in modern polyamorous relationships.* iUniverse.

Cohen, M. T. (2016a). An exploratory study of individuals in non-traditional, alternative relationships: How "open" are we? *Sexuality & Culture, 20*(2), 295-315. https://doi.org/10.1007/s12119-015-9324-z

Cohen, M. T. (2016b). The perceived satisfaction derived from various relationship configurations. *Journal of Relationship Research, 7,* 1-7. https://doi.org/10.1017/jrr.2016.12

Conley, T. D., Matsick, J. L., Moors, A. C., & Ziegler, A. (2017). Investigation of consensually nonmonogamous relationships. *Perspectives on Psychological Science, 12,* 205-232.

Conley, T. D., Moors, A. C., Matsick, J. L., & Zielger, A. (2013). The fewer the merrier?: Assessing stigma surrounding consensually non-monogamous romantic relationships. *Analyses of Social Issues and Public Policy (ASAP), 13*(1), 1-30.

Conley, T. D., Moors, A. C., Ziegler, A., & Karathanasis, C. (2012). Unfaithful individuals are less likely to practice safer sex than openly nonmonogamous individuals. *Journal of Sexual Medicine, 2(9),* 1559-1565.

Conley, T. D., Piemonte, J. L., Gusakova, S., & Rubin, J. D. (2018). Sexual satisfaction among individuals in monogamous and consensually non-monogamous relationships. *Journal of Social and Personal Relationships, 35*(4), 509-553.

Cooney, S. (2018, August 28). What monogamous couples can learn from polyamorous relationships, according to experts. *Time.Com,* 1. https://time.com/5330833/polyamory-monogamous-relationships

Doyle, D. M., & Molix, L. (2014). How does stigma spoil relationships? Evidence that perceived discrimination harms romantic relationship quality through impaired self-image. *Journal of Applied Social Psychology, 44,* 600-610. https://doi.org/10.1111/jasp.12252

Doyle, D. M., & Molix, L. (2015). Perceived discrimination and social relationship functioning among sexual minorities: Structural stigma as a moderating factor. *Analyses of Social Issues & Public Policy*, *15*(1), 357-381.

Easton, D., & Hardy, J. W. (2009). *The ethical slut: A practical guide to polyamory, open relationships and other adventures*. Celestial Arts.

Ferrer, J. N. (2018). Mononormativity, polypride, and the "mono-poly wars." *Sexuality & Culture,* 22(3), 817-836.

Finn, M. D., Tunariu, A. D., & Lee, K. C. (2012). A critical analysis of affirmative therapeutic engagements with consensual non-monogamy. *Sexual and Relationship Therapy, 27*(3), 205-216.

Fowers, B. J., & Davidov, B. J. (2006). The virtue of multiculturalism: Personal, transformation, character, and openness to the other. *American Psychologist, 61*(6), 581-594.

Graham, N. (2014). Polyamory: A call for increased mental health professional awareness. *Archives of Sexual Behavior, 43,* 1031-1034.

Greenberg, L. S., & Goldman, R. N. (2008). *Emotion-focused couples therapy: The dynamics of emotion, love, and power.* American Psychological Association.

Hangen, F., Crasta, D., & Rogge, R. D. (2020). Delineating the boundaries between nonmonogamy and infidelity: Bringing consent back into definitions of consensual nonmonogamy with latent profile analysis. *The Journal of Sex Research, 57*(4), 438-457. https://doi.org/10.1080/00224499.2019.1669133

Haritaworn, J., Lin, C., & Klesse, C. (2006). Poly/logue: A critical introduction to polyamory. *Sexualities, 9*(5), 515-529.

Haupert, M. L., Gesselman, A. N., Moors, A. C., Fisher, H. E., & Garcia, J. R. (2017). Prevalence of experiences with consensual nonmonogamous relationships: Findings from two national samples of single Americans. *Journal of Sex & Marital Therapy, 43*(5), 424-440. https://doi.org/10.1080/0092623X.2016.1178675

Hook, J. N., Davis, D. E., Owen, J., Worthington, E. L., & Utsey, S. O. (2013). Cultural humility: Measuring openness to culturally diverse clients. *Journal of Counseling Psychology, 60*(3), 353-366.

Hutzler, K. T., Giuliano, T. A., Herselman, J. R., & Johnson, S. M. (2015). Three's a crowd: Public awareness and (mis) perceptions of polyamory. *Psychology & Sexuality, 7*(2), 69-87. https://doi.org/10.1080/19419899.2015.1004102

Hymer, S. M., & Rubin, A. M. (1982). Alternative lifestyle clients. *Small Group Behavior, 13*(4), 532-541.

Karpel, A. (2011, July 7). Monogamish, *The Advocate.* http://www.advocate.com/Print_Issue/Features/Monogamish

Knapp, J. J. (1975). Some non-monogamous marriage styles and related attitudes and practices of marriage counselors. *Family Coordinator, 24,* 505-514.

Lehmiller, J. J. (2015). A comparison of sexual health history and practices among monogamous and consensually nonmonogamous sexual partners. *Journal of Sexual Medicine, 12,* 2022-2028. https://doi.org/10.1111/jsm.12987

Lehmiller, J. J. (2018). *Tell me what you want.* Da Capo Press.

McCoy, M. A., Stinson, M. A., Ross, D. B., & Hjelmstad, L. R. (2015). Who's in our client's bed? A case illustration of sex therapy with a polyamorous couple. *Journal of Sex & Marital Therapy, 41*(2), 134-144.

McLean, K. (2004). Negotiating (non)monogamy: Bisexuality and intimate relationships. *Journal of Bisexuality, 4*(1-2), 83-97. https://doi.org/10.1300/J159v04n01_07

Mint, P. (2004). The power dynamics of cheating: Effects on polyamory and bisexuality. *Journal of Bisexuality, 4*(3-4), 55-76.

Mogilski, J. K., Memering, S. L., Welling, L. L. M., & Shackelford, T. K. (2017). Monogamy versus consensual non-monogamy: Alternative approaches to pursuing a strategically pluralistic mating strategy. *Archives of Sexual Behavior, 46,* 407-417. https://doi.org/10.1007/s10508-015-0658-2

Moors, A. C., Conley, T. D., Edelstein, R. S., & Chopik, W. J. (2015). Attached to monogamy? Avoidance predicts willingness to engage (but not actual engagement) in consensual non-monogamy. *Journal of Social and Personal Relationships, 32*(2), 222-240.

Moors, A. C., Matsick, J. L., & Schechinger, H. A. (2017). Unique and shared relationship benefits of consensually non-monogamous and monogamous relationships. *European Psychologist, 22*(1), 55-71.

Moors, A. C., & Schechinger, H. (2014). Understanding sexuality: Implications of Rubin for relationship research and clinical practice. *Sexual & Relationship Therapy*, *29*(4), 476-482. https://doi.org/10.1080/14681994.2014.941347

Perel, E. (2006). *Mating in captivity*. HarperCollins Publishers.

Peterson, F., Bley, J., & Frabotta, R. (2020). *The gender revolution & new sexual health: Celebrating unlimited diversity of the human sexuality hypercube.* Cognella Academic Publishing.

Robinson, M. (2013). Polyamory and monogamy as strategic identities. *Journal of Bisexuality, 13*(1), 21-38.

Rodrigues, D., Lopes, D., & Pereira, M. (2016). "We agree and now everything goes my way": Consensual sexual nonmonogamy, extradyadic sex, and relationship satisfaction. *CyberPsychology, Behavior & Social Networking*, *19*(6), 373-379. https://doi.org/10.1089/cyber.2016.0114

Roman, M., Charles, E., & Karasu, T. B. (1978). The value system of psychotherapists and changing mores. *Psychotherapy: Theory, Research, and Practice, 15*(4), 409-415.

Rubel, A. N., & Bogaert, A. F. (2015). Consensual nonmonogamy: Psychological well-being and relationship quality correlates. *Journal of Sex Research, 52*(9), 961-982.

Rubin, A. M., & Adams, J. R. (1986). Outcomes of sexually open marriages. *The Journal of Sex Research, 22*(3), 311-319.

Rubin, J. D., Moors, A. C., Matsick, J. L., Zeigler, A., & Conley, T. D. (2014). On the margins: Considering diversity among consensually non-monogamous relationships. *Journal für Psychologie, 22,* 1-23.

Schechinger, H. A., Sakaluk, J. K., & Moors, A. C. (2018). Harmful and helpful therapy practices with consensually non-monogamous clients: Toward an inclusive framework. *Journal of Consulting and Clinical Psychology, 86*(11), 879-891. https://doi.org/10.1037/ccp0000349

Seguin, L. J., Blais, M., Goyer, M., Adam, B. D., Lavoie, F., Rodrigue, C., & Magontier, C. (2016). Examining relationship quality across three types of relationship agreements. *Sexualities, 20*(1-2), 86-104.

Serina, A., Hall, M., Ciambrone, D., & Phua, V. (2013). Swinging around stigma: Gendered marketing of swingers' websites. *Sexuality & Culture, 17,* 348-359.

Sheff, E. (2005). Polyamorous women, sexual subjectivity, and power. *Journal of Contemporary Ethnography, 34*(3), 251-283.

Sheff, E. (2014, July 22). Seven forms of non-monogamy. *Psychology Today.* https://www.psychologytoday.com/us/blog/the-polyamorists-next-door/201407/7-different-kinds-non-monogamy

Sprott, R. A., Randall, A., Davison, K., Cannon, N., & Witherspoon, R. G. (2017). Alternative or nontraditional sexualities and therapy: A case report. *Journal of Clinical Psychology, 73*(8), 929-937.

Sue, D. W., Arredondo, P., & McDavis, R. J. (1992). Multicultural counseling competencies and standards: A call to the profession. *Journal of Counseling & Development, 70*(4), 477-486.

Sue, D. W., & Sue, D. (2003). *Counseling the culturally diverse*. Wiley.

Sue, D.W., & Sue, D. (2008). *Counseling the culturally diverse: Theory and practice* (5th ed.). Wiley.

Weitzman, G. (1999, March 12). What psychology professionals should know about polyamory: The lifestyles and mental health concerns of polyamorous individuals. [Web log post]. http://www.polyamory.org/~joe/polypaper.htm

Weitzman, G. (2006). Therapy with clients who are bisexual and polyamorous. *Journal of Bisexuality, 6*(1-2), 137-164.

Whitton, S. W., Weitbrecht, E. M., & Kuryluk, A, D. (2015). Monogamy agreements in male same-sex couples: Associations with relationship quality and individual well-being. *Journal of Couple & Relationship Therapy, 14*(1), 39-63.

Williams, D. J., & Prior, E. E. (2015). Contemporary polyamory: A call for awareness and sensitivity in social work. *Social Work, 60*(3), 268-270.

Woods, S. (2014, September 1). I heard someone describe compersion as "the opposite of jealousy." Huh? *Esquire, 162*(2), 76.

Yarber, W., & Sayad, B. (2010). *Human sexuality diversity in contemporary America* (8th ed.). McGraw Hill.

22

A Liberatory and Intersectional Approach to Sexual Health Care In Partnership With Disability Communities

Julie Lynn Williams

Love Poem to No-One in Particular
By Mark O'Brien
(Poet, activist, disabled, deceased; O'Brien, 1987)

let me touch you with my words
for my hands lie limp as empty gloves
let my words stroke your hair
slide down your back
and tickle your belly
for my hands, light and free flying as bricks
ignore my wishes and stubbornly refuse to carry out my quietest desires
let my words enter your mind
bearing torches
admit them willingly into your being
so they may caress you gently
within

Sex, sexuality, intimacy, and disability, the intersectional human experience that produces pervasive silence among the temporarily abled body (TAB) community (Goodley, 2011), and painful invisibility for those of us who are the disabled. Please note, this author intentionally does not use person-first language, but rather utilizes an identity-first stance reflecting her approach to proud claiming of disability, as it is beautiful. I am honored to write this chapter and utilize identity-first language in defiance of normative suffering language that implicitly suggests disability as an appendage (Andrews et al., 2019; Dunn & Andrews, 2015). This is a language choice that is widely debated both in the literature and in our communities; this author is aware that this is not everyone's stance and respects everyone's individual choice in language and thus, asks that this author's location be understood and respected.

Therefore, I write this chapter proudly identifying myself: I am Dwarf, Hard of Hearing, Queer, and Crip. I am crooked, asymmetrical, and I am dysfluent in movement. I am privileged too. I am White, economically advantaged, employed, and have had the privilege of access to education, healthcare, and more. The fact that I am alive is evidence of my privileges as a 54-year-old diastrophic dwarf. Put simply, I am.

That all being said, a chapter written from this author will indeed attempt to disrupt heteronormative sexual health narratives that have excluded and silenced members of the disability community and offer sexual educators and healthcare providers intersectional and liberatory approaches. This chapter does not accept that expertise lies in the hands of those without disabilities, nor assumes that members of disability community do not and cannot hold position in healthcare. And yet, it remains true that the presence of disability voices in positions of power in healthcare remains underrepresented. Therefore, this author offers a call out and a call in for continued cultivation and recruitment of members of the disability community into positions of administration and power within the healthcare arena. In the meantime, I humbly ask for nondisabled providers to begin to engage in critical analysis of our literature, interventions, and sexual health work for opportunities to dismantle and correct ableism and heteronormativity. I will offer my best attempt in this chapter.

In the pursuit of a liberatory and intersectional approach to sexual healthcare, this chapter will offer ideas on how to join "us" in these efforts to dismantle heteronormativity at both the systems level and direct individual intervention levels. To this end, postmodern concepts from Crip Theory, Liberation psychology, Feminist therapy and Disability-Affirmative Therapy (D-AT) will inform this chapter (Comas-Diaz & Torres Rivera, 2020; McRuer, 2006; Olkin, 2017). This chapter will unfold in the following manner: (a) Debunking and dismantling the grief/adjustment narrative; (b) Provider's impact and the do no harm imperative; (c) Diversity as intersectional; (d) Communities to know and learn from; (e) Interventions/education with partner, partners, and personal-care providers in mind; and (f) References along with additional resources for both practitioners and clients.

In general, sexuality is a term that is predominantly defined by images and narratives of beauty, and abilities privileging constructs such as symmetry, fluidness of movements, and sometimes unnatural almost superhuman sexual feats. Sexuality is also defined by performative expectation confined to constructs of physical intimacy, arousal, and orgasmic outcome. Sexuality framed in this way results in an erasure of asexuality as a viable sexual experience and a sexual life. Asexuality, as a sexual habit, does not preclude the need for ongoing sexual health care. Unfortunately, prevailing normative images and even heteronormative narratives also come with implicit messages of what is healthy, unhealthy, and the bodies that then represent these constructs. Normative parameters of what constitutes sexual functioning further marginalize the disability community, invariably excluding them from sexual health care, dialogues, and sometimes even placing labels of dysfunction and incompetence on them without evidence. Emancipation from these narratives is imperative to sexual health. It is the belief of this author that when oppressive narratives of normalcy are successfully dismantled, one finds the truth and pathway to the most profound liberatory experience necessary for sex positivity.

The human condition represents an intersectional and diverse experience that embodies culture, race, ethnicity, gender, and so many other aspects of what it means to be human. Thus, the pathway to sexual health and well-being is intersectional and diverse in and of itself. The journey to sexual health and wellbeing is informed by the individual's mind, body, spirit, and deepest desires. And yet, the disability experience is often impacted by prevailing historical disability models each of which has the opportunity to either promote or hinder disability liberation. Olkin (2017) reminds us often to collaboratively explore how disability models work with and against a person's well-being. A complete review of the disability models is beyond the scope of this chapter. Therefore, a review of Olkin's (2017) *Disability-Affirmative Therapy: A Case Formulation Template for Clients With Disabilities* is strongly recommended. To provide a very brief overview, however, prevailing disability models include the moral model, which locates disability around moral failing and/or assigned purpose and meaning; the medical model locates disability within the person and the pathology, thus emphasizing adjustment to and correction of disability; and the social model of disability locates disability as a function of social narratives that define "normal," and creates a society privileging able-bodiness. The corrective emphasis, then, focuses on systemic forces and efforts towards inclusion.

Unfortunately, disability models are often used in intervention settings with a focus on "adjustment" to disability, thus implicitly implying a shifting to some state of abnormality and away from a valued state of normalcy. This chapter, however, will challenge prevailing adjustment models, and instead offer contemporary disability liberatory justice models toward sexual healthcare. Approaches to sexual counseling that incorporate the narratives of, and expertise of, disability sexual freedom fighters will be highlighted here.

DEBUNKING AND DISMANTLING GRIEF/ADJUSTMENT MODELS

Typical adjustment models emphasize the impact of disability and/or illness or injury on sexual functioning. Framed in this way, adjustment is conceptualized as a process necessitated by a congenital condition or a change that has occurred that represents a deviation from "normal." A change or deviation then implicitly, if not explicitly, suggests a compromised state of health. As a result, understanding of disability, injury, or illness has resulted in an endless amount of literature offering therapeutic interventions to "help" facilitate acceptance and then adjustment to this abnormal state of being, without addressing the systemic, oppressive, and privileged lenses that shape heteronormative ableism.

The adjustment model may be well intentioned and initially serve a purpose for those newly disabled passing out of TAB status following acute onset of illness and injury. However, it also serves to perpetuate a model of normality, wholeness, and wellness. This potentially creates, if not prolongs, individual suffering. This author also argues that this leaves one more vulnerable in the long run to experience episodic relapsing sadness and distress as a function of exposure to able bodied and heteronormative comparative images and expectancies. If the disabled member is conceptualized as needing to adjust to something that takes away normalcy, it is harder to come out of that in order to then cultivate a sustainable sense of health and well-being without imposing some need for reconciliation known as grief. Additionally, a frame such as this may not be readily inclusive of those who are born with disabilities who have known no other way of "being" and yet have been showered with the normative narrative.

In regard to sexuality and disability, Drexler (2018) refers to the normative narratives as pervasive heteronormative frames that marginalize and silence the voices of disability. She further writes that the heteronormative frames need to be disrupted by nonheteronormative constructs, and offers a reframing of disability sexuality as queer and that which does not conform to heteronormativity and offers liberation.

The typical adjustment narrative is illustrated in the writing of Gill and Hough (2007) who state that acute illness and/or injury can "have profound effects on sexual functioning" (p. 224). They go on to describe an adjustment process that begins with adaptation towards "recovery of lost functions or an improvement of changed functions." It is this very narrative that colludes with the normative framing and then necessitates the adjustment and grief intervention. However, if sexuality was understood as a varied experience, recovery and improvements in functions would not be the expectancies. Rather, the life after onset of disability would be framed as one of discovery and a broadening of one's understanding of sexuality and ability. Consequently, our services need to be targeted in such a way to mitigate heteronormative systemic forces that contribute to the pain and existential suffering that is often experienced in this limited scope of service provision.

As a liberatory act of resistance against unnecessary grief and adjustment, this author puts forward the call to provide interventions that promote awareness of these systemic heteronormative narratives as causes of grief. As such, there is a need to train providers to engage in a journey of discovery towards an unapologetic claiming of one's body as is. Sonya Renee Taylor (2018) stated this beautifully in her work, *The Body is Not an Apology*. The unapologetic sexual liberation of the disabled body is further exemplified in the works *Sins Invalid* (Berne, 2013) and *Disability After Dark* (http://www.andrewgurza.com/homepage). Contemporary disability justice movements suggest adjustment would no longer be a construct if normative models that shroud the sexual experience were exposed, dismantled, and destroyed.

Disability encompasses a vast range of experiences. Therefore, it becomes important for providers to be versed in medical terminology, medical procedures, and related treatments to better understand the disability context. This means that providers need to get used to researching and taking opportunities to engage in ongoing consultations and trainings that review medical treatments. In doing so, providers can be further prepared to challenge the medicalization of the disabled body, and to deepen the therapeutic alliance with disabled clients who often feel burdened with "educating" nondisabled and nonmedical clinicians. Additionally, the ongoing training allows providers to be prepared for the potential for coexisting psychological issues, trauma being a critical construct. For example, for the newly disabled individual and chronically ill individual, posttraumatic stress disorder (PTSD) may be present as a result of the acute medical crisis, ongoing medical crises, intrusive treatment procedures, or the nature of the traumatic injury, resulting in the need for specific treatment for trauma-related psychological needs as well.

Trauma, connected to and subsequently triggered by physical touch, has relevance to intimacy of touch following not only sexual and physical assaults but can also be present as a consequence of medical procedures and intimate personal care services. The presence of trauma should not be confined to the idea of medical maltreatment of inappropriate medical or personal care assistance. Trauma as a byproduct or response to medical procedures and personal care services that are life-saving, necessary, and appropriately done with consent, can nevertheless still be very traumatic. The functions of intense and frequent pain, heightened feelings of exposure and vulnerability, and the duration associated with ongoing medical interventions and personal care routine(s) can be trauma-inducing.

The works of Peter Levine, stemming from his revolutionary book *Waking the Tiger: Healing Trauma* (1997), are highly recommended by this author, as they expand our understanding of trauma. He offers very specific interventions for facilitating healing from trauma, including traumatic medical experiences as they are relevant to sexual intimacy and possibly triggered by intimacy. His work speaks to the importance of understanding the impact of trauma as both a mind-body experience, therefore, interventions need to be targeted via a duality approach. He very boldly posits that healing from trauma cannot be sustained with talk therapy only. Sex educators and clinicians working with disabled communities are advised to practice intentional and consistent ongoing trauma assessments. A template is offered at the end of this chapter to guide providers to incorporate an expanded assessment of trauma that is congruent with unique nuances of medical and personal care-related trauma responses. Trauma that is intrusive and disruptive must be consistently assessed at initial treatment planning sessions. This will determine if trauma work needs to be included in order to appreciate the impact of trauma on sexual health care work and timing of, and order of, treatment.

Sexual abuse is another universal assessment and treatment concern. The disability literature has covered the high rates of sexual abuse within the disability community. For sake of space, and avoidance of not appropriate coverage of all matters involved in sexual abuse, this chapter will not address treatment issues when sexual abuse is present. This author has written in previous works on this and offers providers to reference Williams and Colvin's (2016) chapter, "Coming Together to End Violence Against Women and Girls With Disabilities" which can be found in Miles-Cohen and Signore's edited book *Eliminating Inequities for Women with Disabilities: An Agenda for Health and Wellness*.

This author utilizes a disability-affirmative theoretical (D-AT) approach (Olkin, 2017) when working with clients who have disabilities. As conceptualized by Olkin, D-AT is considered a pan theoretical postmodern critical theory in which disability is incorporated into the case conceptualization in such a way to neither "underestimate" nor "over-inflate" (p. 3) the role disability has played in one's life and find the ways in which disability has informed the individual's life narrative. D-AT is also informed by disability studies, the tenets of feminist therapy, the independent living movement, and the importance of the specific culture of the client. D-AT case conceptualization is developed from an intake process that explores nine areas:

1. The developmental history of the individual (and family) and how disability affected the history;
2. The current sequelae of disability, with an emphasis on pain, fatigue, sleep, and falls;
3. Models of disability (moral, medical, social, biopsychosocial) of the individual, the parents, the partners, and the therapists;
4. Disability in the context of other demographic and cultural variables;
5. The disability culture and community, and the client's knowledge of and interface with this culture and community;
6. How disability affected the person's current social interactions;
7. The experience of microaggressions and the person's responses to these experiences;
8. The management of affective prescriptions (mourning, cheerfulness, bravery) and prohibitions (anger);
9. Current intimacy (sexuality, partnership relationships) and disability within the context of those relationships. (Olkin, 2017, p.5)

PROVIDERS IMPACT AND ROLE: DO NO HARM AND MOVE YOURSELVES OUT OF THE WAY

Providers have a critical role to play as a sojourner to sexual health and ultimately to sexual freedoms within the disability community. To do so in such a way that embodies the guiding ethical principal, "do no harm," providers must first engage in their own essential self-reflections on sexuality and disability. These essential tasks involve becoming clear as to their own intersectional location to sex, sexuality, and sexual health and disability. The silence around sex is real. It remains largely taboo, leaving many to fend for themselves, and this is true particularly within the disability community. The exclusion of disability in sexual health must be addressed before initiation of services by providers. Understanding the diversity of sexual narratives among the disability community can be found in the disability studies literature and in research methodology that has taken a narrative approach.

This author strongly encourages practitioners to start with the work of Drexler (2018), who described the use of ethnographic analysis to better understand oppression of sexual experiences of those with developmental disabilities. Ethnography is an approach to discovery that "seeks to investigate, document and explain culture and structure as manifested in behaviour" (Bressers et al., 2020, p. 226). Drexler's ethnographic research exposed the framing of disability and sexuality in heteronormative themes and by those who have power over disability communities. Drexler referred to examples of this in the *DSM-5* where diagnostic labels are framed as pathological and deviant. Many in the field of disability liberation, yours truly included, argue that it is not enough to be well intentioned. Well-intentioned providers are all drinking the Kool-Aid too and must engage in due diligence as to what they believe and what they have ascribed to when it comes to sex and disability. Sex gets wrapped up into religion, morality, pleasure, pain, and more. When providers are not members of a disability community and sexually diverse communities, the risk of harm is uniquely driven by privileged lenses. Critical analysis as offered by Feminist literature and worldview is needed to look at and disrupt language and practices that convey ableism, homophobia, and misogynistic parameters.

Common beliefs about sexuality and disability are far from liberatory. Many hold the belief that sexuality in disability is perverted. Hence, disability groups are questioned and policed for their sexual urges and feelings. Disabled individuals are questioned more readily and without evidence as to their competence to be a parent, and therefore, exists the manifestation of a belief that disabled should not procreate or be parents. Women with disability are questioned as to their competence around sexuality while at the same time not being offered consistent "well woman" sexual health check-ups. And finally, forced sterilizations are still being performed, more often to women of color with disabilities as well as certain disability groups.

Furthermore, information about sexuality in disability literature is largely about sexual abuse and rarely about sexual pleasure and sexual health. That is not to say that awareness and ongoing work is still needed to better understand, prevent, and support those who are victims and survivors of sexual assaults and abuse. This author devoted a good part of their career prioritizing awareness and interventions, bridging gaps in system care and interventions within disability systems and sexual violence prevention systems. Those efforts are still needed, but when the work stops there at abuse, the focus of care becomes protective and even unintentionally sex prohibitive, lacking in promoting autonomy and sexual expression that is pleasurable and desired.

Disability sexual literature that is inclusive of sexual diversity is also limited. See Olkin for an extensive list of LGBTQ and disability-related articles (Olkin, 2017, pp. 177-179). Olkin offers that disparate coverage of segmented disability groups creates the perception of more valued groups within disability communities (e.g., the proliferation of information regarding sexual health and function available for and about men with disabilities). There is a greater amount of information about spinal cord injuries then other disability groups such as congenital disability groups. The disability hierarchy suggests that disparate research and interventions goes to more valued members in a disability community (e.g., those with acquired disabilities, and those that are seen as previously "able;" therefore, those that hold aspects of ability privilege and value as opposed to disability groups representing congenital disabilities). Disabilities considered invisible disabilities (e.g., those with severe psychiatric disabilities, intellectual differences, and Deaf community members, among others) experience harsher attitudinal judgments from society, like being incompetent, resulting in sexual and reproductive prohibitions.

As we can see, sexual literature is again pervasively based on normative paradigms of sexuality as defined by stages of physiological arousal. Consequently, sexual differences become labeled sexual dysfunction very easily. Asexuality is not even a "thing" in most sexual health conversations. The term is often used as evidence of sexual dysfunction rather than explored as a possible choice and/or sexual difference based on physiological sensations.

Disability alone often creates what has been referred to as an existential angst within providers. It is the one minority status one can acquire at any time; therefore, providers may be confronted with very real reminders as to physical, emotional, and mental vulnerabilities. As a provider, tremendous power to intentionally or unintentionally define and even pathologize disability at the intersection of sexuality is more than a slippery slope. Hence, providers need to consider biases they may hold against and about disability. Implicit biases measurement scales, and even disability attitudinal scales are available which offer providers an opportunity to sit with and challenge their fears and biases (e.g., Harvard Implicit Association Tests: https://implicit.harvard.edu/implicit/takeatest.html).

In sum, providers – be they medical, psychological, and/or sex educators – must do their personal work to avoid doing harm. Diversity training is a must for anyone who will be embarking on a journey working with the disability communities. Moreover, it is recommended that disability as diversity training be sought out that has been written and conceptualized by members of the disability community (Andrews, 2020; Williams, 2019).

DIVERSITY: INTERSECTIONALITY, LIBERATION PSYCHOLOGY, AND FEMINIST THEORY

Diversity is a term that is bandied about with assumed understandings. Typically, diversity is conceptualized as needing to be aware of multiple identity variables such as race, gender, ethnicity, and ability to name just a few. This author will offer that diversity needs to extend beyond a brief benign appreciation of difference as things to learn and value. Rather, diversity consideration must be centered around social and political constructs that inform lived diverse experience. Understanding diverse experiences is not just about understanding different experiences, but it is also about understanding how context as driven by social political forces then creates suffering and does so in varying ways exerting power and taking power. Intersectionality is more than the concept of multiculturalism and multiple identities. Intersectionality refers to the increasing invisibility and erasure of individuals as they hold multiple identities that are devalued (Crenshaw. 1989). It is the synergistic impact of multiple systemic-isms. Providers, therefore, need to appreciate the quote and zeitgeist behind it from feminist writers and therapists: "the personal is political" (Hanisch, 1970). Sexual diversity and gender fluidity are critically important to all humans. Sexual health, education, policies, and more are impacted by heteronormative beliefs. We saw in the year 2019 into 2020 the dangerous impacts of sexual reproductive rights with reduced funding to planned parenthood agencies in the United States (Planned Parenthood Action Fund, 2021). And there are no exceptions for the disability community. Reproductive rights, access to sexual healthcare, forced sterilizations, and policing of sexual behaviors are inherent systemically in disability communities (Krase, 2014).

And yet, we are still in the early stages of understanding, accepting, and celebrating disability as an intersectional diversity variable. The idea that disabled people have sex and have sexual rights is still not fully understood or even appreciated. In 2006, McRuer blew the lid off the pot when he introduced his book *Crip Theory: Cultural Signs of Queerness and Disability*. The use of the term Crip represents a political taking back of the term Cripple, which parallels empowerment theories associated with feminism, queerness, and African American and Latinx cultural movements. McRuer dismantled the ways in which majority culture cultivates the body, sexual identities, and even pleasure in such a way to dominate and make disability as an identity invisible while pathologizing the disability sexual narrative. He spoke to the shared experiences of disability sexuality at the intersections of heterosexism and the coming out process experienced by LGBT communities. And finally, he highlighted the function of invisibility of disability as an identity variable and how it serves to maintain the dominant culture's emphasis on disability as a medical abnormality.

The work of Rohmer and Louvet (2009) painfully illustrated this concept using cartoon images of children gendered as girl or boy and then as Black or White and disabled or nondisabled. The salience as an erasure of disability was made evident with the figure in a wheelchair versus on a bicycle. When participants were asked to describe what they saw, the cartoon figures depicting boy, girl, Black, White child when in a wheelchair were described in one note, disabled or handicapped. All other aspects of the individual were no longer named. Disability, and more specifically the implicit biases held by research participants about disability, resulted in the erasure of the wholeness of the figure.

Understanding diversity therefore, as more than just difference, is critically important to the work of sex educators and providers.

McRuer along with other sexual freedom writers in the Crip community reclaim the narrative of disability and embrace constructs and understanding of queerness as an opportunity to disrupt sexual oppression and to liberate. That being said, the sexual revolution within disability is still new to many and certainly almost absent in sexual health curriculums and provider training. Consequently, the disabled person who is "straight" and, even more so, the Queer Crip has limited access to sexual health support.

However, there is indeed a groundswell of support and education that is happening via a community of disability justice forward thinkers. Cripping the Queer, Feminist Queer Crip, and Black Feminist Crip literature has opened doors to sexual diversity dialogues. Providers often have no idea who these people are and yet they do need to become aware. After all, Garland-Thompson (2002) offers that bringing together disability studies and feminist theory can expand and further develop our wholistic appreciation of the body, sexual narratives, and more. She states, "Feminist disability theory augments the terms and confronts the limits of the ways we understand human diversity, the materiality of the body, multiculturalism, and the social formations that interpret bodily differences" (Garland-Thompson, 2002, p. 16).

COMMUNITIES TO LEARN FROM AND UNIVERSAL SHARED UNDERSTANDINGS

Crips and Crip Theory is concerned with the ways in which neoliberal capitalism (the dominant economic and cultural system as driven by market priorities) has imagined and composed sexual and embodied identities (Bennett, 2007). One example of the communities and projects that represent this powerful reclaiming of the disabled body can be found at Sins Invalid. The description of the effort/project is best described in the words taken directly from Sins website:

> Sins Invalid is a disability justice based performance project that incubates and celebrates artists with disabilities, centralizing artists of color, and LGBTQ / gender variant artists as communities who have been historically marginalized. Led by disabled people of color. Sins Invalid's work explores the themes of sexuality, embodiment and the disabled body, developing provocative work where paradigms of "normal" and "sexy" are challenged offering instead a vision of beauty and sexuality inclusive of all bodies and communities. (https://www.sinsinvalid.org/mission)

Sex educators should also be aware of disability justice work and specific people who are leading this work. For example, No Body Is Disposable is disability justice work of disabled people of color, queer, trans, and gender nonconforming. The names and voices of disability justice activists, writers, and freedom fighters include but are not limited to Patty Berne, Stacey Milbern, Eli Clare, Sebastian Margaret, and Mia Mingus. No Body Is Disposable is a video series providing disability justice tools for activists, educators, and students. Sex educators and providers who are committed to truly understanding the sociopolitical forces that impact and lead to denials of sexual freedoms need to include this work in their training.

Breaking Silences is a community of individuals formed in Ohio who come together as a collective and at the intersections of our multiple identities. This collective formed out of two conferences held to honor sexual freedoms and the work of many who bravely shared their Crip and Queerness, their expertise, and lived experiences at the Breaking Silences 2015 and 2017 conferences (Breaking Silences, Demanding Crip Justice: Sex, Sexuality, and Disability).

From these communities and with intersectionality and liberation being the approach, the author offers the following universal understandings impacting the disability community.

Universal Understandings

1. Sex inclusivity is absent in sex education curriculums and sex care work; thus, recognizing this gap and incorporating it is paramount. Sex inclusivity in disability community means the celebration of all minds and bodies.
2. The medicalization of the body is a shared experience among the disabled, gay, trans, and gender variant communities.
3. Sex educators need to understand intersecting experiences such as pain, fatigue, mobility differences, medication side effects, and fluctuations in disability states as varied narratives, not as variance from normal.
4. Correcting and fixing of disability/individuals/what? is not the path to sexual freedom.
5. Reproductive rights and parenting rights are particularly threatened in the disability community. Therefore, sex educators and providers need to be ready to support and advocate when rights are being violated.
6. The Queer Crip may experience heightened isolation which can increase vulnerability to experience internalized shame. Thus, promoting discovery of these communities and access to disability justice communities mentioned above is a must.
7. There are laws and disability-related offices that at times govern and impact aspects of sexual freedoms around procreation and even consensual sex in residential congregate living facilities. Sex educators and providers need to stay current on each state's regulations and aware of agencies that have power of these decisions (e.g., developmental disability offices, adult protective services). More importantly, be aware of and willing to act as an advocate and support activism in promoting sexual freedoms and sexual rights.
8. Sexual abuse does not happen to all disabled individuals; however, the rates of abuse are high. Therefore, it is important to understand the unique ways and locations of sexual predators. Bridging the gap between disability agencies and sexual violence experts will often fall on the provider and sex educator who is working with the disability community.

Case Application

As the author of this chapter, I want to thank everyone who has honored me with their reparative journeys. The case offered below is not taken from any one person's narrative. The work between therapist and client is too sacred for that. Therefore, for teaching purposes a case narrative has been created with contributions, additions, and subtractions from members of the Crip community and my chosen family.

Client presents as self-identified, Cisgender woman with Spina Bifida and ambulates using a power chair. She is 30 years old, Black, Queer, and presents with depressed and anxious mood. Client requests that She, Her, and Hers pronouns be used and that she identifies as Queer. Client is ready to explore deeper connections with her body, with others, and very much wants to be a mother. Her depression and anxiety come from feelings of uncertainty and fears of rejection from the disability community, the gay community, and Black community.

Client was referred by her primary care medical provider who wrote reason for referral as adjustment to disability. Nothing else. At time of first contact, client expressed irritation and mistrust. Client also expressed surprise that therapist was disabled and commented on disability justice images and quotes all over office. Client expressed "wow, this is a first." When asked what she meant, she said "a doctor with a disability." My response is often, "I am both honored and sad that I am your first disabled therapist."

The informed consent process is modeled to a degree from feminist theorist Laura Brown, explaining in detail the therapeutic approach as well as roles and responsibilities. My clients are offered opportunity to interview "me" as a worthy therapist. What do you need to know about me, my work, and how I approach therapy to offer and create a safe and inclusive environment? To this the client was surprised. I offered to this client my manifesto. I am Professor, Psychologist, Queer, Crip, Hard of Hearing, Dwarf . . . Unapologetic; I will celebrate and honor all minds, all bodies, and all forms of love that is consensual and I strive towards creating a world that is disability liberated. Client smiled and relaxed, offering consent to continue and a willingness "to give it a try."

The typical background information was gathered but for purposes of this chapter, the author will focus in on central issues of intimacy, intersectionality of multiple identities, sexuality, and struggles with incontinence issues during sexual moments.

On initial interview client states that she has never seen a gynecologist or talked with her bowel and bladder specialists about her concern. Consequently, she has practiced secrecy and gone to great lengths to hide and often avoid intimacy. She also shares having very little contact with people who share her intersections as a Black Queer disabled woman. She describes often feeling alone in disability communities, Queer communities, and Black communities. She has not found "home."

She shared that her "education" regarding sexuality was through her mother, who quietly told her that it would take a "very, very special man" to love her. Client remembers perceiving this as "code" for it's NEVER going to happen and if it does, she better accept whoever as a "blessing" and take what she can get because he would be doing her a favor. Client was 14 years old and was beginning to have questions about her sexual preferences and desires. Her sexual vocabulary was limited to gay, queer, straight, and/or bisexual. At that time, she wanted to know more and yet struggled with feelings of shame.

Client also shared that she began her menstrual period at age 13, and shortly after beginning her period she was seen by her lifelong pediatrician who gave her a clean bill of health, patting her on the shoulder and commenting on how she was growing up. However, while client was getting dressed, client's pediatrician began talking with her mother about "long term" planning and the need to seriously consider implications of unwanted pregnancy, genetic transmission, and parenting demands if client became pregnant. Without talking to the client, pediatrician gave mother a number for the nearest university hospital genetic counseling center for people with genetic disabilities. Client remembers hearing the pediatrician say, "They can help you with this."

After the "talk" with her mother and this appointment, she remembers being very confused, anxious, and embarrassed. However, at the time of initial work with therapist, many years later, she was now expressing her anger. She vented to therapist how she had learned nothing about her body or sexual feelings. She was never offered the opportunity to meet with a gynecologist; nor was there any information offered about "safer sex" and/or reproductive choices. It was assumed she would avoid any opportunity to have children. And yet, client very much wanted to be a mother and have her own child.

The client secretly spent years yearning to know more about her body and began searching the web for information; Some was good and some was not so good or helpful. The therapist conceptualized and implemented an integrative approach that included a feminist, liberatory, and Disability-Affirmative approach. Consistent with all these theories, the therapist consistently frames therapy and interventions as "options" and choices – the goal being to create a space where client could find her narrative, her choices, her joy, and ultimately her personal agency.

When initiating care, the therapist offered interventions along 4 vectors as power lines to her center where something got "interrupted" or "erased" or "taken" and needs to be reclaimed. From here, interventions were then implemented, with the client's collaboration and choice as to the related interventions. The four vectors and connected strategies are listed and described below.

1. Information: This process involves exploring who, what, where, and when did you learn about your body, your identities, sex, and sexuality. And then, questions are offered – "Who did you believe? Who hurt you and who have you possibly secretly resisted? What do you want to know? Information is power and offers a pathway to not only know your body and your options but to find your communities and that place you can call 'home'." This involved connecting the client to "disability friendly" gynecologists, specialists in urological care, and reproductive specialists to explore her desire to "make a baby." Moreover, researching with client intersectional communities and exploring readiness to connect, weighing the pros and cons. Finally, dialogues with the client around shared identity variables and those not shared were had. As a White, Queer, Dwarf, I engage in dialogues around the impact of my privileges and power in the room as a means to name it and invite a deepening of trust and respect.
2. Reparation was offered in an effort to acknowledge and to apologize for the lack of information, the assumptions made, and the complete erasure of her intersections as a Black, Queer, Disabled Woman. The reparation was in response to the frequent misinformation that was given to the client about her body's ability to carry a baby to full term; that methods to assist her incontinence can come in the form of getting the correct information from appropriate medical providers and then processing that in session. Reparation was also offered in the form of validation as normalization; shared experiences with other disability community members and again revisiting readiness to connect to forums that are disability liberatory in celebration of our community. Reparation in the use of "Crip Humor" can be healing and empowering, as one is given space to laugh at the limited Able-Bodied experience and their inability to see "our" bodies as liberated with more options, more freedoms, and creativity of living. This humor is not self-deprecating humor but rather humor that weakens the power of ableistic rhetoric about disability and sexuality. Reparative healing can also come from the disability literature as Bibliotherapy. This author uses disability written works, Crip-affirming photography, unapologetic images, and films that share disability sexual liberators and activists. A series of questions and suggestions was offered by this author: Did you ever hear of. . . .? Would you like to borrow this book, movie, or poetry and look up these individuals? Bring your questions to the next session and then let's decide what you will do with these names and ideas towards body liberation and celebration of all bodies.
3. Resistance as a healing construct as well as an empowerment construct is a critical component of intersectional liberatory work. This began in vector one, simply as an introduction to Queer Crip communities who practice and offer forums for disability congruent self-care, and discussions on disability burnout as not "your fault" but the impact of systemic ongoing "erasure." Resistance ultimately becomes unpacked in the realizing and experiencing of pleasure that has often been demonized and ableized at the intersections of Disability, Queerness, Race, and more.
4. Reclamation of the client's body and pleasure came as a combination of finding communities, getting answers that allowed choices around procreation, and ultimately the realization of this desire. Moreover, a deeper connection with a shared and chosen disability community pride allowed for sustained power to continue to navigate a world that is systemically unable to see, celebrate, and support those at the intersections of queerness, disability, race, and gender. By joining online the virtual or in-person disability liberated forums, groups, and dating sites, the client empowered herself to form long-standing friendships and intimate partnerships that serve her well as a buffering system to maintain her power and joy. She has found her home.

Interventions and Prep Work

1. First of all, do not overcomplicate it and yet do not oversimplify it either. As providers who are engaging with good intentions and striving to honor intersectionality, they must strive to maintain the posture of cultural humility and this ought to be a constant dialectic of self-reflective work (Hook et al., 2017). Providers must remember that this is a necessary journey of constantly addressing personally held beliefs and biases about disability and sexuality. The literal expectation of "cultural competence" can serve to impede the actual interventions, as fears of doing it wrong and being politically correct can begin to drive a false sense of "knowing." Hook et al. offer case examples on how to perhaps approach a paradigm shift from cultural competence to an emphasis on personal accountability for lifelong learning and cultural humility instead. Their work embodies what this author considers an honest "leaning in" in clinical supervision and in consultation with colleagues. In sum, they offer a pathway towards how to sustain a posture of humility that doesn't detract from clinical competence but rather enhances competence as it promotes authenticity, in a way that does not suggest settling for inadequate cultural inclusivity. Their work, while not focused on sexual liberation per se, is congruent with breaking taboos and silence, and this provides fertile ground for intersectional and liberatory interventions along with healing.
2. Breathe, and begin practicing ongoing centering-work in whatever way works for you. Specifically, continue to engage in ongoing, compassionate, self-reflective work around your location to sexuality, sex, and disability. Please remember, disability and sexuality are two "things" we all have a location in and potential community membership. Disability is one variable as a function of life, aging, and circumstances, and we can find ourselves members of the disability community at any time throughout our life course. If that day has not arrived at the time of this writing, this author will be waiting with others to welcome you. Our personal lived experiences do not magically leave the clinical room. We bring them into the room and these constructs are forever evolving as we age and develop interpersonally. Our awareness of our boundaries allow us to better center on our clients' needs.
3. Intersectional inclusivity and disability-affirmative work is personal and political. This is not a new idea (Hanisch, 1970). The work begins with your understanding of the context that informs the disability sexual experience.

   Your office layout, whether virtual or in real time, matters too. Right now, try it. Put down this reading and enter your "working" space; take a look around your session room and overall office space. Do not forget to include scrutiny of your virtual space. Ask yourself the hard questions: Who and what does it represent? Who and what is not represented in your décor, pictures, books, and more? Do not forget to think about your entryways, hallways, waiting areas, and bathrooms. Are they accessible, safe, and universal? Finding evidence of your erasure(s) is hard as a function of privileges and implicit biases. We are all drinking the Kool-Aid and we all have them. Therefore, calling on others across differing cultures and disabilities (after you have taken your initial steps to develop your awareness as you examine the spaces you offer services in) is recommended. This is a suggestion for disabled professionals as well, as "we" are not exempt from holding our own assumptions. Once this is done, fix the errors, and continue to engage yourself and the experts from diverse disability community members in this process annually, or as new awarenesses are discovered. Now. (Benton & Overtree, 2012; In the Office . . . Creating a LBG friendly environment: http://www.lesbianhealthinfo.org/community/in_office.htm)
4. Intersectional inclusivity continues in the form of your process, intake forms, and your website. Take a look at your forms. Are they inclusive? How is gender, race, ability, pronouns,

sexuality, and more conveyed? This author incorporates the templates offered by Dr. Laura Brown (http://www.drlaurabrown.com/services/) in the development of her consent for treatment process, as well as Olkin's (2017) templates (D-AT case sample, Chapter 13, pp. 187-197) in her approach to the initial meeting with a client, and has also recently begun to use Olkin's D-AT case template for note taking (p. 189). Reviewing these materials is encouraged.

5. Intersectional inclusivity continues into the sexual history process and what this author likes to refer to as the sexual history dialogue as opposed to "intake," which is a term that feels intrusive, sterile, and cold. Please see the end of this chapter for specific suggestions for inclusivity as reflected in domains to cover, including suggested phrasing, which ought to be shifted and modified in collaboration with your clients.
6. Consider carefully how you approach the intervention, and frame the intervention as a collaborative, discovery process. Perhaps offering the words, "We will find the answers together."
7. Consider your conceptualization of trauma to be intersectional and inclusive to disability. See the end of the chapter for suggestions on trauma specific domains.

CONCLUSION

If you have made it to this paragraph, congratulations. You have reached the end of this author's musings. However, this chapter is certainly not the totality of what is available, but rather, is this author's take on what is available. The author hopes if you were motivated to read this chapter, that you continue to dive deeper into the work of promoting sexual freedoms within the disability community and in partnership with the disability community. There is much work to be done and much more to repair. This author offers a special message to members of the disability community: listen carefully. Please take note and lean in. If you are new to your disability and the disability community, and/or newly finding your disability identity, welcome to the army of those who are fighting to break silences, end the taboos, and promote sexual liberation for all of us while honoring all parts that come together to make us who we are as wholistic and beautiful beings. In this Crip community you will find fierce opinions, passion, love, and compassion, and if you are not already on it – the ride of a fucking lifetime. Most importantly, you are not alone and you are loved.

To our allies . . . hang in there, listen and learn, and know when to get out of our way. Walk, sit, and roll with us, not for us.

Peace out and solidarity.

REFERENCES

Andrews, E. (2020). *Disability as diversity: Developing cultural competence.* Oxford University Press.

Andrews, E. E., Forber-Pratt, A. J., Mona, L. R., Lund, E. M., Pilarski, C. R., & Balter, R. (2019). #SaytheWord: A disability culture commentary on the erasure of "disability." *Rehabilitation Psychology, 64*(2), 111-118. https://doi.org/10.1037/rep0000258

Bennett, A. (2007) A review of queer theory. *Disability Studies Quarterly, 27*(4). ISSN: 2159-8371 (Online); 1041-5718 (Print).

Benton, J., & Overtree, C. (2012). Multicultural office design: A case example. *Professional Psychology: Research and Practice, 43*, 265-269.

Berne, P. (Director). (2013). *Sins invalid: An unashamed claim to beauty* [Film]. New Day Films. https://www.sinsinvalid.org/documentary

Bressers, G., Brydges, M., Paradis, E. (2020). Ethnography in health professions education: Slowing down and thinking deeply. *Medical Education, 54*(3), 225-233. https://doi.org/10.1111/medu.14033

Comas-Díaz, L., & Torres Rivera, E. (Eds.). (2020). *Liberation psychology: Theory, method, practice, and social justice.* American Psychological Association. https://doi.org/10.1037/0000198-000

Crenshaw, K. (1989). Demarginalizing the intersection of race and sex: A Black feminist critique of antidiscrimination doctrine, feminist theory and antiracist politics. *University of Chicago Legal Forum, Vol. 1989, Article 8.* http://chicagounbound.uchicago.edu/uclf/vol1989/iss1/8

Drexler, O. (2018). Disability and queerness: Exploration of disability and sexuality in autoethnography and institutional ethnography. *Michigan Sociological Review, 32,* 133-147.

Dunn, D. S., & Andrews, E. E. (2015). Person-first and identity-first language: Developing psychologists' cultural competence using disability language. *The American Psychologist, 70*(3), 255-263. https://doi.org/10.1037/a0038636

Garland-Thompson, R. (2002) Integrating disability: Transforming feminist theory. *NWSA Journal, 14*(3), 1-32. http://www.jstor.org/stable/4316922

Gill, K., & Hough, S. (2007). Sexual health of people with chronic illness and disability. In L. VandeCreek, F. L. Peterson, & J. W. Bley (Eds.), *Innovations in clinical practice: Focus on sexual health* (pp. 223-244). Professional Resource Press.

Goodley, D. (2011). *Disability studies: An interdisciplinary introduction.* SAGE

Hanisch, C. (1970). The personal is political. In S. Firestone & A. Koedt (Eds.), *Notes from the second year: Women's liberation.* Radical Feminism.

Hollenbach, A. D , Eckstrand, K. L., & Dreger, A. D. (Eds.). (2014). *Implementing curricular and institutional climate changes to improve health care for individuals who are LGBT, gender nonconforming, or born with DSD: A resource for medical educators* [Report by the AAMC Advisory Committee on Sexual Orientation, Gender Identity, and Sex Development]. Association of American Medical Colleges.

Hook, J. N., Davis, D., Owen, J., & DeBlaere, C. (2017). *Cultural humility: Engaging diverse identities in therapy.* American Psychological Association.

Kaufman, M., Silverberg, C., & Odette, F. (2007). *The ultimate guide to sex and disability.* Cleis Press Inc.

Krase, (2014, October 1). History of forced sterilization and current U.S. abuses. *Our Bodies Ourselves.* http:www.ourbodiesourselves.org/health-info/forced-sterilization

Levine, P. (1997). *Waking the tiger: Healing trauma.* North Atlantic Books.

Loeser, C., Pini, B., & Crowley, V. (2018). Disability and sexuality: Desires and pleasures. *Sexualities, 21*(3), 255-270. https://doi.org/10.1177/1363460716688682

McRuer, R. (2006). *Crip theory: Cultural signs of queerness and disability.* New York University Press.

McRuer, R., & Mollow, A. (2012). *Sex and disability.* Duke University Press.

O'Brien, M. (1987). Love poem to no-one in particular. Retrieved from *Guide to the Mark O'Brien papers 1968-1999.* Collection number BANC MSS 99/247c. The Bancroft Library, University of California, Berkeley.

O'Brien, M. (2020). Using an inclusive, sex-positive, gender-neutral approach to taking sexual histories. *JAMA Internal Medicine, 180*(3), 469. https://doi.org/10.1001/jamainternmed.2019.6726

Olkin, R. (2017). *Disability affirmative therapy: A case formulation template for clients with disabilities.* Oxford University Press.

Planned Parenthood Action Fund. (2021). Medicaid and reproductive health. https://www.plannedparenthoodaction.org/issues/health-care-equity/medicaid-and-reproductive-health

Rohmer, O., & Louvet, E. (2009). Describing persons with disability: Salience of disability, gender and ethnicity. *Rehabilitation Psychology, 54*(1), 76-82.

Schmidt, E. (2019). *Usability and feasibility of an enhanced sexual health education program for individuals with intellectual and developmental disabilities* [Doctoral Dissertation, Ohio State University]. OhioLINK Electronic Theses and Dissertations Center. http://rave.ohiolink.edu/etdc/view?acc_num=osu1574716076209766

Schmidt, E. K., Brown, C., & Darragh, A. (2019). A scoping review of sexual health education interventions for individuals with intellectual and developmental disabilities. *Sexuality and Disability, 38,* 439-453. https://doi.org/10.1007/s11195-019-09593-4

Taylor, S. R. (2018). *The body is not an apology: The power of radical self-love.* Berrett-Koehler Publishers.

Tordoff, D. M., Haley, S. G., Shook, A., Kantor, A., Crouch, J. M., & Ahrens, K. (2021). "Talk about bodies": Recommendations for using transgender-inclusive language in sex education curricula. *Sex Roles, 84,* 152-165. https://doi.org/10.1007/s11199-020-01160-y

Williams, J. (2019). Disability as an intersectional diversity variable in the psychology curriculum. In J. A. Mena & K. Quina (Eds.), *Integrating multiculturalism and intersectionality into the psychology curriculum: Strategies for instructors* (pp. 157-168). American Psychological Association.

Williams, J., & Colvin, L. (2016). Coming together to end violence against women and girls with disabilities. In S. E. Miles-Cohen & C. Signore (Eds.), *Eliminating inequities for women with disabilities: An agenda for health and wellness* (243-262). American Psychological Association.

Selected Resources

This is not an all-inclusive list; it has been prepared to acknowledge the potential wealth of information and to motivate the reader to continue the search for personalized information.

*Websites**

Aging and Sexuality Resource Guide (edited by Dr. Antoinette Zeiss)
https://www.apa.org/pi/aging/resources/guides/sexuality
This is an annotated bibliography of journal articles, books, and videos, as well as organizations and information for elders.

American Association of Sexuality Educators, Counselors, and Therapists
www.aasect.org

American Heart Association (sexuality topic)
www.americanheart.org;
https://www.heart.org/en/about-us/diversity-inclusion/pride-with-heart/cardiovascular-health-for-lgbtq-adults

APA Office on Sexual Orientation and Gender Diversity (OSOGD)
http://www.apa.org/pi/lgbt/index.aspx
The mission of OSOGD is to advance the creation, communication, and application of psychological knowledge on gender identity and sexual orientation to benefit society and improve lesbian, gay, bisexual, and transgender people's lives.

Brain Injury Association of America
www.biausa.org;
sa.org_wp-content_uploads_Sexual-Functioning-and-Satisfaction-after-Traumatic-Brain-Injury-.pdf

Chicago Institute of Rehabilitation
https://www.sralab.org/lifecenter/resources/listing-intimacy-fertility-and-sexual-relations-disability

Christopher and Dana Reeve Paralysis Resource Center
https://www.christopherreeve.org/living-with-paralysis/health/sexual-health
This website has a searchable database for disability adjustment topics.

Disability after Dark
http://www.andrewgurza.com/homepage
Andrew Gurza is a Disability Awareness Consultant and Cripple Content Creator. In his work, he seeks to explore how the lived experience of disability feels as it interplays with intersectional communities. By using hashtags like #diSAYbled, #DisabilityAfterDark, #BearinAChair and #KissAQueerCripple, Andrew shares his lived experiences of disability, queerness, sexuality, and body image in a raw, vulnerable, and unapologetic fashion (www.andrewgurza.com/about).

International Society for the Study of Vulvovaginal Disease / The National Vulvodynia Association:
www.issvd.org / www.nva.org

Life on Wheels
www.lifeonwheels.net; https://www.christopherreeve.org/living-with-paralysis/health/sexual-health/video-series-sex-on-wheels
Disability resources from Gary Karp, a person living well with a T12 spinal cord injury. He is a speaker and author who trains rehabilitation professionals and employers about living with a disability.

San Francisco Aids Foundation
https://www.sfaf.org/resource-library/douchies-guide-to-butt-health/

*All websites mentioned in this chapter and all chapters were current at the time of writing.

National Alliance on Mental Illness
https://www.nami.org/Home
National Association of the Deaf
www.nad.org
National Dissemination Center for Children With Disabilities
www.nichcy.org
National Federation of the Blind
www.nfb.org
National Multiple Sclerosis Society
www.nmss.org
The National Spinal Cord Injury Association
www.spinalcord.org
National Stroke Association
www.stroke.org
Paralyzed Veterans of America:
https://www.pva.org (PVA) and offers an authoritative clinical practice guide.
Planned Parenthood Federation of America
www.plannedparenthood.org
The Sexual Health Network (hosted by Dr. Mitch Tepper)
https://www.drmitchelltepper.com/
The Sexual Health Network's website provides easy access to sexuality information, education, counseling, therapy, medical attention, and other sexuality resources for people with disability, illness, or other health-related problems. The Sexual Health Network also provides continuing education and training for health professionals and facilitates educational groups for people with disability or illness.
Sexuality and Disability: History and Practice (Dr. Linda Mona)
www.mypleasure.com;
https://mypleasure.com/pages/sex-and-disabilities-history-practices?_pos=1&_sid=1d74ad16c&_ss=r
Sexuality Information and Education Council of the United States
www.siecus.org
The Society for the Scientific Study of Sexuality
www.sexscience.org

Journals

Journal of GLBT Family Studies, Harrington Park Press, Binghamton, New York (an Imprint of the Hawthorne Press, Inc.). This peer-reviewed journal addresses issues related to being gay, lesbian, bisexual, and transgender and their families. Focus includes parent-child relationships, child development, sibling relationships, family structure, intimate relationships, step families, alternate family structures, and extended family relationships.

Sexuality and Disability, Springer Publishing, New York. This peer-reviewed journal is the most relevant source for scientific articles in this field.

Videos

Berne, P. (Director). (2013). *Sins Invalid: An Unashamed Claim to Beauty.* New Day Films. This documentary explores issues of sexuality and gender, race and class, embodiment and disability.

Scott, C. (Director). (2011). *Scarlet Road.* Paradigm Picture Productions. This documentary explores the life of Australian sex worker who is based in New South Wales (where prostitution is decriminalized) and sells sex to clients who have disabilities.

Sexuality and Spinal Cord Injury. From BC Rehabilitation in Vancouver. (604) 737-6225.
The video is designed for staff members and for training of staff. There may be parts of the video that would be useful for group discussion.

C. J. Alexander & M. L. Sipski (Producers/Narrators; also narrated by Ben Vereen) (1993). *Sexuality Reborn.* Produced by Kessler Institute for Rehabilitation, 1199 Pleasant Valley Way, West Orange, NJ 07052 and available at www.kmrrec.org/KM/nnjscis/sexuality_reborn.php3 or call (973) 243-6812. Explicit videotape highlighting interviews and footage of people with spinal cord trauma who have succeeded in adjusting to their injuries.

Additional Resources, Guidelines, and Templates

Sexual Health Inclusive Dialogue Template

The following bulleted words and topics are offered as guidelines intended to be inclusive, wholistic, and authentic. DO NOT STOP HERE. It is important that providers, allies, and members of our own communities be reminded we have a role in expanding the occupied space beyond oppressive and normative sex narratives.

As a Queer, Crip, Dwarf, Hard of Hearing, White, Professional Psychologist and Professor, I must call myself into this opportunity again and again and encourage all of us to do the same: Sex educators, sex therapists, psychologists, medical doctors, counselors, social workers, disability advocates, and disability activists.

Areas to explore to open the dialogue are provided. Please notice I avoid with intention using the word "other" in order to break a practice of implicitly suggesting a normative and thus pathologizing another's experience. The language and vocabulary of lived sexual experience is infinite and exists on a constantly shifting continuum. Consequently, I try as I might to be open-ended in my approach. Once a service of therapeutic treatment has been initiated and treatment goals established collaboratively, sharing of information and resources that offer my clients room to expand their own experiences with choices and or location of internalized oppressive shaming is continuously offered. The areas below simply offer a starting point.

- How can I respect and support your preferred, safe, and authentic space? How do you identify yourself?
- Gender
- Ethnicity
- Culture
- Language
- Pronouns
- Sexual Identification
- Sexual Experiences and Practices
- Sexual Preferences
- Sexual Traumas come in any form (physical, rape, assault, verbal harassment, denial, prohibitions, etc.)
- Is sex a relational experience for you or not?
- Is asexuality how you define your sexuality?
- If partnership is a part of your sexual narrative, what do you want from your partner? Partners?
- Sexual partners past and current and future?
- Sexual Questions . . . concerns . . . goals?
- Reproductive interests? Questions?
- Sexual informants? Community? Safe places?
- What do you want to know?
- What do you need to know?
- What is your biggest fear?
- What is your biggest hope?
- Do you have questions and/or need information about your sexual health? STIs?
- When was your last sexual health examination with a medical provider? If you have never had a sexual health examination with a medical provider can we discuss this and explore possibilities? Potential benefits and consequences? Fears or hopes in incorporating this into your experience and narrative with intention?

Feedback/Collaboration/Sharing Power

- Is there a question that I have asked that was offensive? Confusing? Unclear?
- Is there a question that I did not ask that leaves an important part of your sexual narrative or needs and wishes unspoken, silent and /or invisible? If so, what is it?

Medical and Personal Care Trauma Responses and and Disability Areas and Constructs to Explore

- What is the nature of your medical interventions and descriptions of personal routines? Explore degrees of intrusiveness.
    - When?
    - How?
    - What?
    - Who?

- Reliability of access and care? Particularly important in personal care routines? Are personal care attendants reliable, respectful of sexual needs, wants and if relevant are personal care attendants able and willing to support preparations needed for sexual activities?
- Frequency?
- Duration?
- Pain?
- Feelings of vulnerability?
- Feelings of aversion?
- Feelings of shame?
- Feelings of anxiety?
- Feelings of anger?
- Do or has any of your historical, and/or current experiences with medical procedures and personal care providers resulted in intrusive memories, nightmares or difficulties establishing feelings of safety and trust?

• Explore with client / consumer and Treatment Planning Needs relevant to sexual health.

References

Andrews, E. E., & Lund, E. M. (2016). Silenced no more: A review of supporting disabled people with their sexual lives [Review of the book *Supporting Disabled People with Their Sexual Lives: A Clear Guide for Health and Social Care Professionals*, by T. Owens & C. de Than]. *Sexuality and Disability, 34*(2), 227-233. https://doi.org/10.1007/s11195-016-9437-9

Asking Essential Sexual Health Questions. National Coalition for Sexual Health. https://nationalcoalitionforsexualhealth.org/tools/for-healthcare-providers/asset/Asking-Essential-Sexual-Health-Questions.pdf

Shapiro, L. (2017) The disabled sexual surrogate. *Reproductive Health Matters, 25*(50), 134-137. https://doi.org/10.1080/09688080.2017.1333894

Wisconsin's Violence Against Women with Disabilities and Deaf Women Project: Disability Rights Wisconsin, Wisconsin Coalition Against Domestic Violence, Wisconsin Coalition Against Sexual Assault (2011). *A Practical Guide for Creating Trauma-informed Disavility, Domestic Violence and Sexual Assault Organizations.* https://www.communitysolutionsva.org/files/Disability_Trauma-Informed-Guide.pdf

Design/Assessment

- Identify specific characteristics (i.e., demographic variables) of your clients and potential clients.
- Identify the specific physical characteristics of the clinic you are practicing in and the effect on the clinic's ability to deliver multiculturally friendly services (e.g., office décor, furniture, artwork, other decorative elements, publications in waiting room, content of printed materials, and website that provides information about the location of facilities. This includes the location of the clinic, the waiting room, the reception desk, and restrooms. Signs need to be both highly visible and easily understandable. Statements regarding fairness: A statement regarding commitment to fairness that is displayed in common areas).
- Accessibility: the degree to which the physical space accommodates the needs of people with a broad range of psychological, cognitive, and physical disorders.
- Identify opportunities for improvement in the physical characteristics of the clinic.
- Prioritize and implement these improvements.

Evaluation/Feedback:

- Develop a process and/or mechanism for gathering customer feedback on the physical design of the clinic.

References

Benton, J. & Overtree, C. (2012). Multicultural office design: A case example. *Professional Psychology: Research and Practice, 43,* 265-269.

Creating a LBG friendly environment. http://www.lesbianhealthinfo.org/community/in_office.htm

Assessing and Ensuring Diversity Inclusive Environments. Wright State University School of Professional Psychology Spring 2017 Grand Round Diversity Integration Event.

23

Sex in Pregnancy and the Family-Centered Perinatal Intervention/Education Model

Mischa Dansby, Racheal L. Johnson, Frederick L. Peterson, Jr., and Heidi Pence

INTRODUCTION

The promotion of discussions between providers and patients regarding sexual relations is a relatively recent part of professional training for healthcare disciplines, even for counselors, nurses, physicians, and psychologists. Despite the promotion of such in professional schools and obvious importance of the topic (especially with patients who are pregnant), many professionals have reservations discussing sex and have difficulty working through their discomfort to have important conversations (Peterson et al., 2020; Risen, 2007).

This chapter is designed to assist readers to build both comfort and confidence discussing sex with patients and sharing sex-positive messages that promote positive health benefits and outcomes for the patients. For example, can you imagine providers advising their pregnant patients that regular sexual relations can help expectant mothers maintain a pregnancy to full term? This type of message is important because there is a general myth among the public that sex during pregnancy will hurt the fetus and increase the likelihood of miscarriage.

A meta-analysis of 59 studies of sex during pregnancy concluded that if a woman does not have a high-risk pregnancy, then sexual intercourse during pregnancy does not hurt the fetus or increase risk of miscarriage and may protect the fetus from early delivery (von Sydow, 1999). In an interesting study of 1,800 pregnant women who were interviewed three times (twice during pregnancy and the last interview postpartum), authors found that women who reported sexual intercourse within the 2 previous weeks were significantly more likely to go full term than women who did not report sexual relations during the same periods (Reamey et al., 1982; Sayle, 2001).

This chapter explores the research that supports positive sexual expression during pregnancy and the perinatal period (when there are no medical contraindications). The psychological perspective of sex during pregnancy is addressed from a psychiatrist's point of view. Success stories of women's perinatal sexual experiences are also shared, some quite humorous (including advice to men in "Breastfeeding for Men 101"). The chapter concludes by providing a positive model of Family-Centered Perinatal Intervention/Education (FCPIE) which has been demonstrated to promote important "right-on-time" health education to expectant couples making their transition to new healthy families (Peterson et al., 1987; Peterson & Peterson, 1993).

TRANSITION THROUGH PREGNANCY INTO PARENTHOOD

(Written by Heidi Pence)

Women have learned from the beginning of history about how pregnancy and childbirth will affect their bodies and life. However, they have hardly ever learned much about sex during pregnancy and the pending transition into parenthood and new family dynamics. As in any family, when it grows, each relationship starts to become more complex as individual commitments become more complex and the roles become more challenging to maintain than they were before pregnancy and birth (see Figure 1).

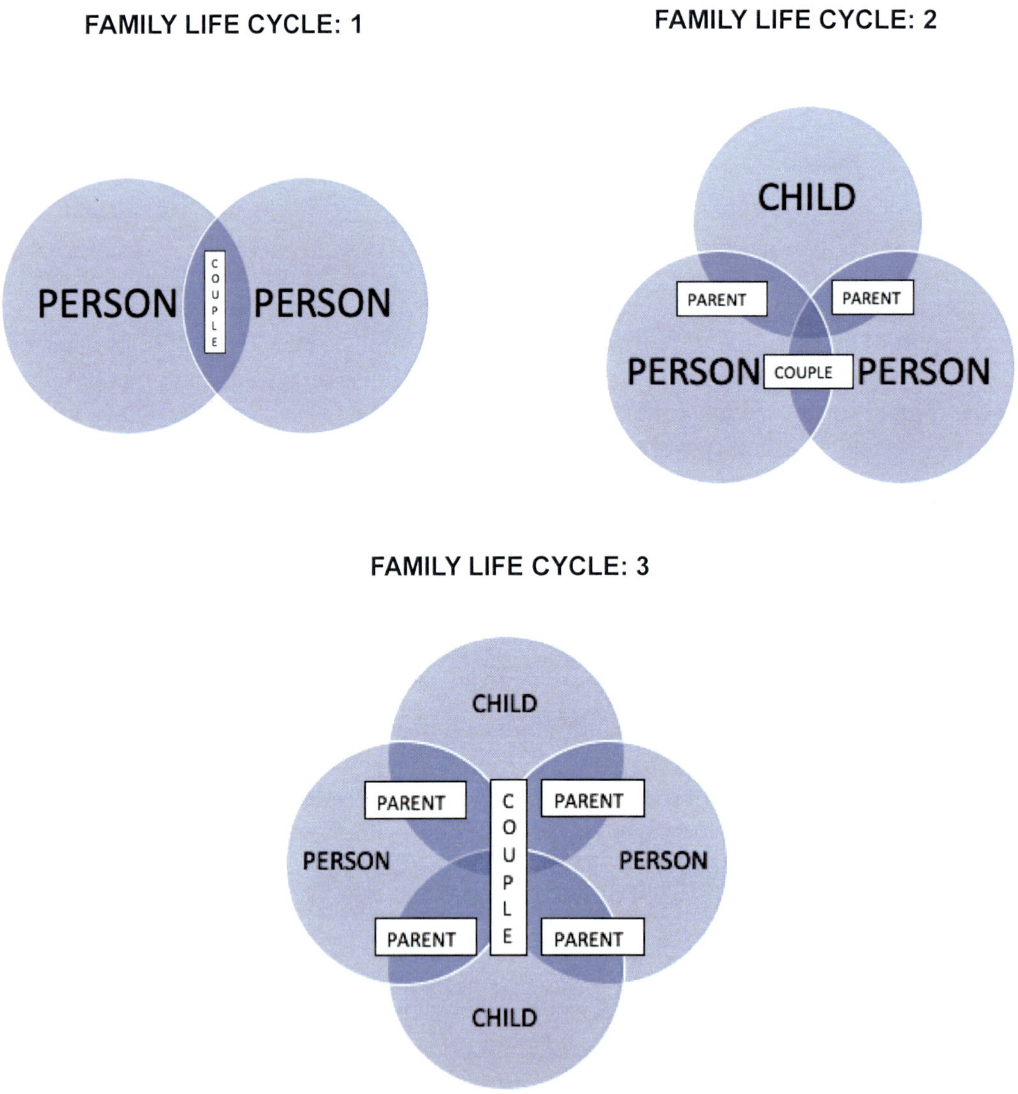

Figure 1. Family Life Cycles.
As families grow from one stage of the family life cycle to another, relationship dynamics become increasingly complex.

As an adult woman, I felt I was prepared for my pregnancy and the birth of my child, but what I was never prepared for (or given much information about) was the family transition or the expansion of my role beyond that of being a mother. My family cycle looked much different than that of Figure 1 (p. 396). I was a single mother learning how to handle an already strained relationship with my daughters' father, all while learning the roles of being an individual and a parent. So, while there are overlapping common experiences between women, each woman's perceptions and narrative is unique to her. Hence, the general model represented in Figure 1 should not always be assumed to be the norm and each expectant mother needs to be treated in a way to respectfully acknowledge her individual needs and worth.

Each family cycle is going to look different whether one is a single parent, a mother having additional children (siblings), or a mother dealing with in-laws and/or step-parents. Each relationship in the family grows from one stage to the next and it is important to learn about the focuses on the multiple roles of each family member. As illustrated later in this chapter, the family-centered perinatal approach goes "beyond the roles of being a parent, but also the roles of being an individual, a lover, and/or an employee" (Peterson & Peterson, 1993, p. 1). The Family-Centered Perinatal Intervention/Education (FCPIE) model can be helpful to expectant mothers with partners but especially for the expectant mothers without supportive partners or family.

THE PSYCHOLOGY OF SEX DURING PREGNANCY, MEDICATION CONSIDERATIONS, AND A PSYCHIATRIST'S PERSONAL EXPERIENCE

(Written by Racheal L. Johnson)

During my training as a psychiatrist, the biopsychosocial approach to patient care was emphasized. For a pregnant patient, this approach helps consider the complexity of her situation and consider different aspects of her care. Biological concerns include medication management and heritability of mental illness. Psychological concerns may revolve around body image, unresolved childhood trauma, feelings of inadequacies, and so forth. Social considerations include safety, family dynamics, support system, and substance use. Her sexual health during pregnancy can be tied to all of these biologic, psychological, and social aspects for holistic care.

Starting with the biologic concerns, psychiatrists are frequently consulted for medication concerns. Pregnancy is no exception. Encouragingly, the vast majority of people simply want what is best for the mother and child. Commonly asked questions include, "Should the medication be stopped? Should I change the medication? How will the medication affect the baby?" While we have guiding principles, care should be tailored to each person and their unique situation. Individual assessments to evaluate the risks versus benefits of any treatment should be thoroughly discussed as part of an informed consent. That being said, let's look at each question with more detail.

Should any medication be stopped in a pregnant patient? It depends. Pregnant patients with mood disorders such as major depression or generalized anxiety disorder are at increased risk for peripartum depression and peripartum anxiety. A mother with untreated depression is at increased risk of having a child with low birth weight, premature delivery, and may have difficulty bonding with her child after birth (Chan et al., 2014). Typically, a Selective Serotonin Reuptake Inhibitor (SSRI) is prescribed for this condition. If a woman has been stable on her medication for mood and would like to stop her antidepressant medication, the medication should be tapered over time and she should be monitored for resurgence of symptoms.

Women who have a psychotic illness are at increased risk of a psychotic episode during pregnancy, potentially leading to the inability to care for themselves or their infant (Odhejo et al., 2017). Women who have bipolar disorder are at increased risk of mania during pregnancy and in the postpartum period (Odhejo et al.). Poor sleep can have a kindling affect for mania.

Should the patient change the medication? It depends. Some psychiatric medications have greater risks for a developing child than others. SSRI medications in general have a similar risk profile, with a few exceptions. Paxil carries an FDA black box warning for cardiac defects and should be avoided in pregnancy in most circumstances.

Zoloft has the best pregnancy profile and is touted as the least likely to cause harm during pregnancy. However, changing an antidepressant medication that is working (such as Zoloft) simply because the patient is pregnant is not recommended. When considering mood stabilizers for patients with bipolar disorder, special consideration should be given to women of child-bearing age (Epstein et al., 2014). Depakote has a black box warning for neural tube defects. This stage of development often occurs prior to the woman's knowledge she is pregnant (Epstein et al., 2014). New studies on Lithium suggest the feared complication of Epstein's anomaly is much lower than previously thought (Poels et al., 2018). Lithium levels are expected to fluctuate at different stages of pregnancy and in the postpartum period, close monitoring is required (Poels et al., 2018).

When considering antipsychotic medications for patients with a psychotic illness or bipolar disorder, only two medications have a Class B pregnancy profile: Latuda and Clozapine. Similar to antidepressant medications, risks versus benefits should be discussed prior to switching from a working medication as patients respond differently to different medications. Is it really in the patient's best interest to switch from a medication she has been stable on for years and risk a potential worsening to her ability to care for herself? Does she have a good support system, people who live in the home that could recognize a decline in functioning and help bring her in for treatment? How does the patient feel about her medications? All of these concerns should be discussed when considering changing medication.

How will the medication affect the baby? Some of the medications with special considerations were mentioned above. In general, SSRI medications during pregnancy carry a risk for premature birth and low birth weight. There may be a slight increase of permanent pulmonary hypertension (Huybrechts et al., 2015). Some infants who are exposed to SSRI medications during development may experience a discontinuation syndrome at birth. This may present as increased fussiness, crying, jitteriness, and so forth, and may last up to a month. When making an informed decision, it is important to remember that untreated depression/anxiety also has increased risk factors. This is not a simple question and should be discussed between the pregnant patient and her prescribing provider in more detail.

What is the heritability of psychiatric illness? In other words, will my baby be affected with the same problems? Some psychiatric conditions have a strong genetic component, such as bipolar disorder, schizophrenia, ADHD, and Autism. Other psychiatric conditions have a moderate genetic component, such as substance use disorders. Anxiety or depression have similar genetic heritability as heart disease or breast cancer. It is important to remember that even if something is highly heritable, it does not mean the child will absolutely have the same condition. We are still learning about the role of epigenetics (the study of changes in organisms caused by modification of gene expression rather than alteration of the genetic code itself), and we do not fully understand the complexity of the human genome (the complete set of genes or genetic material present in a cell or organism). Underlying this biologic question is the psychological fear that mothers may cause harm to their child.

There are many potential psychological concerns that pregnancy can exacerbate or uncover. As a time of transition, many pregnant women struggle with their sense of identity. Pregnant women often think of their own mother during this time. Depending on that experience, they may be fearful of repeating the same mistakes, worry about not living up to their mother, or usurping their mother (Fenster et al., 2009). Underlying body image insecurities may surface. Fear of becoming overweight, feeling undesirable, or fear of losing their romantic partner may occur. If they are a victim of childhood trauma, they may worry about their unborn child's safety. Anger and resentment towards their parents' failure to keep them safe may present during pregnancy. Our culture tends to focus only on the positive aspects of pregnancy, and it may be difficult for pregnant women to discuss any negative thoughts with others surrounding their pregnancy. Being aware and open to discuss the full experience and range of emotions that present with pregnancy can be a very healing experience.

Social aspects in pregnancy include family dynamic, safety, and substance use. Not all pregnancies are planned or wanted. Pregnant women are especially vulnerable and special consideration should be given to how they are living. Is the pregnant woman in a relationship? How does their partner feel about the pregnancy? Who lives in the home? Is there preexisting domestic violence? Domestic abuse may begin or increase during pregnancy.

Substance use and mental health conditions increase risk of domestic abuse. Substance use during pregnancy may cause irreversible harm and should be part of normal screening. Alcohol use during pregnancy is the leading cause of preventable intellectual disability in the United States. Some substances cause a physical dependence, and rapid discontinuation could increase risk of miscarriage while the use of other substances can cause placental abruption resulting in miscarriage. If substance use is identified, education on various treatment options should be discussed.

Other social considerations include the extended family and her plans for childcare. Who else is part of the family unit or support system? Who will be caring for the child after birth? If the mother plans on returning to work, often there is internal conflict between her various responsibilities. Normalizing this conflict can be beneficial to patients. These are just a few of the various social considerations to consider when treating a pregnant patient.

A PERSONAL EXPERIENCE

(Written by Racheal L. Johnson)

Personally, I have had two pregnancies. My first pregnancy was unplanned at 26 years old. While I was married, and having children was part of the eventual plan, it still came as quite the surprise. I prolonged my education as I chose not to expose myself/child to the potential teratogens (an agent or factor which causes malformation of an embryo) routinely found in organic chemistry labs. I knew I wanted to go to medical school and worried how my expanding family may impact that trajectory. I also struggled with my self-image. Obesity runs in my family and I was terrified I would not be able to lose my pregnancy weight.

My self-esteem was further impacted by the changes in my sexual life. Prior to my pregnancy, my spouse and I had an active sexual life. My partner had significant discomfort with sex and pregnancy. Underlying this discomfort was the fear he would hurt our child. It did not matter that the doctors reassured us that sex was safe during pregnancy. Our sex life decreased significantly during my first pregnancy, and I was hurt and angry that something I saw as completely natural made my husband uncomfortable. It was a difficult time in our marriage. After our child was born, the dynamic of relationship continued to evolve. Most of my fears during pregnancy were resolved, and we adapted to life as a family rather than as a couple.

My second pregnancy was later in life, at 38 years old. I was completing a psychiatric residency and I again struggled with my sense of identity. This time, my spouse and I were able to better communicate and I felt much more secure in our relationship. We had already traversed this challenge, and successfully came out on the other side. I saw my body transformation as representations of fertility and youth. I had new fears/concerns as a professional woman with advanced maternal age. I worried about the health of my child more, and about the increased risk of genetic abnormalities. I worried about who would care for my child while I worked and struggled with the guilt that I could not be there for her in the same way I was for my first child.

On a professional level, I am uncomfortable with being seen as vulnerable. At times I overextended myself trying to overcompensate for my upcoming absence also known as maternity leave. Pregnancy can bring out strong reactions from family, peers, and strangers. My pregnancy changed the dynamic within the doctor-patient relationship. Sexual themes were more openly discussed in addition to themes of abandonment, fears of rejection, and frank curiosity about my personal life. Pregnancy meant I was a sexually active female with other important relationships outside of the room. I found myself simultaneously setting firmer boundaries and having more self-disclosure related to my pregnancy.

A few memorable conversations from this recent pregnancy are as follows:

Friend:	"Every time I see you, you're rubbing your belly. Only pregnant people can get away with that. If anyone else was touching themselves that way, it would be seen as sexual." (Rubbing my pregnant belly was quite comforting and often unconscious. I thought of it as holding my baby before my baby was born. Regardless, I like to challenge statements and often use humor as a defense.)
Me:	"How is it not sexual? Isn't pregnancy itself the result of sex?"
Husband:	(who also uses humor) "No, pregnancy is the end of sex."

Therapy patient:	(When I was about 6 months pregnant) "Can you still fit behind the steering wheel?"
Me:	(Using humor) "Yes, and I can promise you I will get bigger."

Upon further discussion, the patient shared how during her pregnancy she eventually had to stop working because she could no longer reach the petals of her car to drive to and from work. Her underlying concern was more related to how much longer I would be able to provide care for her, not my physical appearance.

A stranger in a store:	(Near the same time of 6 months pregnant) "Did you see that poor woman on the news? I just want you to know I am here for you if you need me."

She was referring to a woman who delivered her child alone in a prison cell. This woman felt compassion for me, a stranger, and wanted to let me know I was not alone in the world. I was not expecting to give birth anytime soon, but I chose to appreciate the sentiment behind the statement. Just as everyone experiences pregnancy differently, people respond to pregnancy differently. While natural, it does change who you are and how others react to you.

CLINICAL VIGNETTE – A SUCCESS STORY

(Written by Mischa Dansby)

The following story is based upon actual events but the name of the patient was changed to protect her identity. It is presented in this chapter to provide a positive example of interprofessional collaborative care resulting in what all expectant couples desire: a positive outcome of their pregnancy experience – the birth of a healthy child.

It is also presented to draw attention to the health benefits the patient derived from the inclusion of mental health support. The addition of mental health services to support expectant mothers during the perinatal period is the EXCEPTION rather than the rule for most mothers. This clinical vignette demonstrates the value of the FCPIE model; many of the additional mental health and social support aspects of this patient's perinatal experience are routine "built-in" aspects of a FCPIE class, and done so without any stigma associated with going to a mental health clinic (as this patient did).

Tina was a 22-year-old woman referred to the hospital's mental health clinic by her obstetric care provider who had patient interpersonal concerns. Tina was recently diagnosed with a viable intrauterine pregnancy at 10 weeks gestation. The pregnancy was unintended. She self-identifies as Caucasian of Western European descent, which she discovered through a recent search of her ancestral DNA. After she found out she was pregnant, Tina became curious about her ethnic and cultural background.

Born and raised in a small Midwestern community by a single mother, Tina wanted to be able to provide her offspring with a greater understanding of her lineage, as this was not afforded to her during her upbringing. Spiritually, Tina does not identify with a single religion, but holds a strong belief in God as her higher power and source of strength. Tina enjoys a close relationship with her mother who lives 100 miles away. While Tina discloses her mother was extremely disappointed when she learned of the pregnancy, Tina fully understood her mother's reaction.

As a young, single woman, Tina's mother struggled financially and emotionally to care for her sole child and she did not want this for her daughter. Over time, Tina's mother embraced the pregnancy and continued to be the main source of love and encouragement in Tina's life. Tina was concerned about her own ability to be a good mother. In addition to her mother, Tina had close social support from a neighbor and coworker.

Tina was a single, active-duty Air Force member who worked in the hospital supply and logistics department. She lived on base in the dormitory that houses hospital personnel. Tina had been in a romantic relationship with the father of the baby for 1 year. The baby's father was also an active-duty Air Force member. He was 21 years old at the time of the pregnancy and worked in Security Forces. Tina and the father of the baby contemplated an elective abortion but decided to continue the pregnancy. The couple planned to move into off base housing and live together after the baby was born.

Tina reported a lack of sexual desire due to nausea and was concerned this may have a negative effect on the relationship. Prior to the pregnancy, Tina described her sexual relationship with her boyfriend as mutually satisfying, easily achieving orgasm, and averaging five to seven sexual encounters a week. With the onset of nausea during the pregnancy, she did not feel desirable.

For the sake of her relationship, she believed she should continue to engage in sex, but did not find the experience to be pleasurable. She has been unable to achieve an orgasm with her partner since becoming pregnant and has not attempted self-stimulation due to a lack of desire. Her sexual focus has been maintained on providing pleasure for her boyfriend. She did not feel that he should suffer from a lack of intimacy because she is not feeling desirable or interested in sex. While she did miss the physical energy from a positive sexual experience, she was unsure how to achieve sexual satisfaction given her nausea and general lack of sexual desire.

During her consultation, Tina scored within normal limits on standard measures for symptoms of anxiety and depression. She denied any suicidal or homicidal ideation. Tina's therapist diagnosed her with a mild level adjustment disorder and implemented different interventions to address her concerns. Even though Tina scored within normal limits on initial screening measures, follow-up evaluation employing more sensitive instruments with greater specificity (Beck inventories for anxiety and depression) demonstrated that Tina was having mild-moderate range of these symptoms.

In particular, she was fearful of the "worse thing happening." For Tina, this was the father becoming frustrated with the relationship, choosing to disengage, and not being involved with his child. The "back story" for Tina was her fear that her child would grow up like she did – without the presence and love of a caring father. While much of Tina's concerns were common worries regarding unplanned pregnancies, she was provided in-vivo training to manage her anxiety by building her skill set of breathing and relaxation techniques.

She was also coached in communication skills, particularly related to the importance of expressing her needs and not assuming the boyfriend knew what she is thinking and feeling. In addition, Tina worried that sex during the pregnancy (particularly during later stages) would run a risk of hurting the baby. This was a belief she had heard from other women and accepted as fact. Educational support was provided to help dispel this myth and able her to relax and enjoy her sexual engagement with the boyfriend.

Because the FCPIE class was not available at the medical center where Tina delivered, her therapist thought it would be beneficial to enroll her in the New Parent Support Program (NPSP), which was available as an alternative form of postpartum support. The NPSP helps military expectant parents make a positive transition into parenthood. The nurses and social workers provide home visits and referrals to other resources, as well as separate prenatal and parenting classes.

Tina had multiple factors increasing her risk for sexual dysfunction, including an unintended pregnancy, nausea, reduced sexual desire, and relationship stress. Her therapist recommended she seek evaluation and treatment of her nausea if pharmacologic intervention was desired. The therapist encouraged Tina to explore alternative options to communicate love, affection, acceptance, and intimacy to nurture the couple's relationship.

Tina and the father of the baby attended childbirth education and breastfeeding classes together. The baby's father also attended "Dad's 101" – a course focused on providing fathers with skills to care for newborns through toddlers. Tina spoke with her obstetric care provider regarding the nausea and implemented nonpharmacologic interventions which offered her symptomatic relief. Her prenatal care provider advised her that as the pregnancy progressed, the nausea would improve and her desire for intimacy may return. In addition, Tina was encouraged to openly communicate with her partner regarding intimacy concerns.

Tina and her partner participated in various intimacy-building exercises, which afforded the opportunity to connect without performing sexual acts. Tina found soul gazing and extended cuddle time to be the most rewarding of the exercises. In soul gazing, she and her partner would face each other in a seated position with their knees close to touching and hold eye contact for 3 to 5 five minutes. For extended cuddle time, the couple created a playlist of their favorite slow songs and cuddled as they listened to the entire playlist. Both exercises helped them to reconnect at the end of a busy day.

Additionally, Tina began to see herself once again as desirable and deserving of sexual intimacy. Consistent practice of these intimacy exercises directly contributed to Tina experiencing increased sexual satisfaction. In her third trimester, Tina experienced satisfying orgasmic sexual experiences with her partner and through self-pleasuring. She found that the changes her body underwent were visually stimulating for herself and her boyfriend. She embraced the fullness of her breasts and growing belly and hips, which made her feel more attractive and desirable as a sexual partner.

In preparation for the birth experience, Tina and her partner completed childbirth education classes. As her due date approached, Tina felt exceptionally supported by her partner. With her mother and partner by her side, Tina's pregnancy culminated in the birth of a healthy full-term baby girl. As the demands of caring for a newborn arose, Tina and her partner continued to utilize the intimacy exercises to foster connectedness. The exercises helped the couple maintain the closeness which they both desired.

At the beginning of each pregnancy, the healthcare team in conjunction with the mother is focused on achieving a healthy pregnancy and bringing a healthy baby into the world. Throughout a pregnancy, a multitude of emotional, sexual, and physical changes occur within the woman's body often demanding immediate attention. For Tina, her body reminded her that while she was capable of creating and growing a new life, she did not have to sacrifice sexual desire and personal pleasure.

Equipped with a team of knowledgeable and collaborative health care providers, Tina attained the goal of bringing a healthy baby into her life while enhancing her personal sexual satisfaction. The goals of a healthy pregnancy and sexual satisfaction are not mutually exclusive and should be encouraged. As mentioned, the collaborative care Tina received (addressing her medical, psychological, and sexual health needs) is the exception rather than the rule for expectant mothers. Hopefully, choices for expectant mothers will expand in the future with the option of joining a FCPIE class (where available).

FACTS REGARDING SEX DURING PREGNANCY

Why Do I Feel More Sexual at Times During Pregnancy, and is it Normal?

As a woman's body changes during pregnancy, so can (and usually does) her sexual experience. During pregnancy, the normal blood volume increases to supply the placenta and developing fetus. With the passage of time beyond morning sickness and the increase in blood supply, there often comes the increase in sensations in the majority of a woman's erogenous areas, resulting in easier sexual arousal as well as more frequent and intense orgasms. Orgasms release natural endorphins (the body's feel-good hormones), including oxytocin and other hormones that bring many health benefits.

If Sex is Safe During Pregnancy, Why Would I Not Have Sex?

At the beginning of any first-time mom's pregnancy, there is usually the question of "Will sex hurt my baby?" Sex during pregnancy is generally not only safe for mom, but it is promoted for the health benefits. The majority of obstetricians encourage and prompt sex during pregnancy as long as there are no medical complications. Medical contraindications for why an obstetrician would not encourage sex: Being diagnosed with a "high-risk" pregnancy, preeclampsia, any sexual pain, and the rupture of membranes ("broken water" would be a "Don't Go There" situation because having sex after the water has broken can cause infection for both the mother and fetus).

What is Family-Centered Perinatal Education (FCPIE) and Where is it Offered?

The FCPIE model is a multidisciplinary healthcare intervention (consistent with the integrated model of patient care) that provides perinatal nursing (midwifery when available), health education, and social support to focus on the entire family during the perinatal period for better health outcomes for babies, mothers, and the family. Expectant mothers and their family members participate in a weekly class that takes them through childbirth preparation, the birthing experience, and the postpartum period. FCPIE classes are not commonly available but variations can be and often are created by small groups of dedicated providers and expectant couples who wish to enrich their birthing experiences.

PERINATAL SERVICES TO SUPPORT YOUNG COUPLES BECOMING HEALTHY FAMILIES: THE EVOLUTION OF THE FAMILY-CENTERED PERINATAL INTERVENTION/EDUCATION (FCPIE) MODEL

(Written by Fred Peterson)

Sometimes referred to as "family pie" because of its nurturing qualities, FCPIE is a preventative medicine and interdisciplinary intervention which focuses on the mother and family unit during the perinatal period, and is supportive to other family members as they welcome and integrate their baby into the family system. It is distinct from traditional childbirth education classes and family-centered maternity care by:

1. Addressing the needs of both the expectant mother and her family members whom she decides to include (male partner, female partner, mother, etc.);
2. Being a single perinatal health intervention that addresses the needs of the family ***continuously*** *during both prenatal and postpartum care*;
3. Treating the mother holistically by providing psychological support during the perinatal period without stigma of going to a mental health provider;
4. Celebrating the baby as a new member of the class, extending the social support to mothers through a 5- to 6-month perinatal transition, reducing the sense of isolation, and decreasing the incidence of postpartum depression;
5. Including male and female facilitators to model inclusion of fathers to the work of "welcoming babies to the world" and promoting father-child interaction;
6. Being more consistent with the multidisciplinary model of integrated healthcare as well as adult learning theory in that couples are learning health practices and parenting skills at the time they need them the most; and
7. Incorporating the evidence-based health benefits of Traditional Eastern Medicine with the leading science of Western Medicine through integrating the practices of yoga and tai chi for mothers during the perinatal period.

FCPIE is a multidisciplinary integrated care service (supported by physicians, nurses, midwives, lactation consultants, parenting educators, and many more) focused on the entire family during both prenatal and postpartum. FCPIE builds support for the expecting mother, extends that support system well into postpartum to serve as a buffer against the effects of stress, and provides learning in a timelier manner when expectant parents need and can apply their new learning and skills (Peterson & Peterson, 1993).

Although the amount of FCPIE classes and weeks can be adjusted, the original classes involve 16 to 18 weeks of classes, as seen below. The original research classes (initially named Family-Centered Perinatal Education or FCPE) focused more on health education and support, as described by the following curriculum (Peterson et al., 1987):

Week 1: Orientation, setting realistic expectations, introductions
Week 2: Prepared childbirth training and positive sexuality in pregnancy
Week 3: Prepared childbirth training and problem-solving communication
Week 4: Prepared childbirth training, massages, and affective communication
Week 5: Prepared childbirth training, circumcision, roles of support people
Week 6: Prepared childbirth training and developing baby birthing plans (Family Medical Leave Act)

Week 7: Prepared childbirth training and hospital visits, attachment, and bonding
Week 8: Addressing worries and health benefits of support network (Part I)

BIRTHING BREAK – usually 1 to 2 weeks

Week 9: Sharing birthing stories and introduce baby, breastfeeding consultation
Week 10: Sharing birthing stories and introduce baby, infant care and stimulation
Week 11: Sharing birthing stories and having baby home, dealing with postpartum blues
Week 12: Sharing birthing stories and having baby home, finding time for self and partner
Week 13: Having baby home, engineering social support systems, infant mental health
Week 14: Having baby home, stress management and self-care, sharing responsibilities
Week 15: Having baby home, planning for resuming sex and going back to work
Week 16: Addressing worries and health benefits of support network (Part II) – Celebration

Positive effects of the FCPE classes were demonstrated in both hospital-based and university-based settings. First, the old adage of "if you build it, they will come" was found true as couples had to be turned away after classes filled. The community perceived FCPE classes as an attractive alternative to traditional prenatal childbirth preparation classes. Second, couples who participated had very little attrition and consistently showed up for postpartum classes with their babies. They appreciated the "family focus" of FCPE which included grandmothers, lesbian partners, and boyfriends/husbands in the primary support role. Siblings attended from time to time as well. Third, slightly over 300 family members (151 mothers) participated during a 3-year period. Without screening-out expectant mothers, many (approximately 16%) with high-risk pregnancies, there were no miscarriages, no infants lost, and only six cases of postpartum depression diagnosed (all were provided supportive counseling with positive outcomes). Fourth, FCPE participants (both men and women) overwhelmingly reported their pregnancy and birthing experiences as positive "transitions" into parenthood as opposed to being experienced as a personal crisis.

Additional research results showed interesting changes in self-perception of women and men as they became mothers and fathers. For example, and as expected, new fathers reported increases in their sense of masculinity (think of cigars and chest pounding) from their prenatal scores. What surprised the authors was an associated increase in feelings of femininity by the fathers postpartum because of what they reported as "feelings of awe and tenderness" witnessing the birth of their child and the subsequent "falling in love" process of attachment to their baby.

Alternatively, it is no surprise new mothers reported a postpartum decrease in their sense of masculinity compared to their prenatal scores. What surprised the authors with the new mothers was an absence of an increase in their sense of femininity. Some new mothers cited the reason as the discrepancy between their idealized expectations of motherhood and the lived-experience of being sleep-deprived, physically exhausted, and emotionally drained. As one mother put it, "Sure I feel like a mom, but I don't feel very feminine with my hands in the diaper bucket" (Peterson et al., 1987).

A final observation as to the popularity of the FCPE classes was the repeated emphasis on supporting the primary relationship between the mother and her support person. For example, fathers would get in vivo training on the skills of giving a great foot massage and taken aside to be asked if they had bought flowers that week. Mothers particularly enjoyed sitting in on the fathers' instruction called "Breastfeeding for Men 101" which, among other content, included the following guideline "do's and don'ts" (Peterson, 2000):

Do: BE THERE. No excuses. Breastfeeding success needs a supporting partner. Take advantage of the Family Medical Leave Act to stay at home to support the mother and bond with baby. Defend the mother's right to breastfeed the baby (or pump) wherever and whenever she chooses. Encourage her by telling her she is incredible and you appreciate her making amazing contributions to your baby's optimal development by breastfeeding.

Don't: Ask "Can't you turn those things off?" when her breasts are letting down like rainfall. (This is one of those things mom can't control and may feel embarrassed by, especially during sex. Just make sure she has a towel handy). DO NOT "belly up to the bar" by licking or suckling your partner's free breast when she is feeding the baby on the other breast. (She has an internal switch for going from a nurturing function to an erotic purpose for her breasts. Feeding both you and the baby at the same time can put this system into overload and complicate the resurrection of your sex life). Speaking of sex, DON'T get upset if it takes 6 weeks (or more with a C-section) for your sex life to resume. The hormones involved in breastfeeding can inhibit sexual desire but also help the uterus get back into shape for better sexual responsiveness. Time is needed to heal so DON'T whine and beg like a dog. Take matters into your own hands and let her get her rest. Get a grip on yourself, literally.

The reason the class was discontinued was a professional scandal at the hospital by an obstetrician who lost his license, a resulting sharp decline in referrals to the hospital labor and delivery department, and the third author changing hospitals to take up another line of research.

The "*new and improved*" Family-Centered Perinatal Intervention/Education (FCPIE*)* extends evidence-based health benefits to all mothers but targets reducing risk for at-risk mothers. For example, FCPIE classes include the services of a doula who serves as a powerful extension of support to mothers (and fathers) facing the new experience of birthing their first child.

Also as previously mentioned, FCPIE combines the best of East and West medical traditions by integrating the practices of yoga and tai chi during the perinatal period. According to the Mayo Clinic, prenatal yoga can be a great way to prepare for childbirth. Many expectant mothers look for ways to relax or stay fit and consider prenatal yoga to do so. But then they also learn that prenatal yoga can help them prepare for their labor and promote positive outcomes for the infant's health. Much like other types of childbirth-preparation classes, prenatal yoga is a multifaceted approach to exercise that encourages stretching, mental centering, and focused breathing; these three practices are helpful skills during pregnancy and birth. The Mayo Foundation for Medical Education and Research (MFMER, 2021) states that there is strong support for prenatal yoga as a safe exercise and provides many benefits for pregnant women (and their babies) by promoting:

- Improved sleep;
- Reduced stress and anxiety;
- Increased strength, flexibility, and endurance of muscles needed for childbirth;
- Decreased lower back pain, nausea, headaches, and shortness of breath;
- Bonding with other pregnant women and better prepare expectant mothers for the stress of being a new parent; and
- Reduced risk of preterm birth.

In an Australian study, yoga was found to decrease self-reported distress and increase expectant mothers' perceived skills to assist with their labor and the birth of their baby (Styles et al., 2019). In a fascinating and recent study (*during the COVID-19 pandemic*), investigators studied the potential benefits of yoga in pregnancy-related complications and found significant implications for working women (Nadholta et al., 2020). The authors concluded that yoga can be a safe and preventive intervention as compared to drugs and physical exercise alone. "Yoga, along with usual care, can empower pregnant women in increasing the quality of life by reducing the uncomfortable experiences, stress, anxiety and depression that are pronounced during the COVID-19 pandemic. It is an effective, useful and recommended intervention, which can be prescribed during pregnancy" (Nadholta et al., 2020, p. 275).

Tai chi was also added to the FCPIE as it has a long history of bringing health benefits to those who practice it's "meditative movements" which promote deeper breathing, enhanced relaxation, and greater oxygen saturation of blood for both mother and child. The National Center for Complementary and Integrative Healthcare (a branch of the NIH) defines tai chi as an exercise of slow, gentle movements that shift weight while a person maintains an upright yet relaxed posture and controlled breathing, creating a "moving meditation" (https://nccih.nih.gov/health/taichi/introduction.htm). Many health benefits of tai chi have been well documented by empirical research. Expectant mothers can benefit from them as they progress through the perinatal period. These health benefits include, but are not limited to:

- Pain management (Abbot et al., 2007; Wang et al., 2010b),
- Improved balance and coordination which results in reduced risk for falls (Burschka et al., 2014; Leung et al., 2011),
- Lowering blood pressure (Gallagher, 2003; Jahnke et al., 2010), and
- Strengthening the immune system (Irwin et al., 2003; Yang et al., 2007).

In addition, patients have reported decreased symptoms of stress, anxiety, and depression. Tai chi provides moderate intensity aerobic exercise equivalent to brisk walking and a low-impact form of exercise that is appropriate for a wide variety of individuals, including expectant mothers. A 12-week course of tai chi demonstrated an effect of lowering stress indicators and improving mood (Taylor-Piliae et al., 2006).

A systemic review of tai chi practice indicated a wide-range of benefits including relief from anxiety, stress, and depression (Wang et al., 2010a). Practicing tai chi also facilitates what psychologists refer to as "behavioral activation" and provides an individual a sense of empowerment by doing something one has to do any way (to stay alive) but do so in an intentional manner that brings one the increased health benefits just noted.

SUMMARY

Optimizing a woman's health is the primary objective during pregnancy with the desired outcome of a healthy baby for the start of a new family. Providing quality care and education empowers a woman to fully appreciate the miraculous nature of gestation and birth. Quelling fears and dispelling myths about sexuality during pregnancy fosters a greater opportunity for enhanced sexual health and intimacy. Holistic support during pregnancy is crucial to the health of the woman and the next generation.

Adequate communication between women and their providers about sexual health is often lacking, resulting in women relying only on the advice and experiences of female friends (Johnson, 2011; Murtaugh, 2010). Clinicians must facilitate open discussions and educate women on the potential changes in sexual health in pregnancy and postpartum. Couples should be reassured the changes will gradually recover over time and be educated on alternatives to maintain emotional intimacy and satisfying sexual expression. During a consultation, inquiring about sexual satisfaction in pregnancy should be as common as asking, "What would you like to discuss today?" Healthcare providers should routinely include an assessment of sexual function and sexual practice (Jordan et al., 2014).

As healthcare professionals, we must recognize our biases or limitations and seek educational opportunities to advance our skills. Patients present to us in the most vulnerable states in search of a better understanding of self and we should be ready to assist through their process of healing and exploration.

As the sciences of medicine, nursing, and psychology have evolved, the multidisciplinary integrated care model has become the dominant paradigm regarding best practices for delivery of healthcare to expectant mothers. The authors endeavored to illuminate potential problems that arise in the typical delivery of perinatal care and promote the utilization of comprehensive models such as FCPIE to help prevent and circumvent the challenges that mothers and new families commonly face.

REFERENCES

Abbot, R., Hui, K., Hays, R., Li, M., & Pan, T. (2007). A randomized controlled trail of tai chi for tension headaches. *Evidence-Based Complementary and Alternative Medicine, 4,* 107-113.

Association of Women's Health, Obstetric, and Neonatal Nurses (AWHONN). (1993). *AWHONN's clinical issues in perinatal and women's health nursing*. Lippincott.

Burschka, J., Keune, P., Oy, U., Oschmann, P., & Kuhn, P. (2014). Mindfulness-based interventions in multiple sclerosis: Beneficial effects of tai chi on balance, coordination, fatigue, and depression. *BMC Neurology, 14,* 165.

Chan, J., Natekar, A., Einarson, A., & Koren, G. (2014). Risks of untreated depression in pregnancy. *Canadian Family Physician, 60*(3), 242-243.

Epstein, R. A., Moore, K. M., & Bobo, W. V. (2014). Treatment of bipolar disorders during pregnancy: Maternal and fetal safety and challenges. *Drug, Healthcare and Patient Safety, 7,* 7-29. https://doi.org/10.2147/DHPS.S50556

Fenster, S., Phillips, S., & Rapoport, E. R. (2009). *The therapist's pregnancy: Intrusion in the analytic space.* Routledge.

Gallagher, B. (2003). Tai chi chuan and qi gong. *Topics in Geriatric Rehabilitation, 19,* 72-182.

Huybrechts, K. F., Bateman, B. T., Palmsten, K., Desai, R. J., Patorno, E., Gopalakrishnan, C., Levin, R., Mogun, H., & Hernandez-Diaz, S. (2015). Antidepressant use late in pregnancy and risk of persistent pulmonary hypertension of the newborn. *Journal of the American Medical Association, 313*(21), 2142-2151. https://doi.org/10.1001/jama.2015.5605

Institute for Healthcare Improvement. (2005). *Patient-centered care charter*. Institute for Healthcare Improvement.

Irwin, M., Pike, J., Cole, J., & Oxman, M. (2003). Effects of a behavioral intervention, tai chi chin, on Varicella-Zoster Virus specific immunity and health functioning in older adults. *Psychosomatic Medicine, 65,* 825-830.

Jahnke, R., Larkey, L., Rogers, C., & Etnier, J. (2010). A comprehensive review of health benefits of qigong and tai chi. *American Journal of Health Promotion, 24*(6), e1-e25.

Johnson, C. (2011). Sexual health during pregnancy and the postpartum. *The Journal of Sexual Medicine, 8,* 1267-1284. https://doi.org/10.1111/j.1743-6109.2011.02223.x

Jordan, R., Engstrom, J., Marfell, J., & Farley, C. (2014). *Prenatal and postnatal care: A woman-centered approach.* Wiley.

Lemieux-Charles, L., & McGuire, W. L. (2006). What do we know about health care team effectiveness? A review of the literature. *Medical Care Research and Review, 63*(3), 263-300. https://doi.org/10.1177/1077558706287003

Leung, D., Chan, C., Tsang, H., Tsang, W., & Jones, A. (2011). Tai chi as an intervention to improve balance and reduce falls in older adults: A systematic and meta-analytic review. *Alternative Therapies in Health and Medicine, 17*(1), 40-48.

Mayo Foundation for Medical Education and Research. (2021). Prenatal yoga: What you need to know. *Healthy Lifestyle: Pregnancy Week by Week.* https://www.mayoclinic.org/healthy-lifestyle/pregnancy-week-by-week/in-depth/prenatal-yoga/art-20047193

Murtaugh, J. (2010). Female sexual function, dysfunction and pregnancy: Implications for practice. *Journal of Midwifery and Women's Health, 55*(5), 438-466. https://doi.org/10.1016/j.jmwh.2009.12.006

Nadholta, P., Bali, P., Singh, A., & Anand, A. (2020). Potential benefits of yoga in pregnancy-related complications during the COVID-19 pandemic and implications for working women. *Work, 67*(2), 269-279. https://doi.org/10.3233/WOR-203277

National Association of Complementary & Alternative Medicine. (2014). *Prenatal yoga.* https://www.nacams.org/yoga/disciplines/prenatal-yoga/

Odhejo, Y., Jafri, A., Mekala, H., Hassan, M., & Mahmood, A. (2017). Safety and efficacy of antipsychotics in pregnancy and lactation. *Journal of Alcohol & Drug Dependence, 5,* 267. https://doi.org/10.4172/2329-6488.1000267

Peterson, F. L. (2000). Why are Americans so weird about breastfeeding? *Weekly Impact, 8*(10).

Peterson, F. L., Bley, J. W., & Frabotta, R. (2020). *The gender revolution & new sexual health.* Cognella Academic Press.

Peterson, K., & Peterson, F. (1993). *Clinical issues in perinatal and women's health nursing* Peterson, K., Peterson, F., Blasenak, B., Nicholls, C., & Redman, E. (1987). Strike while the iron is hot: Combining childbirth education, parenting training, and social support. *International Journal of Childbirth Education, 2*(2).

Poels, E. M. P., Bijma, H. H., Galbally, M., & Bergink, V. (2018). Lithium during pregnancy and after delivery: A review. *International Journal of Bipolar Disorders, 6,* 26. https://doi.org/10.1186/s40345-018-0135-7

Reamey, K., White, S. E., & Daniel, W. C. (1982). Sexuality and pregnancy: A prospective study. *Journal of Reproductive Medicine, 27*(6).

Risen, C. (2007). How to do a sexual health assessment. In L. VandeCreek, F. Peterson, & J. Bley (eds.), *Innovations in clinical practice: Focus of sexual health* (pp. 19-33). Professional Resources Press.

Sayle, A. (2001). Sexual activity during late pregnancy and risk of preterm delivery. *Obstetrics and Gynecology, 97*(2).

Styles, A., Loftus, V., & Nicolson, S. (2019). Prenatal yoga for young women: A mixed methods study of acceptability and benefits. *BMC Pregnancy Childbirth, 19,* 449. https://doi.org/10.1186/s12884-019-2564-4

Taylor-Piliae, R., Haskell, W., Waters, C., & Froelicher, E. (2006). Change is the perceived psychosocial status following a 12-week Tai Chi exercise programme. *Journal of Advanced Nursing, 54,* 313-329.

von Sydow, K. (1999). Sexuality during pregnancy and after childbirth: Ametacontent analysis of 59 studies. *Journal of Psychosomatic Research, 47*(1).

Wang, C., Bannuru, R., Ramel, J., Kupelnick, B., Scott, T., & Schmid, C. (2010). Tai chi on psychological wellbeing: Systematic review and meta-analysis. *BMC Complementary & Alternative Medicine, 10,* 23.

Wang, C., Schmid, C., Rones, R., Kalish, R., Yinh, J., Goldenburg, D., & McAlindon, T. (2010). A randomized trial of tai chi for fibromyalgia. *New England Journal of Medicine, 363*(8), 743-754.

Yang, Y., Verkuilen, J., Rosengren, K., Mariani, R., Reed, M., Grubisich, S., & Woods, J. (2007). Effects of a taiji and qigong intervention on the antibody response to influenza in older adults. *American Journal of Chinese Medicine, 35,* 597-607.

24

Navigating Postpartum Sexuality

Ashley N. Grinonneau-Denton

INTRODUCTION

When it comes to human sexuality so many topics are veiled in silence, stigmatized, and considered taboo. Amongst the broad array of topics that fit under the "sexuality umbrella" is that sex during the perinatal period (during pregnancy) is spoken of in a hushed whisper. Then a code of silence is used to frame the postpartum period (or postnatal period) as far as sexuality is concerned. For definition's sake, the postpartum period is defined as anywhere from birth to 6 months after birth (WHO, 2015). This stage is one that is overflowing with what often feels like a copious number of emotions that simultaneously clash and harmonize with one another; thus, creating a unique backdrop of what has been described as both "the best thing that has ever happened to me" and "emotional anarchy" in the space of my office while working with partners and individuals who are traversing the postpartum stage together or respectively.

For the purpose of this chapter, the postpartum period will be explored, along with clinical recommendations that can assist sexual health practitioners in supporting those clients in an effective manner during this unique developmental stage. It is crucial to add another note as well. In an effort to be inclusive of gender-diverse individuals, terms *birthing* person, birthing *persons*, or *birthing partner* will be used to refer to those who are otherwise commonly referred to as *women*, *females*, and *mothers*. Also, the terms *partner*, *partners,* or *nonbirthing person* will be used instead of *husband,* as cisgender and heteronormative biases and relationships show up, all too often, in the space where literature on pregnancy and postpartum are displayed. This results in the exclusion of a very crucial part of the population that identify outside of the female and male gender binary. Disparately, it is worth noting that there is a great paucity of literature representing gender-diverse persons, those in non-monogamous partnerships, sexual and racial minorities, as well as other marginalized groups (i.e., those with physical and intellectual disabilities, etc.) in the postpartum stages. It is encouraged that sexual health practitioners, who wish to utilize the content of this chapter in their clinical work, be mindful of adapting its content in a manner that is relevant to the unique variables of the persons they are working with.

I have worked with a myriad of couples and individuals who have experienced an abundance of joy along with increased emotional and sexual satisfaction throughout pregnancy. I have also heard many a parent vow that their relationship with each other would not change (that much), only to be sorely disappointed to recognize that their once fervent oath is a certain impossibility. After all, bringing a human into the world is no easy task; The impact on all dimensions of a birthing person (and their partner) creates a seemingly spontaneous, existential shift, which is often both joyous and extremely jarring for many. With this said, it is no wonder why 80% of birthing partners experience "the baby blues" and 20% experience significant postpartum depression (McBride et al., 2017). Although bringing a new human into the world for the first time is beyond exciting for most, it is also wrought with the challenges that occur when the former system is thrown out of balance with the addition of a new person, complete with their own distinctive needs. This presence of a new life that flips a birthing person and their partner's former sense of normalcy on its head is bound to shine a light on new challenges and create potential chasms where there were once only small cracks in a relationship's foundation.

Historically, the sexuality of pregnant or recently pregnant birthing persons are topics in empirical exploration that have been underpinned by a social context that has been at war between the concept of sex as recreation versus sex for procreation, with the latter typically being the victor (Buehler, 2018). Though the pregnant person as an archetype has become more revered in recent decades, with accompanying social shifts, the undulations of sexual shame have left their mark. One of the impacts is a dearth of knowledge for new parents on how to create a healthy set of expectations and accompanying behaviors that will keep sexual and emotional intimacy "above water" in the sea of change that new parents can often experience. Although sexual satisfaction naturally ebbs and flows throughout the course of relationships, the postpartum period is an exceptionally vulnerable time for birthing persons as well as their partners due to the surplus of biopsychosocial changes that occur during this developmental interval (Jawed-Wessel & Sevick, 2017).

Specifically, research that focuses on the postpartum stage points to a decrease in sexual satisfaction and intimacy during pregnancy and the postpartum period for partners and the birthing person (Cohen et al., 2019). More specifically, there is often a gradual decline in both sexual desire and satisfaction during pregnancy, with the time it takes to return to a pre-pregnancy sexual baseline around 12 months (Jawed-Wessell & Sevick, 2017). It has also been shown that up to 50-91.3% of birthing partners and nonbirthing partners experience physiological changes that impact components of their sexual health and functioning. Because the challenges that the postpartum period brings often go unaddressed, many new parents find themselves operating under an unrealistic set of expectations when it comes to how they will function during the postpartum period.

The postpartum stage is filled with a plethora of physiological changes that impact all parts of the self. Significant neuroendocrine changes occur postpartum that can contribute to decreased sexual interest during the first 6 to 12 months following childbirth (Rupp et al., 2013). Some of these changes likely occur in the amygdala area of the brain, which is related to sex drive. Birthing partners have been shown to exhibit decreased amygdala responsiveness (Rupp et al., 2013). Elevated prolactin and oxytocin levels associated with breastfeeding can also be associated with low sexual desire in postpartum women (Rupp et al., 2013). In lieu of the surfeit of changes that occur during the postpartum stage, it is not surprising to find that it may take time for new parents to adapt to the many changes that occur during the postpartum period. Although changes in sexual patterns are not fundamentally a problem, long pauses in sexual activity have the potential to impact intimate relationships. Decreased sexual frequency and sexual satisfaction are closely connected with one another (Jawed-Wessel & Sevick, 2017) in conjunction with the general emotional health of the relationship as well.

Experientially, as a sex therapist who works with a multiplicity of folks who come with different identities, orientations, cultural backgrounds, and so forth, there seems to be a universal challenge for all when they attempt to return to any sexual behavior after a long time has passed. To put it simply, we are creatures of habit. Sexual patterns that exist in partnered systems are no exception to this rule. The more time that goes by without priority on one's sex life, the more difficult the journey gets trying to return to their previous level of sexual satisfaction and connection during the postpartum period. Individual therapy, couples' therapy/therapy for partnered systems, and group-oriented approaches that focus on birthing partners and nonbirthing partners have been suggested as proactive approaches that can be taken during pregnancy and the postpartum period to help them on this difficult journey.

It has been shown that birthing persons contribute to the biopsychosocial landscape of a couples' experience of postpartum life in a way that nonbirthing partners do not (Moore Simas et al., 2019). In chorus with all the changes that birthing persons experience during the postpartum stage, factors that contribute to sexual dysfunction and sexual satisfaction (or lack thereof) in birthing persons include current and pre-existing mental health concerns, frequency of sex during pregnancy, personality characteristics, familiarity with partner, history of infertility, chronic illness, pelvic surgeries, former pregnancies, and medications (Shahraki et al., 2018). Amongst the said challenges that arise during the postpartum period, there are other psychosocial challenges that are at risk of occurring during this stage of life including postpartum distress, negative mental health outcomes in male and female-identifying partners, heightened fatigue, feeling overwhelmed, reduction in romantic relationship functioning, and increased conflict in their relationship.

In totality, sexual dysfunction leads to decreased quality of life and dissatisfaction with others, and negatively affects the physical, psychological, social, and emotional health of the birthing person and their partner(s) (Banaei et al., 2016). In this way, the postpartum phase is one in which the birthing person needs the most nurturing and yet, easily, receives the least attention from themselves and their partner(s). Disregarding this issue may lead to a reduced sense of self for the birthing person, their partner, child, and others within their immediate relational system. In an effort to promote a higher level of functioning in birthing persons, their partners, and families, I will include concrete steps and interventions that will apply to birthing persons, their partners, and sexual health practitioners who work with those impacted by the many challenges that are part and parcel to the postpartum phase. With that said, it is important to note there is an obscene scarcity of data to support the specific needs that exist for those who are gender-diverse, sexual minorities, cultural/racial minorities, and other marginalized and oppressed groups. Because of this, I have done my best to consider folks who are not cisgendered, White, and privileged. If the exercises that are displayed in this chapter do not fit your experience or the experience of those you are working with, please modify them as needed to fit your unique needs.

SETTING REALISTIC EXPECTATIONS

The excitement and preparation, in conjunction with no experience with parenting, creates a situation in which first-time parents are often caught unaware by the unrealistic expectations that they have for themselves, their partner(s), and for what actually fulfilling the role of a parent means. From what I have seen in my work with partnered systems, unrealistic expectations are built into the process of being a first-time parent. If there is a lack of planning present, then this sentiment has very little utility. However, if a proactive approach is utilized, then this concept can be very useful for new parents and practitioners that are working with them. With this idea in mind, the following exercise that I have created for first-time parents can help both birthing and nonbirthing partners identify realistic versus unrealistic parenting and relational expectations for their partnerships.

Exercise:
What to Expect After (or When) Expecting

Goal: The goal here is to afford nonbirthing and birthing partners the opportunity to create realistic expectations during pregnancy and/or the postpartum period.

Directions: Partners are requested to ask the following questions (and any other questions that resonate) in order to begin to prepare for the postpartum phase or to re-assess changing needs that occur during the phase.

Physiological:

1. What physiological changes will I experience or have I experienced?
2. How does sexual arousal/desire function differently for me now?
3. What things allow me to be sexually/erotically interested in engaging with my partner(s)?
4. What things allow me to be sexually/erotically disinterested in engaging with my partner(s)?

5. Are there certain types of touch that I desire now/would like to experiment with that seem new during this period?
6. Have you experienced pain or discomfort during the postpartum period during intimate/sexual contact or in your genitals in general?
7. Are there new positions/tools/resources that need to be put in place to make sexual/sensual interaction more physically comfortable?

For those who are breastfeeding:

8. How has the presence of breastfeeding impacted my desire to be sexual/close to my partner?
9. How has breastfeeding changed my concept of my body/partner's body?
10. Is there a way that sensuality with my partner can be integrated with breastfeeding in a way that allows for an increase in feeling closer with your partner?
11. Could changes be made to accommodate more felt support with breastfeeding/to your breastfeeding partner?

Sexual:

1. On a scale of 1-10 (10 being very high and 1 being extremely low), how high would you rate your level of sexual interest?
2. Have you masturbated since the birth of the new baby/babies?
3. Have you and your partner mutually masturbated since the birth of the new baby/babies?
4. Have you and your partner(s) been sexual since the birth of the new baby/babies? If so, how was it?
5. What do you need now to be able to "show up" sexually?
6. Have your needs in regard to sexual initiation changed? If so, how?
7. Have any new fantasies shown up since the baby/babies have been born?
8. How does the concept of autonomy influence/factor into your sexual needs?
9. A way that our "sexual rituals" could change for the better would include ________________.
10. In regard to sexual intimacy, what do you hope to model for your child/children in regard to healthy sexuality?

Emotional:

1. Do you feel different about sexual intimacy with your partner since giving birth/the birth of the new baby/babies?
2. What nonsexual ways of showing nurturance do you need from your partner now?
3. How has sleep impacted your emotional needs in regard to your partner?
4. What new resources need to be put in place to make life more comfortable now that you are a parent, in general?
5. Considering your family-of-origin, what emotional tendencies have shown up for you now that you are a parent?
6. Considering your partner/partners' family-of-origin, what emotional tendencies have shown up for you now that you are a parent?
7. Are there new things that you would like to try sexually that would increase your emotional interest in your partner?
8. Are there things that have occurred between you and your partner(s) that have been meaningful emotionally that have later peaked or diminished your sexual interest?
9. Are there boundaries with other caregivers that need to be set by you and your partner regarding the care of your child/children that would allow you to feel more supported?

PSYCHOLOGICAL AND EMOTIONAL NEEDS

The importance of an autonomous, physical, and emotional sense-of-self for birthing persons is something that is de-prioritized at best, and altogether nonexistent much of the time. Be that as it may, one way in which birthing persons DO focus on themselves is in regard to their physical self-image and the disconnection that they may feel after having a child, regardless of the mode of delivery. The continuum of social standards and prototype for what a birthing person should be is depicted almost always as a female-identifying person, which in and of itself is limiting, and is often less than helpful. One end of the continuum occupies the embodiment of "MILF-dom" ("Mom I'd like to fuck" state of being); and at the other end of the continuum, a "rented womb" that is available to be touched by all who see that it is inhabited (i.e., when a stranger touches the abdomen of a birthing person, often without consent or concern for that person's space or physical body). Oh, the social messages that have been created!

With such an enigma of identity at play during the postpartum season of life, it is no wonder that birthing persons struggle to come to a place of acceptance and contentment in response to their transformed self, physical and otherwise. The objectifying of the birthing person (by self and others) has been shown to create challenges vis-à-vis body shame, concerns about the negative impact of breastfeeding, barriers to breastfeeding, fear of childbirth, disordered eating, greater appearance concerns in mothers, and sexualized behaviors and body surveillance for their children (Beech et al., 2020). As a way to help birthing persons connect with themselves in a more positive way, I have created the following exercise that can help create connection where a deep sense of disconnection is felt both during pregnancy and the postpartum period.

Exercise:

Letter to my Empty Womb / Letter to My Womb / Letter to Your Womb

Goal: To help birthing persons connect with their bodies in a positive way from both a physical and emotional perspective.

Directions: If you are a birthing person and you're currently pregnant and your body is actively going through the changes that come with pregnancy, speak to your body now. If you are a birthing person that is currently in the postpartum stage, speak to your body now. ***Note:*** This activity can be modified to allow partners of birthing persons to affirm their partners during pregnancy or during the postpartum stage as well. Directions will need to simply be modified to fit the scenario that fits your situation/situation of the person(s) you are working with as a practitioner. The steps to take are as follows:

1. Make sure you have a quiet space to reflect and think. If it helps to have a mirror in front of you to be able to view your body, then feel free to sit in front of a mirror if you have the availability to do so.
2. This is a time to give yourself positive affirmations. This is a time to work to accept the things that are challenging you as well. I recommend writing this from a third person point-of-view as if you are speaking to yourself from the outside looking in. This strategy can often create less dissonance when you are working to adopt a more positive narrative with yourself and face the conflict that negative narratives are bringing.
3. You will write a letter to yourself, in whatever order you see fit, about the positive affirmations that you need to help you confront the body images you are experiencing. It is likely that the challenges will be easier to recognize than the affirmative statements will be. If that is true for you, know that it's okay, and that the challenge here is to take as much time to offer yourself at least one affirmation for every challenge/insecurity/negative message/etc. that you are giving to yourself. *Tip*: Using the five senses can be helpful to guide your process. If something else works for you, feel free to try that as well. I have included an example to help illustrate what such a letter may look like. This is also a very helpful activity for those who are struggling with connecting with their child or children and/or who struggle with no longer being pregnant as well.

Dear Birth Goddess,

You are a source of strength and light. In you I see a resilient warrior who often feels like a helpless lonely child. When I hear the messages you give yourself about being fat and not good-enough it saddens me as I know that you have prevailed in ways that even you didn't know existed before you became an actively birthing person. As I look at you and feel the abdomen that holds/held what will be/is now a life, I feel the skin that covers you, supple, flexible, like protective garb that is capable of helping to protect the life that is/was inside. Seeing the strength here makes it easier to ignore the changes to the skin that include stretch marks in ever multiplying forms. Your sense of taste and smell, though changed, has transformed,

> *just like the phoenix within you that is working to rise from the ashes of the war that you are fighting within you. You are strong and resilient even when you don't feel it. The changes that you witness within you are signs of what you are doing and what you have done. I will help you work to be grateful of all the glory that you embody and the wonder that is your ability to weather the storms of this season of your life.*
>
> *Warmly and lovingly,*
>
> *Your Aspiring Stronger Self*

Note to those completing the exercise: This exercise is one that may very well elicit very strong, deeply held emotions. It is important that you are in a safe and grounded space when completing this activity. If you find yourself overwhelmed with the emotion behind doing the above exercise, remember that it is okay to come back to it if you are not ready for the activity at all or in its entirety.

Note to sexual health practitioners: The strength of emotion that can be elicited from this exercise can be very overwhelming for those completing these self-affirmations. If you plan to enact this exercise in a therapeutic space, I recommend making sure there is ample time to prepare, complete, and process the activity. I have found that this exercise is better for some when if it is broken into smaller parts, if need be, versus rushing through it.

THE ROLE OF EMOTIONAL CONNECTION

Despite the excitement that comes with becoming a new parent, it is not unusual for new parents to feel extremely overwhelmed and at a loss for how to create a new structure in a new normal that seems impossible to navigate. In the midst of such feelings, it is common for new parents to feel a sense of sadness, hopelessness, and a loneliness in their relationship with their partner(s) that they have likely never experienced before. With regard to sexual satisfaction and the aforesaid feelings associated with new parenthood, it has been found that new parents who reported more empathy toward their partner and had partners who reported more empathy toward them, also indicated higher sexual satisfaction and more desire to engage sexually with their partners (Rosen et al., 2017).

When new parents have the space to express concern for their partner and try to see things from their partners' point of view, this process may encourage more open communication between partners about their sexual relationship, resulting in more sexual satisfaction for all. Sexual communication may involve discussions of how to adapt or adjust expectations for sexual activity in relation to the new realities of early parenthood. As a therapist that works with dyads and partnered groups, I have found the exercise shared below to be a successful way of exploring new parenthood and can give partners an opportunity to experience mutual empathy.

Exercise:
Increasing and Expanding Empathy

Goal: For partners to increase a sense of dyadic/mutual empathy as a way to feel a deeper emotional connection as well as to create a climate in which sexual desire is prioritized and/or possible.

Directions: The result of this exercise is for each partner to answer all questions and have their emotions and needs honored. If you are in (or working with) a nondyadic, partnered system, make sure that all parties are included in this exercise. Partners will take turns. Each partner will respectively come up with a new part of themselves that they have discovered since becoming a parent/caregiver. The idea here is that this new part and the feelings and needs associated with it will be thoroughly explored. First, one partner will be the *listener* and the other will be the *speaker*, and then both/all parties will then switch after their partner(s) has taken their turn(s). Rinse and repeat until all parties feel honored and have had a chance to play the role of both the *speaker* and *listener.* (***Note for practitioners:*** For those who are working with single parents in any situation, this is an exercise that can be utilized in a manner employing the empty chair technique to give voice, validation, and affirmation to new dimensions of the new parent's lived experience.)

Possible Questions (please modify language if working with single parent):

1. What new belief do you now hold about yourself as a person/partner now that you are parents?
2. What do you feel about this new part?
3. What does that mean to you?
4. Tell me the meaning of this new part and the needs associated with it.
5. Is there a story behind why this is such an important new belief?
6. Does this relate to your history in some way?
7. Does this relate to your history in any way (before you were parents)?
8. What do you want in regard to this part and the associated need(s)?
9. What do you need from me/us in regard to this now that you are parents?
10. Tell me why is this important to you?
11. What is the meaning of your position on this issue?
12. What are all your feelings about this?
13. Are there any feelings you have left out here?
14. What do you wish from me/us here?
15. What would be your ideal dream here?
16. What do you imagine things would be like if you got what you needed met fully and completely?
17. Is there a deeper purpose or goal in this for you?
18. In what way is it central to who you are as a person, to your core identity?
19. Does this relate to some belief or value for you?
20. Is there a fear or disaster scenario if the new need is not honored by me/us?

Notes about this exercise: (a) After completing this activity, by yourself or with those you are working with, it can be useful to go back and re-engage this exercise at a different stage of parenting. Reflecting on the changes that occurred can allow partners to continue to feel connected as the required roles as parents shift with the evolving needs across stages of development. (b) It is highly useful to have partners think of a need that is both emotionally driven and sexually driven and to complete the exercise as many times as needed to cover the respective needs that are expressed.

PHYSIOLOGICAL CHALLENGES

Physiological changes in the postpartum period are inevitable for the birth parent as the changes that happened during pregnancy slow naturally with the baby out of the birthing parent's womb. However, most birthing partners are likely to become more focused on physiological changes and are more likely to feel the impact of postpartum depression and baby blues, which can increase perseverations on bodily changes. One of the most physical tasks that occurs frequently during the postpartum period pertains to birthing partners who breastfeed. Not only is learning to breastfeed with one's child for the first time a completely demanding and all-consuming process which takes up a large store of emotional energy, it is also very demanding on the physical body. Nonbirthing parents may often feel helpless in being able to support their partner. They typically have no physical ability to alternate with their partner, taking on the challenge of breastfeeding themselves. With that said, birthing partners who are breastfeeding are much more likely to have increased desire for physical closeness and sexual intimacy with their partners if they feel emotionally nurtured and supported (Matthies et al., 2019). For this reason, when working with partnered systems during the postpartum stage, I often emphasize the importance of focusing on activities that are more apt to increase spontaneous desire, or in other words, appeal to the emotional hungers of the birthing partner that may need to be satiated. In this section, I have included a checklist that addresses ways in which nonbirthing partners can support their partner who is breastfeeding as well as an intimacy exercise that is aimed at increasing fulfilling intimate experiences during the postpartum period.

Exercise:

Supporting my Breastfeeding Partner Checklist

Goal: This exercise is intended to assist couples and partnered systems during the postpartum period and specifically in regard to breastfeeding.

Directions: Notes about exercise. Both birthing partners and nonbirthing partners are encouraged to add items to the checklist as they see fit (this is in no way to be seen as a one-size-fits-all checklist). This checklist can also be used by sexual health practitioners to have meaningful conversations with couples and partnered systems.

1. Engage in physical nurturing if birthing/breastfeeding partner is up to it (i.e., rubbing shoulders, rubbing feet, caressing typically nonerogenous parts of the body, etc.).
2. Make sure that your partner is comfortable while breastfeeding (i.e., propping up pillows, etc.).
3. Encourage your partner by letting them know that although breastfeeding may be challenging, they are doing a great job.
4. If birthing partner is comfortable, reward them with physical affection after breastfeeding accompanied with some words of encouragement.
5. Ask your partner what they need . . . A LOT!
6. Bring water to your partner while they are breastfeeding. Remember, breastfeeding is dehydrating work and it makes the person manufacturing the milk super hungry!
7. If a breast pump is being used, help your partner by being creative and helping them consider activities that may pass the time. Sometimes sitting with your partner can be enough.
8. Help partner clean breast pump parts, breast pillow, and so forth. Having help like this can help breastfeeding be a less lonely task.
9. Offer to help during the night when baby/babies need to be picked up (if in a bassinet or other room). Even if you go right back to sleep, this can be very helpful to your partner.
10. Prioritize the re-assessing of needs. Make sure to initiate conversations regarding current needs.

Exercise:

Red Light - Yellow Light - Green Light

Goal: Engaging in light, sensual touch can be a way to re-engage intimacy in a nonpressured way. The idea in this exercise is to allow partners to build trust and to focus on nongenitally focused pleasure.

Directions: Set the mood (whatever this means for you). Some ideas may include lighting candles, playing some music, dimming the lights, putting a blanket on the floor or somewhere comfy that is different from where you as partners usually engage in physical affection together. It is ideal if the baby/babies and any other children are free from the space so both you and your partner(s) can be relaxed. Once you are settled, the following steps are suggested:

1. Take off your clothes and lie together, skin to skin.
2. Embrace each other in a long deep hug until you both are able to relax your shoulders, your neck, your entire body into one another. Enjoy this time and do this for as long as you wish. Do not feel the need to rush this in any way.
3. Once you feel nice and relaxed you will each take turns caressing each other's bodies. You can feel free to touch one another's genitals (stay on the outer vulvar region for vulva owners) but not to the point of climax. The idea here is to really explore each other's bodies.
4. The partner that goes first will look to their counterpart(s) to indicate "Red, yellow, or green light" each time the partner who is caressing touches a new part of the body. Green means "stay there," yellow means, "Go and come back later," and red means "Move on from that area." Once the first partner moves from head to toe, partners will switch, rinse, and repeat.

   Note: The next portion of this exercise may make you feel much more vulnerable. If the aforementioned part is all that you and your partner(s) are ready for, then feel free to come back to this next stage at another time and do not proceed further.

5. If each partner is ready for this next step and all have agreed, then it is time to proceed to the more intimate genital exploration. During this portion of the exercise, each partner will take turns looking at one another's genitals, touching them, using the same "Red," "Yellow," and "Green" light directives as above. This time, though, you will touch your partners genitals, moving slowly from one area to the next.

6. Express what you see and feel using only your hands (I love this soft crease right here . . . I love that you trust me enough to let me touch you there, etc.). You will take turns doing this.
7. Once you both have completed the exercise, you are free to enjoy each other as you wish. It is highly encouraged to avoid any penetrative sexual interactions during the first attempts at doing this exercise.

Notes about this exercise: (a) Consistency is key. This exercise is especially useful when it is integrated consistently during the postpartum stage in order to build trust and safety, particularly early on after the baby/babies, before any penetration of any kind occurs. (b) For sexual health practitioners that are using this exercise, it is suggested that you discuss the utility with birthing partners and nonbirthing partners before they engage in the exercise, emphasizing the importance of employing the themes of slow, steady, and consistent while completing it.

CLOSING REMARKS

Due to the vulnerable nature of the postpartum period, it is of utmost importance for sexual health practitioners to assist those that they work with in addressing the multiplicity of issues that will be faced during this unique developmental stage. It is, of course, imperative to allow space to honor the excitement that planning for a new life brings, as well as to explore and prevent potential challenges that often befall new parents.

For those who have the opportunity to begin work with couples and partnered systems during pregnancy, it is highly suggested that a proactive approach be taken to allow aspiring new parents the prospect of circumnavigating some of the challenges that they will ultimately face in the stage of life ahead. This can be done by assisting these parents in creating realistic expectations, preparing for the physiological, emotional, and ultimately, the sexual challenges that are woven through them all.

Encourage proactive planning through some of the experiential activities presented here – all which can be implemented during pregnancy and/or the postpartum period. These exercises will emphasize the need for shared realistic expectations in regard to maintaining sexual activity and desire within consideration of the developmental context of the postpartum stage.

For far too long, postpartum sexuality has been underaddressed within the literature as well as within providers' offices. It is the sexual health practitioner who has the opportunity to create a new set of norms that allows those approaching and moving through the postpartum stage to navigate it in a way that is healthier, more informed, and inclusive of a unique connection to one's sexual self.

REFERENCES AND RESOURCES

Anzaku, A. S., & Mikah, S. (2014). Postpartum resumption of sexual activity, sexual morbidity and use of modern contraceptives among Nigerian women in Jos. *Annals of Medical & Health Science Research, 4*(2), 210-216.

Banaei, M., Tork Zahrani, S., Pormehr-Yabandeh, A., Ozgoli, G., & Azad, M. (2016). Investigating the impact of counseling based on PLISSIT model on sexual intimacy and satisfaction of breastfeeding women. *International Journal of Pharmaceutical Research and Allied Sciences, 5*(3), 489-499.

Beech, O. D., Kaufmann, L., & Anderson, J. (2020). A systematic literature review exploring objectification and motherhood. *Psychology of Women Quarterly, 44*(4), 521-538. https://doi.org/10.1177/0361684320949 81

Brtnicka, H., Weiss, P., & Zverina, J. (2009). Human sexuality during pregnancy and the postpartum period. *Bratislava Medical Journal, 110*, 427-431.

Buehler, S. (2018). *Counseling couples before, during, & after pregnancy.* Springer.

Cohen, M. J., Pentel, K. Z., Boeding, S. E., & Baucom, D. H. (2019). Postpartum role satisfaction in couples: Associations with individual and relationship well-being. *Journal of Family Issues, 40*(9), 1181-1200. https://doi.org/10.1177/0192513X19835866

Jawed-Wessel, S., & Sevick, E. (2017). The impact of pregnancy and childbirth on sexual behaviors: A systematic review. *The Journal of Sex Research*, *54*(4-5), 411-423. https://doi.org/10.1080/00224499.2016.1274715

Matthies, L. M., Wallwiener, M., Sohn, C., Reck, C., Müller, M., & Wallwiener, S. (2019). The influence of partnership quality and breastfeeding on postpartum female sexual function. *Archives of Gynecology & Obstetrics*, *299*(1), 69-77. https://doi.org/10.1007/s00404-018-4925-z

McBride, H. L., Olson, S., Kwee, J., Klein, C., & Smith, K. (2017). Women's Postpartum Sexual Health Program: A collaborative and integrated approach to restoring sexual health in the postpartum period. *Journal of Sex & Marital Therapy*, *43*(2), 147-158. https://doi.org/10.1080/0092623X.2016.1141818

Moore Simas, T. A., Huang, M.-Y., Patton, C., Reinhart, M., Chawla, A. J., Clemson, C., & Eldar-Lissai, A. (2019). The humanistic burden of postpartum depression: A systematic literature review. *Current Medical Research & Opinion*, *35*(3), 383-393. https://doi.org/10.1080/03007995.2018.1552039

Rosen, N. O., Mooney, K., & Muise, A. (2017). Dyadic empathy predicts sexual and relationship well-being in couples transitioning to parenthood. *Journal of Sex & Marital Therapy*, *43*(6), 543-559. https://doi.org/10.1080/0092623X.2016.1208698

Rupp, H. A., James, T. W., Ketterson, E. D., Sengelaub, D. R., Ditzen, B., & Heiman, J. R. (2013). Lower sexual interest in postpartum women: Relationship to amygdala activation and intranasal oxytocin. *Hormones & Behavior*, *63*(1), 114-121. https://doi.org/10.1016/j.yhbeh.2012.10.007

Shahraki, Z., Tanha, F. D., & Ghajarzadeh, M. (2018). Depression, sexual dysfunction and sexual quality of life in women with infertility. *BMC Women's Health*, *18*(1), 92.

World Health Organization. (2015, February 12). *Pregnancy, childbirth, postpartum and newborn care: A guide for essential practice* (3rd edition). https://apps.who.int/iris/bitstream/handle/10665/249580/9789241549356-eng.pdf?sequence=1&isAllowed=y

25

Golden Sexuality: Sex Therapy for Seniors

Carol M. Jaxson-Jager

Grow old along with me, the best is yet to be.
Robert Browning

INTRODUCTION AND PHILOSOPHY

In terms of intimacy in general as well as geriatric health, the topic of senior sexuality is one of the most neglected areas of relationships in the professional health literature. "Old age" is sometimes seen as a repository of wisdom, cultural memories, and tradition. But when it comes to sexual expression, the elderly have been socially segregated from the community and perceived as unattractive, sexless, and even as burdens with mental and physical health issues. As individuals advance in age, there can be increased health concerns. However, older Americans as a whole are frequently viewed as dependent, passive, and usually in need of public assistance.

Aging is a lifelong process that begins at birth and if an individual lives long enough to become "old," they should be applauded for having sustained life's perils rather than demeaned. Thinning hair, sagging skin, mobility issues, digestive problems, and lower energy levels can be used as excuses to exclude the elderly from being seen as sexual beings, and even viewed with distain. The need for intimacy does not wane with age. We all are sexual beings from the "rocking of the cradle to the rolling of the hearse." The need for sexual expression is quite alive, even though society views "Golden Sex" as a "Forbidden Fruit," which should never be eaten (Rae, 2014).

Over half of the adult population in America is over the age of 50 (Mather et al., 2019). Many are challenging the idea of "grandparents in a rocking chair, watching the sun set" concept from a few decades ago. Society is realizing that grandparents can pursue sports like skiing, hiking, and golf. In addition, Grandpa and Nanny may love working out at the gym or starting their own business.

Since there are an increasing number of adults over the age of 50, there are more older couples and individuals seeking higher levels of sexual satisfaction. It is hoped that by reading this chapter you will learn useful strategies to aid you in working with this population and that you will experience how rewarding providing this care can be.

GOLDEN SEXUALITY

Fulfilling sexuality in the golden years can be achieved with individuals who are healthy as well as those with medical issues who have a desire to be sexually active. There are four fundamentally important points of sexuality to review at the start of this chapter.

First, one must have accurate sexual knowledge, which may not always be easy to acquire depending on one's living situation within American culture. There is a lot of erotic stimulation available on prime-time television. However, many Americans learned essentially nothing (or very little) about healthy sexual function as they were growing up. There are few sex-positive curriculums culturally endorsed and used in American schools for sexual health education. Therefore, knowledge about healthy sexual function and expression must be sought individually, while people are developing their unique erotic life. Therapists must incorporate sexual education throughout their work. They must not assume that patients already know basic sexual information. At the same time, therapists need to respect the sexual knowledge older adults may bring with them.

Second, it takes many years to overcome sexual ignorance, stereotypes, and sexually traumatic experiences. Many fundamentalist religions (as well as "mainstream denominations") in American culture discourage full ownership of one's individual sexuality. Religions often label many sexual behaviors as sinful, or at least a misdemeanor against the Divine. Masturbation may be considered a "misdemeanor" but same-sex attraction is definitely a "felony" within some denominations that require excommunication and/or conversion therapy to force the person to reject their attraction for the same sex. Therapists need to be comfortable and skilled navigating respect for religious affiliation and associated beliefs, while at the same time clearly expressing the fact solo-sex and same-sex attraction are considered healthy and normal. If they are not comfortable doing so, they should not be counseling anyone about sexuality. It is also important to keep in mind that it may take years for some individuals to learn to endorse and appreciate their unique sexuality. As a client they have a right to expect your nonjudgmental guidance.

Third, about the time that sexual knowledge, sexual experience, and self-understanding have matured to the level of potential sexual satisfaction, overall health and hormonal physiology may begin to decline (as reviewed in Chapter 4 of this text). Libido, sensual responsiveness, arousal, and ability to reach climax or orgasm can change when hormones may fall below optimal functioning levels. Sex therapy today should not be limited to talking therapy when symptoms of hormonal inadequacy are identified and confirmed by laboratory tests. Restoration of hormonal balance at a level usually found in the 40s can be very helpful for those without medical contraindications. Medications that inhibit sexual response must also be addressed and modified when possible (as discussed in Chapter 5).

Fourth, other blocks to quality of life such as conflict, anger, depression, or performance anxiety require identification (and improvement) if sex therapy is to be effective. Of course, exercise, nutrition, stress management, and general good-health practices are the support structure for golden sexuality. Many seniors believe that the interchange of sexual energy at a deep, even spiritual, level requires the context of respect, love, and appreciation for the beauty and uniqueness of the sexual partner. Whether this happens within long- or short-term relationships, focusing on appreciating the partner, rather than depreciating aspects (or behaviors) of the other, requires maturity, capacity for intimacy, and good communication skills. Seniors who are used to sexual expression only in long-term relationships may find that they need to be open to learning new perspectives and skill sets that can facilitate sexual satisfaction in short-term relationships. Therapists need to keep this in mind and make sure they do not express any judgments from their own value system which a senior client may perceive as disapproving.

SEXUAL HEALTH LITERACY

Today's health care providers often fall short of explaining to clients all of the relevant sexual health topics specific to the client, which may include omission of the diagnostic considerations of the case, appropriate treatment plans, or other risk assessments for their presenting dysfunction. Sexual health literacy includes taking time to actively teach patients what they need to know to resolve their sexual concerns. This includes informing patients so that they can make good choices about how to approach and self-treat their problems. The Sexual Tipping Point model in Chapter 9 is an excellent example of how patient health education can enhance the client's sexual health literacy as well as resolve presenting concerns.

In sex therapy, health literacy also involves demystifying and decreasing sexual shame. Sexual knowledge, sexual self-awareness, and capacity for intimacy all require time and are acquired not just from having conversation, but experiential learning with a sexual partner. Clients may school themselves by reading accurate and positive sexuality guidebooks that inspire as well as educate. There are several texts recommended, including but not limited to:

- *The Guide to Getting it On!* (Joannides, 2004)
- *Come as You Are* (Nagosky, 2015)
- *Mating in Captivity* (Perel, 2006)
- *Read My Lips* (Herbenick & Schick, 2011)
- *The Gender Revolution & New Sexual Health* (Peterson, Bley, & Frabotta, 2020)

For enhanced sexual health literacy, it is helpful for clients to know the five phases of the sexual response cycle and be able to identify which phase of the sexual response cycle is involved in an individual's sexual dysfunction. Understanding the phases of the sexual response cycle is helpful to client care and based on the pioneering sex research by Masters and Johnson (1966), and H. Kaplan (1974). The sexual response cycle begins with desire which is experienced primarily in the brain of the individual which triggers the accumulation of blood in the genitals and other areas of the body (vasocongestion) and contraction of the muscles in the pelvic area and other parts of the body (myotonia).

The ***first phase*** of the sexual response cycle is desire. Individuals spend much more time during this phase of sexual experience than all the other phases combined. The desire phase may last days, months, or years toward a person who becomes the focus of romantic and sexual desire. By comparison, the arousal, plateau, and orgasm phases may last just a few minutes (even in combination). The attributes of sexual desire are considered thoughts, feelings, and fantasies about sex which generate the basis for the next phase of sexual responsiveness – arousal. The thoughts, feelings, and fantasies are often associated with wishing to be near a person, missing them when not in close proximity, wanting to touch them and have their attention, and receiving their affection (including sexual interaction).

The ***second phase*** is the excitement stage (arousal), which is a physiological response to a sexual stimulus (often a desired sexual partner), and typically involving physical stimulation. Studies show that in most 50-year-old males, physical stimulation of the penis is very helpful, if not necessary for achieving erection. Vaginal lubrication in females is also accomplished physiologically and neurologically like erections in males. This physiological arousal (penile erections and vaginal lubrication) is accomplished by the processes of vasocongestion and build-up of sexual/muscular tension. In the arousal phase, individuals show steady progression to a high level of physiological excitement with the entire body activated.

The ***third phase*** is referred to as the plateau stage and is characterized by a period of prolonged pleasure. An individual will enjoy the positive sensual feelings in their body over time while building sexual energy and tension necessary for sexual climax to occur. Men with problems of rapid ejaculation (formally called "premature" ejaculation) often slow down as they age much to the greater satisfaction of themselves as well as their partner(s). The parasympathetic nervous system dominates during the arousal and plateau stages but prepares for the sympathetic nervous system to take over during the next phase.

The ***fourth phase***, orgasm, is the sudden shift into massive sympathetic neuronal discharge in the body. This almost instantaneous shift is marked by uterine contractions and contractions of the pelvic muscles in women. Male orgasm is made up of two stages. The first stage is the emission stage. During emission all of the fluids that contribute to the ejaculate are gathered in the seminal vesicles. Once the emission stage is complete, the second stage, ejaculation, is inevitable and happens almost immediately. Intensified orgasms are one of the benefits that very often occur in working with the sexuality of an older individual or couple. If you are interested in helping couples achieve intensified orgasm, learning and teaching Tantric sexual practices would be a helpful technique. It is good to know and to convey to clients that there is a growing body of research which demonstrates many health benefits (including cardiovascular) as a result of sexual engagement and orgasmic release (see Peterson, 2020, for a review of the health benefits of sexual expression).

The ***fifth phase*** is the resolution or calming down of the system. Males experience a climactic peak, go into resolution, and then have a refractory period. During the refractory period, no amount of sexual stimulation will cause a restart of the sexual cycle. The refractory period gets longer with age. At the age of 60, it may be several hours or days, and by the age of 80, even longer. Women do not experience the same type of resolution, and with ongoing effective stimulation, can have multiple orgasms routinely. Males clearly can have multiple orgasms, but it is an uncommon male who can have several orgasms in an hour like women routinely do. After a satisfying orgasm that is an emotionally and physically fulfilling experience, many women can go for days in a psychological version of the refractory period where they feel satisfied, even though, if effectively stimulated, they could resume the sexual cycle.

SEXUALITY ASSESSMENT FOR OLDER ADULTS

Although healthcare professionals should initiate a conversation about sexuality, a study shows that 63% of 155 physicians did not address sexuality in medical interviews with patients (Tatum et al., 2018). In this study, the main reasons for not addressing sexuality were lack of time, fear of embarrassing the patient, and the resistance to address the subject of sexuality. While physicians may fail to inquire about the sexuality of their older patients, older patients tend to neglect their sexuality due to three main assumptions which are incorrect.

The ***first*** false assumption is that the elderly do not think about sex and are not sexually active. Helgason et al. (1996) however, found that 46% of 70- to 80-year-old men reported having at least one orgasm in the previous month. In a study published in the *New England Journal of Medicine*, Landau & Schumm (2007) found that 30% of elderly women and 60% of elderly men had had sexual intercourse in the last month. The ***second*** false assumption is that sexuality among the elderly, when it does occur, is morally wrong. Often the elderly may feel embarrassed to maintain or discuss their sex life for fear of being thought of as perverted. The ***third*** false assumption is that sexuality in the elderly is awkward and funny to the degree it is the subject of humor and stand-up comedy frequently viewed in night clubs and on television.

Healthcare professionals should learn that sexual activities are expressed within the limitations of chronic health issues along with medications and are part of the normal aging process. Assessment and education of aging adults is indicated, and healthcare professionals are encouraged to take a leading role in opening a discussion of sexuality and providing sexual health education material. Sadly, for multiple reasons, this is not the typical experience of aging clients who recognize they are in need and seek assistance for their sexual health concerns.

When the healthcare professional sees a couple or individual for an initial appointment, the time should be spent gathering enough data to form an overall opinion of the nature of the sexual problem, while communicating caring and competence to the new client. A detailed assessment is critical, regardless of the referral source, the discipline of the practitioner, or the nature of the complaint. If the therapist's time is very limited during standard business hours, the client(s) may be scheduled as the last appointment of the day to allow sufficient time to complete the process.

A helpful assessment strategy that is a significant time-saver is to request the client to bring with them a personal timeline. The timeline is a list of bullet points representing their history of important developmental events such as the year they were born, graduations, marriages, children born, and so on. In addition, clients can also complete and return self-assessments before their appointment for review during the initial consultation. These self-assessments for sexual health and guidelines for clinical assessment are reviewed in detail in Chapters 2 and 3.

During the first interview, the therapist should recognize any discomfort or anxiety as normal behavior in older individuals or couples. This anxiety about sexual matters and discussion is to be expected with older adults but can be seen in younger individuals as well. A therapist wants information that will help determine the needs of the couple or individual. It can be helpful to separate a couple for 10 to 15 minutes for brief individual interviews to allow each person to express themselves more openly. It is essential that the client can share feelings about their attitude toward the sex therapy process, their belief about the attitude of their partner, as well as any questions regarding their presenting problems. When indicated, it is very helpful if the client agrees to a three-appointment assessment process which involves an initial consultation, followed by an in-depth follow-up appointment covering the development history and testing, and culminating in a results-sharing conference (see the therapist guide in Section VI on pp. 579-583 for a sample treatment plan).

The second interview allows the therapist to explore the areas of sexual comfort and discomfort such as nakedness, touch, talking during sex, giving and receiving oral sex, preferred sexual position, or the stimulation necessary for successful climax. The therapist should review the phases of the sexual response cycle with the couple or individual and help them to understand in which phases they are having difficulties. It is recommended that sex therapists require, as part of the assessment, the results of a recent physical exam that is 6 months old or less, and a medical history. A medical history of diseases, medications, and client medical functioning is essential to understanding sexual dysfunction. Of particular interest are lab results for the client's hormone levels, especially when a client is complaining of loss of interest in sex.

Therapists should always inquire if the patient has sought previous therapy for sexual issues, and the outcome of therapy with a previous service provider. The therapist needs to inquire about hormone replacement therapy, the dosage, and form of hormones administered, by which service provider, and dates of the prescription. The therapist should request all information that would be helpful in assisting in the development of a treatment plan.

WHAT TO KNOW ABOUT HORMONES AND HORMONE REPLACEMENT THERAPY (HRT)

Hormones

The function of endocrine glands is to secrete hormones into the bloodstream to communicate and direct activities to organs throughout the body. Hormones affect growth, reproduction, and sexual characteristics (Morley, 2019). In essence, hormones serve as messengers, controlling and coordinating important physiological activities throughout the body. During the aging process, sex hormone production lessens, and this reduction of hormones causes changes in sexual functioning, desire, and arousal.

When levels of the female hormone estrogen reduce with aging, females may experience several distressing bodily changes, such as feeling overheated (hot flashes), night chills in addition to excessive perspiration (night sweats), lessened sexual desire, painful intercourse due to poor vaginal lubrication and thinner vaginal walls, and reduced ability to become aroused. Similarly, the male hormone testosterone lowers and males may also experience distressing changes such as less rigid erections, needing longer to achieve an erection at times, needing more stimulation to achieve and maintain erection and orgasm, shorter orgasms, less forceful ejaculation, less semen ejaculated, and a longer time needed to achieve another erection after ejaculation.

While both aging females and males believe that they are experiencing sexual dysfunctions, they usually are experiencing the normal and expected age-related sexual functioning due to a reduced amount of sex hormones in the system. A therapist must speak with the individual or couple about the normal aging process, review medical information, and help the client(s) understand that the presenting sexual issues may or may not be caused by existing medical issues in addition to sexual concerns, and that their concerns can be addressed either way. Interestingly, male clients may find that "slowing down" physical sexual responsiveness may have positive effects and expand their sexual pleasuring with a partner beyond penile-vaginal intercourse (especially if he has a history of rapid ejaculation).

A reduction of hormones, however, may not be the only reason that a person may have sexual difficulties that affect their ability to have and enjoy sex (National Institutes of Health/National Institute on Aging, 2017). Individuals who visit a therapist for wanting to be able to have and enjoy sex can be affirmed that their interest in sex is normal and healthy, complimented for their initiation to seek consultation, and encouraged that they can enjoy sexual pleasure despite any effects of aging.

Hormone Replacement Therapy (HRT)

Hormone Replacement Therapy is a treatment to relieve the symptoms of menopause such as vaginal dryness, mood swings, night sweats, hot flashes, and reduced sex drive. Some unpleasant symptoms stop by themselves over the years, but HRT can relieve symptoms sooner and is thought to help prevent osteoporosis. Although HRT can make menopause more bearable for some females, there are risks involved, as some types of HRTs may increase the risk of breast cancer. Hence, HRT is not advisable if the client has a history of breast cancer, a history of blood clots, has untreated high blood pressure, has liver disease, or is pregnant. As with many medicines, there are many variations of HRT. Some are taken with other hormones, some tablet form, skin patches, gels, and vaginal creams. HRTs can also have negative effects on some individuals, such as vaginal bleeding, breast tenderness, headaches, nausea, indigestion, or abdominal pain.

HRT can be used by men during andropause, and there are also several options from which to choose. Those include testosterone injections, testosterone patches (applied to back, arms, or buttock), or topical testosterone which is applied to the shoulders, arms, abdomen, thighs, or underarms. Testosterone injections can be self-administered or given through a nurse (usually every 2-3 weeks). Another product (AVEED) is a longer-lasting form of testosterone injection which involves injections every 6 weeks. The risks of testosterone replacement may be fluid retention, acne, and increased urination. More severe risks include breast enlargement, decreased testicle size, worsening of existing sleep apnea, increased cholesterol levels, decreased sperm count, infertility, and increased number of red blood cells which may cause muscle pain, high blood pressure, and blurry vision (Mayo Clinic, 2020).

While there are risks and side effects involved with all medications, a decision to opt for the potential benefits of HRT is best understood to rest within a joint decision-making process between the client and a provider (who has specific prescription privileges and experience prescribing for HRT). Therapists are encouraged to promote the health literacy of their clients by assisting them to understand the risks and benefits as well as the client's specific lab results. It is an uninformed client that just accepts his provider's statement "You are in the normal range, so we are not going to consider HRT." "Normal range" is specific to the individual and "within normal range" for total testosterone serum level in adult men is considered 280-1180 ng/dL (Pagana & Pagana, 2021). If the client's total testosterone is measured at 290 or 300, he is just within the normal range. If told by his provider "don't consider HRT" (and there are no medical contraindications), then the client is not given an opportunity to discuss the possibility of how he might feel better at an elevated level (such as a midrange level of 500-600). A conversation regarding the cost-benefit ratio analysis for an improved quality of life is a valid consideration and should be within the realm of the patient-provider relationship.

INTERVENTIONS

A good guideline for intervening with senor adults is the PLISSIT model (Annon, 1976), which allows the interviewer to further a discussion with older adults in a way that allows the client to feel safe and comfortable about discussing sexuality. This model renders guidelines for therapists to intervene through simple and direct Permission (P) giving, providing Limited Information (LI), Specific Suggestions (SS), or referral of the individual/couple for Intense Therapy (IT).

Therapy for sexual concerns should be determined by the issues presented by the couple or individual; but to help the individual or couple resolve the sexual concern, the therapist will also be addressing emotional responses such as anxiety or depression, anger, guilt, fear of pain, or a sense of loss. In addition, the therapist needs to address the larger context of the relationship, including the sources of distress and couple conflict, perceived rejection, and/or a lack of intimacy. As a result of the intersectionality of these multileveled issues, it is common for therapists to see couples whose presenting complaint is that they have not had sex in several months or years.

In the presence of a sexual impairment, the therapist should address reduced desire, lack of physiological arousal, decreased sexual enjoyment, or when the partner develops an associated sexual impairment. In working with a couple or an individual, the sex therapist should help them recognize that underlying issues may sabotage sexual desire and enjoyment. Because there are literally scores of reasons individuals disclose why they have lost their sexual desire, it is not surprising that the lack of sexual interest is the most common presenting problem to sexual health clinics.

Of particular importance is to identify and discuss any sexual myths the client may have, and work to eliminate these myths as potential factors in a couple's interpersonal conflict. For example, male sexual myths include that a man should have a full hard penis at the drop of a bra (which is inaccurate as well as heterosexist). Due to the many factors that interfere with a man's libido and his ability to have erections, sexual partners at times feel offended if the man struggles to get or maintain an erection. In short, the partner takes the lack of instant erection "personally" without due consideration of his level of stress, alcohol consumption, medication effects, or dozens of additional factors. Other myths regarding sexual performance interfere with the quality of sex satisfaction, such as real men do not have sexual problems, real men can always "perform" during sex, or real men do not talk about feelings or emotions. Ironically, a man focusing more intensely on the quality of his erection is the best way for him to lose an erection.

While these may seem like significant deterrents to healthy and enjoyable sex for men, there also seem to be more sexual myths placed on women. The greater number of sexual myths regarding females is consistent with the historical pattern of pathologizing of, and suppression of, female sexual expression through the American institutions of law, medicine, and education (Peterson, 2020). Some female sexual myths include that sex is only for women under the age of 40, that sex is really for reproduction, that it is a man's job to initiate sex, that women should not sweat or lose control during sex, that she should always be lady-like during sex even during orgasm, that women should be able to squirt (ejaculate) if they are really enjoying an orgasm, that pregnancy and delivery reduce a woman's response, and that if a woman cannot have an orgasm quickly, there is something wrong with her.

Of course, some of the most dangerous sexual myths are the rape myths that perpetuate the rape culture commonly found in America, especially on college campuses (these include variations of "no" does NOT mean "no" when women do not give consent). This is the "short list" of sexual myths about women and it is imperative to evaluate your clients for their sexual health literacy and potential interference from sexual myths. General male and female myths include: Real sex means penile-vaginal intercourse, that sex is only good if both partners have thunderous orgasms (at the same time), that any sexual contact should lead to sex, that you should know what your partner wants without having to ask, and that fantasizing about someone else means she or he is not happy with the relationship. Section VI in this book contains a patient handout of the most common sexual myths, titled "A Healthcare Professional's Guide to Contemporary Sexual Myths" (pp. 607-612).

To the surprise of many mental health professionals, most of the interventions employed to resolve sexual concerns are the same techniques used by general counselors and therapists to address other relationship issues. Sex therapy is just another a type of talk therapy that is utilized for treating sexual issues and therefore has goals and "homework" that is more often focused on sexual health goals.

Sex therapists are mental health professionals who have obtained specialized training and are able to deal with more complicated sexual health problems that more general interventions do not resolve. The sex therapist is trained in specific methods to help clients find means to meet their sexual needs. Like other areas of specialized training and practice, practitioners are invited to consider sex therapy training to expand their practice and enjoy learning new areas of practice. If you are interested in this training, consult the website for the American Association for Sexuality Educators, Counselors and Therapists (AASECT): www.aasect.org

TYPES OF TECHNIQUES USED TO ADDRESS SEXUAL CONCERNS

Relaxation Training is learning to refocus attention to relax the body and focus the mind on breathing and awareness of other body sensations. These skills also include progressive muscle relaxation, breathing with the diaphragm, and guided visualization. Being able to relax the mind and body is critically important to expand one's comfort zone relative to sexual thoughts, feelings, and behaviors that traditionally have caused muscular tension, anxiety, and self-criticism (even self-condemnation).

Mindfulness involves learning a skill set which allows one to focus on the present moment and not being judgmental about thoughts and sensations when they occur. The goal is to calmly acknowledge and accept one's feelings, thoughts, and bodily sensations to facilitate a peaceful state of mind and body (see Chapter 11 in this text by Dr. Denton).

Guided Sexual Imagery/Fantasy is the process of discussing and normalizing a variety of sexual fantasies, having the client write out their own erotic stories, encouraging exploration of the fantasies with self or partner stimulation.

Sexual Communication is talking about sexual feelings and thoughts with a sexual partner, such as sexual needs, physical affection, eye contact, discrepancies between partners histories of emotional or sexual abuse, and creating a ritual or pattern of sex communication that works for both.

Directed Masturbation involves comfort with looking at and touching oneself. Once that is accomplished, then mirror exercises are used for viewing genital and entire body area. The client can self-stimulate, feel sexy, and focus on what is positive about themselves, determining what "blocks" are present. The client adjusts to body image issues, religious and or cultural background, and dealing with negative sexually related cognitions (such as eliminating negative self-criticisms).

Cognitive Restructuring involves having the client identify thoughts and/or beliefs that are problematic about sexuality, then learn to normalize the negative feelings of distress, anxiety, fear, and disappointment. Finally, the therapist helps the client challenge and eventually change the content of the problematic thought process. The therapist provides the client with appropriate education, helps client stick to the facts (no emotional reasoning), identifies cues that increase chances of misinterpretation, helps the client decatastrophize, and encourages the client to keep a diary of thoughts, feelings, and outcomes.

Correcting Problematic Thoughts (also part of cognitive restructuring) helps the client identify thoughts/beliefs that are problematic about sexuality such as:

- Emotional reasoning (what I feel is the reality)
- Maximization or minimization (exaggerating or reducing)
- Shoulds/Musts (musterbating) "I must not fantasize about my girlfriend's friend. . . ."
- Filtering (focus on negatives, and ignore positives)
- Catastrophizing (expectation of the worse outcomes)
- Excitatory or inhibitory factors - Generating a list of conditions or factors which positively or negatively affect desire and or arousal (i.e., context, energy level, appropriateness, mood, what kinds of emotion and sexual stimulation are needed, relative strength or inhibitory factors, faulty belief) that challenge sexual communication and penetration-based sexual script (sex does not end because of a lost erection)

Sensate Focus

This technique was popularized by Masters and Johnson and is a series of behavioral exercises that a couple can do together in order to enhance intimacy and connection. This technique has seven elements that are the foundation of this technique:

- Mutual responsibility between partners for addressing sexual needs and concerns
- Information and education about sexual function and sexual activity
- Willingness to change attitudes about sex
- Getting rid of sexual performance anxiety
- Helping couples improve communication about sex and sex techniques
- Reducing problematic behavior and sex roles in the relationship
- Structured homework assignments

Sensate Focus is very helpful with clients to learn experientially and for assisting clients to focus on their immediate body sensations (getting out of their heads and self-criticisms which inhibit enjoyment of the present experience). Instructions for clients to complete Sensate Focus touching exercises are in Section VI of this text (pp. 589-593, "Sensual Pleasuring Through Sensate Focus Exercises" by Dr. Bley).

CONCLUSION

Although there are growing attempts to address the issues of aging in America, older adults continue to experience being pushed to the side of mainstream society in a general way and, specifically, socially stigmatized as sexual beings and even "de-sexed" as human beings. Unless someone needs money and is soliciting contributions, or wants them to babysit, seniors often feel ignored as fellow

Americans. Older citizens are often "overgeneralized" by frequent portrayals in advertising as having health issues, needing assistance in living, or preparing for death. In short, they are seen more as burdens to others rather than humans being with natural and healthy needs to love and be loved.

As senior citizens, older adults are often retired and have time to do the things they enjoy, such as traveling, volunteering, and biking to name a few activities. If health issues become more dominant in a person's life, sexual issues can arise which may cause self-image distortion, anxiety, depression, arousal issues, vaginal dryness, erectile function, or ejaculatory ability. These experiences can cause relationship issues with a partner or oneself.

Aging is a lifelong process, as is the need for intimacy and sexuality. Older adults continue to want to express their sexual and intimacy needs, despite reduced functioning. Older adults who want to address their sexual and intimacy needs may more likely contact a general mental health professional than a sexual health professional just because there are relatively very few sex therapists by comparison. You are encouraged to do what you can to increase your sense of comfort and confidence assisting senior adults who present at your practice with sexual concerns and questions. You have already started by reading this text, and especially this chapter, which addresses the sexual health needs of senior adults.

When in need of additional guidance, you are welcome to contact a certified sex therapist for consultation on a particularly challenging case. Secondly, you may wish to gain specialized training or even become certified yourself as a sex counselor or therapist. Sex therapists are mental health professionals of various disciplines (typically counselors, therapists, social workers, psychologists, and nurses) trained in sexuality issues and meet national certification requirements that are set by AASECT. Certified sex counselors and therapists are easy to find through the AASECT website.

Sexual issues are ongoing throughout one's lifespan and can become especially problematic when an individual becomes older because of other health issues. Sexuality is at the heart of a person's being and is a means of connectedness with others. Many older adults want to be intimately connected, emotionally and/or sexually. Being connected to others is an important aspect of overall health, not just emotional wellbeing. You can help a client reach the goal of accepting and enjoying their own being, or to be a part of someone else's life. As mental health professionals (and sex therapists), we are privileged to be able to help individuals and couples enjoy Golden Sexuality as a value-added, health-enhancing, and cherished aspect of later life.

REFERENCES

Alman, I. (2020, May 15). How long should sex actually last? *Psychology Today*. https://www.psychologytoday.com/us/blog/sex-sociability/202005/how-long-should-sex-actually-last

Annon, J. (1976). The PLISSIT Model: A proposed conceptual scheme for the behavioral treatment of sexual problems. *Journal of Sex Education and Therapy, 2,* 1-15.

Blair, O. (2017, February 17). Using supportive furniture and Viagra: A sex therapist's guide to sex for the elderly. *The Independent.* https://www.independent.co.uk/life-style/love-sex/sex-therapy-elderly-old-men-women-positions-viagra-support-aid-a7584366.html

Bradway, K. E., & Beard, R. L. (2015) "Don't be trying to box folks in": Older women's sexuality. *Affilia: Journal of Women and Social Work. 30*(4), 504-518.

Butarro, T., Koeniger-Dononhue, R., & Hawkins, J. (2014). Sexuality and quality of life in aging: Implications for practice. *The Journal for Nurse Practitioners, 10*(7), 480-485. https://doi.org/10.1016/j.nurpra.2014.04.008

Davis, L. M. (2007). Golden sexuality: Sex therapy for seniors. In L. VandeCreek, F. Peterson, & J. Bley (Eds.), *Innovations in clinical practice: Focus on sexual health.*(pp. 261-276). Professional Resource Press.

Goodman, H. (2014). For women, sexuality changes with age but doesn't disappear. *Harvard Health Blog*. https://www.health.harvard.edu/blog/for-women-sexuality-changes-with-age-but-doesnt-disappear-201402137035

Gurvinder, K., Subramanyam, A., & Pinto, C. (2011). Sexuality: Desire, activity and intimacy in the elderly. *Indian Journal of Psychiatry, 53*(4), 300-306.

Helgason, A., Adolfsson, J., Dickman, P., Arver, S., Fredrikson, M., Göthberg, M., & Steinbeck, G. (1996). Sexual desire, erection, orgasm and ejaculatory functions and their importance to elderly Swedish men: A population-based study. *Age and Ageing, 25*(4), 285-291. https://doi.org/10.1093/ageing/25.4.285

Herbenick, D., & Schick, V. (2011). *Read my lips.* Rowman & Littlefield Publishers.

Joannides, P. (2004). *The guide to getting it on!* UNKNO.

Kaplan, D. B., & Berkman, B. J. (2019). Intimacy and older adults. *Merck manual, professional version.* https://www.merckmanuals.com/professional/geriatrics/social-issues-in-older-adults/intimacy-and-older-adults

Kaplan, H. S. (1974). *The new sex therapy: Active treatment of sexual dysfunctions.* Brunner/Mazel.

Lindau, S., & Schumm, P. (2007). A national study of sexuality and health among older adults in the U.S. *New England Journal of Medicine, 357*(8), 762-774.

Masters, W., & Johnson, V. (1966). *Human sexual response*. Little Brown.

Mather, M., Scommegna, P., & Kilduff, L. (2019). *Fact sheet: Aging in the United States.* Population Reference Bureau. U.S. Government. https://www.prb.org/resources/fact-sheet-aging-in-the-united-states/

Mayo Clinic. (2020). *Testosterone therapy: Potential benefits and risks as you age*. https://www.mayoclinic.org/healthy-lifestyle/sexual-health/in-depth/testosterone-therapy/art-20045728

McCarthy, B. (2005). *Sex therapy for middle age and older adults*. Alexander Street Press.

Morley, J. (2019). Endocrine function. *Merck manual.* https://www.merckmanuals.com/home/hormonal-and-metabolic-disorders/biology-of-the-endocrine-system/endocrine-function.

Nagoski, E. (2015). *Come as you are.* Simon and Schuster.

National Institutes of Health. (2017). *Sexuality in later life*. National Institute on Aging. https://www.nia.nih.gov/health/sexuality-later-life

Pagana, K. & Pagana, T. (2021). *Mosby's manual of diagnostic and laboratory tests.* Mosby.

Perel, E. (2006). *Mating in captivity.* Harper.

Peterson, F. (2020). Health benefits from sexual expression. In F. Peterson, J. Bley, & R. Frabotta, *The gender revolution and new sexual health* (pp. 148-174). Cognella Academic Press.

Peterson, F., Bley, J., & Frabotta, R. (2020). *The gender revolution and new sexual health.* Cognella Academic Press.

Rae, R. (2014). Forbidden fruit in the golden years: Elderly sexuality. *Journal of Geriatric Mental Health, 1,* 8-13.

Rheaume, C., & Mitty, E. (2008). Sexuality and intimacy in older adults. *Journal of Geriatric Nursing, 29*(5), 342-349. https://doi.org/10.1016/j.gerinurse.2008.08.004

Rogers, P. (2019). Sex and aging. *Healthline.* https://www.healthline.com/health/healthy-sex-and-aging

Tatum, P., Talebreza, S., & Ross, J. (2018). Office-based evaluation of sexual function and complaints. *American Family Physician, 97*(12), 776-784.

University of Chicago Medical Center. (2010). Life is shorter for men, but sexually active life expectancy is longer. *Science Daily.* www.sciencedaily.com/releases/2010/03/100309202927.htm

Watters, Y., & Boyd, T. V. (2009) Sexuality in later life: Opportunity for reflections for healthcare providers. *Sexual and Relationship Therapy, 24*(3-4), 307-315. https://doi.org/10.1080/14681990903398047

Wilson, L. (2018). A guide to a fulfilling sex life for seniors. *UNC Health Talk.* https://healthtalk.unchealthcare.org/a-guide-to-a-fulfilling-sex-life-for-seniors/

Section V

Sexual Compulsivity and Sex Offending

26

An Introduction to Paraphilias With Special Focus on "Traveler" Sex Offenders*

Ronald DeLong, Frederick L. Peterson, Jr., and David Miller

INTRODUCTION

Our understanding of paraphilias, and especially pedophilia, has evolved tremendously over the last several decades as evidenced by the development of sexual science – particularly in the field of sex offender assessment and treatment. In addition, there has been a rise in professionalism within the field to integrate current research into practice, create standard guidelines to assist clinicians, and organize professional associations to advance the field of clinical sexology in general as well as in sex offender assessment and treatment. Examples of professional associations include, but are not limited to, the Society for the Scientific Study of Sexuality (SSSS; founded in 1966), Society for Sex Therapy and Research (SSTAR; founded in 1975), the Association for Treatment of Sex Abusers (ATSA; founded in 1984), and the International Association for the Treatment of Sex Offenders (IATSO; founded in 1998).

The topic of paraphilias used to be considered a clinical enigma limited to psychoanalytical explanations and accompanied by a prevailing public sentiment of "lock 'em up and lose the key" 50 years ago. Today, the study of paraphilias (including pedophilia) now has evidence-based treatments that demonstrate that sex offenders can, and do, change their behavior for the better when provided (and many times mandated) the right therapy with the right intensity, duration, and social environment (Peterson et al., 2020). Paraphilias are characterized by intense arousal to atypical circumstances involving sexual-type behavior. As demonstrated by the Sexual Expression Cube (see Chapter 7), sexual behavior is an immensely varied phenomenon that can range from the tender, intimate, and erotic to the pornographic, bizarre, and illegal.

Of course, not all unusual sexual behaviors are problematic, and even fewer requiring intervention and treatment. However, some paraphilias do require intervention when specified sexual impulses are acted upon in ways that can lead to harm to the self or others. The evaluation and treatment of those who have been diagnosed with a paraphilic disorder (and who have been deemed a risk of harm to others) requires awareness, sensitivity, and competence as a provider including, but not limited to, sex-specific training in sexual variations (and sex offender treatment), an understanding of mandatory reporting laws and regulations involving confidentiality, and a capacity to empathize with those who are traditionally denied understanding and effective treatment.

*The current authors acknowledge the 2007 contribution of Gene Abel, Markus Wiegel, and Candice Osborn in a previous publication entitled *Innovations in Clinical Practice: Focus on Sexual Health* (2007; VandeCreek, Peterson, & Bley, Editors) upon which this chapter draws from yet it is extensively updated. (During the COVID-19 pandemic, attempts to reach Dr. Abel and coauthors concerning revising their original chapter were unsuccessful.)

This chapter emphasizes several key points about paraphilic behaviors that are not necessarily understood, or even accepted, within the general population as well as the mental health and law enforcement communities. To do so, a review of several types of paraphilic disorders is provided. Furthermore, a detailed examination of client evaluation and treatment issues allows for an introduction to the "how-to's" when clients present with paraphilias. This chapter is not meant to be a comprehensive coverage of all aspects of such evaluations and treatment. Instead, the authors clarify several topics that will assist providers to have greater comfort and confidence when responding clinically to clients involved in paraphilic behaviors.

A LIMITED REVIEW OF THE HISTORY OF THE TERM PARAPHILIA AND TYPOLOGIES

The term "paraphilia" represents a clinical concept with an interesting history going back to the beginning of psychiatry with Richard von Kraft-Ebbing, who published the first classification of sexual behaviors that were pathologized because they were considered, at that time, moral sins against God and society (Peterson et al., 2020). His book, *Psychopathia Sexualis* (1886/1892), is considered the first modern psychiatric classification of sexual behaviors, defining them as mental illnesses if they caused harm to others or oneself, which seems reasonable. However, at the time, masturbation was considered a disease leading to disability (even insanity) and requiring treatment, especially for youth. A diagnosis of masturbation as disease (MAD) was referred to as Onanism, Self-Abuse, and other names in medical texts of the era (and all the way into mid-20th century). Same-sex attraction and behavior was listed as an illness by Kraft-Ebbing and remained so for nearly a century until declassified by the American Psychiatric Association in 1974. Kraft-Ebbing drew his conclusions from observing people's behavior who had been placed in early asylums and, living in a time before the advent of the scientific method, confused correlation with causation. Essentially, most sexual activities that did not have a possibility of producing babies were pathologized by Kraft-Ebbing, including many such behaviors that are today considered "usual and customary" in the kink community and often considered normal in many heterosexual marriages. American psychiatrist Martin Kafka (2006) has written, "Sexual disorders once considered paraphilias (e.g., homosexuality) are now regarded as variants of normal sexuality" (p. 23). For a more in-depth coverage of MAD (masturbation as disease) and the medical pathologizing of what is considered normal sexual behaviors today, please see the readings on the history of sex in *Science in the Bedroom* (Bullough, 1994), *The Destroying Angel* (Money, 1985), and *The Gender Revolution & New Sexual Health* (Peterson et al., 2020).

While Kraft-Ebbing got the ball rolling in terms of the early classification systems for what we now call paraphilia, many have contributed to the study of what have been historically called sexual perversions and sexual deviations. The term comes from the Greek παρά (para) "beside" and φιλία (-philia) "friendship, love." Paraphilias (experiences of intense sexual arousal to atypical objects, situations, or individuals) have wide-ranging variations: from common forms of transvestism and fetishes, to esoteric sexual interests of falling in love with (and marrying) a roller coaster (LeVay et al., 2015), to dangerous forms of lust murder (Purcell & Arrigo, 2006). Two decades after the publication of *Psychopathia Sexualis,* the term paraphilia (paraphilie) was coined by an early sexologist in Austria (Friedrich Krauss in 1903), and it was first used in English another decade later (in reference to Krauss) by American urologist and prolific writer William J. Robinson (Janssen, 2014). The term paraphilia also appears in Robinson's *Medical Sex Dictionary* (1933), as does the term "self-abuse," referring to the disease of masturbation. The term paraphilia was introduced into the *Diagnostic and*

Statistical Manual of Mental Disorders (3rd ed. [*DSM-III*]; American Psychiatric Association, 1980) to replace the archaic term of sexual deviation.

In a valuable study of the prevalence of paraphilias by Abel and Bradford (2005), the records of 561 individuals were examined who had collectively committed over 290,000 sex acts. The majority of the reported acts were exhibitionism, frottage, child sexual abuse of boys outside the family, and voyeurism. Surprisingly, acts of rape, incestuous sexual molestation of boys, bestiality, sadism, sexual abuse of girls outside the home, public masturbation, and fetishism were infrequently reported. These data reflect what various clients reported doing and do not reflect what typically brings them in for evaluation or treatment. The most common reasons adult males seek evaluation is for accusations of child sexual abuse (32%), voyeurism (15%), and public exposure (11%). Adolescent males seek evaluation for accusations of child sexual abuse (58%); fetishism (23%); voyeurism (16%); obscene phone calls, frottage/rape, and phone sex (each 15%); and exhibitionism (11%). Adult females seek evaluation primarily for accusations of child sexual abuse (18%). Adolescent females seek evaluation for accusations of child sexual abuse (46%), making obscene phone calls (17%), fetishism (11%), and frottage/rape (10%). Although frottage (sexual touching of another without their permission) and voyeurism (window peeping) commonly occur, the individuals involved in this activity infrequently appear in the clinic for evaluation because voyeurs are infrequently apprehended, and frottage behavior is usually ignored because the police may view it as a nuisance crime (unless it involves the touching of a child) (Abel & Bradford, 2005).

Within the *Diagnostic and Statistical Manual of Mental Disorders* (5th ed. [*DSM-5*]; American Psychiatric Association, 2013), paraphilic disorders are classified into two individualistic schemas, or groups. The first group is based upon anomalous activity preferences and are subdivided into two separate factors. The first factor, referred to as courtship disorders, are labeled as such due to their resemblance to distorted views of human courtship behavior (voyeuristic disorder, exhibitionistic disorder, and frotteuristic disorder). The second factor, listed as algolagnic disorders, involve the presence of pain and suffering (sexual masochism disorder and sexual sadism disorder). The subsequent schema, or group, of paraphilic disorders focuses on anomalous target preferences, thus deviating from traditional standards within normal society. Said disorders within this specific group include one directed at other humans, specifically victims under the age of 13 (pedophilic disorder) and two directed elsewhere (fetishistic disorder and transvestic disorder) (American Psychiatric Association, 2013). The following sections will review some of the most common paraphilias encountered in clinical practice.

SPECIAL FOCUS: "SOLICITATION / INTERNET TRAVELER" SEX OFFENDERS

With the onset of the internet in the 1990s, our way of life with computers has become more informed as well as mainstream. At the touch of a few keys, we are able to obtain massive amounts of information in order to complete tasks, order food, find a date, seek pornography, or engage in bullying. Even worse, our children are subjected to inappropriate and/or sexual solicitations by an adult or even an adolescent. Offenders have been able to formulate, develop, and execute a "more progressive and clandestine methodology" regarding ways to contact and establish a relationship with a potential victim (DeLong et al., 2010). The ability to make contact with potential child or adolescent victims has become more available and easier to access. With the ease of online access, children and adolescents can engage in conversations with other peers, prosocial chat rooms, or with other adults who focus on reading and evaluating their vulnerabilities in order to solicit possible sexual information with the possibility of leading to a sexual encounter.

By "trolling" the innumerable array of chat rooms, social media, and other various options of online social contacts, offenders have a "smorgasbord" of possibilities of contacting and engaging in the "pick and choose arena" of victims in order to establish what would be considered for them a "safe" choice of victim selection (DeLong et al., 2010). However, such offenders are not a homogeneous group but do appear to demonstrate variable characteristics, yet making them align with a cluster of behavioral patterns thereby permitting some understanding of their modus operandi.

Research has identified some types of internet offenders (Alexy et al., 2005; Babchishin et al., 2011; Briggs et al., 2011; Wolak et al., 2010) that range in their interactions from solicitation, child pornography, and traveling to meet potential child victims. This broad-based focus would appear to demonstrate the utilization of opportunities available to the online offender and the array of potential activities in order to obtain their desired goal. However, child pornography, for instance, can be utilized as a tool of persuasion and setting up the potential victim by lessening the child's defenses and normalizing the identified behavior wished by the offender (Elliot & Beech 2009; Krone 2004). Child pornography can also be the sole desired object of sexual gratification and pleasure (deviant fantasy interest, coping mechanism, curiosity, etc.) rather than its utilization to "a means to an end" (Seto, 2012a; Seto & Eke, 2015; Seto et al., 2010).

Another use of the internet would be the facilitation of the commercialization of sexual exploitation of children (e.g., sex trafficking of juveniles and the distribution of child pornography) (Durkin & DeLong, 2012). Thus, the internet has become the main impetus of the child sexual offender as well as the commercial exploiter of a variety of deviant interests, including sex as well as financial (DeLong & Durkin, 2012). Not surprisingly, governmental resources have focused more on internet child pornography and arrests of online sex offenders, for child-exploitive materials have been increasing exponentially (Seto, 2012b).

SPECIAL FOCUS: BACKGROUND ON "SOLICITATION / INTERNET TRAVELER" SEX OFFENDERS

As identified, the internet can be a haven for those seeking information regarding all types of subjects, interests, and instruction. The destructive element of this mode of interaction would focus on the solicitation of children by adults. Research has been revealing the degree and depth regarding the use of the internet for sex-offending purposes. According to the second National Juvenile Online Victimization Study, the Internet Crimes Against Children (ICAC) task forces (along with their affiliates and other federal agencies) reported and identified 1,981 arrests for online sex offenses (Mitchell & Jones, 2013). A random sampling from this study ($n = 794$) of other agencies (educated and trained to conduct ICAC cases) reported 1,001 arrests along with a random sampling ($n = 1,425$) of other U.S. agencies that reported 340 arrests, noting that although the internet has been a productive and viable tool for a variety of uses, it has notably been utilized as a destructive and flagrant means of harm to minors with regard to sexual abuse and their naïvety, curiosity, and means of social support and connection (DeHarta et al., 2017; Mitchell & Jones, 2013).

Further noted in DeHarta et al. (2017) were the findings of the second Youth Internet Safety Survey (YISS-2) in 2004 which identified one in seven (13%) of the youths surveyed had been sexually solicited. Per this research, "sexually solicited" was defined as "youth being asked to engage in sexual activities or sexual talk or give personal sexual information" (DeHarta et al., 2017, p. 84). Also reported was 27% of the solicited youths were requested to send sexual photographs of themselves (Wolak et al., 2006). Adults were defined as persons 18 years or older which demonstrated 39% of the solicitations reported. Further revealed were almost half (49%) of the aggressive sexual solicitations were conducted by adults. "Aggressive sexual solicitations" were defined as requests for offline contact via email, telephone, or in person. Alexy et al. (2005) identified research addressing three categories of internet sex offending against children:

1. *Traders* – 59% of this type traded and/or collected child pornography.
2. *Travelers* – 22% of this category solicited children online to meet in person for sex.
3. *Combined* – 19% of the combination included those who engaged in both types of behaviors. Although not inclusive, it has been noted that these offender types could be involved in several different sorts of sex offending, including prior solicitation, but have utilized the internet as another and possibly more effective means of contacting potential victims, child pornography viewers/collectors only, and those who have succumbed to the use of the internet as a means of meeting children but have not had any such contact in the past (first time users). (Hansen, 2006)

According to Malesky (2007), his study of a Federal Bureau of Prison Sex Offender Treatment Program presented findings which noted that the preferred methods of contact with potential victims of sex offenders were via chat rooms, then from online profiles and bulletin boards. Further noted was the high percentage use of chat rooms (80%) with approximately 71% of the offenders successfully meeting and having sexual contact with a child victim. Also identified was the age and motivation of the offender – adult men who did not attempt to hide or conceal their age or sexual intent when communicating with a potential child victim (Wolak et al., 2010).

Of particular importance was the identification of those who traveled to meet minors, specifically, through undercover sting operations. They were usually older males, more often from middle-class backgrounds, and who typically did not have a criminal, violent, or sexually deviant history (Wolak et al., 2010). Unlike travelers who set up to meet their victims, online solicitation offenders focus on engaging a victim online, but typically do not set up to meet their victim, thus producing a lower risk potential (Seto et al., 2012). Further noted was the victim typically knows their offender and understands the offender's intent is sexual (Wolak et al., 2012).

The offender would usually engage in grooming tactics and behaviors to feign a romantic relationship in order to successfully complete a sexual encounter (Tener et al., 2013). These relationships are characterized by the offender as consensual, nonforcible, and the victim typically reported their relationship with the offender was one of a love interest (Tener et al., 2013). Because the typical victim was an adolescent, contact offenders, in general, are generally not pedophiles as portrayed via the media and other common beliefs.

Defining the differences of online solicitors of potential victims, the group who "travels" would indicate a higher level of risk since they not only establish a relationship with their online victim, but also go as far as establishing an actual in-person meeting for the purpose of a sexual encounter. With regard to the strategic methodologies of this group, Mitchell et al. (2005) identified a generalized dynamic in which the traveler established their modus operandi:

1. They utilize the computer to access numerous potential victims within a short period of time.
2. They are able to maintain a sense of power and control through anonymous interactions with others.

3. They engage in nonphysical or sexual (hands-off) contact with potential victims, thereby allowing them to develop a relationship which encourages a false sense of trust.
4. This allows the offender to remain anonymous and assists them in the grooming and assessing of potential victims.

Qualye et al. (2006) also identified that this offender group further experienced immediate gratification which was/is a strong influence for sex offenders to utilize the internet in order to avoid negative circumstances and feelings such as boredom, anxiety, and depression.

Mitchell et al. (2010) further reported that solicitation of potential victims have been sought via internet communication platforms such as gaming sites, chat rooms, and social networking sites which are typically populated by children or adolescents. The use of deception (i.e., identifying self as a child or adolescent) would typically be utilized in order to develop a relationship thereby establishing a level and degree of trust. Once developed, the offender could persuade the targeted individual to join a private communication mode (i.e., email, instant messenger, text message, etc.) in order to further isolate and continue to develop and assuage the victim into a potential meeting. As the development of technology has increased, the use of cell phones has become more mainstream to obtain direct/isolated contact – particularly useful once the relationship has progressively matured (Briggs et al., 2011; Mitchell et al., 2007; Whittle et al., 2014).

SPECIAL FOCUS: ONLINE GROOMING PATTERNS OF "SOLICITATION / INTERNET TRAVELER" SEX OFFENDERS

The term "grooming" would seem to be a ubiquitous term within the context of offending behavior with regard to "setting up" a potential victim in order to build trust and control over them for whatever goal the offender may be seeking (i.e., sexual, monetary, etc.). Children and adolescents consistently share the same wants and needs for attention and affection, with adolescents considered to have more sexual curiosity (Peterson et al., 2020). Hence, the ability for an online offender to manipulate, shape, and develop online relationships would be substantial; not only would it provide similar emotional needs of the offender, but also include a variety of opportunities to target, exploit, and leverage the offender to seek and have access to several victims at one time. Cybertip.ca (Canada's national tip line for reporting the online sexual exploitation of children; 2021) identified and classified 645 reports from the Department of Justice Canada of online grooming as "luring" children, an attempt made by offenders to gain access to children. Of those reports:

- 25% involved victims 13 years old or under, with the youngest being 7 years old
- 48% involved victims 14-17 years old
- 22% of incidents occurred on Snapchat
- 23% of incidents occurred on Instagram, Facebook, or Facebook Messenger
- 12% of incidents occurred on an online gaming platform

Olson et al. (2007) identified a common model of solicitation in which minors are introduced to the grooming process, and progress from an introductory stage to actual introduction and contact with the identified offender. The lead author has taken the liberty to further breakdown this process into digestible stages for interpretation purposes. The process typically includes:

1. ***Introduction phase.*** The offender obtains a position in which interaction with the potential victim provides some type of direct communication or initial greeting (Leatherman, 2009). The use of low stress introduction topics would include age, sex, location, hobbies, or other nonsexual interests.
2. ***Communication phase I.*** The offender typically engages the victim in positive yet seemingly caring communication in order to "desensitize" the victim from such things as sexual language and sexual acts into a seemingly nonthreatening vernacular (i.e., "play").
3. ***Communication phase II.*** As the offender continues to utilize less-threatening language, communication progresses to the use of slang, abbreviations, net speak, and emoticons/emoji which are typical of such online communications. The offender further lessens the threat to the victim by incorporating youthful and consistent language for online age group members (e.g., kewl) thereby producing and rendering the sexual exchange as less threatening. Further noted was the use of flattery; minor sexual comments and the beginning of addressing the victim's sexual interests (within a casual manner); and playing games of confusing messages in order to test the victim's willingness to respond favorably to their comments (which sends a message of cooperation and acceptance of the offender). Comments such as, "I'm not good enough for someone like you," "I'm too old for you," and so on, are examples of such communication strategies.
4. ***Approach phase.*** The offender has developed a more trusting relationship thereby taking greater liberties with regard to sexual acts online. Sexual interactions and potential attempts to meet the victim tend to occur at this phase. The offender will typically engage in sending explicit sexual pictures or videos, even utilizing direct online contact via a webcam for immediate access and real-life sex with the victim. This process could also include the teaching and coaching of how to masturbate; performing other sexual acts through instruction, as well as the performance of exhibition; and possibly requesting future continuous sexual online feeds to the offender. Also in this phase would be the time for the offender to establish an actual meeting time and place to further the sexual relationship to in-person experiences.

Other tactics have further been identified by Cybertip.ca (2021) which noted several common techniques in which online offenders utilized to entice and gain the trust of their potential victim(s):

- Falsely identifying themselves online as a peer (e.g., child from another school, connected through sport, friend of a friend, or known to the child in some way)
- Flattery/compliments/support
- Promise of gifts, money, tablets, drugs, alcohol
- Pitting the parents against the child (e.g., your parents are too strict, your parents don't understand you)
- Exchange of sexual pictures to make victim more comfortable in sending sexual pictures/videos in return
- Take pictures with or without the child's knowledge while live-streaming. This is often followed by the use of extortion to control the child and/or threatening to share the material unless the child produces additional sexual images/videos
- Threats, intimidation, and harassment

Further investigating this sexual offending behavioral process, other studies have noted specific motivational reasons for engaging in these behaviors, thus identifying a more nuanced understanding of the offender's modus operandi (Kloess et al., 2017). Briggs et al. (2011) described a dichotomous subtype of offenders (*contact driven and fantasy driven*) who utilized internet communications to entice a child/adolescent into a sexual relationship. Such communication types consist of chat rooms, dating sites, social media, and so forth, in which the offender would establish a rapport with the identified victim in order to set up some type of sexual exploitation.

A contact-driven offender focused on and was motivated by setting up a potential physical meeting with a targeted victim for the purpose of sexual contact. A fantasy-driven offender was predominately focused with online sexual interactions and activities specifically for sexual gratification. However, it is possible that the fantasy-driven offender may arrange an in-person meeting for the continuation of their online sexual interactions. These are based on the offender's fantasies and behaviors during his online exchanges with the victim (with items central to his fantasies, like clothing, particular sexual acts, etc.).

As identified, an online offender's patterns of grooming behaviors are based on thoughts and fantasies which are central to the offender's key sexual interests (Webster et al., 2012). Such patterns consist of:

1. ***Intimacy-seeking offenders.*** These offenders portend they have a romantic and consenting relationship with the child. Their pattern consists of talking and developing a relationship in order to know more about them before meeting them for a physical encounter.
2. ***Hypersexual offenders.*** These offenders have been identified as being highly sexualized. Their interest lies on engaging in sexual talk and fantasy without concern about getting to know or developing a relationship with the child.
3. ***Adaptable offenders.*** These offenders tend to focus on an eclectic approach of utilizing different personas and identities in order to adapt their behavior to that of the child. This would permit them to be chameleonic in their ability thereby adjusting to the victim's behavior and needs without identifying a specific type other than being young. These offenders also will utilize child pornography as a facilitating tool in the process, but not necessarily desire or motivated to seek a physical encounter with the child.

Linguistic practices have also been noted with regard to the particular verbiage and mannerisms of communication. These manipulative communicative styles are especially interesting since they consist of written text rather than in-person communication. Olson et al. (2007) identified a communication theory regarding online offenders who utilize a technique which entraps the victim and lures them into an ongoing sexual relationship. By setting up a framework which allows the (child) victim to believe that sexual talk and sexuality is advantageous for them, the offender will be able to engage in sexual relations and mask it as "normal" and "appropriate." This process would be highly coercive, presented in a favorable manner in order to gain the victim's cooperation and compliance.

Overall, various forms of grooming are available and needed in order to successfully complete the sexual goal or intention of the offender. By focusing on a systematic process, an offender can obtain access and evaluate the vulnerability of the potential victim whether they are online or in person. Thus, the type of offender will be revealed through these behavioral patterns and other identified information, especially as it pertains to their modus operandi.

SPECIAL FOCUS: ONLINE SOLICITATION OFFENDER TYPOLOGIES

Several typologies have been identified since the inception of the internet and its use for sexual purposes. The purpose of a typology has been to formulate a classification of observable characteristics regarding an offender and which ones fit a particular set of sexual and nonsexual behaviors that tend to establish an identified victim (Lanning, 2001). Furthermore, typologies tend to permit the order and classification of different types of crime, criminals, and victim, as well as to simplify and make sense of complex realities. As the evolution of the internet continues, sexual offenders continue to be understood, and the differentiation between types is necessary in order to ascertain their motives, intent, and specific distinctions. By developing and refining these classifications, a more defined understanding of the specific patterns and behaviors can be developed for different groups of sexual offenders (online solicitation vs. child pornography or a combination) and their different motivations (contact-driven vs. fantasy-driven).

Online offenders typically consist of child pornography viewers, collectors, along with those who focus on interacting and setting up the child or adult into an in-person meeting. Alexy et al. (2005) and Webster et al. (2012) identified that the role of pornography has been utilized by some of the online offenders, but that this has expanded to those who travel to meet their victim and may use pornography as a grooming prop to obtain access to the identified victim.

Pedophilia and Sexual Abuse of Minors

Many individuals who face accusations of sexually abusing a minor (and who have become involved with the judicial system) are often mandated to complete a psychosocial evaluation. Therefore, it is essential to have a clear understanding of the diagnostic criteria for pedophilia. The category of child sexual abuse is not an official psychiatric diagnosis (multiple determinations of child abuse are included under both T and Z codes within the *DSM*), but is defined as any sexual act, involving a child, that is intended to provide sexual gratification to a parent, caregiver, or any other individual.

Within the *DSM* classification system, examples of sexual abuse involve fondling a child's genitals, penetration, incest, rape, sodomy, and indecent exposure. It further includes *noncontact exploitation* of a child by a parent, caregiver, or any other individual (American Psychiatric Association, 2013). Some individuals may have sexually abused a child but are not pedophiles, generally because they have not carried out this behavior for longer than 6 months, do not have sustained sexual interest in children, or they are involved in child abuse for strictly financial reasons (such as producing or distributing child pornography). It is believed that most, but not all, pedophiles attempt to carry out child sexual abuse. Pedophiles who have sexual urges and fantasies involving sex with children may not have actually sexually abused a child. If the client admits to sexual abuse, the provider needs to not only get as much detail as possible regarding the duration, frequency, and kinds of sexual acts reported, but must also keep state mandatory reporting laws in mind.

Cases of suspected child sexual abuse necessitate a clinician having a clear understanding of and ability to identify individuals with pedophilia. This topic is exceedingly important, because research by Abel and Harlow (2002) indicates that those who meet the criteria for pedophilia in the *DSM* commit 95% of the acts of child molestation, compared to 88% of all the victims of child sexual abuse. In a large group of 4,000 adult child sexual abusers, 65% met the *DSM-IV-TR* criteria for pedophilia. Because this one psychiatric illness constitutes such a large percentage of the acts of child molestation, it is critical to identify potential pedophiles so that treatment can proceed rapidly, protecting potential victims and protecting pedophiles from themselves.

Regarding paraphilic interest in children, the terms *pedophilia* and *child molestation* represent related, but separate, phenomena. Said differently, the men (and sometimes women) engaged in these activities are separate but overlapping populations (Abel et al., 2007; Camilleri & Quinsey, 2008). The pedophilic individual will express sexual interest in young children (usually prepubertal or early pubertal children) that is intense and enduring. He may or may not ever actually commit a sex offense by sexually touching a child or viewing child-oriented pornography; so, it is imperative that the provider "go there" by asking specifically related questions in a neutral and nonjudgmental manner in order to increase the likelihood of disclosure.

A second key point is that intense sexual interest in prepubertal children (pedophilia) is different from men's sexual interest in older teenagers (ephebophilia). Adults who have a sexual interest in adolescent, postpubertal children (such as a 16-year-old who displays secondary sex characteristics) are biologically, sociologically, and psychologically common. Of course, today, it is a sex crime for adults to pursue minors and engage in sex with them (unless, of course, you marry them; see below). How common is adult sexual attraction to adolescents? Very common. One indication of how common this phenomenon is relates to simply observing the great uptick in convictions for child pornography over the last 2 decades (much of the imagery, if not most, involve sexually exploited teenage girls). Another indication is to look at the related phenomena of child marriages. If a minor gets married, and at least one of the two individuals are not at least 18 years old, then it is called child marriage and legal in most states. Between 2000 and 2015, there were over 200,000 child marriages in the United States, with the vast majority of them involving teenage girls marrying adult men (Tsu et al., 2017).

Child molestation does involve a contact sex offense of a child by an adult, but the sex offender may or may not have a pedophilic disorder. It is important to note this difference because the clear majority of contact sex offenses against children are committed by men with pedophilic disorder (Abel et al., 2007). Regarding the type of assessment strategies used in the evaluation of sex offenders, evaluating risk levels for recidivism, and the types of treatment approaches employed, the ability to accurately diagnose pedophilia and differentiate nonpedophilic offenders is also important.

Fetishism

Individuals with a sexual fetish rarely present themselves for treatment, because, in many cases, the pursuit of the sexual fetish does not disturb them (unless they are blocked and/or unable to access their object of desire). Sexual fetishists usually come to clinical attention in two ways. First, an individual's partner may discover the fetish (that has been hidden from the partner) or the individual may attempt to convince his or her partner to participate in the fetish. When the partner either finds the sexual fetish upsetting or refuses to participate despite repeated efforts by the client, the couple may present for couples counseling or individual sex therapy. Second, a sexual fetish may come to light in the course of assessing another sexual behavior for which the client is primarily seeking an assessment. One study found that sexual fetishism was a secondary diagnoses in 33% of individuals with a primary diagnosis of bestiality, 25% of individuals engaging in obscene phone calls, 22% of individuals with pedophilia, 20% of transvestites, and 11% of those involved in voyeurism (Abel & Osborn, 1992). Just about any object or body part can become the focus of a sexual fetish. However, sexual fetishes often focus on clothing, such as underwear or lingerie; certain materials, such as rubber or leather; and particular body parts (partialism), such as feet, legs, or hair (Laws & O'Donohue, 1997). A fetish may also focus on more unusual items, such as jewelry, balloons, their partner smoking cigarettes during sex, and so on. Persons with a sexual fetish engage in a variety of behaviors with the fetish object to achieve sexual arousal and orgasm, including fondling, stroking, wearing, smelling, or sucking the object while masturbating or engaging in sexual activity with a partner. Some individuals require the presence of the fetish object, actually or in fantasy, in order to become aroused, and are not able to become sexually aroused or reach orgasm without the fetish object. Individuals with sexual fetishes have, in some studies, been found to have higher than average levels of sexual arousal or an increased capacity for developing conditioned sexual arousal (Bailey, 1991). Although most individuals do not come in contact with the legal system as a result of their fetish, when it does happen it is usually as a consequence of the person attempting to steal the fetish object. More frequently, the diagnosis of a sexual fetish disorder (which, according to the *DSM-5* criteria, requires significant distress or impairment in social, occupational, or other important areas of functioning) results in relationship conflicts arising from the person insisting the fetish be incorporated into sexual activity with the partner.

Bestiality

Bestiality is frequently considered the realm of sexual jokes but should be considered a serious problem if it causes an individual (or the partner) distress. It is thought to be not that uncommon among pubescent adolescents who are motivated to sexually experiment with arousing themselves by involving a family pet. It is also believed to be more common among rural populations than city dwellers, perhaps due to the frequent exposure of farm animals mating and easy access to the same. Usually, this adolescent experimenting extinguishes itself with maturation and coupling with a human sexual partner. Sometimes, bestiality can become a long-term pattern even when the individual does couple with a human sexual partner.

Bestiality is a clinical concern because an individual who can maintain sexual arousal while having a sexual encounter with an uncooperative animal can disassociate from much of the realities of such activity. Therefore, of all of the aforementioned paraphilias, bestiality is most likely to lead to disclosures or discovery of other categories of paraphilic behavior. Such an individual can ignore the consequences to victims or other, more violent, types of sexual acts.

Compulsive Internet Sexual Behavior

Cybersex (via Twitter, Snapchat, Private Message/Direct Message [PM/DM], Grindr, WhatsApp, webcams, etc.) is any web-based communication where you can send sexually explicit images and communication. These forms of technology facilitate new forms of sexual "e-affairs" that cause major relationship conflict when discovered. They are very popular forms of sexual expression in today's high tech world because of the facilitating factors of accessibility, the affordability, and the perceived anonymity people believe they have (discussed below). Occasionally, catfishing is also a problem behavior, which is when a person "reels-in" another person into an emotional and sometimes sexual (online) relationship that is based on deception. Catfishing involves creating an online presence using another person's imagery or personal information – so common that there is a popular television show by the same name (Peterson et al., 2020).

Use of the internet to meet people and to initiate romantic and/or sexual relations has now become considered the "new norm" in the information age in which Americans live. However, an individual's use of this technology can become repetitive, excessive, and even compulsive involving pornography, sex chat rooms, and attempts to meet and be sexual with underage individuals. About 20% of all internet users engage in some form of online sexual activity (Cooper et al., 2000). For the vast majority of these individuals, internet sexual behavior is mainly recreational or educational and does not cause problems. However, for about 17%, internet-related sexual behavior becomes problematic and compulsive (Cooper et al., 2000). Much like individuals with other types of compulsive behaviors, these individuals were characterized by an increased appetite, desire, or tolerance for internet sexual behaviors; denial or minimization of negative consequences; repeated unsuccessful attempts to stop or limit online sexual activities; continuing to engage in internet sexual activities despite negative consequences; and interference in offline relationships as well as feelings of distress, guilt, and shame. Individuals with compulsive internet sexual behaviors reported spending an average of 15 to 25 hours per week pursuing online sexual activities (Cooper et al., 2000). As with all paraphilic sexual behaviors, men use the internet for sexual activity more frequently than women (Cooper et al., 2002).

Telephone-sex lines, erotic magazines, and adult movie theaters have transformed to an endless supply of pornographic material available to anyone who owns a computer with internet. Other paraphilic behaviors are promoted through the utilization of internet technology, as pornographic sites include a multitude of fetish options, thus promoting sexual gratification for individuals outside of the traditional norms of society without judgment. Internet characteristics include a sense of anonymity, ease, affordability of access, the ability to repent oneself as they see fit, and the availability of a wide range of ever-updated sexual materials (Beard, 2005). This transformation has been life altering, but has ultimately led to problematic issues, specifically involving the promotion of compulsive and illegal activity.

The negative consequences resulting from online sexual activities, particularly when they take on compulsive qualities, can be devastating and far-reaching. One study found that of individuals who engage in internet-related sexual behaviors, 5.8% access the internet for sexual reasons exclusively from work, while another 12.7% reported accessing the internet to engage in online sexual behaviors both from work and from home (Cooper et al., 1999). Thus, 20% of men and 12% of women are using work computers for at least some portion of their internet sexual activities (Cooper et al., 2000). Individuals who view pornography at their work site are involved in a very problematic behavior, because most major companies have hired security personnel or installed computer software that scan the use of company computers to identify those looking at or exchanging erotica or pornography. Because this behavior is against company policy, immediate dismissal is very possible and, although most cases of internet pornography are not criminal actions, the loss of a job and positive letters of reference can have significant repercussions for the individual.

In accordance with the *DSM-5* (American Psychiatric Association, 2013), characteristics of paraphilic disorder involve intense and recurrent urges pertaining to a variety of subjects deemed taboo by traditional society. For the majority of society, online paraphilic materials are largely ignored and dismissed (Balbreath et al., 2002). However, for those who meet criteria for a paraphilic disorder, the online medium serves as a welcomed opportunity to seek out and explore their sexual deviation (Balbreath et al., 2002). The internet possesses an infinite amount of pictures, stories, and movies akin to any diverse type of sexual behavior. Due to the anonymity of these sites, individuals will remain without help until a situation occurs where they are discovered by the authorities, a family member, a coworker, or, in rare cases, the individual decides to self-disclose (Galbreath et al., 2002). Until then, individuals utilize the internet to interact with other personalities with similar interests, thus rationalizing their behavior through shared experiences (Kicaburun & Griffiths, 2018). This is especially true as it pertains to voyeurism through the availability of "spy cameras," exhibitionism through the creation of inappropriate texting and picture sharing, and other fetish-type behavior. Although limited data exists due to the nature of its existence, one can assume that the creation and adherence to the dark web has promoted harmful sexually deviant behavior through unchallenged streamlined activity (Galbreath et al., 2002). This has led to not only the discovery of new paraphilic interests in some individuals, but has also served to cultivate activity among those with a preexisting tendency for such behavior (Balbreath et al., 2002). Further research suggests there is a connection with problematic internet use and deviant personality traits that include psychopathy, narcissism, and sadism, all of which are conducive to paraphilic type comportments (Kicaburun & Griffiths, 2018).

When assessing someone with potential compulsive internet sexual behaviors, it is important to quantify the number of hours an individual spends pursuing sexual activities via the internet. Cooper and colleagues (1999; 2004) have found that individuals who spend 11 hours or more per week in sexual activities on the internet experience greater distress and interference, and tend to be more sexually compulsive than those who spend less than 10 hours per week. It is typical for clients who are confronted by a significant other about these nonparaphilic sexual compulsions to at first deny and minimize them and then to promise never to do the behavior again; but months later, they frequently revert to their sexually compulsive behaviors. Besides quantifying the number of hours a client spends on these activities, it is also important to gather details about the types of online activities in which they are involved (e.g., chat rooms, online erotica, newsgroups, etc.) as well as the content of the online sexual stimuli.

Voyeurism

Most individuals find it arousing to watch a sexual partner undress or to look at a naked sexual partner. When this viewing is done without the knowledge or consent of the person being watched, it becomes problematic. Doing so while watching a stranger on the internet is essentially the basis of the majority on commerce within the multibillion dollar industry we refer to as the "porn industry." The careful assessment of voyeurism is particularly important because it may represent a "gateway paraphilia" for some individuals. Although not all voyeurs engage in more severe forms of paraphilic behavior, some research indicates that voyeurism tends to develop prior to other paraphilias such as exhibitionism or frotteurism (Abel & Rouleau, 1990; Freund & Watson, 1990). Individuals with voyeuristic sexual interests frequently prefer this to looking at pornography because voyeurism involves a relationship, albeit a one-sided or imagined one, with a real person (Laws & O'Donohue, 1997). Voyeurs rarely watch females who are known to them. The voyeuristic behaviors may be exciting to the client because it involves watching something personal and intimate, violating taboos, or the risk of getting caught. These individuals have been found to possess poor social skills, be less assertive, experience sexual dysfunction, and have deficits in sexual knowledge (Marshall, Eccles, et al., 1991).

As noted, there is some degree of voyeuristic sexual fantasies and interest that is considered normative. The assessment of voyeurism should therefore focus on the extent to which it has become a preoccupation or compulsive behavior. A diagnosis of voyeurism may be appropriate when it dominates a person's sexual fantasies and behaviors, supplants and interferes with the normal progression of courtship, or when it causes the person distress. A provider should assess the amount of time the client spends fantasizing about, seeking out opportunities for, and engaging in voyeuristic sexual behaviors. Clinicians can assess the degree of compulsiveness by asking whether the person has ever unsuccessfully tried to stop these behaviors. Paying careful attention to the antecedents and consequences of the voyeuristic behavior can provide some insight into the function of the behaviors for the person, such as emotion regulation which is frequently associated with a behavior becoming compulsive. Finally, voyeurism should not be dismissed as a victimless crime, but should serve as a warning sign to assess the degree to which it has escalated to other behaviors such as exhibitionism, frotteurism, stalking, and potentially rape.

Exhibitionism

There is a high degree of overlap between exhibitionism and other paraphilias, including voyeurism, public masturbation, frotteurism, obscene phone calls, and child sexual abuse. Of course, today's internet serves to promote the act of exhibitionism through the exchange of pictures and videos to both expecting and unsuspecting parties. As is usually the case in individuals with paraphilias, exhibitionists conceal their sexual behavior from friends and family and do not talk to their victims. Therefore, they do not appreciate how others see their behavior and, instead, interpret it in a way that is supportive of repeating the exhibitionistic behavior.

There could be a legitimate debate whether exhibitionism or voyeurism is the most commonly committed paraphilia. However, per research by Abel and others (Abel & Bradford, 2005; Cox & McMahon, 1978), relative to the numbers of exhibitionistic acts that are committed, only a small percentage of exhibitionists actually seek out evaluation. Like many other paraphilias, exhibitionism tends to begin during the mid-teen years or during the mid-20s (Abel & Rouleau, 1990; Smukler & Schiebel, 1975). It tends to be predominantly a male disorder, although limited reports of female exhibitionists exist (Fedoroff et al., 1999). However, the targets of exhibitionism tend to be exclusively female. Exhibitionists can expose their genitals from a variety of environments; some exhibit (generally only to a small number of individuals) in public settings, from their car, or from their own home or other buildings. The reaction an exhibitionist expects from his victim can range from shock and fear to sexual approval and reciprocation (Laws & O'Donohue, 1997). Individuals who expose their genitals tend to have similar demographic backgrounds to persons in the general population. In addition, exhibitionists do not seem to have a specific psychological profile or evidence of a distinguishable sexual arousal profile on objective measures (Marshall & Hall, 1995; Marshall, Payne et al., 1991). When assessing exhibitionism, it is particularly important to determine the underlying motivations; that is, to assess the function of the behavior through its antecedents and consequences. Because exhibitionists have a very high frequency of exhibitionistic acts prior to their seeking treatment, they have a high recidivism rate posttreatment (Marshall, Eccles, et al., 1991). In general, a person with a lengthy history of a paraphilic behavior has a greater likelihood of recidivism than someone with a paraphilia whose frequency is low. The laws in most states are no longer treating exhibitionism as a nuisance crime because of the relative high frequency of acts of exhibitionism and significant recidivism rates posttreatment. A provider should also consider this paraphilia as serious because re-arrest can have profoundly negative consequences to the community and the exhibitionist. In addition, it is important to assess individuals with this paraphilia carefully, because about 30% exhibit exclusively to children or minors and may be at risk for sexually abusing minors.

Frotteurism

The *DSM-5* describes frotteurism as deriving sexual excitement from rubbing up against or touching other individuals without their knowledge. This is done frequently in crowded places such as subways. Freund and colleagues (Freund et al., 1997; Freund & Watson, 1990) consider frotteurism as one of the courtship disorders. Individuals with frotteuristic sexual interest frequently are also involved in other paraphilic behaviors – voyeurism and exhibitionism, in particular (Freund et al., 1997). Like clients who engage in voyeuristic or exhibitionistic sexual behavior, clients engaging in frotteurism will have done so on numerous occasions. The paraphilia frotteurism should be distinguished from more severe grabbing of female breasts, buttocks, and genitals that are better conceptualized as sexual assault or sexual harassment. Asking the client whether the persons he is touching are aware that his actions are for sexual arousal may be helpful in this respect. When assessing this disorder, it is important to obtain as clear a description of the frequency of such behaviors, the locations where they generally occur (on a bus or subway), and the types of behaviors involved (e.g., rubbing genitals against another person, touching another person's hair, genital area, etc.). Because a client may be reticent to fully admit the frequency of such behaviors, it may be helpful to ask how frequently he rides the subway or bus, and to determine whether he is spending more time there than necessary to allow for additional opportunities to engage in frotteurism. It is also important to determine the degree to which these acts occur impulsively as opposed to being planned, as well as how frequently the activity is associated with the utilization of alcohol and other substances.

Transvestism

The topic of transvestism can be controversial among advocates of gender nonconformity and nonbinary gender identities. However, the important distinction is that transvestism is defined as a paraphilic disorder upon which intense *sexual arousal* stems from wearing clothes originally designed for the opposite gender. The actual wearing of clothes does not constitute a disorder in and of itself, rather when an individual's urge to do so can lead to a substantial distress or impairment within their everyday life (American Psychiatric Association, 2013). An individual with transvestic disorder traditionally exhibits a comorbidity; specifically, some form of anxiety or depression due to the impact of the said disorder (pertaining to specific consequences).

The act of cross-dressing is typically common within the male population but can occur in both sexes and often starts during childhood or adolescence. To be diagnosed with this particular disorder, an individual must experience a strong arousal from the thought, or act, of wearing at least one piece of clothing meant for the opposite sex (American Psychiatric Association, 2013). It is important to note that transvestic-type behavior is not traditionally synonymous with gender dysphoria, or even autogynephilia, to which one can originate pleasure from imagining being of the opposite gender.

Sexual Masochism and Sadism

The topic of consensually giving and receiving pain and/or humiliation for sexual pleasure has evolved significantly over the last 2 decades as the kink community has become more visible and has demanded recognition as a legitimate form of sexual expression. Most acts of masochism and sadism occur within the context of a committed and consensual relationships or as a result of internet chat rooms bringing together individuals with these common interests. When such behavior is mutually enjoyable and consensual between those involved, it does not constitute a problematic behavior. It is exceedingly unusual for masochism and sadism to be performed against an unwilling partner, although sadistic acts are extensively reported in the media.

Consensual forms of Bondage/Discipline/Sadomasochism (B&D, S&M) need to be distinguished from sadistic rape, lust murders, and sexually sadistic criminal behavior. It is estimated that only 5% to 10% of rapists meet the diagnostic criteria for sadism (Abel et al., 1988). Most rapists are not sadists and use only as much force and violence as is needed to gain compliance from their victims, albeit in their own distorted perception (Freund & Watson, 1990; Prentky & Knight, 1991). In addition to issues of anger, power, and dominance, most cases of rape (including acquaintance or date rape) are characterized by a lack of inhibition of arousal in response to outward signs of distress and suffering by the rape survivor, rather than an increased arousal to the suffering of the victim (Lohr et al., 1997). The distinguishing characteristic in lust murders is the fact that the sexual arousal is derived from the killing. Sexually sadistic criminals, who are often the subjects of high-profile reports in the media, tend to be rare. Data from 30 cases collected by the FBI indicate that, in nearly all of the cases, the offenses were carefully planned (Dietz et al., 1990). Commonly, victims were abducted, held captive for more than 24 hours, tortured, and, in 73% of the cases, were murdered. The preferred sexual activities included sexual bondage, anal rape, forced fellatio, and insertion of foreign objects. In many such cases, the individuals have profoundly narcissistic personality traits and many meet criteria for antisocial personality disorders. Sexually sadistic criminals and stalkers tend to be particularly dangerous, and it is strongly suggested that the average therapist not attempt to assess or treat this type of individual. Such individuals should be referred to a qualified and experienced forensic psychiatrist.

LEGAL VS. ILLEGAL PARAPHILIA BEHAVIORS – DISCUSSION OF CHILD PORNOGRAPHY

The majority of paraphilic-type behaviors are legal and could arguably be considered a healthy, albeit extraordinary, way of expressing sexual interests. As noted previously, examples of this include transvestic acts and even sadomasochism when practiced between two adults within the bounds of safe and consensual behavior. However, other forms of sexual behavior are extremely harmful to self and others, specifically acts that harm unsuspecting individuals under 18 years of age. Simply put, sexual behaviors should not cause a significant amount of distress upon others, especially others who have not provided consent. Those behaviors that do cause distress should be identified and corrected, thus minimizing the damage potentially caused to others.

As mentioned, the creation of the internet has provided a platform that promotes both legal and illegal sexual activity. Acts considered taboo are promoted and easily obtained throughout the dark web medium in an anonymous fashion. This is especially true as it pertains to pedophilia and child pornography. At the 2011 National Strategy Conference on Combating Child Pornography, then Attorney General Eric Holder said, "*Unfortunately,* we've . . . seen a historic rise in the distribution of child pornography, in the number of images being shared online, and in the level of violence associated with child exploitation and sexual abuse crimes. Tragically, the only place we've seen a decrease is in the age of victims. This is – quite simply – unacceptable [emphasis added]." Because of greater emphasis on combating child pornography, there have been increasing numbers of prosecutions. The number of arrests for child pornography in the United States tripled between 2001 and 2010 (Seto, 2013). Hence, there is an increased need for comprehensive assessments that include objective measures, particularly because there is a common notion that all individuals who view child pornography are eventually going to commit a contact sex offense against a child.

Increased attention to battle child abuse is extremely important, and all available law enforcement resources should be directed towards saving children being harmed and trafficked. Child abuse most often occurs in the home, but with the advent and availability of the internet, predators can also effectively solicit children online and travel to them for the purposes of committing a sex offense: so-called "travelers" (DeLong et al., 2010) discussed earlier in this chapter.

However, and this is another important note, the notion that all people who look at child pornography are at high risk for attempting to have sex with children (become a traveler) is just not accurate. Some people look at many different types of online pornographic images and never intend to act in such a way that reflects the content of the pornography (i.e., watching a video of a person having sex with an animal). Perhaps a better explanation would be people who view online films regarding the Holocaust. Some viewers may be considered individuals who want to learn about genocide and teach their children about it with the hope of never seeing another example of genocide in their lifetime. Some viewers watch it only because it is a high school or college assignment. However, there may be some viewers who watch the film for the purpose of criticism and picking it apart because they are Holocaust deniers. There may even be dangerously deviant viewers who watch the film footage because they enjoy sadistic fantasies of planning a future genocide.

At a law conference of judges and attorneys discussing the topic of judicial sentencing of individuals convicted in child pornography cases, forensic psychiatrist Fred Berlin (who testified in many famous cases, including the Jeffrey Dahmer case) presented on the topic of pedophilia and child pornography. Dr. Berlin shared that the reason people watch child pornography is all about the *intent of the viewer*. He used an example of people who enjoy being scared by watching horror movies. "Fans of horror movies don't want to be in one," he explained (Berlin, 2015). Knowing the intent of a person for viewing pornography may be important clinically, but perhaps more important to the court is, what does the intent of viewing mean in terms of an individual's risk for committing a contact sex offense?

Some people view different types of porn out of curiosity, some view child pornography because it is sent to them and they didn't know what it was, some view it because of severe obsessive-compulsive disorder, some view it as a stress response to the objectification of children killed in war, some view it as a means of self-punishment to prove how depraved they are, and some pedophiles view it because they do find it sexually arousing (Peterson et al., 2020).

After conducting a long-term study of a large group of men who had been convicted of possession of child pornography, leading researcher of sex offender behavior Michael Seto stated (in his 2012 testimony to the U.S. Sentencing Commission) that less than 5% (2.1%) of men arrested for online child pornography went on to commit a contact sex offense against a child. Understanding the difference in risk factors between men arrested for online child pornography and men arrested for having sexual contact with children is exceedingly important.

For example, if a man arrested for child pornography possession is evaluated and found to not demonstrate sexual interest in children or be a risk of harm to any child, then he may be granted an alternative sentence that better serves the community as well as his rehabilitation. If that same man can serve a sentence of incarceration during weekends and be allowed to work his regular job during the week, he can then serve his time, still pay his debt to society (including taxes), and continue to support his family. Such judicial judgments in sentencing have been made in appropriate cases that present very low risk of recidivism or commitment of a sexual contact offense. Of course, child pornography is illegal expressly because of the abuse children experience in the production of it. It should be illegal, and its use should be prosecuted. But the intent of the viewer's use of pornography makes a big difference in terms of the risk for either repeating the crime or committing a contact offense. If a person does show evidence of pedophilic interest and he is determined to be at risk of harm to others, then treatment is often provided during incarceration. The treatment is typically more intense, more frequent, and longer in duration during incarceration. If treatment is on an outpatient basis, probation or parole stipulations exist and they must be integrated into the treatment program. Community monitoring occurs as well with sex offenders regularly reporting to their probation officer, sometimes wearing electronic ankle monitors.

When an individual is struggling with illegal paraphilic behavior, there is a general stereotype of all sex offenders as having "high and frightening" recidivism rates, a phrase often cited in court decisions, including the Supreme Court (J. Barna, PhD, JD; personal communication, March 20, 2015 at Gilvary Symposium [Sentencing on Pornography Cases], School of Law, University of Dayton, Dayton, Ohio). The notion of "high and frightening" recidivism rates reflect a common attitude that all sex offenders will commit another sex crime so it's better to keep them in prison. There is certainly a small subset of sex offenders who are resistant to treatment, are violent in nature, and continue to be dangerous to others. These are the hardened criminals who do fit the stereotype. And they are the reason that 20 states have special civil commitment laws (as controversial as they are) that allow judges to keep some sex offenders incarcerated after they have served their sentence, albeit they remain incarcerated in treatment centers with locked doors and razor wire (Mears, 2010).

However, the research clearly supports the view that sex offender treatment is effective, that most sex offenders do change for the better, and that only a minority of sex offenders are reconvicted for sex crimes. Well-known sex crime researchers Hanson and Morton-Bourgon conducted a large scale meta-analysis of recidivism rates of adult sex offenders and found a rate of 14% over 5 to 6 years. Recidivism rates usually increase the longer the period the sex offender is studied, and when they expanded their period of review to 15 years, the recidivism rates for adult sex offenders are estimated to increase to 24% (Hanson & Morton-Bourgon, 2005).

EVALUATING CLIENTS

When a provider is faced with assessing an individual with paraphilic behavior, especially a potential behavior that could be determined by the judicial system to be a sex offense, it is most ideal to collect information from as many sources as possible, including alleged victims if they are willing to be interviewed or have already made written statements that are part of the police record. Many times accusations are made but there is not enough evidence to substantiate a prosecutor moving ahead with charges, but the parties may be involved with visitation and/or custody disputes related to the accusations of sexual misconduct by the accused. Whenever there is a custody fight and a court requests an evaluation of the alleged perpetrator, it is ideal to request the court to order an expanded evaluation to include the individual making the accusation. Even better is to get permission to evaluate both parents as well as the child(ren) who are alleged to be victimized. The following story is a true account of such a request of the court and the expanded scope of evaluation. It is a cautionary story of ruling out a paraphilia by collecting sufficient and overwhelming evidence:

> A mother of two boys made allegations that the father of the children had sexually abused her sons, based on her observations of the boys after their return from visitation with the father. Her observations had to do with how the children (5 and 7 years old) would wet the bed, were "acting odd," and did not want to talk to their mother about their visit with the father. In addition, she stated she observed the children "grabbing at their bottom" and would sometimes be seen to "rock their pelvis" when laying on the floor in what she considered an overtly sexual manner. The mother stated her belief that the children had been sexualized by sexual abuse by the father and that the father was a pedophile. She filed complaints against the father with the police and children's protective services, causing an immediate interruption of the boys having visitation with the father. He was allowed to have a 2-hour weekly visitation with the boys under supervised conditions. The court ordered an evaluation of the father but then approved a request to have both parents included in the evaluation. Upon initiation of the assessment, it was learned that the boys were in treatment for posttraumatic stress disorder (PTSD) with a local counselor who worked closely with the local child protective services. It also came to light that the mother believed not only the father but also the paternal grandfather was abusing the boys. Sheriff and social work reports stated that both the children denied ever being touched inappropriately by their father or anyone else. The boys stated the same under evaluation by the provider conducting the assessment and did not appear fearful or anxious of the father when observed together during the evaluation. Psychological testing and diagnostic interviewing of the father was within normal range (using the MMPI-2 and MCMI-III) with the exception of his anger regarding restricted parenting time. There was no evidence of any prior criminal history, sexual compulsive behavior, or use of pornography. There was no evidence of sexual interest in children as evidenced by objective measures taken outside the awareness of the father (see the Abel Assessment for Sexual Interest [AASI] described in Chapter 3, pp. 40-41). There were no signs of other paraphilic behavior either. Psychological testing and diagnostic interviewing of the mother revealed an unfortunate history of being sexually abused as a child as well as an adult (but not by the father of the children). The mother met the diagnostic criteria for PTSD and stated that she wondered from time to time if she had PTSD but never had previously engaged in mental health services. It did not appear that she was consciously intending to create false allegations of abuse against the father (or grandfather). Rather, she appeared to "see signs of trauma" where there was none due to her history of abuse. The mother even appeared relieved to know that she had PTSD and could pursue treatment for herself. The judge in the case ordered the boys to be withdrawn from treatment and resume the shared parenting.

Of course, all allegations of abuse of children should be taken seriously and investigated to protect children with an abundance of caution. Evaluation of any client who presents with alleged or confirmed problematic sexual behaviors or paraphilias requires a comprehensive assessment involving multiple topic areas. Beyond assessing the specific behavior with which the client presents, the evaluation needs to include obtaining informed consent, identifying all additional paraphilic as well as nonparaphilic sexual behaviors, objectively measuring sexual interests and arousal, mapping cognitive distortions, and assessing the client's general sexual functioning and sexual knowledge.

Additionally, it is important to include an assessment of the client's social and assertiveness skills, substance use issues, relationship functioning, and medical/physical history at some point in the overall evaluation. Many of these topics can be assessed provisionally while obtaining a thorough and comprehensive initial history from the client. A crucial difference between an assessment of paraphilic sexual behaviors and other forms of psychopathology is the need to obtain information from clients who are most often defensive, angry, isolated, filled with self-reproach, and motivated to minimize, distort, and misrepresent their sexual behaviors. As a result, it is crucial to review all possible collateral materials carefully prior to the first interview with the client, and the provider should request, in writing, all available materials regarding the accusations. In most evaluation settings, time for conducting clinical interviews is limited, and employing questionnaires and psychological tests (such as the MMPI-2 and MCMI-III) can facilitate completing a thorough assessment in a limited amount of time. Evaluation of sexual arousal and sexual interests may also require the use of specialized objective measures (such as those used in the AASI or measures using penile plethysmography). Most providers do not have (nor want to have) the necessary training, knowledge, or experience to conduct such comprehensive assessments. It is at these occasions when it is appropriate to refer a client to a sex-specific therapist or evaluator.

REFERRING CLIENTS TO A SEX-SPECIFIC THERAPIST

When a provider determines that a client needs to undergo sex offender-specific therapy, it is important to know the difference between traditional therapists and sex offender-specific therapists. Traditionally, general outpatient weekly therapy is not particularly effective at dealing with serious chronic paraphilias (Abel & Harlow, 2002). Sex-specific therapists experienced in treating sex offenders have unique training, qualifications, and evaluative/treatment skills not only for working with clients, but also to protect the general public from individuals with paraphilias who pose a significant risk. When referring a serious sex offender, there are several characteristics that a sex-specific therapist should have.

First, the therapist should have the necessary experience treating the type of paraphilia being referred. Second, a therapist should have the ability to include (and should regularly use) objective measures of sexual interest and arousal as part of the initial assessment, as well as to evaluate treatment outcomes. If the therapist does not have the necessary training or equipment to do objective sexual interest testing, the therapist should have a working relationship with another evaluator who can provide such testing. Third, if a provider is not able to prescribe psychopharmacological medications themselves, they should be able to work with a prescriber and be knowledgeable about issues involved with relevant medications to reduce sexual drive and desire (e.g., monitoring of hormone levels or liver functioning). Fourth, in addition to using medication to reduce paraphilic sexual arousal and interests, the therapist should employ behavioral treatments that directly reduce such sexual interests, such as covert sensitization, aversion, or satiation therapies. Fifth, the therapist's treatment package should contain cognitive-behavioral and relapse prevention therapy modules and skills training. And last, it is recommended that the therapist preferably be a member of the Association for the Treatment of Sexual Abusers (ATSA) or the International Association for the Treatment of Sex Offenders (IATSO).

CONCLUSION

An intensely interesting aspect of the work of forensic mental health professionals is assisting clients to recover from and manage the adverse consequences which follow a paraphilic sex offense. Each case is like a mystery to solve: assisting the individual to discover their intent and motivations for engaging in such problematic behavior; getting in touch with their pain and confusion they have created; helping their family (if any) have hope for positive change; and assisting the individual build the skills to walk a path that leads to what most people want in life – health, a sense of purpose, meaningful relationships, and of course being a law-abiding citizen.

Whether the paraphilic behavior is legal or illegal, much of the process of recovery is the same: there must be a recognition and acceptance that the problematic behavior can no longer be tolerated, and effective resolution of causative factors must occur. Then, the process of rebuilding the individual's life and relationships can begin.

The recognition of their problem comes in many forms. Sometimes it is forced upon a person by the law, by their failing health, or by a partner walking out after many requests for change have been ignored. This recognition can lead to connection with others through reaching out for help. Most times, individuals do not proactively ask for help because they are paralyzed by fear and an overwhelming dread of having what is secret brought out to the light. It is this fear and anxiety that keeps people trapped in their dilemma, and continues to perpetuate the cycle of the paraphilic behaviors. Maladaptive coping, isolation, and fear fuel most problematic sexual behavior (including paraphilias); but connection to relationships (with self and others, including sex-specific therapists) is what promotes recovery and health.

REFERENCES

Abel, G., Becker, J., Cunningham-Rathner, J., Mittelman, M., & Rouleau, J. (1988). Multiple paraphilic diagnoses among sex offenders. *Bulletin of the American Academy of Psychiatry and the Law, 16,* 153-168.

Abel, G., & Bradford, J. (2005, May 21-26). *The assessment of child sexual abusers* [Paper presentation]. American Psychiatric Association 158th Annual Meeting, Atlanta, GA.

Abel, G., & Harlow, N. (2002). *The Abel and Harlow Stop Child Molestation Prevention Study* (rev. text ed.). Child Molestation Research and Prevention Institute. https://www.bishop-accountability.org/specialtopics/abuse-data/2002-04-Abel-Harlow-Child.pdf

Abel, G., Jordan, A., Hand, C., Holland, L., & Phipps, A. (2001). Classification models of child molesters utilizing the Abel Assessment for Sexual Interest. *Child Abuse and Neglect, 25,* 703-718.

Abel, G., & Osborn, C. (1992). The paraphilias: The extent and nature of sexually deviant and criminal behavior. *Psychiatric Clinics of North America, 15,* 675-687.

Abel, G., & Rouleau, J. (1990). The nature and extent of sexual assault. In W. L. Marshall, D. R. Laws, & H. E. Barbaree (Eds.), *Handbook of sexual assault: Issues, theories, and treatment of the offender* (pp. 9-12). Plenum.

Abel, G., Wiegel, M., & Osborn, C. (2007). Pedophilia and other paraphilia. In L. VandeCreek, F. Peterson, & J. Bley (Eds.), *Innovations in clinical practice: Focus on sexual health* (pp. 157-175). Professional Resource Press.

Alexy, E., Burgess, A., & Baker, T. (2005). Internet offenders: Traders, travelers, and combination trader-travelers. *Journal of Interpersonal Violence, 20*(2), 804-812. https://doi.org/10.1177/0886260505276091

American Association of Sex Educators, Counselors and Therapists. (2016). AASECT position statement on sex addiction. https://www.aasect.org/position-sex-addiction

American Psychiatric Association. (1980). *Diagnostic and statistical manual of mental disorders* (3rd ed.).

American Psychiatric Association. (2013). *Diagnostic and statistical manual of mental disorders* (5th ed.). https://doi.org/10.1176/appi.books.9780890425596

Babchishin, K. M., Hanson, R. K., & Hermann, C. A. (2011). The characteristics of online sex offenders: A meta-analysis. *Sexual Abuse: A Journal of Research and Treatment, 23*(1), 92-123. https://doi.org/10.1177/1079063210370708

Bailey, K. (1991). Human paleopsychopathology: Implications for the paraphilias. *New Trends in Experimental and Clinical Psychiatry, 7,* 5-16.

Beard, K. (2005). Internet addiction: A review of current assessment techniques and potential assessment questions. *CyberPsychology and Behavior, 8,* 7-14.

Beitchman, J., Zucker, K., Hood, J., DaCosta, G., Akman, D., & Cassavia, E. (1992). A review of the long-term effects of child sexual abuse. *Child Abuse and Neglect, 16,* 101-118.

Berlin, F. (2015, March 20). *The paraphilias with an emphasis on pedophilia and viewers of child pornography.* [Presentation]. Gilvary Symposium (Sentencing on Pornography Cases), School of Law, University of Dayton, Dayton, Ohio.
Braun-Harvey, D., & Vigorito, M. (2016). *Treating out-of-control sexual behaviors – Rethinking sex addiction.* Springer.
Briggs, P., Simon, W., & Simonsen, S. (2011). An exploratory study of internet-initiated sexual offenses and the chat room sex offender: Has the internet enabled a new typology of sex offender? *Sexual Abuse: A Journal of Research and Treatment, 23,* 72-91.
Bullough, V. L. (1994). *Science in the bedroom: A history of sex research.* Basic Books.
Camilleri, J., & Quinsey, V. (2008). Pedophilia: Assessment and treatment. In D. Law & W. O'Donohue (Eds.), *Sexual deviance: Theory, assessment, and treatment* (pp. 183-212). Guilford.
Carnes, P. (2001). *Out of the shadows: Understanding sexual addiction* (3rd ed.). Hazelden Press.
Centers for Disease Control and Prevention (CDC). (2014). Prevalence and characteristics of sexual violence, stalking, and intimate partner violence victimization: National Intimate Partner and Sexual Violence Survey. *American Journal of Public Health, 105*(4), e11-e12.
Coleman, E. (2011). Impulsive/compulsive sexual behavior: Assessment and treatment. In J. Grant & J. Potenza (Eds.), *Oxford handbook of impulse control disorders* (pp. 375-388). Oxford University Press.
Cooper, A. (2002). *Sex and the internet. A guidebook for clinicians.* Brunner-Routledge.
Cooper, A., Delmonico, D., & Burg, R. (2000). Cybersex users, abusers, and compulsives: New findings and implications. *Sexual Addiction and Compulsivity, 7,* 5-29.
Cooper, A., Delmonico, D., Griffin-Shelly, E., & Mathy, R. (2004). Online sexual activity: An examination of potentially problematic behaviors. *Sexual Addiction and Compulsivity, 11,* 129-143.
Cooper, A., Griffin-Shelly, E., Delmonico, D., & Mathy, R. (2001). Online sexual problems: Assessment and predictive variables. *Sexual Addiction and Compulsivity, 8,* 267-285.
Cooper, A., Morahan-Martin, J., Mathy, R. M., & Maheu, M. (2002). Toward an increased understanding of user demographics in online sexual activities. *Journal of Sex and Marital Therapy, 28,* 105-129.
Cooper, A., Scherer, C., Boies, S., & Gordon, B. (1999). Sexuality on the internet: From sexual exploration to pathological expression. *Professional Psychology: Research and Practice, 30,* 154-164.
Cox, D., & McMahon, B. (1978). Incidents of male exhibitionism in the United States as reported by victimized female college students. *International Journal of Law and Psychiatry, 3,* 453-457.
Cybertip.ca (2013). http://www.cybertip.ca/en/child-sexual-abuse/grooming/#fn1
DeHart, D., Dwyer, G., Seto, M. C., Moran, R., Letourneau, E., & Schwarz-Watts, D. (2017) Internet sexual solicitation of children: A proposed typology of offenders based on their chats, e-mails, and social network posts. *Journal of Sexual Aggression, 23*(1), 77-89. https://doi.org/10.1080/13552600.2016.1241309
Delmonico, D., & Griffin, E. (2014). *Sexual addiction: Assessment, management, and treatment.* Routledge.
Delmonico, D., Griffin, E., & Moriarty, J. (2001). *Cybersex unhooked: A workbook for breaking free from compulsive online sexual behavior.* Hazelden Educational Press.
DeLong, R., & Durkin, K. (2017). Internet-facilitated child sexual exploitation crimes. In M. Khosrow (Ed.), *Encyclopedia of information science and technology* (4th ed., pp. 1366-1375). IGI Global.
DeLong, R., Durkin, K., & Hundersmarck, S. (2010). An exploratory analysis of the cognitive distortions of a sample of men arrested in internet sex stings. *Journal of Sexual Aggression, 16*(1), 1-12.
Department of Justice Canada. (2013) *Sexual offending against children and youth.* Government of Canada. http://www.canada.ca/en/news/archive/2013/02/sexual-offending-against-children-youth.html
Dietz, P., Hazelwood, R., & Warren, J. (1990). The sexually sadistic criminal and his offenses. *Bulletin of the American Academy of Psychiatry and the Law, 18,* 163-178.
Dockterman, E. (2018, May 14). Can bad men change? Inside sex offender treatment. *Time.* https://time.com/magazine/us/5272326/may-21st-2018-vol-191-no-19-u-s/
Durkin, K. F., & DeLong, R. L. (2012). Internet crimes against children. In Z. Yan (Ed.), *Encyclopedia of cyber behavior* (pp. 799-806). IGI Global. https://doi.org/10.4018/978-1-4666-0315-8.ch066
Elliott, I, & Beech, A. (2009). Understanding online child pornography use: Applying sexual offense theory to internet offenders, *Aggression and Violent Behavior, 14*, 180-193.
Fedoroff, J., Fishell, A., & Fedoroff, B. (1999). A case series of women evaluated for paraphilic sexual disorders. *The Canadian Journal of Human Sexuality, 8,* 127-140.
First, M. B. (2014). DSM-5 and paraphilic disorders. *Journal of the American Academy of Psychiatry and the Law, 42*(2), 191-201. http://jaapl.org/content/42/2/191

Freund, K., Seto, M., & Kuban, M. (1997). Frotteurism and the theory of courtship disorder. In D. R. Laws & W. O'Donohue (Eds.), *Sexual deviance: Theory, assessment, and treatment* (pp. 111-130). Guilford.

Freund, K., & Watson, R. (1990). Mapping the boundaries of courtship disorder. *Journal of Sex Research, 27,* 589-606.

Galbreath, N., Berlin, F., & Sawyer, D. (2002). *Paraphilias and the internet.* In A. Cooper (Ed.), *Sex and the Internet: A guidebook for clinicians* (pp. 187-205). Brunner-Routledge.

Hansen, C. (2006). *Prominent men caught in Petaluma sting.* https://undercover.hosting.nyu.edu/s/undercover-reporting/item/12853

Hanson, K., & Morton-Bourgon, K. (2005). The characteristics of persistent sexual offenders: A meta-analysis of recidivism studies. *Journal of Consulting and Clinical Psychology, 73*(6).

Holder, E. (2011, May 19*) Transcript: Attorney General Eric Holder remarks on combating child exploitation.* National Strategy Conference on Combating Child Exploitation, San Jose, California. https://www.bet.com/article/7mfd7g/eric-holder-remarks-on-combating-child-exploitation

Janssen, D. (2014). How to "ascertain" paraphilia? An etymological hint. *Archives of Sexual Behavior, 43*(7), 1245-1246.

Kafka, M. (1997). Hypersexual desire in males: An operational definition and clinical implications for males with paraphilia and paraphilia-related disorders. *Archives of Sexual Behavior, 26*(5), 505-526. https://doi.org/10.1023/a:1024507922470

Kafka, M. (2006). Therapy for sexual impulsivity: The paraphilias and paraphilia-related disorders *Psychiatric Times, 13*(6), 23.

Keighley, K. (2017). Police-reported crime statistics in Canada, 2016. *Juristat, 37*(1). Statistics Canada. https://www150.statcan.gc.ca/n1/pub/85-002-x/2017001/article/54842-eng.htm

Kicaburun, K., & Griffiths M. (2018). The dark side of internet: Preliminary evidence for the associations of dark personality traits with specific online activities and problematic internet use. *Journal of Behavioral Addictions, 7*(4), 993-1003. https://doi.org/10.1556/2006.7.2018.109

Klein, M. (2011). *America's war on sex: The continuing attack on law, lust, and liberty* (2nd ed.). Praeger.

Kloess, J., Seymour-Smith, S., Hamilton-Giachritsis, C., Long, M., Shipley, D., & Beech, A. (2017). A qualitative analysis of offenders' modus operandi in sexually exploitative interactions with children online. *Sexual Abuse: A Journal of Research and Treatment, 29,* 563-591.

Krone, T. (2004). A typology of online child pornography offending. *Trends & Issues in Crime and Criminal Justice, 279,* 1-6.

Lanning, K. (2001). *Child molesters: A behavioral analysis.* https://www.missingkids.org/content/dam/missingkids/pdfs/publications/nc70.pdf

Laumann, E., Gagnon, J., Michael, R., & Michaels, S. (1994). *The social organization of sexuality: Sexual practices in the United States.* University of Chicago Press.

Laws, D., & O'Donohue, W. (Eds.). (1997). *Sexual deviance: Theory, assessment, and treatment.* Guilford.

Leatherman, A. (2009). Luring language and virtual victims: Coding cyberpredators' online communicative behavior [Technical report]. Ursinus College.

LeVay, S., Baldwin, J., & Baldwin, J. (2015). *Discovering human sexuality* (3rd ed.). Sinauer Associates.

Levenson, J., Brannon, Y., Fortney, T., & Baker, J. (2007). Public perceptions about sex offenders and community protection policies. *Analyses of Social Issues and Public Policy, 7*(1).

Ley, D. (2018). Compulsive Sexual Behavior Disorder in ICD-11: What does this mean, for advocacy against sex addiction diagnosis? *Psychologytoday.com.* https://www.psychologytoday.com/us/comment/973268

Lohr, B., Adams, H., & Davis, J. (1997). Sexual arousal to erotic and aggressive stimuli in sexually coercive and noncoercive men. *Journal of Abnormal Psychology, 106,* 230-242.

Malesky, L. (2007). Internet sexual activity: A comparison between contact and non-contact child pornography offenders. *Journal of Sexual Aggression, 16,* 181-195.

Mark, K., Janssen, E., & Milhausen, R. (2011). Infidelity in heterosexual couples: Demographic, interpersonal, and personality-related predictors of extra-dyadic sex. *Archives of Sexual Behavior, 40,* 971-982. https://doi.org/10.1007/s10508-011-9771-z

Marshall, W., Eccles, A., & Barbaree, H. (1991). The treatment of exhibitionists: A focus on sexual deviance versus cognitive and relationship features. *Behaviour Research and Therapy*, 29, 129-135.

Marshall, W., & Hall, G. (1995). The value of the MMPI in deciding forensic issues in accused sex offenders. *Sexual Abuse: A Journal of Research and Treatment, 7,* 205-219.

Marshall, W., Payne, K., Barbaree, H., & Eccles, A. (1991). Exhibitionists: Sexual preferences for exposing. *Behaviour Research and Therapy, 29,* 37-40.

Mears, B. (2010). Supreme Court: Sex offenders can be held indefinitely. *CNN.* http://www.cnn.com/2010/CRIME/05/17/scotus.sex.offenders/index.html#:~:text=Washington%20(CNN)%20%2D%2D%20The%20U.S.,sexually%20dangerous%22%20in%20the%20future

Millon, T., Davis, R., & Millon, C. (1997). *Millon Clinical Multiaxial Inventory-III Manual* (2nd ed.). National Computer Systems.

Mitchell, K., Finkelhor, D., Jones, L., & Wolak, J. (2010). Use of social networking sites in online sex crimes against minors: An examination of national incidence and means of utilization. *Journal of Adolescent Health, 47,* 183-190.

Mitchell, K., Finkelhor, D., & Wolak, J. (2005). The internet and family and acquaintance sexual abuse. *Child Maltreatment, 10*(1), 49-60. https://doi.org/10.1177/1077559504271917

Mitchel, K., Finkelhor, D., & Wolak, J. (2007). Youth internet users at risk for the most serious online sexual solicitations. *American Journal of Preventive Medicine, 32,* 532-537.

Mitchell, K., & Jones, L. (2013). *Internet-facilitated commercial sexual exploitation of children.* Crimes Against Children Research Center, University of New Hampshire.

Mitchell, K., & Jones, L., Finkelhor, D., & Wolak, J. (2011). Internet-facilitated commercial sexual exploitation of children: Findings from a nationally representative sample of law enforcement agencies in the United States. *Sexual Abuse: A Journal of Research and Treatment, 23*(1), 43-71. http://unh.edu/ccrc/pdf/CV201.pdf

Mitchell, K., Wolak, J., & Finkelhor, D. (2005). Police posing as juveniles online to catch sex offenders: Is it working? *Sexual Abuse: A Journal of Research and Treatment, 17,* 241-267.

Mitchell, K., Wolak, J., Finkelhor, D., & Jones. L. (2012). Investigators using the internet to apprehend sex offenders: Findings from the Second National Juvenile Online Victimization Study, *Police Practice and Research, 13*(3), 267-281. https://doi.org/10.1080/15614263.2011.627746

Money, J. (1985). *The destroying angel: Sex, fitness and food in the legacy of degeneracy theory, Graham Crackers, Kellogg's Corn Flakes, and American health history.* Prometheus Books.

Olson, L., Daggs, J., Ellevold, B., & Rogers, T. (2007). Entrapping the innocent: Toward a theory of child sexual predators' luring communication. *Communication Theory, 17*(3), 231-251. https://doi.org/10.1111/j.1468-2885.2007.00294.x

Peterson, F., Bley, J., & Frabotta, R. (2020). *The Gender Revolution & New Sexual Health.* Cognella Academic Press.

Pratarelli, M., & Browne, B. (2002). Confirmatory factor analysis of internet use and addiction. *CyberPsychology and Behavior, 5,* 53-64.

Prentky, R., & Knight, R. (1991). Identifying critical dimensions for discriminating among rapists. *Journal of Consulting and Clinical Psychology, 59,* 433-443.

Purcell, C., & Arrigo, B. (2006). *The psychology of lust murder: Paraphilia, sexual killing, and serial homicide.* Academic Press.

Qualye, E., Vaughn, M., & Taylor, M. (2006). Sex offenders, internet child abuse images and emotional avoidance: The importance of values. *Aggression and Violent Behavior, 11,* 1-11.

Robinson, W. (1933). *Medical sex dictionary.* The Eugenics Publishing Company.

Schultz, D., & Schultz, S. (2004). *The history of modern psychology.* Wadsworth/Thompson Learning.

Seto, M. (2012a, February 6). *Child pornography offender characteristics and risk to reoffend.* Testimony to the United States Sentencing Commission, Washington, DC.

Seto, M. (2012b). Is pedophilia a sexual orientation? *Archives of Sexual Behavior, 41*, 231-236.

Seto, M. (2013, October 30-November 2). *Assessment and treatment of internet sex offenders* [Paper presentation]. The Annual Conference of the Association for the Treatment of Sex Abusers, Chicago, IL, United States.

Seto, M., & Eke, A.. (2015). Predicting recidivism among adult male child pornography offenders: Development of the Child Pornography Offender Risk Tool (CPORT). *Law and Human Behavior, 39,* 416-429.

Seto, M., Reeves, L., & Jung, S. (2010). Motives for child pornography offending: The explanations given by the offenders. *Journal of Sexual Aggression, 16,* 169-180.

Seto, M., Wood, J., Babchishin, K., & Flynn, S. (2012). Online solicitation offenders are different from child pornography offenders and lower risk contact sexual offenders. *Law and Human Behavior, 36,* 320-330. https://doi.org/10.1037/h0093925

Smukler, A., & Schiebel, D. (1975). Personality characteristics of exhibitionists. *Diseases of the Nervous System, 36,* 600-603.

Snyder, H. (2000). *Sexual assault of young children as reported to law enforcement: Victim, incident, and offender characteristics.* U.S. Department of Justice, Office of Justice Programs. Justice National Center for Juvenile Justice. https://bjs.ojp.gov/content/pub/pdf/saycrle.pdf

Sugrue, D. (2007). Sexual addiction/compulsivity: Diagnosis and treatment. In L. VandeCreek, F. Peterson, & J. Bley (Eds.), *Innovations in clinical practice: Focus on sexual health* (pp. 177-196). Professional Resource Press.

Tener, D., Wolak, J., & Finkelhor, D. (2013). A typology of offenders who use online communications to commit sex crimes against minors. *Journal of Aggression, Maltreatment & Trauma, 44*(3), 319-337.

Tsu, A., Nolan, D., & Amico, C. (2017, July 6). Child marriages in America by the numbers. *Frontline* (Public Broadcasting System). http://apps.frontline.org/child-marriage-by-the-numbers/

von Kraft-Ebbing, R. (1892). *Psychopathia sexualis.* (C. Chaddock, Trans.). F.A. Davis Company. (Original work published 1886)

Webster, S., Davidson, J., Bifulco, A., Gottschalk, P., Caretti, V., Phan, T., . . . Craparo, G. (2012). *European online grooming project, final report, European Union.* European Commission Safer Internet Plus Programme. https://www.academia.edu/23987615/European_Online_Grooming_Project_-_Final_Report

Weiss, R. (2013). *Cruise control: Understanding sex addiction in gay men* (2nd ed.). Gentle Path.

Whittle, H., Hamilton-Giachritsis, C., & Beech, A. (2014). "Under his spell": Victims' perspectives of being groomed online. *Social Sciences, 3*(3), 404-426. https://doi.org/10.3390/socsci3030404

Wolak, J., Finkelhor, D., Mitchell, K. (2012). *Trends in law enforcement responses to technology-facilitated child sexual exploitation crimes: The third National Juvenile Online Victimization study (NJOV-3).* Crimes Against Children Research Center.

Wolak, J., Finkelhor, D., Mitchell, K., & Ybarra, M. (2010). Online "predators" and their victims: Myths, realities, and implications for prevention and treatment. *American Psychologist, 63*(2), 111-128.

Wolak, J., Mitchell, K., & Finkelhor, D. (2006). *Online victimization of youth: Five years later.* National Center for Missing and Exploited Children. http://unh.edu/ccrc/pdf/CV138.pdf

27

Do Men Use Pornography as a Maladaptive Coping Behavior? An Inquiry, Case Studies, and Best Practices

Frederick L. Peterson, Jr., Zane Ferguson, Emily Chriswell, Molly Peters, and Bran Allen

INTRODUCTION

In mental health clinics across America, men have been presenting themselves (often at the insistence of their wives) with complaints of using pornography to an extent that it is ruining their relationships, their health, and even their careers. Many times, but not always, these men also have coexisting problematic sexual behaviors. These behaviors include, but are not limited to, behaviors such as excessive masturbation (to the diminishment of or substitution for relational sex), marital affairs (traditionally called infidelity or cheating), cybersexing and/or e-affairs (any of the web-based systems in which sexually explicit images and communication can be sent and received), and miscellaneous sexual behaviors including visiting massage parlors (usually with sexual contact), employing sex workers (in person or online), frequenting strip-clubs or adult XXX book stores (with or without sexual contact), and sex tourism (visiting abroad expressly for sexual purposes). There are also paraphilic sexual behaviors (some legal and some not) that can be very harmful to spouses, children, and others (Peterson et al., 2020).

Pornography use (sexually explicit material specifically intended for sexual gratification) refers to depictions of people or behaviors intended to be sexually arousing and is closely related to complaints of partners when it has adverse effects on relational sex. Pornography has additional concerns regarding the sexual objectification of women, partners feeling like they cannot compete with the professional models depicted, and some spouses seeing pornography use as a form of infidelity. Obviously, pornography is extremely common in our increasingly technology-based culture, and in the opinion of the authors, has unfortunately overtaken school-based education and parental instruction as the most common form of sex education in America (Peterson et al., 2020).

The increased use of internet pornography has also raised concerns among some regarding a cultural desensitization and normalization of child sexual abuse (Lanning, 2001). With the advent of the internet, the use of pornography has exploded concurrent to the general population due to the "3A's" – access, affordability, and (perceived) anonymity (Cooper, 2002). In addition, the advent of "porn tube" streaming services (in 2006) that do not require downloading are also believed to have accelerated the use of online pornography as a "super normal stimulus" and has even been theorized as a potential contributory factor in the development of sexual dysfunction in men under 40 (Park et al., 2016).

It was estimated that about one-third (36%) of all internet users visit at least one adult sexually oriented website per month and the average user of online pornography sites does so 7.7 times per month (Stone, 2017). The U.S. government, including all branches of the military, has spent nearly 70 years banning many forms of obscenity and pornography (with mixed results) and does so for many understandable reasons (e.g., prevention of sexual harassment and hostile work environments), but especially the prevention of sexual exploitation of children (Stone, 2017).

This contribution focuses on the clinical concerns of men when they seek help from mental health professionals, voluntarily or otherwise, related to their use of pornography. The authors present two case studies which illustrate the compulsive and problematic use of pornography. The first case study is about a man named Doug who finds the fabric of his life unraveling through the compulsive use of legal pornography. In the second case study, the authors explore how legal pornography users can transition to become sex offenders through the use of child sexually oriented materials (child pornography). The second case study also addresses the special issues of combat military personnel and veterans, which the authors conceptualize the use of pornography as a maladaptive coping behavior to stress. Finally, treatment guidelines from best models are presented for providing therapy to pornography (both legal and illegal) users. The primary question explored in this chapter: Do men use pornography (including child-oriented images) as a maladaptive coping behavior? While it is acknowledged that women and adolescent girls use pornography, men are believed to be the primary consumers. Stone (2017) reports that one of three visitors to sex-related websites are estimated to be female. However, for simplicity sake, this chapter will use male examples and pronouns for pornography users.

PROBLEMATIC USE OF PORNOGRAPHY

There has been a general increase in the level of "acceptance" in the use of pornography in the general population and even some mental health professionals may ask, "What is the problem with legal porn?" Legal use of pornography (no child images) can create serious adverse disruptions in many areas of men's lives as well as with the lives of their partners and family members. Potential disruptions in men's lives can occur across seven domains of health and include the following effects, depending upon the individual man and his partner's personal value system:

- **Emotional Health** – Some users of pornography may experience shame, remorse, embarrassment, humiliation, and guilt. Partners, children, and some family members may feel a sense of betrayal, confusion, anger, shame, embarrassment, and humiliation. The most severe emotional consequences (e.g., when children discover pornography on dad's PC) include extreme anxiety or depression requiring hospitalization to avoid suicide.
- **Relational Health** – This includes potential relationship conflict and marital discord, decreased relational sex with partner, separation from spouse and children, isolation from family and friends who turn against the individual, loss of reputation, and sometimes relocation to start their life over. If the pornography is found on a laptop by minor children in the home, further relational and emotional complications can result.
- **Physical Health** – Men who compulsively use porn are not as likely to engage in healthy activities (such as maintaining an exercise program) and are more likely to lose sleep to the detriment of their overall health, including daytime fatigue and lowering their immune response. If men start going beyond the limits of using pornography to actual contact, of course, sexually transmitted infections (for men and their partners) become a risk as well as being assaulted during encounters for anonymous sex.

- **Financial Health** – There are direct costs of purchasing pornography and indirect costs of mental health therapy, medical health care, and attorneys for relationships that end in divorce.
- **Spiritual Health** – There may be dissonance or misalignment between spiritual/religious beliefs and the use of pornography, resulting in self-perception as "unforgiven, freak of nature, or being a sinner/condemned."
- **Vocational Health** – This is related to but different from financial health. Vocational health issues involve tardiness due to the use of porn, loss of a license for violation of professional boundaries, or the risk of losing employment from on-the-job use.
- **Legal Health** – Besides involvement with attorneys for divorce proceedings, this domain usually involves the use of child pornography with resulting prosecution and/or imprisonment for solicitation or possession of child pornography.

Any one of the areas of health can be devastating to an individual and his family, but usually the use of pornography adversely impacts several areas of health at the same time, making the whole experience feel overwhelming. A crisis occurs typically from the discovery, by the partner, of secret use of pornography (and sometimes additional forms of sexual behavior). In addition and often simultaneously, significant relationship conflict occurs when pornography use diminishes relational sex with the partner or it becomes a complete substitute to the frustration of their partner. As noted previously, partners also sometimes feel like they cannot compete with the level of sexual attraction of porn star models; they argue against unrealistic depictions of sexual behavior and the resulting erroneous expectations, and object to the sexual aggression toward and sexual objectification of women (Peterson et al., 2020).

CASE STUDY I: A PROFESSOR'S COMPULSIVE USE OF LEGAL PORNOGRAPHY*

Doug came into the clinic in a crisis period of his marriage and career caused by his use of pornography, other sexual acting out, and depression. He was married to a beautiful woman whom he loved named Eve. Doug was a well-respected academic and had written several books on topics regarding the criminal justice system. He was a 40-year-old man with many blessings, yet was unhappy in his life. He started drinking more over the last couple years, and was secretly viewing pornography. Doug and Eve went through a terribly tragic event that led to Doug becoming severely depressed, and he increased his drinking as well as his use of pornography. All of these maladaptive behaviors were strategies he used to cope. This tragic event also served as a catalyst for Doug disclosing to Eve that he had been hiding a history of childhood sexual abuse.

A traumatic event occurred which involved Eve's brother (Juan) who was diagnosed paranoid schizophrenic and was sometimes threatening to her. Doug's mother-in-law was concerned that Juan was getting worse and wanted to visit him for a wellness check. Doug accompanied his wife Eve and his mother-in-law to Juan's apartment and found him in an agitated state with suspicious thoughts concerning the family's motives for the visit to his home. Doug asked to use the restroom and while Doug was down the hallway in the bathroom, Juan produced a handgun and shot Eve in the chest at point blank range. Juan then proceeded to shoot his mother. Doug heard the shots and came out to see what Juan had done, saw the two bodies on the floor and ran out the back door thinking both his wife and mother-in-law were dead and that he was next. As is sometimes said, miracles do happen and the bullet that entered Eve barely missed all her vital organs and, after the initial shock of being shot in

*This case study is based upon true events. Names have been changed and some details omitted to protect the privacy and identity of those who gave permission for this story to be shared for teaching purposes.

the chest, Eve crawled over to her mother and started performing CPR (Eve had medical training). The mother laid there, nearly dead in a pool of blood, but saw Juan aiming to shoot Eve a second time – this time directly in the head while Eve was doing CPR on the mother. In the last moments of the mother's life, she tried to protect her daughter by picking up her purse and hugging Eve around the neck with it. Juan fired the second shot at Eve. The bullet, intended to enter Eve's brain, was found weeks later as it had lodged in the checkbook within her mother's purse. In the meanwhile, Doug had called the police and the brother was arrested.

Over time, Eve recovered and somehow they survived as a couple. They had both sought out counseling support and the marital therapist they worked with referred Doug to the lead author for individual therapy to address his pornography use, depression, and drinking. Doug sat in the consultation office slumped over in what appeared to be the personification of shame. He held his head hanging down in his hands, eyes to the floor, and barely able to speak. After a few moments, Doug spoke just above a whisper and explained that his life had spiraled out of control in a circle of drinking, pornography, and sexual avoidance of his wife. Earlier that week, Eve found a flirty text on her phone that invited her to meet Doug for a drink after work. The text was intended for someone else. Eve told Doug to move out of the house, their children cried for days, and Doug decided to commit to do whatever he could to save his marriage.

Doug told a story of a life falling apart characteristic of men caught up in repeating cycles of compulsive pornography use spinning further out of control. He explained he felt adrift in life, moving away from the people and things he always held most dear in his heart. There was an overwhelming sense of powerlessness and confusion mixed with guilt and embarrassment. Doug's story covered a decade of slow-growing distance in his marital relationship and a growing "cancer" of secret use of pornography. He described himself and Eve as religiously faith-based and were virgins when they married. Before the shootings, Doug reported that those years together with Eve were the best period of the marriage. Over the course of their next 10 years, he experienced a diminishing closeness with Eve as his best friend, less sexual intimacy, and getting bored with the routine of his life as a professor, despite his love for his wife and children. Of course, Doug (as well as his wife) was also experiencing posttraumatic stress disorder (PTSD) because of the shootings.

Doug watched online pornography and masturbated, not only as a rationalized supplement to the lessening amount of sex he was having with Eve, but also to escape the shame of abuse. Increased masturbation is a common compensating strategy used when a partner is less interested in sex. It is usually not a problem except when masturbation becomes paired with pornography and shrouded in secrecy. However, Doug started using masturbation as a substitute for relational sex with Eve and the couple began to increasingly avoid sex over time, creating a low sex/no sex marriage.

The combined pornography and masturbation escalated when their communication stopped and Doug's secret activity facilitated the construction of a double life. Eve once caught him viewing his pornography and insisted on marital counseling, to which Doug acquiesced. As a result, things appeared to improve temporarily but Doug had only made external changes to appease her and stay in the marriage. He did not acknowledge or make internal changes regarding his emotionally restricted life. He did not talk about his PTSD or his growing sense of depression. He also did not acknowledge his increased drinking. No meaningful internal changes occurred with his emotional state, poor self-perception, or his lack of purpose in life. So, after a year, the couple had lost any benefit from the marital counseling and regressed back into a pattern of emotional/sexual avoidance.

This was where Doug failed himself, Eve, and his family. Part of his shame was his history of sexual abuse, which no one knew about except he and his abusive sister. She was 5 years older than Doug and able to physically beat and sexually abuse him. The abuse went on for years until he hit puberty and was able to knock her down by punching her in the face. The abuse stopped but the denial in his family system continued (even after he had previously complained to his parents that he was getting beat up and sexually abused by the sister). As a child, Doug created a denial system that allowed him to function as if the abuse never happened, and this served as a basis for compartmentalizing his abuse. As an adult, Doug began thinking that he could also compartmentalize a double life of pornography use without consequences to his marriage, family, or himself.

Eve came to a consultation apparently just to make sure she had an opportunity to help her husband by providing information that would enable the therapist to understand Doug from her perspective. Eve got to talk alone without her husband present (he was asked to wait in another room). She was a beautiful young woman a few years Doug's junior. Her eyes were red and tearful. She appeared to be full of pain, betrayal, and anguish. It had been just a few days since, once again, she discovered evidence of her husband's second life. She had an aura of being shell-shocked. Eve made it clear that her being there was not to be seen as "standing by her man" and that she had given herself a gift of not pressuring herself to make any immediate decision about the marriage. She was explicit regarding the possibility that she may not choose to continue the relationship.

Her immediate input from the start was both appreciated and critical to the treatment outcome for Doug, if not the couple. By being there, she provided invaluable input as to the extent of the problem and what consequences were a result of his secret pornography use. She also informed herself by asking questions about what the treatment for her husband was about and how it was different than the counseling they had previously tried. In addition, she was given support to take care of herself and get treatment for her own PTSD. She was invited to call with any information about her husband's behavior that she thinks may be relevant to his treatment.

During the course of meeting with this couple, it was the first time any therapist in the clinic had ever had to physically step between a husband and wife. Why? Because Eve could not control her anger and was physically wailing on Doug around the head and shoulders. She was told that her feelings were valid and understandable yet she would have to refrain from violence. She was told that Doug would be the primary focus of treatment, but as long as the marriage had a potential for being preserved, their relationship would be the second client in the treatment room. Eve agreed that she needed her own source of support to help her sort out her feelings, deal with her PTSD, and come to a decision regarding the marriage. Therefore, she agreed to receive her own short-term individual counseling with another therapist to help her deal with her anger and impulses of violence toward Doug, and learn to effectively manage her symptoms of PTSD.

Doug was almost at rock-bottom. His marriage was likely over, he was separated from his children, and he worried about how much his professional reputation had been damaged. While Doug had developed himself professionally through his writing as a consultant to the criminal justice system, his specific area of expertise was the investigation and prosecution of sex crimes. Beyond getting himself healthy and saving his marriage (for real this time), Doug was very concerned about his children. He was worried about whether or not the children could understand what was going on and the changes related to his living separately. For a short while, he did not see his children at all and then started to see them only with another supervising adult present.

The reason for this was that Eve was blindsided by the discovery of his double life and was really questioning how well she knew Doug. Basically, she wondered that if she did not know about all the secret pornography for such a long time, what else does she not know about her husband? She started to question if the children were safe from harm when they were in his care. The first author employed specialty assessments which included objective measures of sexual interest to determine if Doug demonstrated any evidence of sexual interest in children. These tests were negative (showing an absence of sexual interest in children). This was reassuring to Eve and the couple worked out a visitation schedule by which Doug could maintain a significant and emotionally meaningful connection with the children.

Doug's crisis stabilized for the time because he now had some hope from re-establishing contact with his children and Eve was not immediately moving to end the marriage. He saw grace in Eve taking a "wait and see" approach to her decision-making. Doug obsessed about how he had brought himself to a place that was so distant from where he wanted to be. He kept thinking about how his life was not perfect, but so much better a few years ago when his marriage, family, and career were intact. What had his life come to? Now, he felt like a pathetic, lonely man in a dumpy apartment wanting to masturbate to porn. Doug admitted to seeing himself as a poisonous influence in his family's life and seriously thought that they would be better off without him. He felt that he had no one to call who would want to talk to him or cared if he lived or died. In fact, he convinced himself there were many people who wished that he would kill himself. Doug was a man without any sense of worth.

Through a combination of individual and group therapy, Doug was given guidance to reflect on his internal life and sort out the factors that brought him to such a miserable place in his life. Through his emotional exploration, he gained insight into the factors that helped put him on his path of self-destruction. During the course of treatment, Doug developed a sense of safety and supportive structure to explore long-standing issues that he had traditionally ignored and pushed to the edge of his consciousness. He came to understand that these factors were not excuses for his sexual acting-out but were factors in the development and maintenance of his sexually compulsive use of pornography. For Doug, his individual mix of contributing factors included:

- Sexual and physical abuse as a boy by his older sister for several years
- Developing a compulsive use of pornography as a teenager that continued into his marriage
- Having doubts about being masculine enough and a good-enough lover
- Self-beliefs about needing to be in control and non-emotional as a man
- Witnessing a fatal shooting of his mother-in-law and near fatal shooting of his wife
- Having an undiagnosed case of severe clinical depression and PTSD
- Drinking excessively and experiencing disinhibition of behavior
- Guilt from previous sexual indiscretions that were unknown to his wife
- Not having communication skills to resolve marital resentments
- Feeling he was condemned by God for being an "abomination" in his mind.

Doug joined a men's sexual health group that brings together men who struggle with their personal challenges and search for personal health. As unlikely as it seems, the men's group starts out as a collection of strangers who slowly create a safe space to speak honestly about their sexual compulsions without fear of judgment or attack, admit their shortcomings and disappointments in themselves, and face the hurt they have caused others. Once men reach both a sense of safety and honesty, they have an opportunity to begin healing themselves, making amends, and rebuilding relationships. Doug was a rather traditional fellow and very hesitant to join in the mix of conversation, so he sat and listened for several weeks.

He saw that for some men, it was too late when they found their way to the group. He learned that those men had to deal with too much anger, suspicion, and hopelessness after they faced the fact that whatever life still remained in the relationship had been damaged beyond resuscitation. Doug heard stories of men with partners in their marriage or business who had already passed their point of no return. The group could only help those men find a way to make the unbearable a bit more bearable by finding ways to manage the loneliness, guilt, and pain of personal ruin so they could get past the point of wanting to die and could start to build a new life.

Doug also witnessed other men who had begun the process of recovery. He hoped to replicate a similar salvation of his own marriage and career. Some men are slow to lay down the burden of secrecy and begin rebuilding trust with their partners (as well as with themselves). Doug witnessed men starting to make authentic changes within themselves, not just for window dressing in the marriage. Fortunately, he found most men lucky enough to come into the group while there was still time for healing to take hold. Like Doug, most of them were fortunate to have partners willing to suspend any decision to exit the relationship until they could judge for themselves if the man was making genuine changes for the better.

Doug found that the men hold confidential what they hear in group and that this trust with each other is of paramount importance. He discovered that trust was the essence of the safe space which allowed sharing of painful details of their lives. In one group meeting, Doug watched as a man share some of the details of his personal dilemma, a marriage on the rocks that was in crisis after his wife discovered his inappropriate email communications on his personal laptop with a woman at work. This rang a bell for Doug as he felt the shame in the man's words.

Although Doug sometimes felt confused, he began to feel a profound appreciation for where he was. Doug was surprised when Tony (another group member) shared a bit of twisted wisdom when Tony spoke of his history of lying about his secret life to his wife. Tony shared that his marriage never started to heal until he decided that it was more important to be honest than be married! This statement struck fear into Doug's heart but Tony explained that the more he lived "in the light" with honesty, the more healing could happen in his marriage and the more likely he would be able to save not only himself but his family.

Finally, Doug had an opportunity to speak and shared a few details of why he was joining the group. The common joke is "What are you in for?" He shared as much as he was comfortable disclosing since he was the new guy, saying that he wished to do everything he could to make things right with his wife. However, there was one thing she requested of him that Doug dreaded and could not bring himself to do, and that was going to a Sex Addicts Anonymous (SAA) group as part of his recovery program. Doug had heard a couple of the men mention that they attended SAA but explained that he was too ashamed of what he had done to his life and family. He could not think of how talking about it in a public meeting could help. He was also fearful of being identified by someone that he works with at the university (like a student) or someone who attends the same church. Another man in the group (Carlos) reached out to Doug by saying he remembered having the same fears and that Carlos also had a job that was very much in the public eye. He offered to meet Doug before the Saturday morning meeting and attend the meeting together.

Doug realized he was in the middle of a group of men who were committed to improving their own health as well as the collective health of each other. This, of course, was a key step in improving the health of their marriage and family. He was not sure what was going to happen in additional groups but his initial apprehension melted away to a positive anticipation to return and learn. He did not know all the how-to of repairing his life and relations with his family. He only felt hope about being in the right place to learn. Doug accepted Carlos' invitation.

No matter what additional challenges Doug would face, sexual in nature or otherwise, he learned that walking a path of health is a balancing act of the right amounts of the right ingredients at the right times. The ingredients are love, peace, faith, and wisdom. All four of these ingredients are the basic building blocks of his relationship with himself and his wife. Love encompasses acceptance and compassion for oneself as well as others. Peace involves finding ways to quiet the noise of past trauma and finding one's center. Faith means hope and the belief in the resiliency of the human spirit. Wisdom knows that each of us, as life itself, are full of paradox and contradiction, yet we can decide to make the right choices to rebuild a life (with others) that may not be perfect but is damn well worth living.

In time, Doug found the right amount of the right healing ingredients in time to save himself and his marriage. He added liberal amounts of three additional and critical elements: promoting a sense of safety, exercising transparency, and making a friend of accountability. He no longer was depressed and having thoughts of self-destruction but instead appreciated his daily life with his wife and children. Over time, a shift occurred within Eve from "How could you do this to me?" to "How can we move forward together?" They became focused on making a new normal which was satisfying to both of them. The marital relationship grew past the hurt and betrayal to a focus on living in the present and sharing enjoyment of each other's company as well as pleasure in touching one another. They discovered a renewed sense of themselves individually, as a couple, and as a family.

TREATMENT FOR COMPULSIVE USE OF LEGAL PORNOGRAPHY

The recovery process from compulsive use of pornography will be discussed in two sections. The first addresses providing assessment and treatment to men (like Doug) who are involved with ongoing relationships that they wish to repair and preserve. These types of cases are by far the majority of men who seek out treatment (even if they are doing so under pressure from their partners at first) and most often involve compulsive use of legal pornography. The second type of case management discussed is with men who are viewing pornography involving sexually exploitive images of children (discussed after the Case Study II). These men rarely present themselves to treatment voluntarily and are coming to the attention of mental health providers primarily in court-ordered treatment programs.

When there is recognition that compulsive use of (legal) pornography is causing problems in a relationship, couples often choose to seek professional consultation and may engage in treatment with the hope of conflict resolution. The recovery process can take many paths depending upon the particular circumstances of their situation. These details are as varied as the types of sexual behaviors that compel people to seek professional help, yet a key factor is whether the partner to the pornography user wishes to stay in the relationship. There is no strict right or wrong in terms of making this decision as each person must make their own choice in accordance with their own personal values. However, there are a few guidelines that are helpful to consider, including the history of the relationship, the amount of emotional investment one has in the other person, and what the desired outcomes are for each individual. When the partner chooses to stay in the relationship (at least to see if there are signs of improvement in the short term), then a key factor in the recovery process is activated for the man who has been viewing pornography because there is a greater likelihood that the man will engage in treatment.

The partner's decision to stay, whether they stay long-term or not, usually provides motivation for change as the man understands that he has made serious mistakes, has hurt others by his actions, and wants to do what he can to be a healthier individual. If the partner immediately decides the relationship is over, it is a whole other story and the man may often continue on a path of self-destruction until he hits rock bottom in pick-up bars, a hospital, incarcerated, or in the morgue. When there is an alignment of factors that allows the recovery process to occur, it may often start with relapse, an expected part of the path to health. Of course, this requires hope, commitment, and determination of the individual to continue to pursue higher levels of health. If he hasn't hit bottom or paid enough in significant damages to his life (as well as others), then he is likely to continue the same behavior that created his problems. He may possibly completely wreck their lives and even get to a point of wanting to end it all.

It takes even more hope, patience, and grace for the partners of pornography users, especially those who choose to preserve their relationship with these men. Wives and partners find themselves in states of shock, betrayal, and with a whirlwind of intense emotions when they discover the secret life of husbands and boyfriends. There is often an absence of support available to these partners. Even when partners seek out support, they are sometimes confronted with judgments, misinformation, and advice they don't want to hear such as "he will never change and the only rational thing to do is to divorce him immediately." This may be true for men who refuse to acknowledge they have a problem and who continue to engage in sexual compulsivity. Unfortunately, wives and partners are sometimes told directly (or it is indirectly implied) that their problems are due to "not doing enough to make their man happy in the bedroom." In these domestic situations, one person is never responsible for the choices of another.

Many men who compulsively view pornography do actually change for the better when they receive the right support. For any mental health provider to play fortune teller and tell distraught partners that there is no hope of change is a professional disservice. At the same time, wives and partners who want to realize relationship repair should expect their husband/boyfriend to create accountability and transparency as part of their recovery. Accountability and transparency are requirements for men who want to do all they can to preserve a marriage. Every partner of a man who is sexually acting out secretly (by any variation) needs to be able to receive several disclosures which can help facilitate a decision (at least temporarily) to stay and heal the relationship. These disclosures include, but are not limited to, three key points: (a) an explanation of why and how their sexual compulsivity developed, (b) the explanation be delivered in a way that is acceptable to the partner (no blaming the partner), and (c) inherent in the explanation are the reasons why the partner would possibly believe they will not re-experience pain and anguish repeatedly if they decide to stay in the relationship.

Sometimes the typical counseling services available in the community are sufficient to resolve matters using some of the guidelines mention above. However, many times there is a "regression to the mean" and a return to the compulsive behaviors within just months of the cessation of counseling. An intensive multimodal treatment approach is often needed, especially when the pornography use has proven to be a repeated cycle of the man being caught, submitting to counseling, and then going back to compulsive viewing. In these cases, an intensive outpatient treatment approach for compulsive use of pornography is recommended (Peterson et al., 2020) and to contain at least five of the following seven components:

1. A sexual health and mental health evaluation that involves input from the partner, review of the history of pornography use (including types used and motivations for use), psychological testing, and separately solicited desired outcomes. Employing objective measures for the assessment of an individual's sexual interest patterns is helpful in ruling out any pedophilic interest (Abel et al., 2007).
2. Individual counseling for the man with compulsive use of pornography that emphasizes the explanation to the partner (mentioned above) and effective planning/execution of relapse prevention.
3. Participation in a professionally led men's sexual health group that promotes transparency and accountability; a positive model of male sexuality; and prosocial skills to live a mission-guided, healthier life.
4. Marital and/or relationship counseling with an emphasis on communication training, making amends, re-establishing trust, and healing the relationship.
5. Consideration and utilization of pharmacological treatment options, including psychotropic medications to decrease anxiety and depressive symptoms as well as voluntarily lowering libido and initiation of sexual activity.
6. Individual or group counseling for the partners of the men with sexually compulsive behaviors in order to support their healing and decision-making.
7. Optional yet recommended participation in a community-based support group such as Sex Addicts Anonymous (SAA), Sex and Love Addicts Anonymous (SLAA), Celebrate Recovery (CR), or a similar support group that a man can attend on any given day he chooses.

NOVELTY-SEEKING SYNDROME

Legal Pornography Use Can Facilitate Use of Illegal Pornography

Of key interest to sex offender researchers is the question of how pornography viewing becomes compulsive in nature and how use of legal pornography can progress to riskier behaviors such as viewing more deviant and illegal child pornography. Research done by Park et al. (2016) reported that habitual consumption of pornography can lead to increased tolerance and the need for more extreme material. In the study, Park and his associates reviewed basic reinforcement of behavior (through the brain-based reward systems) which encourage organisms to remember and repeat critical behaviors, such as sex, eating, and socializing. The study asserts that chronic internet pornography use may become a self-reinforcing activity and an individual's reward system can become vulnerable to pathological learning. The study's authors propose that this self-rewarding system can be particularly impactful for adolescents, creating two significant potential consequences: A greater risk of what appears to be an addiction-like or compulsive nature to the viewing of pornography, and greater potential future use of deviant pornography such as bestiality and child pornography.

In the same study, Park and associates compared subjects with "pornography addictions" to those who have drug addiction and found they have similar brain reactions. An example of this would be the amygdala's reaction when a predicting picture is shown just before the pornography image. Similar reactions have been seen to occur when drug users are exposed to cues connected to their drug of choice (such as pictures of drug paraphernalia). The researchers also observed decreased ventral striatal-PFC coupling in both pornography and drug users, which is related to impulse control. Beside the neurobiology of having the feel-good chemical experience in the brain (essentially the pleasure principle of "if it feels good do it"), the strong effects of operate conditioning cannot be underestimated as a reinforcement of sex-seeking behavior (Hoffmann, 2007). This phenomenon is often seen by clinical professionals who work with online pornography sex offenders who have been convicted of possession of child pornography. A common clinical observation drawn from hundreds of assessments of histories of pornography users is something referred to as the "novelty-seeking syndrome."

Novelty-seeking syndrome (Peterson et al., 2020) is a process by which a user of pornography starts watching erotic content of interest (legal pornography) for a period of time until desensitization and normalization occurs, at which point the content seems not as exciting as it used to be for the individual. There is then a greater risk of searching for different content that might be considered more exotic or erotic (as well as extreme) that may potentially bring more intense levels of sexual arousal (novelty-seeking). Some researchers have taken notice that many online sex offenders describe progressing from legal to illegal child pornography as an "escalating process" that can be explained by the visceral effects of sexual arousal. Winder et al. (2015) assert that when an individual becomes sexually aroused by viewing legal pornography, he is more likely (less able to control his sexual urge) to click on risky "pop-ups," search for more deviant stimuli (such as content with younger aged people or more violence), and ignore potential consequences of his behavior (getting caught or the harming of a child). The concept of novelty-seeking syndrome is also supported by empirical studies using nonoffending samples. For example, after subjects were stimulated by viewing legal pornography, they tended to show a greater willingness to engage in sexual activity with an underage female (Ariely & Loewenstein, 2006) and engage in sexually coercive behavior (Boufard & Miller, 2014).

USE OF ILLEGAL PORNOGRAPHY AND COMMITTING SEX OFFENSES

While viewing internet pornography is relatively common and the viewers of child pornography are believed to be a smaller subset of overall pornography use, the prevalence of viewing child pornography may be higher than is commonly believed. While this paper does not directly address the topic of treatment of contact sex offenders, an interesting study from Germany sheds light on the prevalence of child pornography use. Dombert and colleagues (2016) examined self-reported accounts of sexual interest in prepubescent children among men living in Germany (n = 8,718). Approximately 5% (5.5% or 479) of the men surveyed reported at least one form of pedophilic interest. These included both contact offenses and noncontact offenses, with 1.7% of respondents indicating the use of child pornography exclusively and 0.7% reporting child pornography use as well as contact sexual offenses against children. These findings are of special interest in that they come from a self-reported sample and are close to the estimated prevalence of pedophilic disorder in the *DSM-5* – an estimated 3% to 5% of the general male population based mostly on criminal sex-offender statistics (American Psychiatric Association, 2013).

Acquiring the ability to repress sexual arousal is important in men who are at risk of committing contact sex offenses. However, research has shown that many sexual offenders are unable to suppress their sexual arousal (Babchishin et al., 2017). Additionally, the role of sexual arousal plays a part in decision-making relative to engaging in a sex offending act. Ariely and Loewenstein (2006) found that activities which were not arousing (when the men were not sexually aroused) became sexually charged and appealing when the men were sexually aroused. Hence, the state of sexual arousal which is already in place is likely an important factor in a man being more susceptible to find a sexual stimulus arousing that he would normally not be aroused by (such as pornography of a contact sex offense).

It is essential to note that there are important differences in the characteristics of child pornography offenders and child sexual contact offenders. Contact offenders are more likely to have antisocial tendencies whereas internet-only offenders have lower antisocial tendencies (Babchishin et al., 2018). The risk of recidivism is an important factor to consider when looking at child sexual offenders. Contact offenders who also viewed child pornography are more likely to reoffend (Seto & Eke, 2005). The recidivism rates for contact offense in mixed offenders is 6% as opposed to the 2% recidivism rates for noncontact offense by internet-only offenders (Babchishin et al., 2014).

A pertinent issue when discussing sexual offenses against children is that of acquired pedophilia. Gilbert and Focquaert (2015) describe acquired pedophilia as the onset of pedophilic behaviors post-brain disturbance or injury. Their research revealed a case study involving a man who began sexually abusing children after experiencing brain trauma from a motorcycle accident, although he had typical adult-oriented sexual interests prior. They cited various other cases of nervous system impairment and the onset of paraphilic sexual urges, including interest in pornographic images of children. How then, might traumatic brain injuries in combat veterans (which is fairly common, especially concussion injuries) possibly affect an injured veteran's likelihood to engage in the use of child pornography? Full discussion of this topic is beyond the scope of this chapter and future research is needed on the relationship between combat veteran's TBI with concussion injuries and pornography use.

VETERAN USE OF PORNOGRAPHY AS A MEANS OF COPING WITH STRESS

Background for Case Study II

The relationship between warfare and sex is as old as war itself and historically manifests in many ways, including use of local prostitution by foreign soldiers, armies having their own "comfort women" (sexual slavery), and use of rape as a weapon to terrorize civilian populations (Hirschfeld, 1937). With the advent of print, soldiers could carry their own favorite forms of erotic drawings, "girly magazines," and sexually oriented stories which became usual and customary possessions for soldiers far from home. Starting in the 20th century (1902), military organizations began addressing the risks of using "sex" as a means of dealing with the stress of being a soldier or sailor. "Blue book" guides started to include information regarding the risks of "venereal diseases" (known today as sexually transmitted infections) and warning that "VD" can "knock out fighting men as efficiently as enemy bullets" (*The Bluejackets' Manual*; United States Navy, 1944).

There has been much written on the topic of soldiers using coping behaviors to deal with the stress of war (such as alcohol and drug use), but little written on the topic of veterans' maladaptive use of pornography (and other compulsive sexual behaviors) as a means to avoid the traumatic memories of combat (Howard, 2007). However, an interesting case study by Michael Howard explored a veteran's use of sexually compulsive behavior as a means of distraction for traumatic combat memories. He found that treating the compulsive sexual behavior alone would not be a satisfactory form of treatment. Instead, in situations where there is trauma that drives the compulsive sexual behavior, it is most important to treat the trauma first (Howard, 2007). Howard asserts that if the trauma is left untreated, the offender is likely to substitute one compulsive behavior for another.

Another case study regarding combat veterans and sex offenses against children was examined by Burgess and colleagues (2008). A Vietnam veteran was found not guilty of possession of child pornography based on reason of insanity. His defense claimed that the genital mutilation in children he was exposed to during his combat tour contributed to the development of his compulsive use of child pornography. He was, however, found guilty of engaging in sexual conduct with a minor. Future research could be useful in examining any potential relationships between physical injury in combat or moral injury during war with any increased vulnerability of pornography and/or sex offending. The second case study (about an Army medic) in this chapter attributes both exposure to combat and exposure to child pornography in the combat zone as contributing factors in his subsequent use of child pornography after separation from the military.

Discussion of Moral Injury, Suicide Risk, And Online Pornography Among Veterans

When considering the use of pornography as a possible maladaptive coping behavior among veterans, the discussion must include the topic of moral injury as well as combat trauma. Moral injury is defined as the negative affect and characterization of the symptoms resulting from the perpetration of, the witnessing of, or the failure to prevent the behaviors that violate one's beliefs of right and wrong (Litz et al., 2009). Despite this term being generalizable to all people, there has been previous research on the prevalence of moral injury symptoms being found in combat veterans. The symptoms of moral injury include, but are not limited to, difficulty connecting with others, reduced impulse control, and loss of religiosity/faith (Howard, 2007; Vargas et al., 2013). These factors can contribute to a three-fold increased risk for suicide among veterans.

Veterans have been found to account for 20% of all suicides in the United States (Cesur, 2013; Stern, 2014) while veterans are only 7.6% of the U.S. population (National Conference of State Legislatures, 2019). These findings lead to research into negative effects of military service that may not be characterized by PTSD but nonetheless contribute to maladaptive coping methods and socially deviant behaviors like drug use, compulsive sexual behaviors (including use of pornography), and isolation (Howard, 2007; Stern, 2014). Despite the fact that treatment is available to returning veterans, current approaches in therapy continue to fall short (Litz et al., 2009). Current mental health resources (e.g., those provided by the Department of Defense and the Department of Veterans Affairs) are clearly insufficient in terms of accessibility, frequency, intensity, and the "right fit" (matching to veteran's need) as evidenced by the high rate of suicides among veterans.

A study led by Kraus et al. (2017) found that of the over 800 post-deployment respondents, more than 13% of males reported some degree of sexual compulsivity. Despite the fact that there was no differentiation between internet-based sexual compulsivity and in-person sexual compulsivity, the study identified the prevalence of sexual compulsivity in post-deployment veterans and exemplifies the need for further research into their post-deployment sexual behaviors. A study of the prevalence of compulsive sexual behaviors led by Smith et al. (2014) found that 16.7% of a veteran sample (n = 258, all with deployments) reported engaging in compulsive sexual behaviors.

Feeling unable to connect with others can often lead to a keen sense of social isolation. According to Young (2008), isolation has been found to be positively correlated with sexual compulsivity centered on internet use. This differentiation was found by identifying a lack of reported sexually compulsive behaviors prior to the development and what could be referred to as post-deployment compulsive sexual behavior. Young (2008) goes on to suggest that online sexual behavior, both deviant and otherwise, is done in response to moments of high stress or tension. This directly applies to the case study at hand as individuals returning from combat, having undergone moral injury and/or displaying symptoms of PTSD, expressing feelings of continued distress regarding experiences while deployed (Howard, 2007; Stern, 2014). Further, in a study of over 250 men, it was found that of those who reported that they engage in compulsive sexual behavior, 97.7% also met the diagnostic criteria for PTSD (Smith et al., 2014).

Reduced impulse control (resulting in compulsivity) in regard to sexual behavior has been found to be a significant predictor of online sexual offending (Gillespie et al., 2016), thereby providing support to the theory that reduced impulse control may be a predictor of online sexual offending. In addition, there has been evidence of an increase in the rate of sharing of pedophilic pornographic files which leads to the risk of being exposed to previously unwanted material when entering sexually oriented websites (Wild et al., 2019).

". . . As long as it was only online, it was okay" (Young, 2008). This excerpt is from a series of 22 case studies. This attitude, combined with findings from Schorr et al. (2018), clearly identify how deployments can alter individuals' moral alignment and can lead to the initiation of deviant online sexual behavior. Further support is found in the identification of distorted attitudes being a significant predictor of online sexual offending (Gillespie et al., 2016). Moral injury symptoms include alterations to moral alignment and loss of faith (Howard, 2007; Vargas et al., 2013). As the following case study exemplifies, some veterans describe moral injury as "losing one's moral compass" and as a contributing factor to using pornography, especially child-oriented, sexually exploitive materials.

CASE STUDY II: MALE VETERAN USING ILLEGAL PORNOGRAPHY*

Max is a man in his 40s who grew up in a middle-class intact family. He was one of four siblings and described his childhood as somewhat emotionally turbulent. However, he denied any type of emotional, physical, or sexual abuse during his development. He felt cared for and loved by his parents yet was in trouble on a regular basis with the usual conflicts with his father during adolescence. But before his teenage years, Max admitted that he would get in trouble for his aggression and picking on his siblings and peers. While he was picked on by bullies, Max stated that he was also a bully at times, once picking on his brother to the point of dislocating his brother's shoulder.

Max was a bright child intellectually. But as he got older, he skipped school and had more "blow-ups" with his father who was in a leadership position in the school system that Max attended. At 14 years of age, he started smoking cigarettes, then marijuana, and drinking alcohol whenever he had the chance. Max reported that he estimated being grounded about 60% of his high school years.

Max started masturbating about age 12 on a regular basis and said he never got in trouble during his youth because of his sexual behavior. He reported that he felt a sense of shame regarding sex due to his Catholic upbringing. He started dating at age 16 and lost his virginity the next year with his first long-term girlfriend. He broke up with this girlfriend when he went off to college. Since then, he has had only short-term relationships that occasionally are sexual.

His use of pornography started in junior high school and continued unabated through his adolescence. His viewing of pornography focused exclusively upon adults portrayed in consensual sexual

*This case study is based upon true events. Names have been changed and some details omitted to protect the privacy and identity of those who gave permission for this story to be shared for teaching purposes. Details of this story may be distressing and/or triggering to some readers.

activities. While he was in his 20s, he joined the U.S. Army and became a medic. He served in combat on two separate deployments in Iraq, each 12 months long. It was during this time that Max reported seeing child pornography for the first time. Per his account, pornography (including child pornography) was commonly used by military personnel in the combat zone when soldiers are at base camp or aid stations. Max stated he started viewing pornography as a way to unwind and reduce tension during his first deployment, much the same way he did when he was a teenager.

He started viewing sexual images of children later in his first tour, after developing a sense of depersonalization and symptoms of combat-related PTSD. After constant levels of high arousal from firefights and witnessing many deaths (American, combatant, and civilian), Max became "apathetic to life." During combat, he would sometimes step out of his armored vehicle to return fire without even wearing his helmet. He was becoming increasingly desensitized to seeing death around him and objectifying Iraqi people as enemies (and potential targets). He reported that many of the combatants killed were 13- to 14-year-old boys, including a 12-year-old boy that "tried to blow us up." His viewing of pornography escalated during his second tour.

The entire combat experience changed Max's sense of reality. He was in a world where he would routinely see dead bodies, including dead children. His experience was that every day could be his last, as it was for many others whose deaths he witnessed. The usual rules of right and wrong were suspended. As he continued to survive his combat experience, his sense of depersonalization increased. As he felt he was becoming less and less the human being that he once was, the objectification of others intensified towards Iraqi adults and children.

Max remembers being particularly affected by an encounter in which he was atop of his Humvee in the gunner's seat and firing upon what appeared to be a suicide bomber in a car coming toward his unit. After firing at the vehicle, it was discovered that the occupants were dead, including a 9-year-old girl and her parents. An intense sense of guilt and dread broke through his emotional numbing whenever he had reoccurring thoughts that he was responsible for the young girl's death.

During later periods of his deployments, Max stated that he started sleeping very randomly and he would experience "daydreams" in which he would have very intrusive thoughts and images of violent events. He thought he might be on the brink of hallucinating at times. He stated that there were times when viewing child pornography that his thoughts would return to the 9-year-old-girl and many other incidents where children were killed. His use of pornography was cyclical. At times of highest stress is when he would seek out child pornography. Max stated, "I loathed myself; I'd be disgusted and physically ill. I wouldn't eat or sleep and remain awake ruminating of the injuries and deaths of children during my deployments."

Max related that after his discharge from the Army and about 6 weeks after his return to the United States, he resumed his viewing of child pornography during cycles of self-disgust when he would seek it out. These cycles usually ran every 3 to 4 months. He tried to reconstruct his life as a civilian by getting accepted to medical school and then practice as a physician. However, his medical studies were impaired by his continued sense of depersonalization and dissociative episodes. He would describe times when he was in a lecture hall during a class, having intrusive thoughts of combat events, and then "coming back to the present and noticing time had elapsed."

His plans to complete medical school were aborted when the FBI identified his personal computer as one involved in viewing and receiving child pornography. He was arrested when his home was raided by a SWAT team and he was taken into custody. Rather than resisting his arrest or even being upset by the raid, Max felt relieved. He stated "I didn't realize that I really wanted to be caught. I was so ill, exhausted mentally and physically from hating myself, that being arrested seemed like a great weight had been lifted from me."

It appeared that Max saw himself as a "monster out of control" and his cyclic use of child pornography was evidence of his depravity and moral bankruptcy. Being arrested was a "natural course of action" of society to put him in check and rightly punish him for his transgressions. His Catholic upbringing and religious convictions were not nearly enough for him to commit to not killing himself. While Max seriously considered ways he could end his life, he could not accept the amount of harm his death would cause his parents, particularly his mother. Max's perceived need for punishment was so strong that it compromised his ability to assist his attorney to defend him in court.

With his parent's and attorney's encouragement, Max decided to enter therapy to try to find an alternative path to health. If he was not going to submit to suicide, he also did not want to have his parents watch a "slow-motion self-destruction." Only after months of subsequent sex-specific therapy would Max consider doing anything that might assist his attorney to seek anything less than maximum sentencing. Max was diagnosed with major depression and combat-related PTSD.

Max was assessed to be at low risk for reoffending (by using child pornography) because he loathed his use of it and saw any potential relapse as giving up on life and dealing a crushing blow to his parents, who he feared could not sustain the stress. Max was also considered not to be a risk for making a contact sexual offense with a minor. Men convicted of using child sexual exploitation materials for the first time and have no other criminal record (of any kind) are estimated to have a low risk of making a contact sex offense. Babchishin et al. (2018) report a recidivism rate for this group as 0% to 2% for committing a contact sex offense. A leading researcher of sex offense recidivism, Michael Seto, testified before the U.S. Sentencing Commission in 2012; he quoted a similar low risk of recidivism (of men convicted of using child pornography and no other crimes), which was 2.1% for going on to commit a contact sex offense.

Max had voluntarily completed 2 of the 3 years of a sex offender treatment program before his case even came to trial within a federal district court. The specific details of his sex offender treatment are beyond the scope of this chapter but, suffice it to say, treatment centered around weekly group therapy meetings. Fortunate for Max, his case was assigned to a judge who took interest in veterans and the traumatic experiences they sometimes endure while serving their country. The judge took careful review of arguments from both the prosecutor and defense as well as calling for expert testimony (without involvement of either prosecutor or defense). He saw cause for the uncommon use of variance in his sentencing of Max and subsequently sentenced him to no time in federal prison but rather stipulations of probation which included finishing the sex offender treatment program which he had already started. He was ordered to pay restitution to the survivors of child sexual exploitation who were filmed (as children) in the child pornography videos which Max had viewed (totaling nearly $50,000). Several other standard stipulations were made as part of his probation period, which was ordered to last 5 years.

BEST PRACTICE CONSIDERATIONS IN TREATING MEN WITH COMPULSIVE USE OF CHILD PORNOGRAPHY

Multiple obstacles are faced when trying to find best treatment models for child pornography and maladaptive pornography users. As a cautionary note, the following recommendations are drawn from conflicting research conclusions and problems with the way research sometimes categorize child pornography users in the same group as contact sex offenders. Also, the research on the treatment of all pornography users is considered constrained due to the stigma associated with (a) sexuality in general, (b) paraphilia even more, and (c) pedophilia being the most stigmatized - including those who use child pornography (Seto & Ahmed, 2014). Relevant research on the treatment of men who use child pornography has much overlap with the previous recommendations of maladaptive legal pornography users. However, the recommendations are more in-depth (specific in terms of type and intensity), involve community supervision, and require a greater need for integrated services within a comprehensive program. As a review, they include:

1. A sexual health and mental health evaluation that involves in-depth review of the types of pornography used and motivations for its use, psychological testing, and objective measures of sexual interest patterns. Employing objective measures for the assessment of an individual's sexual interest patterns is helpful in differentiating men who are pornography users with pedophilic interest from those users of child pornography who do not have pedophilic motivations (Abel et al., 2007; Seto & Ahmed, 2014).
2. Individual counseling for the man with compulsive use of pornography that emphasizes effective planning/execution of a health maintenance and relapse prevention plan, treatment of psychiatric comorbidities, and an introduction of positive models of male sexuality (Babchishin et al., 2014). Smith et al. (2014) found evidence showing there is a significant correlation between PTSD, childhood trauma, and compulsive sexual behavior. This suggests that the treatment of the sex offender's own trauma could result in improvement of the maladaptive coping mechanisms or, at the very least, the effects of the trauma should be considered during further research of treatment practices. Some of the specific topics addressed during individual treatment are the same as those addressed during group treatment, as delineated below.
3. Participation in a professionally led men's sexual health group that promotes transparency and accountability, a positive model of male sexuality, and prosocial skills to live a mission-guided, healthier life, which is similar to the Good Lives Model of sex offender treatment (Ward & Gannon, 2006) as well as the Internet Sex Offender Treatment Program (I-SOTP) of the United Kingdom (Middleton, Mandeville-Norden, & Hayes; 2009). The latter has been described as having six critical components of treatment (both individual and group) which include (a) motivation to change, (b) functional analysis of online offending behavior, (c) attitudes and beliefs, (d) interpersonal deficits, (e) self-regulation skills, and (f) relapse prevention skills and setting new life goals.
4. Consideration and utilization of pharmacological treatment options, including psychotropic medications to decrease anxiety and depressive symptoms as well as voluntarily lowering libido and initiation of sexual activity. These treatment options have been found to be helpful for serious sex offenders and go beyond typical use of SSRI medications to the use of antiandrogens (Thibaut et al., 2010).
5. When appropriate (in instances of the online sex offender having significant others), marital and/or relationship counseling with an emphasis on communication training, making amends, re-establishing trust, and healing the relationship. This component of treatment is not a primary focus for sex offenders; however, relationship stability may contribute to a lower risk of recidivism during the post-release years of opportunity for pedophilic sex offenders to re-offend (Prentky, Knight, & Lee, 1997).

OTHER TREATMENT CONSIDERATIONS

Beier et al. (2014) used a multimodal treatment plan called Prevention Project Dunkelfeld that included aspects of cognitive-behavioral therapy, pharmacology, psychology, sexology, relapse prevention, self-regulation, aspects of the Good Lives Model, self-monitoring, coping strategies, and developing empathy for their victims. A preliminary *t*-test analysis was used in this study to see if the treatment group improved in areas such as loneliness, sexual self-regulation, emotional coping, and empathy. After 1 year of the treatment, a significant improvement was found in all the areas stated above. However, a follow-up study was conducted by Mokros and Banse (2018) that found the opposite to be true when using a different sample. Their research revealed little to no improvement in the subjects which leads to a contradiction in the research of the effectiveness within the Dunkelfeld program. There were several limitations to both of these studies, including small statistical power.

Wild et al. (2019) conducted a review of existing *web-based treatment approaches* used in other mental health environments and conclude with a recommended treatment option for sexual offenders. They emphasize that the risk, need, and responsivity principles that are typically applied within CBT for online and contact offenders could be applied to the online-only treatment. The article goes further into detail about the advantages and disadvantages of online use as well as how one should go about setting up an online therapeutic setting. It should be made clear that there is a lack of solid evidence that supports any treatment option working effectively against relapse of the contact and online offenders.

Seto and Ahmed (2014) argue for the need to have an individualized treatment option for online offenders and push for continuing the treatment perspective for symptom management instead of a cure for pedophilia. They differentiate four different types of online offenders:

1. Offenders who are sexually attracted to children
2. A hypersexual compulsive type that should have treatment focused on sexual regulation
3. The risk-taker type
4. Those that view the pornography out of curiosity or other nonpedophilic reasons

Therefore, the specific best practice treatment interventions used must be matched to the specific type of offender to enhance treatment outcomes.

Internet-only offenders were found to have difficulties in mood regulation as well as difficulties with interpersonal functioning (Magaletta et al., 2012). These findings suggest that the differences in the characteristics of the offenders play an important role in the treatment of the offenders. It is likely problematic for treatment programs to provide the same treatment intervention to both internet-only sex offenders and those who have committed contact sex offenses.

Traits that differentiate online offenders from contact offenders could be a key component to developing effective treatment. Often, two types of problems arise in the research. First, all online sex offenders viewing child pornography are assumed to meet the diagnostic criteria for pedophilic disorder. Second, the two types of offenders (online and contact types) are treated as one and the same during therapeutic recovery. Henshaw et al. (2017) explored the literature that shows child pornography offenders are younger, Caucasian, educated, poorly socially adjusted, less likely to have a history of sexual or physical abuse, and a lower likelihood of substance abuse. They also saw that, when compared to contact offenders, child pornography offenders were unlikely to have prior offenses, had more empathy towards their victims, had less distorted thinking towards their offending, had higher levels of loneliness, and demonstrated higher levels of preoccupations with fantasies.

It is suggested that mental health professionals address the online offender's high level of sexual preoccupation, deviant sexual interest, and interpersonal deficits during treatment. One such program in the United Kingdom, the Internet Sexual Offender Treatment Program, focuses on online-only offenders. The aims of the program consist of motivations for changing behavior, analyzing the offending behavior, victim awareness, emotional self-regulation, addressing compulsive internet use and sexual deviancy, and relapse prevention (Henshaw et al., 2017).

Webb et al. (2007) further emphasize the difference between online and contact offenders by showing evidence pulled from offenders' files in three different London rehabilitation centers. The evidence revealed that contact offenders have higher levels of psychopathic traits, more distorted views on sexual assault, and a negative association with supervision.

For the most severe offenders, a luteinizing hormone-releasing hormone agonist could be used as an effective treatment to decrease sexual urges and behaviors (Turner & Briken, 2018). However, this would not be a recommended treatment for all offenders. Cognitive behavioral therapy is the most common practice for treating child sexual offenders. There are limitations when it comes to implementing therapeutic treatments. Many therapists refuse to treat child sexual offenders due to lack of training and because they may currently be treating victims of sexual assault (Wild et al, 2019).

SUMMARY

The development of effective treatments for men's use of pornography is an evolving field contributing to our understanding of not only how to best help men not engage in these behaviors which can hurt and exploit others, but also how best to protect society by lowering rates of recidivism for users of child pornography. Of course, treatment of sex offenders using child pornography is a high research priority; therefore, evidence-based recommendations are more easily found for treatment of sex offenders involved in child pornography than patients who are involved with legal pornography. However, there are three main points this chapter offers for consideration by general mental health professionals.

First, this chapter addressed users of legal pornography as another chapter more directly focuses on assessment and treatment of contact sex offenders or those who attempt to importune (see Chapter 26). Most readers of this text are more concerned with what to do with their clients involved with legal pornography and the relationship conflicts that can result. It is important to include users of child pornography in this chapter to address the relationship between legal and illegal pornography, especially aspects of the *novelty-seeking syndrome*. Of course, all users of legal pornography are not affected the same way and it is not suggested that any person using legal pornography for a long time is inevitably going to start using child-oriented pornography. However, it is clear that most users of child pornography report that they started with legal pornography and also state that they eventually have sought increasingly more taboo sexual imagery leading to child pornography.

Second, there is sufficient evidence for the assertion that men use pornography as a maladaptive coping behavior whether they are using legal or illegal pornography. It is now understood that motivations for pornography use (even child pornography) vary among users and effective treatment for these men is both individualized specific to their motivations. Included in this assertion is that men use child pornography for different reasons. While use of child pornography is wrong and all sexual exploitation of children should be prevented and/or prosecuted, research supports the view that the vast majority of these users of child pornography sites do not go on to commit contact sex offenses.

Third, the inclusion of the topic of child pornography in this chapter is informative in terms of drawing inferences as to how to treat men who use legal pornography, even though there is far less research on treatment of men seeking treatment secondary to their use of legal pornography. Many treatment recommendations have been presented in this chapter to hopefully provide clinicians with greater comfort, confidence, and understanding to assist men (and couples) who are seeking counseling to resolve their personal and relational issues regarding pornography use.

As a final guide for clinicians, a tool is offered as a means of assisting men to focus on many of the key aspects of living a healthy life and preventing the continued cycles of pornography use. The *Personalized Health Maintenance and Relapse Prevention Plan* addresses some of the "best practices" discussed in this chapter. The utility of this tool can be helping men recognize how maladaptive their behavior is, understanding their underlying needs relayed to pornography use, and assisting them to make more healthy (adaptive) behavioral choices. It is recommended as a starting point for men seeking professional help to improve their lives. The next page explains the tool, but for the full tool, see pages 597-600.

Personalized Health Maintenance and Relapse Prevention Plan*

Having a specific written plan to be healthy is more effective if it is organized (on paper) and shared with others for accountability rather than just having some ideas rolling around in your head (even good ideas) regarding how to have a healthier life. This plan can be especially helpful to avoid and deal with triggers that lead you to act in a self-defeating (even self-destructive) manner. It can be used to avoid and/or prevent a relapse of many types of self-harm behavior, including the use of alcohol and drugs, sexual acting out, or suicidal thoughts and behaviors. This plan also goes beyond relapse protection by assisting individuals to walk a path of intention and healthy daily living. It is recommended that drafting a personalized health maintenance and relapse prevention plan contain the following ten components:

1. Create a *Personal Mission Statement* clarifying your sense of purpose in life.

2. Identify what your "bottom lines" are that you do not want to cross/be part of your healthy life.

3. Identify triggers for acting out (both emotional and situational triggers).

4. Inventory your healthy coping behaviors – both "Tried and True" as well as "Expanding the Toolbox" behaviors.

5. Based on your personal map of social relationships, create a *Personal Mission Support Team.*

6. Create a "Prediction Relapse Scenario" identifying "warning" thoughts, feelings, and behaviors.

7. Develop a *Personal Model of Positive Sexuality.*

8. Create a time management schedule for structuring preferred recovery and health maintenance practices.

9. Create a reinforcement schedule by which you reward yourself in healthy and positive ways for effective execution of your plan and practices.

10. Rate your level of satisfaction with the *Big Wheel of Health and Well-Being* scale at the beginning of your efforts (as a baseline measure) and after 1, 3, and 6 months of healthy practices. For those seeking to enhance their sexual health as well, you can rate your levels of satisfaction in the same way using the *Sexual Health and Well-being Satisfaction* scale.**

---

* By Dr. Frederick L. Peterson, Clinical Psychologist at the 88th Medical Operations Readiness Squadron, Wright-Patterson Air Force Base. For the full tool, go to pages 597-600.

** Both of these questionnaires can be found in Section VI of this text as well as in the introductory chapters of *The Gender Revolution & New Sexual Health* by Peterson, Bley, and Frabotta (2020).

REFERENCES

Abel, G., Wiegel, M. & Osborn, C. (2007). Pedophilia and other paraphilias. In L. VandeCreek, F. Peterson, & J. Bley (Eds.), *Innovations in clinical practice: Focus on sexual health* (pp. 157-175). Professional Resource Press.

American Psychiatric Association (2013). *Diagnostic and statistical manual of mental disorders* (5th ed.). https://doi.org/10.1176/appi.books.9780890425596.

Ariely, D., & Loewenstein, G. (2006). The heat of the moment: The effect of sexual arousal on sexual decision making. *Journal of Behavioral Decision Making, 19*(2), 87-98. https://doi.org/10.1002/bdm.501

Babchishin, K., Curry, S., Fedoroff, J., Bradford, J., & Seto, M. (2017). Inhibiting sexual arousal to children: Correlates and its influence on the validity of penile plethysmography. *Archives of Sexual Behavior, 46*(3), 671-684. https://doi.org/10.1007/s10508-017-0952-2

Babchishin, K., Hanson, R., & Vanzuylen, H. (2014). Online child pornography offenders are different: A meta-analysis of the characteristics of online and offline sex offenders against children. *Archives of Sexual Behavior, 44*(1), 45-66. https://doi.org/10.1007/s10508-014-0270-x

Babchishin, K., Meridian, H., Bartels, R. & Perkins, D. (2018). Child sexual exploitation materials offenders. *European Psychologist, 23*(2),130-143. https://doi.org/10.1027/101 6-9040/a000326

Beier, K., Grundmann, D., Kuhle, L., Scherner, G., Konrad, A., & Amelung, T. (2015). The German Dunkelfeld Project: A pilot study to prevent child sexual abuse and the use of child abusive images. *The Journal of Sexual Medicine, 12*(2), 529-542. https://doi.org/10.1111/jsm.12785

Bradford, J., Kingston, D., Ahmed, A., & Fedoroff, J. (2010). Commentary: Sildenafil in phallometric testing - An evidence-based assessment of sexual offenders. *Journal of the American Academy of Psychiatry and the Law, 38*(4), 512-515.

Burgess, A., Mahoney, M., Visk, J., & Morgenbesser, L. (2008). Cyber child sexual exploitation. *Journal of Psychosocial Nursing & Mental Health Services, 46*(9), 38-45. https://doi.org/10.3928/02793695-20080901

Cesur, R., Sabia, J., & Tekin, E. (2013). The psychological costs of war: Military combat and mental health. *Journal of Health Economics, 32*(1), 51-65. https://doi.org/10.3386/w16927

Cooper, A. (2002). *Sex and the internet: A guidebook for clinicians.* Brunner-Routledge.

Dombert, B., Schmidt, A., Banse, R., Briken, P., Hoyer, J., Neutze, J., & Osterheider, M. (2016). How common is men's self-reported sexual interest in prepubescent children? *Journal of Sex Research, 53*(2), 214-223. https://doi.org/10.1080/00224499.2015.1020108

Falligant, J., Alexander, A., & Burkhart, B. (2017). Risk assessment of juveniles adjudicated for possession of child sexual exploitation material. *Journal of Forensic Psychology Practice, 17*(2), 145-156. https://doi.org/10.1080/15228932.2017.1270640

Fedoroff, J. (2018). Can people with pedophilia change? Yes they can! *Current Sexual Health Reports, 10*(4), 207. https://doi.org/10.1007/s11930-018-0166-1

Frankfurt, S., Debeer, B., Morissette, S., Kimbrel, N., Bash, H., & Meyer, E. (2018). Mechanisms of moral injury following military sexual trauma and combat in post-9/11 U.S. war veterans. *Frontiers in Psychiatry, 9.* https://doi.org/10.3389/fpsyt.2018.00520

Gannon, T., & Polaschek, D. (2005). Do child molesters deliberately fake good on cognitive distortion questionnaires? An information processing-based investigation. *Sexual Abuse: Journal of Research and Treatment, 17*(2), 183-200. https://doi.org/10.1007/s11194-005-4604-z

Gilbert, F., & Focquaert, F. (2015). Rethinking responsibility in offenders with acquired paedophilia: Punishment or treatment? *International Journal of Law & Psychiatry, 38,* 51-60. https://doi.org/10.1016/j.ijlp.2015.01.007

Gillespie, S., Bailey, A., Squire, T., Carey, M., Eldridge, H., & Beech, A. (2016). An evaluation of a community-based psycho-educational program for users of child sexual exploitation material. *Sexual Abuse: A Journal of Research and Treatment, 30*(2), 169-191. https://doi.org/10.1177/107906321663 9591

Grantz, K. (2007). Commentary on the Mental Health Advisory Team IV Operation Iraqi Freedom final report. *Traumatology, 13*(4), 46-49. https://doi.org/10.1177/1534765607309944

Henshaw, M., Ogloff, J., & Clough, J. (2017). Looking beyond the screen: A critical review of the literature on the online child pornography offender. *Sexual Abuse, 29*(5), 416-445. https://doi.org/10.1177/1079063215603690

Hirschfeld, M. (1937). *Sexual history of the world war: From reports collected by the Institute for Sexual Science.* Falstaff.

Hoffmann, H. (2007). The role of classical conditioning in sexual arousal. In E. Janssen (Ed.), *The psychophysiology of sex* (pp. 261-273). Indiana University Press.

Howard, M. (2007). Escaping the pain: Examining the use of sexually compulsive behavior to avoid the traumatic memories of combat. *Sexual Addiction & Compulsivity, 14*(2), 77-94. https://doi.org/0.1080/1072 0160701310443

Jones, E. (2018). Moral injury in time of war. *The Lancet, 391*(10132), 1766-1767. https://doi.org/10.1016/s0140-6736(18)30946-2

Kaplan, M. (2015). Taking pedophilia seriously. *Washington & Lee Law Review, 72*(1), 75-170. https://scholarlycommons.law.wlu.edu/wlulr/vol72/iss1/4/

Kraus, S., Martino, S., Potenza, M., Park, C., Merrel, J., & Hoff, R. (2017). Examining compulsive sexual behavior and psychopathology among a sample of postdeployment U.S. male and female military veterans. *Military Psychology, 29*(2), 143-156. https://doi.org/10.1037/mil0000147

Kraus, S., & Sweeney, P. (2019). Hitting the target: Considerations for differential diagnosis when treating individuals for problematic use of pornography. *Archives of Sexual Behavior, 48*(2), 431-435. https://doi.org/10.1007/s10508-018-1301-9

Lanning, K. (2001).*Child molesters: A behavioral analysis.* https://www.missingkids.org/content/dam/missingkids/pdfs/publications/nc70.pdf

Lewis, R. (2018). Literature review on children and young people demonstrating technology-assisted harmful sexual behavior. *Aggression and Violent Behavior, 40,* 1-11. https://doi.org/10.1016/j.avb.2018.02.011

Litz, B., Stein, N., Delaney, E., Lebowitz, L., Nash, W., Silva, C., & Maguen, S. (2009). Moral injury and moral repair in war veterans: A preliminary model and intervention strategy. *Clinical Psychology Review, 29*(8), 695-706. https://doi.org/10.1016/j.cpr.2009.07.003

Lykins, A., Cantor, J., Kuban, M., Blak, T., Dickey, R., Klassen, P., & Blanchard, R. (2010). The relation between peak response magnitudes and agreement in diagnoses obtained from two different phallometric tests for pedophilia. *Sexual Abuse: A Journal of Research & Treatment, 22*(1), 42-57. https://doi.org/10.1177/1079063209352094

Macleish, K. (2018). On 'moral injury': Psychic fringes and war violence. *History of the Human Sciences, 31*(2), 128-146. https://doi.org/10.1177/0952695117750342

Magaletta, P., Faust, E., Bickart, W., & Mclearen, A. (2012). Exploring clinical and personality characteristics of adult male internet-only child pornography offenders. *International Journal of Offender Therapy and Comparative Criminology. 58(*2), 137-153. https://doi.org/10.1177/0306624x12465271

McCarthy, M. (2017). An exploration of moral injury as experienced by combat Veterans. *Dissertations & Theses, 317.* https://aura.antioch.edu/cgi/viewcontent.cgi?article=1324&context=etds

McConaghy, N. (1997). Science and the mismanagement of rapists and paedophiles. *Psychiatry, Psychology and Law, 4*(2), 109-123. https://doi.org/10.1080/13218719709524905

Middleton, D., Mandeville-Norden, R., & Hayes, E. (2009). Does treatment work with internet sex offenders? Emerging findings from the internet sex offender treatment programme (i-SOTP). *Journal of Sexual Aggression, 15*(1), 5-19. https://doi.org/10.1080/13552600802673444

Mokros, A., & Banse, R. (2019). The "Dunkelfeld" project for self-identified pedophiles: A reappraisal of its effectiveness. *The Journal of Sexual Medicine, 16*(5), 609-613. https://doi.org/10.1016/j.jsxm.2019.02.009

National Conference of State Legislatures. (2019). Suicide prevention: NCSL Task Force on Military and Veterans Affairs. www.ncls.org>research>military-and-veterans-affairs>ncsl-task-force

Ogle, A., Reichwald, R., & Rutland, J. (2018). Psychological impact of remote combat/graphic media exposure among US Air Force intelligence personnel. *Military Psychology, 30*(6), 476-486. https://doi.org/10.1080/08995605.2018.1502999

Park, B., Wilson, G., Berger, J., Christman, M., Reina, B., Bishop, F., & Doan, A. (2016). Is internet pornography causing sexual dysfunctions? A review with clinical reports. *Behavioral Sciences, 6*(3), 17. https://doi.org/10.3390/bs6030017

Peterson, F., Bley, J., & Frabotta, R. (2020*). The gender revolution & new sexual health: Celebrating unlimited diversity of the human sexuality hypercube*. Cognella Academic Publishing.

Prentky, R., Knight, R., & Lee, A. (1997). Child sexual molestation: Research issues. National Institute of Justice Research Report. NCJ Number: 163390.

Price, M., Strachan, M., Ruggiero, K., & Acierno, R. (2012). Combat experiences, pre-deployment training, and outcome of exposure therapy for post-traumatic stress disorder in operation enduring freedom/operation Iraqi freedom veterans. *Clinical Psychology & Psychotherapy, 20*(4), 277-285. https://doi.org/10.1002/cpp.1768

Purcell, N., Griffin, B. J., Burkman, K., & Maguen, S. (2018). "Opening a door to a new life": The role of forgiveness in healing from moral injury. *Frontiers in Psychiatry, 9*, Article 498. https://doi.org/10.3389/fpsyt.2018.00498

Schiffer, B., Amelung, T., Pohl, A., Kaergel, C., Tenbergen, G., Gerwinn, H., . . . Walter, H. (2017). Gray matter anomalies in pedophiles with and without a history of child sexual offending. *Translational psychiatry*, *7*(5), e1129. https://doi.org/10.1038/tp.2017.96

Schorr, Y., Stein, N., Maguen, S., Barnes, J. B., Bosch, J., & Litz, B. (2018). Sources of moral injury among war veterans: A qualitative evaluation. *Journal of Clinical Psychology, 74*(12), 2203-2218. https://doi.org/10.1002/jclp.22660

Seto, M. (2001). The value of phallometry in the assessment of male sex offenders. *Journal of Forensic Psychology Practice, 1*(2), 65. https://doi.org/10.1300/J158v01n02_05

Seto, M. (2012). *Child pornography offender characteristics and the risk to reoffend.* Testimony to the United States Sentencing Commission (February 6, 2012), Washington, DC. https://www.ussc.gov/sites/default/files/pdf/amendment-process/public-hearings-and-meetings/20120215/Testimony_15_Seto.pdf

Seto, M., & Ahmed, A. G. (2014). Treatment and management of child pornography use. *Psychiatric Clinics, 37*(2), 207-214. https://doi.org/10.1016/j.psc.2014.03.004

Seto, M., & Eke, A. (2005). The criminal histories and later offending of child pornography offenders. *Sexual Abuse: A Journal of Research and Treatment, 17*(2), 201-210. https://doi.org/10.1007/s11194-005-4605-y

Smith, P., Potenza, M., Mazure, C., McKee, S., Park, C., & Hoff, R. (2014). Compulsive sexual behavior among male military veterans: Prevalence and associated clinical factors. *Journal of Behavioral Addictions, 3*(4), 214-222. https://doi.org/10.1556/jba.3.2014.4.2

Stern, J. (2014). PTSD: Policy issues. *Psychoanalytic Psychology, 31*(2), 255-261. https://doi.org/10.1037/a0036008

Stone, G. (2017). *Sex and the constitution: Sex, religion, and law from America's origins to the twenty-first century.* Liveright Publishing Corporation.

Studer, L., & Aylwin, A. (2006). Pedophilia: The problem with diagnosis and limitations of CBT in treatment. *Medical Hypotheses, 67*(4), 774-781. https://doi.org/10.1016/j.mehy.2006.04.030

Thibaut, F., De La Barra, F., Gordon, H., Cosyn, P., & Bradford, J. M. (2010). The World Federation of Societies of Biological Psychiatry (WFSBP) guidelines for the biological treatment of paraphilias. *World Journal of Biological Psychiatry, 11*(4), 604-605.

Turner, D., & Briken, P. (2018). Treatment of paraphilic disorders in sexual offenders or men with a risk of sexual offending with luteinizing hormone-releasing hormone agonists: An updated systematic review. *The Journal of Sexual Medicine, 15*(1), 77-93. https://doi.org/10.1016/j.jsxm.2017.11.013

United States Navy. (1944*). The bluejackets' manual* (12th ed.). United States Naval Institute.

Vargas, A., Hanson, T., Kraus, D., Drescher, K., & Foy, D. (2013). Moral injury themes in combat veterans' narrative responses from the National Vietnam Veterans' Readjustment Study. *Traumatology, 19*(3), 243-250. https://doi.org/10.1177/1534765613476099

Ward, T., & Gannon, T. A. (2006). Rehabilitation, etiology, and self-regulation: The comprehensive good lives model of treatment for sexual offenders. *Aggression and Violent Behavior, 11*(1), 77-94. https://doi.org/10.1016/j.avb.2005.06.001

Webb, L., Craissati, J., & Keen, S. (2007). Characteristics of internet child pornography offenders: A comparison with child molesters. *Sexual Abuse: A Journal of Research and Treatment, 19*(4), 449-465. https://doi.org/10.1007/s11194-007-9063-2

Wild, T., Fromberger, P., Jordan, K., Müller, I., & Müller, J. (2019). Web-based health services in forensic psychiatry: A review of the use of the internet in the treatment of child sexual abusers and child sexual exploitation material offenders. *Frontiers in Psychiatry, 9, 763.* https://doi.org/10.3389/fpsyt.2018.00763

Wilson, R., Looman, J., Abracen, J., & Pake, D. Comparing sexual offenders at the Regional Treatment Centre (Ontario) and the Florida Civil Commitment Center. *International Journal of Offender Therapy and Comparative Criminology, 57*(3), 377-395. https://doi.org/10.1177/0306624X11434918

Winder, B., Gough, B., & Seymour-Smith, S. (2015). Stumbling into sexual crime: The passive perpetrator in accounts by male internet sex offenders. *Archives of Sexual Behavior, 44*(1), 167-180. https://doi.org/10.1007/s10508-014-0302-6

Yandell, M. (2018). Moral injury and human relationship: A conversation. *Pastoral Psychology, 68*(1), 3-14. https://doi.org/10.1007/s11089-018-0800-x

Young, K. (2008). Understanding sexually deviant online behavior from an addiction perspective. *International Journal of Cyber Criminology, 2*, 298-307. https://www.proquest.com/docview/89228141

28

Assessment and Treatment of Active-Duty Members With Compulsive Sexual Behaviors

Frederick L. Peterson, Jr., Keith Happawana, Regina D. Shillinglaw, and William Wall

INTRODUCTION

Compulsive sexual behavior (CSB), also known as problematic sexual behavior (PSB), describes a cluster of features that may include sexual fantasies, urges, and related behaviors that are distressful and lead to impairment in daily functioning (Derbyshire & Grant, 2015). These features may present as paraphilic (i.e., fetishism, exhibitionism, pedophilia), nonparaphilic (i.e., sexual behaviors such as compulsive masturbation, use of pornography, or acts with others), or a combination of the two (Kraus et al., 2016). As noted elsewhere in this text, CSB is not formally acknowledged in the *Diagnostic and Statistical Manual of Mental Disorders* (5th ed.; *DSM-5*) due to difficulty with establishing formative criteria (Derbyshire & Grant, 2015), but diagnostic criteria have been proposed in the form of a hypersexual disorder (American Psychiatric Association, 2013).

It is important to note that the most recent draft of *The International Classification of Diseases* (*ICD-11*; World Health Organization, 2019) does depict such a diagnosis. Within this draft, CSB is characterized as a pattern of inability to control sexual impulses and consequent behavior, even if the outcomes are adverse and undesirable (Ley, 2018). Due to current limitations in formal diagnostic recognition of CSB, research pertaining to the detrimental effects of CSB can be difficult to find in literature, particularly within military populations.

CSB occurring within a military context is recognized, yet is primarily cited as comorbid features secondary to mental disorders (e.g., posttraumatic stress disorder, major depressive disorder, anxiety-related disorders) and also as secondary to post-deployment adjustment. Since CSB has not been as heavily analyzed in isolation, intervention recommendations are lacking (Howard, 2007; Smith et al., 2014). As current studies call for better intervention approaches for military members and veterans with CSB (Kraus et al., 2017; Smith et al., 2014), the case studies presented within this chapter are aimed to provide intervention recommendations both from a psychotherapeutic and pharmacologic perspective.

---

*The descriptions of group treatment and case studies contained in this chapter have been carefully altered to protect identities of individuals while maintaining the key points of treatments and outcomes. Contents of this chapter do not represent any specific DOD information and do not reflect DOD policy or actual clinical information.

MEN'S SEXUAL RESPONSIVENESS IN THE BRAIN AND COMPULSIVE SEXUAL BEHAVIOR

Men's sexual response involves several regions in the brain that are critical for effective erectile development necessary for successful sexual engagement. There has to be sufficient activation of the parasympathetic nervous system to allow relaxation and erectile response to occur. The hypothalamus plays an important role in regulating erections by acting as a center of integration for multiple erotic input to the brain (Pfaus, 2009). More specifically, a man's response to the inherent rewards of sexual pleasure is primarily moderated by the mesolimbic dopamine pathway, receiving and integrating excitatory ("let's get it on") input and inhibitory ("let's not") input from all sources of erotic input, including other limbic structures (amygdala, hippocampus) and the prefrontal cortex (Volkow et al., 2011).

Even more specifically, the hypothalamic nuclei facilitate erections by receiving erectile-facilitating input from the mesolimbic dopamine pathway - the ventral tegmental area (VTA), and the nucleus accumbens (NAc) (Melis & Argiolas, 2011). The VTA-NAc circuit forms the core of a broader, more complex set of integrated circuits commonly called the "reward system" of the brain (Alcaro et al., 2007). Hence, dopamine signaling in the reward system plays a central role in sexual arousal, sexual motivation, and penile erections (Andersson, 2011; Pfaus, 2010).

The neurobiology of CSB is not well defined, particularly due to nonsubstantive terminology and disagreement on whether CSB is considered an addictive behavior, a form of obsessive-compulsive behavior (separate from the addiction model), and/or another form of self-defeating pleasure-seeking phenomena. However conceptualized, there is support for understanding this behavior is associated with increased activation of the anterior cingulate, ventral striatum, and amygdala (among other aspects of what is considered the "pleasure and reward circuits" of the brain). The activation of these brain structures has been noted in men with CSB over men who do not have CSB. Furthermore, men with CSB have the same functional connectivity abnormalities noted in brain studies of men with drug addictions (Kraus et al., 2016).

In addition, the use of dopamine replacement therapies and selective serotonin reuptake inhibitors (SSRIs) have been demonstrated as effective, even if only temporarily, in reducing the frequency and intensity of CSB. This suggests that CSB may be driven by deficient mesolimbic dopaminergic functioning and anxiety-reduction mechanisms (Gola & Potenza, 2016; Voon et al., 2014). As a more long-term solution, group therapy catered to those complaining of CSB has been demonstrated effective as well (Hook et al., 2008). There is research support for the assertion that effective therapeutic interventions for assisting men with CSB may best involve the combined use of medication and therapy. Implementation of these theoretical approaches will be elaborated upon in this chapter's case studies.

TREATMENT OF ACTIVE-DUTY MEN WITH COMPULSIVE SEXUAL BEHAVIORS (CSB)

Discussion of the treatment of active-duty personnel with CSB will include general treatment considerations (including medication); key points related to individual treatment, especially with active-duty personnel diagnosed with PTSD (including health maintenance and relapse prevention); and the utilization of group treatment with a focus spotlight on the Men's Sexual Health Group.

Generally, the use of medication is often considered an important aid to men wanting to feel better and gain control over their behavior. Medications are more often employed as a concurrent treatment to counseling when an individual has one or more of the following circumstances: (a) He has been diagnosed with a mood and/or anxiety disorder at a moderate to severe level of symptoms; (b) He has engaged in a long-term, well-established pattern of problematic sexual behavior which results in serious life consequences; (c) He wants to diminish the intensity of his libido/urge so he is not thinking about sex as often; and (d) He has failed other general treatment approaches, such as marital counseling.

Regarding psychotherapy, it is generally recommended to use individual Cognitive Behavior Therapy (CBT), which runs concurrently with group treatment (discussed later in detail). During CBT, it is helpful to look for the client's stuck points like "I am not good enough" or "I am a disgusting person and do disgusting things." There should be an emphasis on deconstructing the validity of negative self-beliefs. In addition, effective planning, skill development, and execution of a relapse prevention plan and a positive model of male sexuality is recommended (Babchishin et al., 2014; Peterson et al., 2020).

Regarding the focus within individual psychotherapy on relapse prevention, Sugrue (2007) recommends the following components of an effective relapse prevention plan:

- Sexual behaviors in inner circle (compulsive behaviors I must stop).
- Sexual behaviors in middle circle (dangerous behaviors I must avoid).
- What is at stake if I don't control my behavior?
- What do I have to gain by maintaining control of my sexual behavior?
- Ways to take better care of myself.
- Ways to take better care of my relationships.
- Circumstances that should put me on alert.
- Early signals of pending relapse.
- In case of emergency, know what my safety plan is, which includes my mantra, whom to call, my most effective control techniques, and my psychological "first-aid" kit.

Expanding beyond immediate relapse prevention into the realm of health maintenance, Peterson et al. (2020) offer a 10-point plan for health maintenance and relapse prevention:

1. Develop a personal mission statement regarding one's sense of purpose.
2. Identify what your "bottom lines" are that you do not want as part of your healthy life.
3. Identify triggers for acting out, both emotional and situational.
4. List healthy coping behaviors, "Tried and True" as well as "Expanding the Toolbox."
5. Create a "Personal Mission Support Team" from your social network.
6. Create a "Prediction Relapse Scenario" to identify warning signals of relapse.
7. Aspire toward the Model of Positive Male Sexuality (see next page).
8. Use time management for scheduling for preferred "recovery practices."
9. Establish a reinforcement schedule by which a reward system promotes positive behaviors of recovery practices and healthy lifestyle choices.
10. Rate your levels of satisfaction using standardized measures (the Big Wheel of Health questionnaire and/or the Sexual Health Functioning Continuum) at the beginning of your efforts (as a baseline measure) and after 3, 6, and 12 months of health practices. (The Big Wheel of Health questionnaire and the Sexual Health Functioning Continuum are both described later in the chapter and are included in Section VI).

What is the Model of Positive Male Sexuality? The model is a set of 12 characteristics that men can aspire to for their own personal growth and daily practice. It is helpful to supportively challenge men to possess as many of the following characteristics as they can to achieve overall positive male sexuality (remembering the goal is progress, not perfection):

1. Feelings of self-worth as a man (integration of positive male identity).
2. Sense of self-security with an internal locus of control so a man does not feel like he must prove his masculinity to others.
3. Commitment to the principles and practices of consensual sex.
4. Acceptance and appreciation of a positive sexual self-image.
5. Ability to avoid and/or recover from cyclic patterns of PSB (CSB).
6. Ability to positively practice self-pleasuring in a healthy manner.
7. Communication and intimacy skills to experience emotional closeness with others.
8. Openness to continuously learning how to be a better sexual partner based on his partner's sensual/sexual interests and preferences.
9. Active exercise to be healthy and well via the Big Wheel of Health.
10. Tolerance and acceptance of others who are different from himself.
11. Understanding that sexuality is another form of communication that serves an overall goal of meaningful and emotional connection.
12. Understanding and practicing the value of lifelong learning regarding the unique aspects of positive sexuality at every stage of life.

As illustrated below, the Model of Positive Male Sexuality can be conceptualized as a goal continuum to assess progress at various points during treatment:

Model of Positive Male Sexuality

To what extent do you experience the following:

(0-10 subjective scoring with 0 = never and 10 = almost always)

1. Feelings of self-worth as a man (integration of positive male identity).

   0-- 5 ---10

2. Sense of self-security with an internal locus of control so I do not feel like I must prove my masculinity to others, male or female.

   0-- 5 ---10

3. Commitment to the principles and practices of consensual sex.

   0-- 5 ---10

4. Acceptance and appreciation of a positive sexual self-image.

   0-- 5 ---10

5. Ability to avoid and/or recover from cyclic patterns of problematic sexual behavior.

   0-- 5 ---10

6. Ability to positively practice self-pleasuring in a healthy manner.

   0-- 5 ---10

7. Communication and intimacy skills to experience emotional closeness with others.

   0-- 5 ---10

8. Open to continuously learning how to be a better sexual partner based on his partner's sensual/sexual interests and preferences.

   0-- 5 ---10

9. Active exercise to be healthy and well via the Big Wheel of Health.

   0-- 5 ---10

10. Tolerance and acceptance of others who are different from himself.

    0-- 5 ---10

11. Understanding that sexuality is another form of communication that serves an overall goal of meaningful and emotional connection.

    0-- 5 ---10

12. Understanding and practicing the value of lifelong learning regarding the unique aspects of positive sexuality at every stage of life.

    0-- 5 ---10

GROUP TREATMENT: THE MEN'S SEXUAL HEALTH GROUP

(called the "Men's Group")

As noted earlier, concurrent individual and group modalities are considered best practice treatment when available and/or viable. A special group treatment was established to assist active-duty personnel who presented themselves to the Mental Health Flight seeking help with their compulsive sexual behaviors. Men were screened to exclude any with active psychotic symptoms as well as personality disorders that could be disruptive to the group process. All participation in the group was voluntary, but men were asked to come to at least 10 meetings before deciding to leave the group, abide by the group rules concerning confidentiality, and to speak to others (as well as be spoken to) by first names rather than rank. The goals of the Men's Sexual Health Group are to (a) develop positive sexual identity, (b) decrease the frequency and intensity of compulsive sexual behaviors (to point of elimination), (c) decrease levels of anxiety and depression, (d) decrease the sense of individual social/emotional isolation, and (e) promote development of positive male sexuality.

The Mental Health Flight initiated a Men's Sexual Health Group with program evaluation measures included. As with any mental health clinic, the Mental Health Flight utilized a scheduling program for appointments and printed appointment information for patients. To use positive affirming language and to minimize social stigma, appointments were simply listed as the "Men's Group." Further description of the pilot Men's Group follows:

- Men were assessed at baseline and at 12 weeks for symptom levels.
- Weekly meetings of 90 minutes duration started in October 2019.
- There were eight active-duty members (seven USAF and one Army).
- Ages ranged from 23 to 59 with an average age of 33 (four were in their 20s).
- Rank varied with Airman and Sergeants (E3-E6), two Captains, one Major.

- Marital status varied with six married and two single.
- Partner status varied as well, with six partners/spouses willing or wanting to stay in the marriage and two partners/spouses wanting to separate and/or leave the marriage.
- Education: One HS, two some college, two associate degrees, three MS degrees.
- Sex Orientation (sex designation): All cisgender men.
- Sexual Orientation: six self-describe as heterosexual, two identify as bisexual.
- Sex Role Orientation: five identify as traditional masculinity, three androgynous.

What the men were most concerned about and what they described as their motivation to join the group were listed as: Their uncontrollable urge to masturbate, sexual thoughts toward female friends, having less sex with their partner, living in a no sex/low sex marriage (with desire discrepancy between partners), wanting to be noticed by women, having affairs, self-described porn addiction and fetish interests, anxiety about most everything sexual, and worries regarding returning to voyeuristic behavior (not presently doing). The desired outcomes the men wished to achieve as a result of joining the men's group were listed as: Control of urges to sexually act out, remove porn/masturbation from their life, be able to say no to sexual advances from others, be a strongly supportive husband, have a healthy self-esteem, be a better father for their children, have a more "normal sexual mind," and have a larger penis (evidently written by a man with a sense of humor).

The most common self-identified behaviors considered a problem by the men included: Masturbating with online pornography (6), masturbating with pornography resulting in less sex with a partner (5), masturbating with pornographic magazines and DVDs (4), masturbating with erotic literature (3), masturbating using webcams (3), masturbating using chat rooms (3), sexting nude photos of self (2), sex via a professional relationship (2), masturbation in public spaces (1), voyeurism (1), exhibitionism (1), sexually touching a sleeping person (1), and having sexual affairs.

Reevaluation of the men's anxiety and depressive symptoms after 3 months of treatment demonstrated significant improvement. Employing repeated measures using the Beck Anxiety Inventory (BAI) showed a group baseline mean of 24.2 decreasing to 7.5 (over 12 sessions). Employing repeated measures using the Beck Depressive Inventory (BDI) showed a group baseline mean of 33.0 decreasing to 15.7 (over 12 sessions). Overall, the men reported decreases in the frequency and intensity of their compulsive sexual behaviors. Six men reported "significant improvement" and two men reported "moderate improvement."

Limitations of the pilot group study/evaluation included low numbers of participants and not being able to parse out treatment effects between individual, group, and medication interventions. In addition, it is unknown if clinical improvements would be sustained after treatment ended. The strengths of the evaluation demonstrated that "If you build it, they will come." That is to say, active-duty personnel will come to the Mental Health Flight for treatment of these types of personal concerns. Several inferences could be made, including (a) personal need is greater than the influence of stigma as a barrier to seeking services, (b) potential for research was demonstrated, and (c) this specialty treatment served as a valuable training experience for residents as well as social work interns.

Case Study 1: The Recruiter

Bryan, a 35-year-old heterosexual White male, serves as an active-duty army staff sergeant and recruiter, which is well known as a highly demanding and stressful position. He has completed three different assignments and two deployments, both of which were to combat zones with hostile enemy fire. Bryan was also well regarded by his superiors, as noted by a military record which has been listed as "outstanding," all the way up to his most recent incident (discussed below), and he has been an honor graduate from every school he has attended. In terms of relevant history, psychiatric history is unremarkable for treatment and medical history includes a prior vasectomy. Substance abuse was not noted or found to be an area of challenge for Bryan. He grew up in the East Coast, the army has been his primary career, and he is married (first marriage) with four children.

Bryan was initially seen in primary care behavioral health due to difficulties with managing what he called "my pornography and sex addictions." He was then referred to a sexual health specialist due to concerns related to CSB. At intake, Bryan described longstanding difficulties with CSB, and went on to detail how he would chronically masturbate to pornography when he was younger, when deployed, and feeling distress. He experienced a lack of control when doing so. He was able to maintain a normal life, despite these difficulties, until he recently initiated advances with another woman he was involved with as a recruiter. Bryan noted that he did not have the intention of beginning a relationship with this woman (he instead was receiving enjoyment from the explicit conversations they were having), and once this woman realized that Bryan was not interested in a relationship, she reported harassment to his superiors. Bryan was found to be in violation of the uniformed code of military justice. He was punished by a 6-month suspended demotion to sergeant (rank would not be permanently lost if he showed good behavior), he was moved to a different location, and a $2,000 specialty repay was collected. From a mental health perspective, Bryan wanted to work on better managing his challenges. He was referred to both a men's CSB group (which was facilitated by the same provider) and for psychiatric medication management.

The group was formatted around open discussion for problem areas anyone was experiencing related to CSB. Time was managed to ensure all members had a chance to participate, and all members were given a chance to share any closing thoughts toward the end of each session. Bryan was an active participant throughout sessions and openly described much of the challenges that he was facing, because "It is great to see that I am not the only one. I feel like I can tell you all anything." He began by noting that he was working on repairing his marriage, as his wife was profoundly hurt and upset with what Bryan did but she chose to stay with him. He was prescribed Paxil (10 mg) around the time group therapy began, and noted a few weeks later that he was feeling improvement, and that he had his first positive interaction with his wife since the incident. He continued to show improvement and even got two puppies, which he noted were positive additions to the family despite the puppies negatively affecting sleep quality and quantity.

Over a period of 3 months, Bryan continued to show improvements in groups, but did note that the initial Paxil dose was no longer as effective. The dosage was increased to 20 mg, from which Bryan noted decreased libido (which he described as "a good thing"). Another side effect was that while Bryan could achieve erections, he could no longer climax. He was able to manage and reconcile this challenge with his wife (group members worked with him on how to have the discussion). Paxil was eventually increased again to 30 mg due to deteriorating benefits, when he reported difficulties with irritability (however, some of the irritability was attributed to sleep difficulties).

Overall, Bryan went on to show recovery and stability, which was also recognized by his command who returned his rank, gave him a new assignment out of state, and a future deployment overseas. He rebuilt his marriage with his wife and has not had any additional incidents since.

Screeners over the sessions show marked decreases in depressive and anxiety symptoms (from severe to mild), and Bryan reported that he felt that he was doing better with managing his difficulties. On the Beck inventories for measuring symptom levels of anxiety and depressive symptoms (range of scores are 0-63, with <10 within normal range and 30+ as severe range for anxiety and depressive symptomology, respectively), he scored in the severe range for both at baseline assessments, with the anxiety score of 47 and the depression score of 56. After 3 months of treatment, he scored 12 and 17 respectively for anxiety and depressive symptoms, which would indicate mild symptomatology and marked improvement. He also opted to be an advocate for bringing men's groups to other bases, and noted dissatisfaction that such treatment options are not more readily available for members affected by CSB. In terms of treatment effects, Bryan described the medication as being helpful for decreasing distress and allowing him to better participate in group therapy, and he attributed more long-term behavioral change to skills and strategies learned from group. Bryan eventually moved on to the new assignment, and continues to reach back from time to time to share that he is doing well.

Case Study 2: The Officer

Capt Z is a married, African American active-duty military officer in his early 30s who voluntarily sought treatment in the Mental Health Flight due to anxiety, occupational problems, and marital problems associated with an acute situational stressor. Capt Z was referred by another psychologist in the clinic who was unable to continue treatment with him due to a deployment. The transfer was taking place after only a few sessions and it was, therefore, not disruptive to treatment. Capt Z was amenable to the referral.

The referral information stated that Capt Z was seeking treatment due to anxiety, relationship disruption, and potential job threats due to a situation in which he was possibly being blackmailed secondary to his involvement with online pornography. Assessment and interview revealed that Capt Z had a long history of pornography use dating back to his preteen years. In general, he described his use of pornography as a gradually increasing habit beginning around age 10. Initially, he consumed "normal porn," and as time passed and he advanced through puberty, he viewed more diverse types of pornography with a gradual progression in his mid-20s to a particular interest and affiliation with fetish chat rooms involving dominance and submission. Capt Z described efforts to cut back on the pornography-related behavior at various points in his life, most notably once he was married. However, he admitted that he ultimately returned to the behavior during periods of stress and sexual dissatisfaction.

Over the several years prior to seeking treatment, Capt Z's connection with some of the fetish chat rooms had deepened, and he had been contacted by organizers of the chat room to contribute money for a "sex club" that was reportedly being developed within the United States. The claim was that this club would offer members access to sexual activity in line with their particular interests in exchange for financial dues and fees. Since Capt Z had never found a reliable in-person outlet for his sexual interests, this idea was very appealing to him, and he began sending money. Over a period of approximately 18 months, Capt Z sent around $40,000 to contribute to the start-up of the sex club with the expectation and promise that he would be a member. Over time, he reported that the requests for money continued even after giving so much, and he became suspicious. When he challenged the legitimacy of the sex club plans, his contacts became coercive with the eventual threat that they would tell his family and employer about his involvement if he did not send more money. Realizing that he was being blackmailed, Capt Z made the decision to be forthright and honest with his wife and his military commander, and this led to multiple consequences including their recommendation that he seek mental health care. However, he did not feel coerced into mental health treatment per his report; he stated openly that he needed help managing the anxiety associated with the situation and wanted to address the underlying issues that he had been experiencing with pornography use over the years.

Occupational consequences that occurred after he told his commander about the situation were numerous and substantial. In fact, it is remarkable that Capt Z was able to salvage his career. Since Capt Z holds a Top Secret Clearance, this clearance was immediately suspended temporarily while an investigation ensued. To hold a Top Secret Clearance, one must maintain consistent reliability and good judgment. Also, there is a requirement that those with high security clearances do not put themselves in situations which make them vulnerable to forces, organizations, or individuals who may be a threat to national security. Clearly, in Capt Z's case, he had violated all of these requirements. Many military leaders may have chosen to permanently revoke his Top Secret Clearance, and this would have possibly ended his military career. However, Capt Z had been a valuable asset to his unit, and his commander was willing to let the investigation determine the final outcome. Not surprisingly, the investigation found that Capt Z was the victim of a blackmail scheme from another country, and he had been targeted through his use of legal pornography (from his personal computer). The investigating organization proceeded with attempting to identify and prosecute the perpetrators, but Capt Z reported that this had not been successful. No charges were brought against Capt Z by the military.

In addition to the uncertainty of Capt Z's military future at the time, he experienced shame since his commander and a few other leaders in the organization knew what he had done. He felt embarrassed about having his sexual interests known to others, and he felt an appropriate sense of guilt for having broken the rules of holding a Top Secret Clearance. Finally, Capt Z felt embarrassed for being "gullible" and robbed of a substantial amount of money. In retrospect, he could see clearly how the perpetrators had manipulated him with far-fetched and untrue information.

Relationship consequences following the disclosure of the attempted blackmail were also significant. Not surprisingly, Capt Z's wife was angry that he had contributed money without her knowledge, especially to a cause that was not consistent with their marital agreement. He reported that they had a traditional monogamous heterosexual relationship with no engagement in mutual pornography or fetish activity. Interestingly, he indicated that his wife had never really complained too much about his use of pornography unless it became "too frequent." However, his interest in fetish-type activity was not supported by her at all (she had not known about it previously), and she reportedly told him that "he needed to get that problem fixed" by attending therapy. Surprisingly (to him), she decided to stay in the marriage while he "worked on the problem." He also experienced shame about what had happened, and a sense of guilt for not being honest with her about his online sexual behavior.

An important point relevant to this case is that, at the time of his referral to mental health services, there were no providers in the clinic who were trained in providing treatment to address specific sexual disorders. Therefore, a referral was made to an off-base provider in the local area who had training in such problems and was able to take the insurance provided by the military for reimbursement. However, Capt Z's military-affiliated provider checked in with his USAF mental health therapist monthly to ensure he was getting care off base for his primary problems, to assess his deployability on an ongoing basis, and to teach him mood management and relationship skills. The parameters of these areas of focus were discussed with Capt Z, and he expressed understanding. Although his specific problematic sexual behaviors were not the target of treatment, the USAF therapist regularly inquired about his duty performance, marital satisfaction, and adherence to military regulations regarding the use of government computers and his Top Secret Clearance (Capt Z had never used his government computer inappropriately, including for pornography). In addition, his overall functioning and coping skills were a focus of treatment.

The USAF therapist saw the patient for 34 sessions over the course of 18 months. Treatment focused on helping him cope with the Office of Special Investigation (OSI) investigation process, addressing the marital difficulty he was experiencing, and helping him understand some of the factors that contributed to his use of pornography over time. Capt Z came into treatment with some helpful strengths such as high motivation for change, intelligence, transparency, ample unit support, and adequate marital support for seeking care. However, it was clear early on that he had learned early in his life to prioritize the needs of others over his own and to cope with conflict primarily through avoidance and acquiescence, especially in personal relationships.

Capt Z had been raised by very traditional immigrant parents, and while his mother was emotionally supportive, his father was highly critical throughout his childhood and even with Capt Z as an adult. He recalled coping with this by trying to please his father to avoid criticism and not challenging him when he was critical and emotionally abusive to him. To date, that was how he responded when his father criticized his job, his parenting, and so forth. While there was no physical abuse in his history, the emotional abuse from his father was a daily experience.

Capt Z described discovering pornography at a time when the internet was fairly new and when he was beginning to experience an interest in sex. The easy access to pornography made it a quick learning curve in terms of accessing an outlet for sexual desires, and he was able to keep this hidden for years. Gradually, he sought more intense and unusual sexual content as mentioned before, and over time, his time spent on the computer with pornography became his primary outlet for sexual gratification, distraction, and entertainment. As an adult, a contributing factor was that his wife (they had been married for 10 years and had a 1-year-old child when he started treatment) was very rigid in how she approached most aspects of their life (sexual activity, parenting style, leisure time), and he felt that he had no voice in how their life progressed. For example, she did not believe that time away from their child was needed, and she expected all of the leisure time to be spent together as a family. As other examples, she did not approve of him having a night out with friends on a monthly basis and she requested that his gym time occur before his workday rather than after his workday so he could be home by 5:00 p.m. daily. Capt Z had come to use pornography in his adolescence and adulthood as a coping factor, and he perceived it as one of the two aspects of his life that were "his." Of note, exercise was the other one and he enjoyed going to the gym.

It seemed that his care with the off-base provider was not progressing as well as hoped. While he experienced some remission/lessening of pornography use (he had completely terminated use of chat rooms), he still had periods of increased use which corresponded to elevated stress and feelings of being unappreciated at home. In a fortunate coincidence, a new provider was hired in the Mental Health Flight around that time who had substantial expertise in treating sexual compulsivity. The decision was made (collaboratively, with the patient) to withdraw the patient from off-base care by the general psychologist and have his treatment be managed entirely by this new, military-affiliated provider.

At the time Capt Z's care was transferred to the new provider, he had gained a substantial amount of insight into the historical, recent, and maintaining variables for his anxiety and relationship problems. In addition, he could see how sexual compulsivity had become one of his main tools for managing these challenges. Further, he was able to place this behavior in the context of his upbringing which included cultural factors of valuing family relationships and harmony as well as the context of entering puberty during a time of an explosion of availability of online pornography. He identified that engaging in behavioral change involved making the unfamiliar choice to be more assertive (exposure) over time, yet he was not sure he was willing to do that on a regular basis. His ability to clearly state this ambivalence reflected progress because the most passive and acquiescent approach would have been to agree to "try." Capt Z conducted several cost-benefit analyses about this, and at the time of referral, Capt Z was excited about having the opportunity to work with the gaining provider who had particular expertise in his presenting problem. He was hopeful that the work they had done together would set the stage for success in more specifically targeting sexual compulsivity.

After significant treatment (that Capt Z characterized as very helpful), his care was transferred for specialty sex-specific treatment that focused upon his CSB. He then started to participate concurrently in both individual and group treatment focused on his sexual compulsive behavior. He reported that the group therapy was value-added, as he had never been in the presence of a group of men where he felt he could talk about anything without fear of judgment. In fact, Capt Z disclosed that he was sexually abused as a boy and discussed how he felt that those experiences contributed to the development of his CSB.

Captain Z was given the Beck inventories for measuring symptom levels of anxiety and depressive symptoms (range of scores are 0-63, with <10 within normal range and 30+ as severe range for anxiety and depressive symptomatology, respectively). Since he had already received significant treatment before joining the Men's Group, Capt Z's scores were considerably lower than they would have previously been. He scored 8 on the anxiety measure (BAI) and 17 on the depression measure

(BDI) at baseline assessment. After 3 months of treatment, his scores continued to decline with 3 on the BAI and 4 on the BDI, which would indicate mild symptomatology and marked improvement.

Capt Z felt like he had "turned his life around" and was ready to start a new chapter in his marriage as well as his career. He brought his wife to an appointment for her to report directly on her perception of how things have changed for her and the family. Capt Z's wife stated that she was considering leaving her husband when she was told what all had happened with the loss of $40,000 and his sexual behaviors on the pornography site. She decided to postpone her decision and see what kind of changes her husband made and if they would be sustained. During this time, she saw the efforts he made at receiving treatment, felt the relationship continued to heal, and decided to have a second child (she was pregnant). The Capt and his family transferred to another Air Force base when he accepted a new position and a second opportunity to live a healthier life and enjoy a marriage without hiding CSB secrets.

DISCUSSION

Working with active-duty personnel with presenting concerns of problematic sexual behaviors has its own distinct considerations yet related to treatment for Veterans already separated from the military. The primary question is one of medical readiness for world-wide deployability, and sexual compulsive behaviors sometime contribute to a patient being determined unfit or unsuited for military service.

An example would be a major who asked for help regarding his "self-described sex addiction" to pornography but was told there were no counseling services available for his concern. Three years later and after eight career deployments, he was separated for use of child pornography. In addition, the *Military Times* published several examples of active-duty personnel who were either separated and/or incarcerated for their compulsive use of pornography ("Addicted to online porn," 2013).

Based upon research review and clinical experience, the authors recommend that outpatient treatment services be made more widely available for active-duty personnel with compulsive sexual behaviors. It is also recommended that such services involve a combination of *at least five of the following seven components*:

- A comprehensive sexual health and mental health evaluation that involves input from the partner, as well as objective measures for the assessment of an individual's sexual interest patterns, to see if there is any question regarding sexual interest in children (Abel et al., 2007).
- Individual counseling that emphasizes the effective planning and execution of relapse prevention, and an introduction of positive models of male sexuality (Babchishin et al., 2014; Peterson et al., 2020).
- Participation in a professionally led men's sexual health group that promotes accountability, a positive model of male sexuality, and prosocial skills to live a mission-guided, healthier life.
- When appropriate, marital and/or relationship counseling with an emphasis on communication training, reestablishing trust, and relationship repair.
- Utilization of pharmacological treatment options, including psychotropic medications, to decrease anxiety and depressive symptoms as well as voluntarily lowering libido and initiation of sexual activity.
- Individual or group counseling for partners of the men with CSB/PSB to support the partner's healing.

- Participation in community-based groups such as a Sex Addicts Anonymous (SAA) or Celebrate Recovery (CR) so men can get support any time needed.

Of course, as the case examples exemplified, treatment of active-duty personnel often involves planning or preparation for deployment into hostile environments. General Order 1, which covered all deployed troops in Operation Enduring Freedom and Operation Iraqi Freedom, prohibited use of pornography as well as alcohol consumption. In both cases, there were significantly high numbers of breaches by which Command did not order any subsequent nonjudicial punishment. While there was some effort to minimize introduction of alcohol and pornography, both were transported by contractors, in many cases along the same supply lines as other war material travel. Digital access to the internet widely available in MWR (Morale, Welfare, and Recreation) Internet Cafés and other access points created pathways for access to all forms of pornography. Pornography was often copied onto CDs, flash drives, and other portable devices which could be shared among other military members. Indigenous members also became suppliers of pornography. There is no doubt that the pornography available included all varieties, including child pornography.

Clinical experience of Department of Defense and Department of Veterans Affairs mental health professionals, when treating combat Veterans with PTSD, often demonstrates a strong relationship between attempts to manage traumatic memories of combat and whatever preexposure behaviors were present in the Veteran's life, including use of tobacco, alcohol, and pornography in any form. These preexposure coping (albeit unhealthy) behaviors created the conditions of treatment where the upstream drivers (combat trauma exposure) need to be addressed first in treatment. As the PTSD condition improved in symptom management, patient reports of compulsive and compensatory behaviors generally decreased.

"Therapeutic Continuums" can be useful in helping patients understand the degree of impact their deployment experiences had on them, as well as (later) measure their progress in their treatment goals. One variety of such "therapeutic continuums" is the "Big Wheel of Health" measure described in Section VI (pp. 575-578) of this text. It is made up of 25 items across 8 domains of health which are all rated on a 2-point continuum. This therapeutic continuum is in the form of a self-assessment questionnaire which serves as a basis for a structured interview and intervention for increasing the patient's awareness of the impact of his problematic sexual behavior. It also measures treatment progress.

A briefer (and perhaps more direct) use of a "Sexual Health Functioning Continuum" is offered by William Wall, a retired Lt. Colonel with specialty training in sex offenses and combat deployments. His therapeutic continuum employs collaborative completion of each domain of health, described below. The patient is asked the extent of impact each of their self-identified problematic sexual behaviors (such as his use of pornography) has on his life and to plot the impact from low impact (healthy) to high impact (unhealthy). The completion of the Sexual Health Functioning Continuum below usually generates greater patient insight, therapeutic discussion, and a means of measuring treatment progress.

Emotional Health

0 (healthy) --------------------------------- 5 -----------------------------------10 (Unhealthy)

Relational Health

0 (healthy) --------------------------------- 5 -----------------------------------10 (unhealthy)

Physical Health

0 (healthy) --------------------------------- 5 -----------------------------------10 (unhealthy)

Financial Health

0 (healthy) ---------------------------------- 5 ------------------------------------10 (unhealthy)

Spiritual Health

0 (healthy) ---------------------------------- 5 ------------------------------------10 (unhealthy)

Vocational Health

0 (healthy) ---------------------------------- 5 ------------------------------------10 (unhealthy)

Legal Health

0 (healthy) ---------------------------------- 5 ------------------------------------10 (unhealthy)

When working with active-duty personnel and Veterans, it is helpful to explore combat-related trauma along with the identity continuums of "predeployment self," "deployed self," and "postdeployment self." It is important to pay attention to thoughts and behaviors present in these different domains, and noting the presence of behaviors in the "postdeployment self" that were not present before being exposed to combat trauma.

A similar pattern emerged in the "postdeployment self" which consisted of increased compensatory behavior and negative self-appraisals. These behaviors were usually not present in the predeployment history and narrative, particularly when PTSD, depression, and moral injury were noted in the "postdeployment self." Pornography can be used to avoid traumatic memories, but more likely it is employed to reinforce reward pathways and experience positive emotions (versus the negative emotional turmoil often associated with traumatic combat memories).

The purpose of this chapter was to promote the availability of sexual health services to active-duty personnel who may present with concerns of problematic sexual behavior, including use of pornography. A brief summary of brain science related to sexual compulsive behaviors was presented along with treatment recommendations associated with clinical interventions for associated behaviors.

Two case studies were offered as examples of how these services, when available, can be of assistance to service members in terms of making "course corrections" to preserve their military career as well as saving their marriage. References were made to adverse examples of what can happen when such services are not available (the Major prosecuted for child pornography, the example highlighted by the *Military Times*, and the Army medic case study from Chapter 27 of this text).

Details of a men's group were provided to demonstrate how such a treatment service has viability and utility within an active-duty environment. In short, one question this chapter answered is: Will active-duty personnel with distress concerning sexual health problems (especially pornography) overcome the barrier of social stigma associated with coming to the Mental Health Flight? The answer: "If you build it, they will come."

REFERENCES

Abel, G., Wiegel, M., & Osborn, C. (2007). Pedophilia and other paraphilia. In L. VandeCreek, F. Peterson, J. Bley (Eds.), *Innovations in clinical practice: Focus on sexual health* (pp. 157-175). Professional Resource Press.

Addicted to online porn – X-rated internet explosion wreaks havoc with troops' careers, lives. (2013, March 6). *Military Times*. https://www.militarytimes.com/2013/03/06/addicted-to-online-porn-x-rated-internet-explosion-wreaks-havoc-with-troops-careers-lives/

Alcaro, A., Huber, R., & Panksepp, J. (2007). Behavioral functions of the mesolimbic dopaminergic system: An affective neuroethological perspective. *Brain Research Review*, 56, 283-321.

American Psychiatric Association. (2013). *Diagnostic and statistical manual of mental disorders* (5th ed.). https://doi.org/10.1176/appi.books.9780890425596

Andersson, K. (2011). Mechanisms of penile erection and basis for pharmacological treatment of erectile dysfunction. *Pharmacology Review,* 63, 811-859.

Babchishin, K. M., Curry, S. D., Fedoroff, J. P., Bradford, J., & Seto, M. C. (2017). Inhibiting Sexual arousal to children: Correlates and its influence on the validity of penile plethysmography. *Archives of Sexual Behavior, 46*(3), 671-684. https://doi.org/10.1007/s10508-017-0952-2

Babchishin, K. M., Hanson, R., & VanZuylen, H. (2014). Online child pornography offenders are different: A meta-analysis of the characteristics of online and offline sex offenders against children. *Archives of Sexual Behavior, 44*(1), 45-66. https://doi.org/10.1007/s10508-014-0270-x

Cooper, A. (2002). *Sex and the internet: A guidebook for clinicians.* Brunner-Routledge.

Derbyshire, K., & Grant, J. (2015). Compulsive sexual behavior: A review of the literature. *Journal of Behavioral Addictions*, 4(2), 37-43. https://doi.org/10.1556/2006.4.2015.003

Edwards, W., & Coleman, E. (2004). Defining sexual health: A descriptive overview. *Archives of Sexual Behavior, 33*(3), 189.

Gola, M., & Potenza, M. (2016). Paroxetine treatment of problematic pornography use: A case series. *Journal of Behavioral Addictions, 5*(3), 529-532. https://doi.org/10.1556/2006.5.2016.046

Hook, J., Hook, J., & Hines, S. (2008). Reach out or act out: Long-term group therapy for sexual addiction. *Sexual Addiction & Compulsivity, 15*(3), 217-232.

Howard, M. (2007). Escaping the pain: Examining the use of sexually compulsive behavior to avoid the traumatic memories of combat. *Sexual Addiction & Compulsivity, 14*(2), 77-94. https://doi.org/10.1080/10720160701310443

Kraus, S., Martino, S., Potenza, M., Park, C., Merrel, J., & Hoff, R. (2017). Examining compulsive sexual behavior and psychopathology among a sample of postdeployment U.S. male and female military Veterans. *Military Psychology, 29*(2), 143-156. https://doi.org/10.1037/mil0000147

Kraus, S., & Sweeney, P. (2019). Hitting the target: Considerations for differential diagnosis when treating individuals for problematic use of pornography. *Archives of Sexual Behavior*, *48*(2), 431-435. https://doi.org/10.1007/s10508-018-1301-9

Kraus, S., Voon, V., & Potenza, M. (2016). Neurobiology of compulsive sexual behavior: Emerging science. *Neuropsychopharmacology: Official Publication of the American College of Neuropsychopharmacology, 41*(1), 385-386. https://doi.org/10.1038/npp.2015.300

Ley, D. (2018). Compulsive sexual behavior disorder in ICD-11. *Psychology Today, 24.*

Melis, M., & Argiolas, A. (2011). Central control of penile erection: A re-visitation of the role of oxytocin and its interaction with dopamine and glutamic acid in male rats. *Neuroscience Biobehavorial Review*, 35, 939-955.

Peterson, F., Bley, J., & Frabotta, R. (2020). *The gender revolution and new sexual health: Celebrating unlimited diversity of the human sexuality hypercube.* Cognella Academic Press.

Pfaus, J. (2009). Pathways of sexual desire. *Journal of Sexual Medicine, 6,* 1506-1533.

Pfaus, J. (2010). Dopamine: Helping males copulate for at least 200 million years: Theoretical comment on Kleitz-Nelson et al. (2010). *Behavioral Neuroscience, 124,* 877-880.

Smith, P., Potenza, M., Mazure, C., McKee, S., Park, C., & Hoff, R. (2014). Compulsive sexual behavior among male military veterans: Prevalence and associated clinical factors. *Journal of Behavioral Addictions, 3*(4), 214-222. https://doi.org/10.1556/jba.3.2014.4.2

Stone, G. (2017). *Sex and the constitution: Sex, religion, and law from America's origins to the twenty-first century*. Liveright Publishing Corporation.

Sugrue, D. (2007). Sexual addiction/compulsion: Diagnosis and treatment. In L. VandeCreek, F. Peterson, & J. Bley (Eds.), *Innovations in clinical practice: Focus on sexual health* (pp. 177-196). Professional Resource Press.

Volkow, N., Wang, G., Fowler, J., Tomasi, D., & Telang, F. (2011). Addiction: Beyond dopamine reward circuitry. *Proceedings of the National Academy of Sciences of the United States of America, 108,* 15037-15042.

Voon, V., Mole, T., Banca, P., Porter, L., Morris, L., Mitchell, S., . . . Irvine, M. (2014). Neural correlates of sexual cue reactivity in individuals with and without compulsive sexual behaviours. *Public Library of Science One, 9*(7), e102419. https://doi.org/10.1371/journal.pone.0102419

World Health Organization. (1992). *The ICD-10 classification of mental and behavioural disorders: Clinical descriptions and diagnostic guidelines.* https://apps.who.int/iris/handle/10665/37958

World Health Organization. (2019). *International statistical classification of diseases and related health problems* (11th ed.). https://icd.who.int/

29

Consulting With Courts On Sex Crime

Richard Rothenberg, Elizabeth Sarnoski, Pamela Broderick, and Christopher Marett

INTRODUCTION

Mental health professionals are sometimes asked to examine an individual and offer an assessment of the likelihood of a repeat sexual offense. This can be challenging given that such assessments generally occur outside the setting in which the actual behavior in question would manifest. For instance, the risk assessment may be based on an office interview or on behavioral observations made in a locked, controlled environment when the actual ultimate question is the probability of the behavior manifesting in the uncertainty of a community setting (Melton et al., 2018). Despite this limitation, courts request risk assessments to assist with maintaining public safety and to ensure an appropriate restrictive level of care (Marett & Mossman 2017; Melton et al., 2018). There are three broad approaches to clinical risk assessments: clinical judgment, structured professional judgment, and actuarial tools.

THREE APPROACHES TO RISK ASSESSMENT

Traditionally, mental health professionals estimated risk through their use of clinical judgment, in which the professional would review any data believed to be relevant. Such data could include previous treatment history, the criminal complaint, laboratory work, collateral history, and a clinical interview. The practitioner would then evaluate the acquired information and render a judgment regarding risk of reoffense (Marrett & Mossman, 2017). While this approach permits flexibility, it generates poor interrater reliability. This is likely due to the idiosyncratic process of gathering and weighing information used by individual evaluators (Bengtson & Lângström, 2007; Hanson & Morton-Bourgon, 2009).

In contrast, the second category of risk assessment tools is "structured professional judgment." This approach requires evaluators to consider specific empirically based indicators. A structured professional judgment tool is typically scored, though the score does not generate a specific risk category. Rather, the overall risk determination is left to the evaluator. This style of assessment allows for some clinically salient input that accounts for variables not relevant to the initial study population while requiring assessment of and accounting for empirically derived risk factors (Marett & Mossman, 2017; Melton et al., 2018; Skeem & Monahan, 2011).

Finally, actuarial risk assessments utilize specific data points that are calculated in a specific manner to generate a risk assessment. Because the data used to generate the assessment is collected and used in a specific manner as dictated by the assessment manual, the interrater reliability is generally improved (Hanson & Morton-Bourgon, 2009). However, the structure results in limited flexibility and a loss of opportunity to insert clinically germane information that is not otherwise accounted for in the actuarial assessment (Melton et al., 2018; Skeem & Monahan, 2011). Both actuarial assessment and structured professional judgment outperform unstructured clinical judgment (Hanson & Morton-Bourgon, 2009; Skeem & Monahan, 2011).

EXPRESSION OF RISK

Risk assessment is best expressed in terms of prognosis and probability rather than diagnosis and dichotomous "risky" or "not risky" solutions (Helmus & Babchishin, 2017; Marett & Mossman, 2017; Skeem & Monahan, 2011). Further, it is important to define a target outcome and time frame (e.g., the "risk of committing a sexual offense in the next 5 years"). Because the statement of risk is probabilistic, it is important to have a basic understanding of relevant statistics (Mossman, 1994). Sensitivity is a measure of the probability of having a positive test in the context of the behavior having occurred. This is typically represented as "true positive rate," or the number of individuals the test predicted would have risky behavior and did indeed have the behavior divided by all those who did have the behavior. Specificity measures the probability of a negative test result accurately identifying those who indeed did not have the measured behavior. The positive predictive value assesses how many of the risky people were correctly identified using the test by dividing the true positive (those who were predicted to have the behavior and did) by the sum of the true positive and the false positive (those who were predicted to have the behavior but did not). Similarly, negative predictive value assesses the probability that a negative test correctly identified the absence of the behavior or risk from all those who the test predicted as negative or not risky. The use of these statistics in understanding the usefulness of the risk assessment tools is impacted in part by the prevalence or base rate of outcome behavior (e.g., violence) in the population.

In addition, use of a particular assessment does not yield an inherent "risky" or "not risky" determination but rather yields a value that represents risk on a continuum. Changing the cutoff value for "risky" versus "not risky" alters the relationship between sensitivity and specificity (Helmus & Babchishin, 2017; Marrett & Mossman, 2017). For instance, if the cut-off threshold for risk were such that all individuals convicted of a sex offense were required to remain in the hospital or incarcerated for the rest of their lives, the sensitivity for correctly predicting who would reoffend and need to be kept in the hospital would be 100%. However, the specificity (the number who were not at risk to reoffend and were appropriately released) would be extremely low. Conversely, if the cut-off for the assessment resulted in all sex offenders being released, the specificity would be high while the sensitivity would be low (Mossman, 1994). While the ideal assessment would be 100% sensitive and 100% specific, few, if any, psychological assessment tools reach this level of performance.

The Receiver Operator Curve (ROC Curve; see Figure 1) helps demonstrate the relationship between sensitivity and specificity by graphing the sensitivity (the true positive rate) against 1-specificity (the false positive rate). This allows the evaluator to assess the inherent tradeoffs between sensitivity and specificity for a given tool (Mossman, 1994). Based on the context, the best probability threshold for a positive test can be selected. Any value on the straight line where sensitivity = 1-specificity, or false positive rate, indicates that the predictive capability of the tool was no better than chance. Values below this line indicate that the discrimination capability of the tool between non-reoffenders and offenders is worse than chance and values above this line indicate the discrimination capability is better than chance. The area under the curve (AUC) represents the predictive power of the tool. In addition to understanding the tradeoff between sensitivity and specificity, AUCs of two assessments can be used to determine which model is likely to offer the most accurate prediction

(Mossman, 1994). However, AUCs cannot account for variation in follow-up intervals (Helmus & Babchishin, 2017). Other commonly used statistics to evaluate recidivism rates include Harrell's C, which is similar to AUC, but allows for data comparison despite variation in follow-up times (Helmus & Babchishin, 2017). Cohen's d is a measure of effect size and is measured by calculating the number of standard deviations between two means (Helmus & Babchishin, 2017).

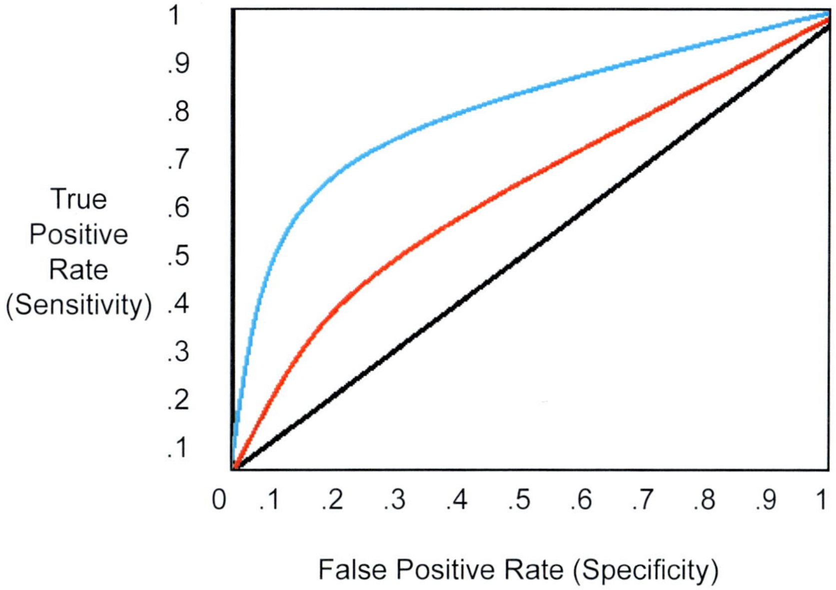

Figure 1. Example Receiver Operator Curve

While the above statistics measure discrimination, calibration is emerging in the literature, though without consensus to date (Helmus & Babchishin, 2017; Singh, 2013). Calibration compares the measured result of the tool in one sample (in this case the recidivism rate per cutoff score contained in the norms) with the measured result, observed recidivism rate at that score in a second sample. In an ideally calibrated test, the two distributions will match exactly (Helmus & Babchishin, 2017). Common measures of calibration include the chi-square test which measures the correspondence between the expected and observed rate though it does not provide an effect size (Helmus & Babchishin, 2017). The E/O index, the ratio between expected recidivists and observed recidivists, can provide an effect size (Helmus & Babchishin, 2017). The best possible calibration will occur with the result of 1 as in the expected recidivists and observed recidivists were equal (Helmus & Babchishin, 2017).

Other commonly used statistics include the number needed to detain (NND) which is the number of offenders that need to be detained or otherwise isolated from the community to prevent one episode of sexual re-offense (Buchanan & Leese, 2001). The number needed to safety discharge is the number of offenders that would need to be discharged prior to expecting a repeat offense (Singh, 2013). These concepts are impacted by the underlying base rate but help provide a clinically useful interpretation of statistical information.

The above variety of assessments provides a potential menu of options for clinicians evaluating sexual recidivism risk, but there is a wide variation in how clinicians employ each tool. Neal and Grisso (2014) surveyed 434 international forensic evaluators about their last two forensic evaluations and found that 74.2% had used one tool or more in their assessment process. Of those who used tools, the average number of tools used was four. This survey was not specific to the evaluation of sex offenders, but of those who had completed a sex offense risk evaluation, 96.9% reported using a structured tool (Neal & Grisso, 2014). The Static was the most commonly used assessment (65.6% of sex offender risk evaluations) followed by SVR-20 (13.6%) and STABLE, SORAG, VRAG which were each used less than 10% of evaluations in this study.

A study by Kelley et al. (2020) surveyed clinicians regarding their assessment use when evaluating sexual offender risk and found that the majority (82.4%) used an actuarial assessment while 30.8% used a structured professional judgment (SPJ) tool (Kelley et al., 2020). The Static-99R was the most common assessment used overall. A significant majority (89.4%) of respondents reported using the newest version of the selected actuarial tool. The majority (58.0%) used only one static risk instrument in their evaluations while a large minority used two or more. The majority of respondents reported using only one normative source for the Static-99/99R, though the process used to select the norm was relatively evenly split between clinical judgment, other idiosyncratic "matching methods," using only the "routine" norm, and using an actuarial method to determine reference group selection. Criminogenic needs were less frequently assessed, but the STABLE-2007 was the most commonly used by about half of the participants, followed by the SVR-20. Of the participants who measured treatment gains, the STABLE-2007 was most common at about 30% which was followed by the SOTIPS (Sex Offender Treatment Intervention and Progress Scale) at 14.4% and VRS-SO at 13.3%. Approximately a third (36.1%) did not feel that there was enough empirical support to measure treatment gains using any of the instruments. Specific measures of protective factors were infrequently used but when used, the structured assessment of protective factors was the most common (10%). The majority of assessors (60%) reported using "empirically guided assessment." Kelly et al. (2020) concluded that the most common current practice in evaluated sexual recidivism risk was to use new static actuarial instrument, a measure of criminogenic needs and a qualitative description of protective factors.

RISK ASSESSMENT TOOLS

Sexual offense recidivism risk assessment instruments vary in their scope and the elements they include. Some research suggests that actuarial instruments are the most accurate (Hanson & Morton-Bourgon, 2009) in estimating risk of sexual offense recidivism, though structured professional judgment tools are also superior to a clinician's judgment alone. In practice, it is common for assessments to include both structured professional judgment and actuarial instruments. Although general psychological testing can be valuable for assessment of an individual's general mental health functioning and psychopathology, it may not be useful for assessment of sexual reoffending risk.

STRUCTURED PROFESSIONAL JUDGMENT TOOLS

A commonly utilized structured professional judgment instrument is the Hare Psychopathy Checklist – Revised (PCL-R). The PCL-R is a 20-item symptom rating scale that is used to diagnose psychopathy and pairs a semistructured interview with a review of the individual's records and history (Hare, 2003). Psychopathy is a personality pattern associated with risk of sexual offense recidivism. The relationship between PCL-R scores and results of actuarial tools specifically designed to predict sexual reoffending is modest (Murrie et al., 2012). Although total PCL-R scores are often used in forensic reports and testimony, research suggests that some components of the PCL-R are more predictive than others. PCL-R items are divided into two factors: Factor one includes an interpersonal facet and an affect facet, and factor two includes an impulsive lifestyle facet and an antisocial behavior facet. Meta-analyses have shown that factor 2, specifically the antisocial behavior facet, is a significantly stronger predictor of violence and sexual recidivism (Hawes et al., 2013). Additionally, high PCL-R scores indicate higher risk of severe violence but have a weaker association with overall sexual recidivism. Due to this, those who commit rape tend to score high on the PCL-R relative to those who perpetrate other offenses (Rowlands et al., 2017). The PCL-R's predictive value may be associated with the evaluator's level of training specific to using the PCL-R, and thus, research findings of the PCL-R's validity may not generalize to the field (Murrie et al., 2012).

Another useful structured professional judgment instrument is the Sexual Violence Risk-20 (SVR-20). The SVR-20 is a 20-item checklist of studied risk factors for sexual offense which does not assign a final score or risk level (Boer et al., 1997). The SVR-20 is the second most widely used instrument for assessment of sexual recidivism risk behind the Static-99, discussed below.

ACTUARIAL TOOLS

Commonly utilized actuarial instruments include the Static-99, Static-2002R, Rapid Risk Assessment for Sexual Offense Recidivism (RRASOR), Sexual Offender Risk Appraisal Guide (SORAG), and the Minnesota Sex Offender Screening Tool – Revised (MnSOST-R). The Static-99 and the Static-2002R are the most widely used and most researched measures for assessing sexual recidivism risk among sexual offenders. The Static-99 includes ten items related to offense information and offense history. The Static-2002R is a revised vision of the Static-99. The Static-2002R differs in that it has 14 items, subscales to aid interpretation, and more standardized coding rules (Hanson, 2002). These revisions were intended to increase clarity regarding common points of confusion for evaluators. The coding manual increased from a two-page Static-99 manual to a 50-page manual for the Static-2002R, which includes scoring and interpretation examples (Boccaccini et al., 2017). The RRASOR is composed of four items and has similar coding to the Static-9. The SORAG has been shown to have good discriminatory power but not across all sexual offenses. The SORAG is especially good at assessing risk for child molesters. The MnSOST-R is a 16-item instrument based on research with incarcerated male sexual offenders (Epperson et al., 2003). Revisions are common in actuarial risk assessment instruments as refinements to existing tools occur as more research data becomes available (Ozkan et al., 2020).

Table 1: Comparison of Assessment Approaches*

Assessment Approach	Explicitly Identifies Risk Factors	Measures Risk Factors	Combines Risk Factors and Yields Final Risk Estimate	Examples
Clinical Judgment				
Standard List of Risk	X			
Structured Professional Judgment	X	X		SVR-20, RSVP, PCL-R
Actuarial	X	X	X	SORAG, RRASOR, Static 2002R, MnSOST-R

*Adapted from Skeem and Monahan (2011).

Research on head-to-head comparisons of actuarial instruments has shown that the Static-2002R, SORAG, RRASOR, and MnSOST-R all have a moderate level of predictive accuracy, but some instruments may perform differently for assessing risk of different sexual offenses. For violent or serious sexual offenses, the accuracy of the Static-2002R and the SORAG were significantly superior to the RRASOR and the MnSOST-R. Head-to-head comparison did not suggest that one actuarial instrument outperformed others across the board (Langton et al., 2007).

Although actuarial instruments are sometimes considered superior to structured professional judgment instruments, they are not without potential flaws. The predictive value of actuarial instruments can be jeopardized by incorrect scoring or interpreting, not recognizing test limitations, or overemphasizing risk scores in the presence of other information. Additionally, actuarial instruments have been criticized for lack of inclusion of dynamic risk factors that may alter recidivism risk. Research has shown that accounting for situational risk factors (e.g., active substance use or relationship stress) increases predictive accuracy (Rowlands et al., 2017). Inclusion of these dynamic risk factors is a strength of some structured profession judgment instruments, like the SVR-20.

Adolescent and female offenders are special populations to consider regarding assessment of sexual reoffending risk. All of the assessment instruments discussed thus far are validated for male adults. Instruments validated for male adolescents aged 12 to 18 years include the Juvenile Sex Offender Assessment Protocol (J-SOAP-II) and the Estimate of Risk of Adolescent Sex Offense Recidivism 2.0 (ERASOR 2.0). The J-SOAP-II may be better suited for one-time risk assessments, whereas the ERASOR 2.0 may be better suited for conducting repeated risk assessment during treatment to assess progress (Boer et al., 1997). There are no risk assessment instruments validated for female sexual offenders. The low base rate for female sex offender leads to an overestimation of risk when instruments are used that are validated for male offenders.

There is no gold standard risk assessment instrument for sexual offense recidivism. Important factors to consider when choosing a risk assessment instrument include the evaluator's experience and training with the instrument, the target population and limitations of the instrument, and the time of administration of the instrument. For example, the PCL-R requires several hours to complete and should be administered and scored by a clinician with adequate training and experience. Review of the instrument's manual is essential as it will outline the target population for the instrument, the limitations of the instrument, and will assist the evaluator in determining if the instrument is appropriate for the assessment in question. Another example is the MnSOST-R which is based on incarcerated male sexual offenders, and thus it would not be an appropriate instrument for risk assessment of an individual in an outpatient treatment program. Table 1 on page 499 summarizes the main approaches to risk assessment and reviews examples of each.

HOW COURTS USE EXPERT TESTIMONY

The primary role of an expert witness is to "assist the trier of fact to understand the evidence" (*Federal Rules of Evidence, Rule 702,* 2010). Ideally, expert testimony provides objective information to the judge and/or jurors to help them make decisions regarding the case. A study by Otto and Petrila (2006) showed that no expert testimony on future risk of sexual recidivism had been excluded by the courts. Yet other research shows that while some courts are required to closely evaluate the scientific validity of expert testimony, they have shown little willingness to do so when the testimony concerns the risk of sexual recidivism (Krauss & Scurich, 2013). One possible explanation for the courts' lack of consideration concerning testimony related to the risk of sexual recidivism is motivated reasoning. Motivated reasoning refers to the biased search and processing of information to reinforce some goal extrinsic to decision accuracy (Carlsmith et al., 2007). In other words, people seek out information that is congruent with their preferred outcome. When presented with information, they tend to selectively credit or discredit that information depending on whether it supports their preferred outcome. Reasonable people can and will disagree about the quality of a given risk assessment. Yet crediting or discrediting the assessment based on its outcome can only reinforce preexisting desires and goals, which does little to promote informed decisions (Krauss & Scurich 2013).

In 2016, the authors of the Static-99 made a significant change in terms of how they categorize and consequently communicate risk to other individuals. Previously, the status quo in risk assessment had been for scale developers to translate scores into risk level in ways that were poorly defined and difficult to compare across measures. This problem often led to similar scales placing the same offenders into different categories (Barbaree et al., 2006; Jung et al., 2013; Mills & Kroner, 2006). Compounding this confusion is the fact that different professionals may also have very different interpretations of what labels like "low," "moderate," and "high" mean (Hilton et al., 2008; Monahan & Silver, 2003; Slovic et al., 2000). To help address this problem, the United States Council of State Governments Justice Center assembled a group to develop standardized risk levels for general offenders. The new risk levels for the Static-99R and Static-2002R were developed in line with the Justice Center's proposed risk levels and informed by empirically based risk communication metrics: percentiles, risk ratios, and recidivism estimates (Hanson et al., 2017).

Jurors' Perception

A study by Boccaccini et al. (2014) revealed nearly all jurors (91.9%) reported they needed to hear testimony from experts to make good decisions in regard to Sexually Violent Predators (SVP). A majority of these individuals (69.4%) also indicated these experts were "very good" at predicting whether someone would commit a sexual offense in the future. In general, the research (Guy & Edens 2003; Turner, 2011) documents that jurors involved in SVP cases view defense experts as less influential than State experts. Despite the fact defense experts may be viewed as less influential than State experts and their opinion may not differ greatly from the opposing expert's, they can serve an important counterbalancing role. This counterbalancing role allows them to frame information and communicate to the jury and/or judge in a manner to help support their position even though the information itself may not necessarily change. Scurich and John (2011) found that mock jurors were much less likely to decide that a patient needed to be civilly committed when they were told that there was a "26% probability of violence occurring" as opposed to a "74% probability of violence not occurring." Further, gender may play a role in how a juror perceives risk testimony. Men rate clinical testimony at a significantly higher dangerous score while in experiential mode, and actuarial testimony higher while in a rational mode. This difference is not observed in women (Lieberman et al., 2007).

Judges' Interpretation

In bench trials, it is difficult to determine how the judge or magistrate will use the information provided by expert witnesses. Although most jurisdictions have clear rules and standards of evidence related to expert witness testimony (e.g., those outlined in the *Daubert* and *Frye* standards), there is no such standard determining how a judge or magistrate may weigh the information presented to them. Each judge or magistrate may weigh the information presented to them differently based on their own personal beliefs and experiences related to sex offenders. In addition, other factors such as media coverage of a case and the current political climate may also influence a decision made by the judge/magistrate despite the information presented to them by an expert witness. Ultimately, experts can offer their opinion based on their evaluation to the court, but the judge/magistrate makes the final decision regarding the disposition of the case which may or may not be consistent with the opinion and recommendations offered by the expert witness.

Jury/Public Perception and Mismatch With Data

Few words in our society engender such a strong emotional reaction as "sex offenders." This strong emotional reaction from people can lead to misperceptions and/or reinforce already preexisting misconceptions regarding this particular group of individuals (King & Roberts, 2017). This continued emotional panic associated with registered sex offenders leads to15 legislations based on fear and public outcry rather than facts and research. Research (Craun & Theriot, 2009; Katz-Schiavone et al., 2008; Levenson et al., 2007) has shown that the general public holds incorrect beliefs or endorsed myths about sex offenders, which likely stems from fear or misrepresentation of sensational cases in the media.

A common misconception regarding sex offenses is that their occurrence is steadily increasing, particularly those involving child victims and unknown perpetrators (Anderson & Sample, 2008; Fuselier et al., 2002; Galeste et al., 2012; Mears et al., 2008; Pickett et al., 2013; Quinn et al., 2004). The study by Levenson, Brannon, et al. (2007) found that over three quarters of the participants believed the rate of sexual crimes were increasing by almost 30%, when in fact the official statistics and victimization data are from the Bureau of Justice and Federal Bureau of Investigation are significantly lower than those observed prior to the mid-1990s (Bureau of Justice Statistics, 2003; Ferguson & Hartley, 2009). Craun and Theriot's (2009) research found that their participants were more concerned about a child being sexually victimized by a stranger than someone they know despite the fact that the research shows that vast majority of sex offenders are relatives, family friends, or neighbors of their victims (Douard, 2007; Janus, 2006). An ongoing problem in providing accurate information and data related to sexual assault/abuse is the fact that these types of crimes continue to be underreported.

One of the most common myths in regard to sex offenders are that they are chronic recidivists (Mancini & Mears, 2010) who cannot be rehabilitated (Galeste et al., 2012; Levenson, 2003; Quinn et al., 2004; Sample & Bray, 2006; Sundt et al., 1998). However, the research has consistently shown that the recidivism rate for sex offenders is lower than other offenders who have committed other types of crimes (Hanson & Morton-Bourgon, 2009; Helmus et al., 2012; Tewksbury et al., 2012; Zimring et al., 2007). Although sex offenders are more likely to recidivate with a sexual offense, the risk remains relatively low, and they are actually more likely to recidivate with a nonsexual offense than a sex offense (Babchishin et al., 2016; Bureau of Justice Statistics, 2002; Hanson & Bussière, 1998; Tewksbury et al., 2012). The research has also shown that certain sex offender treatment models can be effective in reducing recidivism, specifically for younger offenders (Hanson et al., 2002; Kim et al., 2016; Schmucker & Lösel, 2015).

Many myths and misconceptions regarding the motivation of sex offenders have been perpetuated without examining the available facts and data. For example, there is the "abused-abuser hypothesis," where many individuals believe that sex offenders were sexually abused as children and continue this cycle of abuse by becoming sex offenders themselves. A longitudinal birth cohort study by Leach and colleagues (2015), however, found very few sex offenders with a confirmed history of sexual abuse and no significant relationship between past victimization and future abuse. The increasing prevalence of pornographic material on the internet has also contributed to a misconception that sexually explicit materials may contribute to sexual victimization by feeding into the misogynistic idea of women as objects of sexual gratification of men (Dworkin, 1981). Yet multiple studies have contradicted this assertion by finding there is no relationship between viewing pornography and misogynistic attitudes (Barak et al., 1999; Baron, 1990; Davies, 1997). In addition, the research available shows low support for pornography as an influential factor in sex crime commission (Gentry, 1991; Kutchinsky, 1991; Linz et al., 2004).

Another common misconception regarding sex offenders are that they are all male. More recent research and data provides evidence the prevalence of female sex offenders may be higher than initially thought. The Bureau of Justice Statistics conducts the National Crime Victimization Survey (NCVS), a household survey on violent crime incidents including rape and sexual assault. An analysis of the 2010-2013 NCVS data on rape and sexual assault found that female perpetrators (acting without male coperpetrators) were reported in 28.0% of rape/sexual assault incidents involving male victims and 4.1% of incidents involving female victims (Temple et al., 2017). Similar to male-perpetrated sexual victimization, female perpetration of sexual abuse is underreported to officials (Denov, 2003; Mendel, 1995).

In general, members of the community have demonstrated high level of support for policies such as registration, notification, and residence restrictions based on their belief that such policies are effective in preventing sexual victimization (Comartin et al., 2009; Levenson et al., 2007; Schiavone & Jeglic, 2009). Although these policies and procedures related to sex offender registration and notification are intended to decrease recidivism, the research indicates their effects were modest (Prescott & Rockoff, 2011; Shao & Li, 2006) or had no significant impact on recidivism (Sample & Kadleck, 2008; Sandler et al., 2008; Tewksbury & Jennings, 2010; Veysey et al., 2008). Despite the fact that 90% of the public is aware that they have access to online sex offender registries, only slightly more than one third of the public reports ever accessing this information (Anderson & Sample, 2008; Kernsmith et al., 2009).

Clinical Vignette

Mr. Smith is a 63-year-old man who had been convicted of second degree criminal sexual conduct approximately 17 years ago while living in Michigan. He had been required subsequently to register as a sexual offender in the state of Michigan. Upon moving to Ohio, he had been required to register as a sexual predator. He has petitioned the Court for reclassification of his sexual offender registration requirements.

Mr. Smith denied any formal sexual education while a child. During my interview with Mr. Smith, he reported first becoming sexually active at age 14. He engaged in oral and vaginal intercourse with a female neighbor who was approximately 1 or 2 years older than he was at the time. Mr. Smith described having numerous sexual relationships with other women. Some of these sexual relationships were more casual and occurred out of happenstance and convenience rather than as part of a long-standing romantic relationship. He also talked about having some long-term girlfriends and romantic relationships which involved oral and vaginal intercourse. He acknowledged not always being faithful to his wife both while they were dating and during the course of their marriage. For a period of time, he received sexual favors from women in exchange for crack cocaine.

Mr. Smith denied engaging in the sexual activity cited in the index offense. He defined the situation as a misunderstanding and a product of discrimination. The victim, he explained, was a neighbor that came over to his house to play with his daughter frequently. He had drunk alcohol and smoked marijuana at the time of the index offense. By Mr. Smith's account, the victim came into the house to use the bathroom, and he claimed to have had little contact with her while in the house. The victim's mother, on the other hand, accused Mr. Smith of locking the door to prevent her daughter from leaving, then proceeding to engage in sexual activity with her. Mr. Smith denied any sexual contact with the identified victim, but he was later arrested based on the accusations of the victim's mother and the victim's statements to the police. He maintained that he was arrested because he was African American and the identified victim and her mother were Caucasian.

Mr. Smith claimed no rape kit had been completed for the identified victim. He said his lawyer advised him to accept a plea bargain because of the jury makeup and he would likely lose the case even though he denied engaging in any type of sexual activity with the identified victim. Mr. Smith talked about accepting the plea bargain in order to "stay out of jail." Initially, Mr. Smith was placed on probation after accepting the plea bargain, but he eventually served 3 years in prison after committing a probation violation.

The police documentation suggests Mr. Smith lured the victim into his house by offering her candy. The victim indicated Mr. Smith then "touched" her, pointed to her buttocks and vagina, then proceeded to digitally penetrate both her anus and vagina. She said that Mr. Smith then told her not to tell anyone what happened. In a later police interview, the victim also alleged Mr. Smith engaged in anal and vaginal intercourse with her during this same encounter.

As part of this evaluation, the examiner completed the Minnesota Multiphasic Personality Inventory-2 (MMPI-2) and the Static-99R. On the Static-99R, Mr. Wilson received a total score of -2, which placed him in the **low** category for risk of sexual reoffending. In studies of the Static-99R, offenders from routine correctional samples with scores of -2 sexually reoffended at a rate of 1.3 percent in 5 years with a 95% confidence interval of 1.0% to 1.8%. At the time of this assessment there were no statistics or information available regarding the rate of sexual recidivism beyond 5 years. The examiner also cited a study by Hanson (2002) in his report which provides evidence that with Mr. Smith's increasing age, the research suggests a decrease in deviant sexual drives, improvement in self-control, and decreased opportunity for sexual offense recidivism. Based on the evaluation, the examiner opined that Mr. Smith was at a low risk of sex offense recidivism. The examiner testified in court to his findings and the court ruled that Mr. Smith was not a sexual predator. Rather, he was adjudicated as an offender with a registration period of 10 years in Ohio, for which he would receive time credited for time spent in Michigan and for the time he had already lived in Ohio.

CONCLUSION

When mental health professionals are asked to evaluate risk of sexual offending, they have a broad armamentarium of tools at their disposal. Generally, actuarial tools and structured professional judgment tools are preferred for their greater performance over clinical judgment. Estimations of risk can be presented in a variety of formats, though the contemporary trend is toward empirical rather than categorical communication. Experts should be aware of the potential biases of juries and judges and tailor their communication responsively. Further, it is important to address common misconceptions regarding sexual offending when presenting risk testimony.

REFERENCES

Anderson, A., & Sample, L. (2008). Public awareness and action resulting from sex offender community notification laws. *Criminal Justice Policy Review, 19,* 371-396. https://doi.org/10.1177/0887403408316705

Babchishin, K. M., Hanson, R. K., & Blais, J. (2016). Less is more: Using Static-2002R subscales to predict violent and general recidivism among sexual offenders. *Sexual Abuse: Journal of Research and Treatment, 28*(3), 187-217. https://doi.org/10.1177/1079063215569544

Barak, A., Fisher, W., Belfry, S., & Lashambe, D. (1999). Sex, guys, and cyberspace: Effects of internet pornography and individual differences on men's attitudes toward women. *Journal of Psychology and Human Sexuality, 11*(1), 63-91. https://doi.org/10.1300/J056v11n01_04

Barbaree, H. E., Langton, C. M., & Peacock, E. J. (2006). The factor structure of static actuarial items: Its relation to prediction. *Sex Abuse, 18*(2), 207-226. https://doi.org/10.1177/107906320601800207

Baron, L. (1990). Pornography and gender equality: An empirical analysis. *The Journal of Sex Research, 27*(3), 363-380.

Bengtson, S., & Långström, N. (2007). Unguided clinical and actuarial assessment of re-offending risk: A direct comparison with sex offenders in Denmark. *Sexual Abuse: A Journal of Research and Treatment*, *19*(2), 135-153. https://doi.org/10.1177/107906320701900205

Boccaccini, M. T., Murrie, D. C., & Turner, D. B. (2014). Jurors' views on the value and objectivity of mental health experts testifying in sexually violent predator trials. *Behavioral Sciences and the Law, 32,* 483-495.

Boccaccini, M. T., Rice, A. K., Helmus, L. M., Murrie, D. C., & Harris, P. B. (2017). Field validity of Static-99/R scores in a statewide sample of 34,687 convicted sexual offenders. *Psychological Assessment, 29*(6), 611-623.

Boer, D. P., Hart, S. D., Kropp, P. R., & Webster, C. D. (1997). *Manual for the Sexual Violence Risk – 20: Professional guidelines for assessing risk of sexual violence.* The Mental Health, Law, and Policy Institute.

Buchanan, A., & Leese, M. (2001). Detention of people with dangerous severe personality disorders: A systemic review. *Lancet, 358,* 1955-1959.

Bureau of Justice Statistics. (2002). *Bureau of Justice Statistics 2002: At a Glance.* https://bjs.ojp.gov/content/pub/pdf/bjsg02.pdf

Bureau of Justice Statistics. (2003). *Compendium of Federal Justice Statistics 2003.* https://static.prisonpolicy.org/scans/bjs/cfjs03.pdf

Carlsmith, K., Monahan, J., & Evans, A. (2007). The function of punishment in the "civil" commitment of sexually violent predators. *Behavioral Sciences & the Law, 25,* 437-448. https://doi.org/10.1002/bsl.761

Comartin, E., Kernsmith, P., & Kernsmith, R. (2009). Sanctions for sex offenders: Fear and public policy. *Journal of Offender Rehabilitation, 48,* 605-619. https://doi.org/10.1080/10509670903196066

Craun, S. W., & Theriot, M. T. (2009). Misperceptions of sex offender perpetration: Considering the impact of sex offender registration. *Journal of Interpersonal Violence, 12,* 2057-2072. https://doi.org/10.1177/0886260508327706

Daubert v. Merrell Dow Pharmaceuticals, 509 U.S. 579, 113 S.Ct. 2786 (1993).

Davies, K. A. (1997). Voluntary exposure to pornography and men's attitudes toward feminism and rape. *The Journal of Sex Research, 34*(2), 131-137. https://doi.org/10.1080/00224499709551877

Denov, M. (2003). The myth of innocence: Sexual scripts and the recognition of child sexual abuse by female perpetrators. *Journal of Sex Research, 40,* 303-314. https://doi.org/10.1080/00224490309552195

Douard, J. (2007). Loathing the sinner, medicalizing the sin: Why sexually violent predator statutes are unjust. *International Journal of Law and Psychiatry, 30,* 36-48. https://doi.org/10.1016/j.ijlp.2006.04.004

Dworkin, A. (1981). *Men possessing women.* The Women's Press.

Epperson, D. L., Kaul, J. D., Huot, S., Goldman, R., & Alexander, W. (2003). Minnesota Sex Offender Screening Tool-Revised (MnSOST-R) technical paper: Development, validation, and recommended risk level cut scores. https://rsoresearch.files.wordpress.com/2012/01/ia-state-study.pdf

Federal Rules of Evidence, Rule 702. (2010).

Ferguson, C. J., & Hartley, R. D. (2009). The pleasure is momentary . . . the expense damnable? The influence of pornography on rape and sexual assault. *Aggression and Violent Behavior, 14*(5), 323-329. https://doi.org/10.1016/j.avb.2009.04.008

Frye v. United States, 293 F. 1013 (D.C. Cir 1923).

Fuselier, D. A., Durham, R. L., & Wurtele, S. K. (2002). The child sexual abuser: Perceptions of college students and professionals. *Sex Abuse, 14*(3), 271-280. https://doi.org/10.1177/107906320201400306

Galeste, M. A., Fradella, H. F., & Vogel, B. (2012). Sex offender myths in print media: Separating fact from fiction in U.S. newspapers. *Western Criminology Review, 13,* 4-24.

Gentry, C. S. (1991). Pornography and rape: An empirical analysis. *Deviant Behavior, 12,* 277-288.

Guy, L. S., & Edens, J. F. (2003). Juror decision-making in a mock sexually violent predator trial: Gender differences in the impact of divergent types of expert testimony. *Behavioral Sciences & the Law, 21,* 215-237. https://doi.org/10.1002/bsl.529

Hanson, R. K. (2002). Recidivism and age follow-up data from 4,673 sexual offenders, *Journal of Interpersonal Violence, 17*(10), 1046-1062.

Hanson, R. K., Babchisin, K. M., Helmus, L. M., Thornton, D., & Phenix A. (2017). Communicating the results of criterion referenced prediction measures: Risk categories for the Static-99R and Static-2002R sexual offender risk assessment tools. *Psychological Assessment,* 29(5), 582-597.

Hanson, R. K., & Bussière, M. (1998). Predicting relapse: A meta-analysis of sexual offender recidivism studies. *Journal of Consulting and Clinical Psychology, 66,* 348-362. https://doi.org/10.1037/0022-006X.66.2.348

Hanson, R. K., Gordon, A., Harris, A., Marques, J., Murphy, W., Quinsey, V., & Seto, M. (2002). First report of the collaborative outcome data project on the effectiveness of psychological treatment for sex offenders. *Sexual Abuse, 14*(2), 169-194. https://doi.org/10.1177/107906320201400207

Hanson, R. K., & Morton-Bourgon, K. (2006). The characteristics of persistent sexual offenders: A meta-analysis of recidivism studies. *Journal of Consulting and Clinical Psychology, 73,* 1154-1163. https://doi.org/10.1037/0022-006X.73.6.1154

Hanson, R. K., & Morton-Bourgon, K. E. (2009). The accuracy of recidivism risk assessments for sexual offenders: A meta-analysis of 118 prediction studies. *Psychological Assessment, 21*(1), 1-21.

Hare, R. D. (2003). *The Hare Psychopathy Checklist–Revised* (2nd ed.). Multi-Health Systems.

Hawes, S. W., Boccaccini, M. T., & Murrie, D. C. (2013). Psychopathy and the combination of psychopathy and sexual deviance as predictors of sexual recidivism: Meta-analytic findings using the Psychopathy Checklist–Revised. *Psychological Assessment, 25*(1), 233-243.

Helmus, L. M., & Babchishin, K. M. (2017). Primer on risk assessment and the statistics used to evaluate its accuracy. *Journal of Black Psychology, 44*(1), 169-194. https://doi.org/10.1177/0095798420928194

Helmus, L., Hanson, R. K., Thornton, D., Babchishin, K. M., & Harris, A. J. R. (2012). Absolute recidivism rates predicted by Static-99R and Static-2002R sex offender risk assessment tools vary across samples: A meta-analysis. *Criminal Justice and Behavior, 39,* 1148-1171. https://doi.org/10.1177/0093854812443648

Hilton, N. Z., Carter, A. M., Harris, G. T., & Sharpe, A. J. B. (2008). Does using nonnumerical terms to describe risk aid violence risk communication? Clinician agreement and decision making. *Journal of Interpersonal Violence, 23*(2), 171-188. https://doi.org/10.1177/0886260507309337

Janus, E. S. (2006). Failure to protect: America's sexual predator laws and the rise of the preventive state. *Criminal Justice Review, 33,* 255-256. https://doi.org/10.1177/0734016808316821

Jung, S., Pham, A., & Ennis, L. (2013). Measuring the disparity of categorical risk among various sex offender risk assessment measures. *Journal of Forensic Psychiatry & Psychology, 24*(3), 353-370. https://doi.org/10.1080/14789949.2013.806567

Katz-Schiavone, S., Levenson, J., Ackerman, A., & Jay, M. (2008). Myths and facts about sexual violence: Public perceptions and implications for prevention. *Journal of Criminal Justice and Popular Culture, 15*(3), 291-311.

Kelley, S. M., Ambroziak, G., Thornton, D., & Barahal, R. M. (2020). How do professionals assess sexual recidivism risk? An updated survey of practices. *Sexual Abuse, 32*(1), 3-29.

Kernsmith, P. D., Comartin, E., Craun, S. W., & Kernsmith, R. M. (2009). The relationship between sex offender registry utilization and awareness. *Sexual Abuse: Journal of Research and Treatment, 21*(2), 181-193. https://doi.org/10.1177/1079063209332235

Kim, B., Benekos, P., & Merlo, A. (2016). Sex offender recidivism revisited: Review of recent meta-analyses on the effects of sex offender treatment. *Trauma, Violence & Abuse, 17*(1), 105-117. https://doi.org/10.1177/1524838014566719

King, L. L., & Roberts, J. R. (2017). The complexity of public attitudes toward sex crimes. *Victims & Offenders, 12*(1), 71-89.

Krauss, D. A. & Scurich, N. (2013). Risk assessment in the law: Legal admissibility, scientific validity, and some disparities between research and practice. *Behavioral Sciences and the Law, 31,* 215-229.

Kutchinsky, B. (1991) Pornography and rape: Theory and practice? Evidence from crime data in four countries where pornography is easily available. *International Journal of Law & Psychiatry, 14*(1-2), 47-64. https://doi.org/10.1016/0160-2527(91)90024-H

Langton, C. M., Barbaree, H. E., Seto, M. C., Peacock, E. J., Harkins, L., & Hansen, K. T. (2007). Actuarial assessment of risk for reoffense among adult sex offenders: Evaluating the predictive accuracy of the Static-2002 and five other instruments. *Criminal Justice and Behavior, 34*(1), 37-59.

Leach, C., Stewart, A., & Smallbone, S. (2015). Testing the sexually abused-sexual abuser hypothesis: A prospective longitudinal birth cohort study. *Child Abuse & Neglect, 51,* 144-143. https://doi.org/10.1016/j.chiabu.2015.10.024

Levenson, J. S. (2003). Policy interventions designed to combat sexual violence: Community notification and civil commitment. *Journal of Child Sexual Abuse: Research, Treatment, & Program Innovations for Victims, Survivors, & Offenders, 12*(3-4), 17-52. https://doi.org/10.1300/J070v12n03_02

Levenson, J. S., Brannon, Y. N., Fortney, T., & Baker, J. (2007). Public perceptions about sex offenders and community protection policies. *Analyses of Social Issues and Public Policy (ASAP), 7*(1), 137-161.

Levenson, J. S., D'Amora, D. A., & Hern, A. L. (2007). Megan's Law and its impact on community re-entry for sex offenders. *Behavioral Sciences and the Law, 25,* 587-602.

Lieberman, M. D., Eisenberger, N. I., Crockett, M. J., Tom, S. M., Pfeifer, J. H., & Way, B. M. (2007). Putting feelings into words: Affect labeling disrupts amygdala activity in response to affective stimuli. *Psychological Science, 8*(5), 421-428. https://doi.org/10.1111/j.1467-9280.2007.01916.x

Linz, D., Paul, B., Land, K., Williams, J., & Ezell, M. (2004). An examination of the assumption that adult businesses are associated with crime in surrounding areas: A secondary effects study in Charlotte, North Carolina. *Law & Society Review, 38,* 69-104. https://doi.org/10.1111/j.0023-9216.2004.03801003.x

Mancini, C., & Mears, D. (2010). To execute or not to execute? Examining public support for capital punishment of sex offenders. *Journal of Criminal Justice, 38,* 959-968. https://doi.org/10.1016/j.jcrimjus.2010.06.013

Marett, C. P., & Mossman, D. (2017). From baseball to courtroom: How baseball explains risk assessment. *Psychiatric Annals, 47*(9), 443-448.

Mears, D., Mancini, C., Gertz, M., & Bratton, J. (2008). Sex crimes, children, and pornography: Public views and public policy. *Crime & Delinquency, 54,* 532-559. https://doi.org/10.1177/0011128707308160

Melton, G. B., Petrila, J., Poythress, N. G., Slobogin, C., Otto, R. K., Mossman, D., & Condie, L. O. (2018). *Psychological evaluations for the courts: A handbook for mental health professionals and lawyers* (4th ed.). Guilford Press.

Mendel, M. P. (1995). *The male survivor: The impact of sexual abuse*. Sage.

Mills, J. F., & Kroner, D. G. (2006). The effect of discordance among violence and general recidivism risk estimates on predictive accuracy. *Criminal Behaviour and Mental Health, 16*(3), 155-166. https://doi.org/10.1002/cbm.623

Monahan, J., & Silver, E. (2003). Judicial decision thresholds for violence risk management. *International Journal of Forensic Mental Health, 2,* 1-6.

Mossman, D. (1994). Predictions of violence: Being accurate about accuracy. *Journal of Consulting and Clinical Psychology, 62*(4), 783-792. https://doi.org/10.1037/0022-006X.62.4.783

Murrie, D. C., Boccaccini, M. T., Caperton, J., & Rufino, K. (2012). Field validity of the Psychopathy Checklist-Revised in sex offender risk assessment. *Psychological Assessment, 24*(2), 524-529.

Neal, T. M., & Grisso, T. (2014). Assessment practices and expert judgment methods in forensic psychology and psychiatry: An international snapshot. *Criminal Justice & Behavior, 41*(12), 1406-1421.

Otto, R. K., & Petrila, J. (2006). Admissibility of expert testimony regarding recidivism in sexually violent predator proceedings. In A. Schlank (Ed.), *The sexual predator law and public policy, clinical practice* (Vol. 3; pp. 2-1–2-11). Civic Research Press.

Ozkan, T., Clipper, S. J., Piquero, A. R., Baglivio, M., & Wolff, K. (2020). Predicting sexual recidivism. *Sexual Abuse, 32*(4), 375-399.

Pickett, J., Mancini, C., & Mears, D. (2013). Vulnerable victims, monstrous offenders, and unmanageable risk: Explaining public opinion on the social control of sex crime. *Criminology, 51*(3), 729-759. https://doi.org/10.1111/1745-9125.12018

Prescott, J. J., & Rockoff, J. E. (2011). Do sex offender registration and notification laws affect criminal behavior? *Journal of Law and Economics, 54*(1), 161-206.

Quinn, J. F., Forsyth, C. J., & Quinn, C. M. (2004). Societal reaction to sex offenders: A review of the origins and results of the myths surrounding their crimes and treatment amenability. *Deviant Behavior, 25*(3), 215-232. https://doi.org/10.1080/01639620490431147

Rowlands, M. T., Palk, G., & Young, R. M. (2017). Psychological and legal aspects of dangerous sex offenders: A review of the literature. *Psychiatry, Psychology and Law, 24*(6), 812-824.

Sample, L., & Bray, T. (2006). Are sex offenders dangerous? *Criminology & Public Policy, 3*(1), 59-82. https://doi.org/10.1111/j.1745-9133.2003.tb00024.x

Sample, L., & Kadleck, C. (2008). Sex offender laws legislators' accounts of the need for policy. *Criminal Justice Policy Review, 19,* 40-62. https://doi.org/10.1177/0887403407308292

Sandler, J. C., Freeman, N. J., & Socia, K. M. (2008). Does a watched pot boil? A time-series analysis of New York State's sex offender registration and notification law. *Psychology, Public Policy, and Law, 14*(4), 284-302. https://doi.org/10.1037/a0013881

Schiavone, S. K., & Jeglic, E. L. (2009). Public perception of sex offender social policies and the impact on sex offenders. *International Journal of Offender Therapy and Comparative Criminology, 53*(6), 679-695. https://doi.org/10.1177/0306624X08323454

Schmucker, M., & Lösel, F. (2015). The effects of sexual offender treatment on recidivism: An international meta-analysis of sound quality evaluations. *Journal of Experimental Criminology, 11*(4), 597-630. https://doi.org/10.1007/s11292-015-9241-z

Scurich, N., & John, R. S. (2011). The effect of framing actuarial risk probabilities on involuntary commitment decisions. *Law and Human Behavior, 35,* 83-91. https://doi.org/10.1007/s10979-010-9218-4

Shao, L., & Li, J. (2006). *The effect of sex offender registration laws on rape victimization.* Unpublished Manuscript.

Singh, J. P. (2013). Predictive validity performance indicators in violence risk assessment: A methodological primer. *Behavioral Sciences & the Law, 31*(1), 8-22. https://doi.org/10.1002/bsl.2052

Skeem, J. L., & Monahan, J. (2011). Current directions in violence risk assessment. *Current Directions in Psychological Science, 20*(1), 38-42. https://doi.org/10.1177/0963721410397271

Slovic, P., Monahan, J., & MacGregor, D. G. (2000). Violence risk assessment and risk communication: The effects of using actual cases, providing instruction, and employing probability versus frequency formats. *Law and Human Behavior, 24*(3), 271-296. https://doi.org/10.1023/A:1005595519944

Sundt, J. L., Cullen, F. T., Applegate, B. K., & Turner, M. G. (1998). The tenacity of the rehabilitative ideal revisited: Have attitudes toward offender treatment changed? *Criminal Justice and Behavior, 25*(4), 426-442. https://doi.org/10.1177/0093854898025004002

Temple, J., Choi, H. J., Reuter, T., Wolfe, D., Taylor, C., Madigan, S., & Scott, L. (2017). Childhood corporal punishment and future perpetration of physical dating violence. *The Journal of Pediatrics, 194,* 233-237. https://doi.org/10.1016/j.jpeds.2017.10.028

Tewksbury, R., & Jennings, W. G. (2010). Assessing the impact of sex offender registration and community notification on sex-offending trajectories. *Criminal Justice and Behavior, 37*(5), 570-582. https://doi.org/10.1177/0093854810363570

Tewksbury, R., Jennings, W., & Zgoba, K. (2012). A longitudinal examination of sex offender recidivism prior to and following the implementation of SORN. *Behavioral Sciences & the Law, 30,* 308-328. https://doi.org/10.1002/bsl.1009

Turner, D. B. (2011). *Juror perceptions of the influence of expert witness testimony in Texas sexually violent predator civil commitment hearings* [Doctoral dissertation). Retrieved from ProQuest Dissertations and Theses. (Accession Order No. 3484779)

Veysey, B., Zgoba, K., & Dalessandro, M. (2008). A preliminary step towards evaluating the impact of Megan's Law: A trend analysis of sexual offenses in New Jersey from 1985 to 2005. *Justice Research and Policy, 10,* 1-18. https://doi.org/10.3818/JRP.10.2.2008

Zimring, F. E., Piquero, A. R., Jennings, W., & Hays, S.A. (2007). The predictive power of juvenile sex offending: Evidence from the Second Philadelphia Birth Cohort Study (June 21, 2007). http://dx.doi.org/10.2139/ssrn.995918

30

Man's Search for Redemption: Masculinity, Gay Identity, and the Psychology of Incarceration

By the late Gerald "Jerry" Myers

Edited by Judith Skillings With an Introduction and Post-Epilogue by Frederick L. Peterson, Jr.

What is to give light must endure burning.
Viktor Frankl

AN INTRODUCTION

In the spring of 2019, a colleague handed me a package with a manuscript somebody had sent him. He was up-to-his-ears busy and asked if I would be interested in looking over what the sender had in mind. I took the package and set it on my ever-growing "to-read" pile. Weeks later, I opened it up to find a manuscript and letter that were going to change how I taught my courses at Wright State University. The letter was written by a man named Mr. Jerry Myers and explained that he had earned a college degree, conducted research on sex offenders, and had written a book – all while he was in prison. Through the help of a friend and volunteer, Karen Thimmes, Mr. Myers would send written pages to Karen who would word-process them into an extraordinary story, which is now the abbreviated chapters before you. The original manuscript was well over 100 pages and beyond the scope of this book. However, I believe Mr. Myers' story has strong value for students in professional training, mental health providers, and law enforcement professionals. Hence, a shortened version of his story is included here with an invitation to any reader to contact me to get a copy of his full manuscript.

I believe Mr. Myers' story is important to be published for several wide-ranging reasons which the author did not have any intent of addressing. This point may be one of the leading reasons the story is so remarkable. Mr. Myers did not set out to make any grand commentary about contemporary social issues. He simply described the details of his life and in doing so, challenged stereotypical thinking many people have regarding those labeled sex offenders as well as those who serve time in prison.

It is my hope that the public in general can gain insight to themselves from his narrative, but this hope may be overoptimistic and unrealistic. At first, the average individual may not want to identify with Mr. Myers or recognize his basic human needs such as to be safe, to belong, and to love as well as be loved (needs we all have). What I am certain of is the value this story has to individuals in clinical training within the helping professions. Going inside Mr. Myers' narrative provides a window into the workings of an individual divided within himself – to some degree a common experience within most of us; and an individual who wants to change for the better in some physical, emotional, or spiritual way – again, like most of us.

Mr. Myers has written a memoir, *Man's Search for Redemption*, which is by far the most interesting manuscript I have read in several years. Because his entire memoir is beyond the scope of this book, only the essential core story is presented here. It captures a fascinating combination of interweaving themes which comprise the social fabric of America in the later 20th century. These themes describe:

- What it was like growing up gay during the 1950s when Senator Joe McCarthy not only led the charge of the *Red Scare* search for communists in the U.S. government but concurrently manufactured the *Lavender Scare*, which was obsessed with identifying and excising homosexual individuals from government employment. What most Americans do not realize is that, while it took a decade to reel in the outrageous civil liberty violations of the Red Scare prong of McCarthyism, the silent majority of Americans allowed the Lavender Scare prong of McCarthyism to go unchecked for many decades. This memoir describes what it was like for a man with same-sex attraction to come to understand himself before there was any such thing as a public, positive gay identity.
- A fascinating mid-20th century point-of-view *study of gender* and the effects of a rigid and strongly enforced binary system. This memoir is a story of mid-century masculinity in America, in which a confused young man chose to fly into hyper-masculinity to become a "tough guy" who would never be questioned about his sexuality. Going to jail was worn as a badge of courage and revered by his peers.
- An inside perspective on the *psychology and sociology of incarceration*, with remarkable details of the "caste system" within American prisons and how those identified as sex offenders were routinely exposed to humiliating and extreme stressors. For example, prisoners identified as sex offenders routinely were paraded in front of the general prisoner population with cat calls and other humiliations as well as being subject to prisoner-on-prisoner violence with guards' tacit approval. Within this culture, Mr. Myers describes his struggle against his life-force being drained from him in prison, and his strategies to not only stay sane but improve his mind.
- An *activist-participant perspective on the first state-wide sex offender treatment program* in Ohio. Mr. Myers sought help for his need for treatment by writing scores of scholars and authorities in psychology and human behavior (including the likes of B. F. Skinner). When there were no treatment options in prison, Mr. Myers brought a "right to treatment" lawsuit against the Ohio prison system, earned a degree in psychology from Ohio University, and conducted original research on sex offenders. Mr. Myers was literally "part and parcel" of the birth of the field of sex offender treatment within Ohio prisons and was witness to the concurrent "Treatment Movement" that was sweeping across the country during the final decades of the 20th century.

I formed a partnership-of-sorts with Mr. Myers in which I agreed to contribute historical and professional context to *Man's Search for Redemption*. I became fully devoted to doing all I could to support the publication of his manuscript, as it is a value-added aspect of my work as a professor and therapist. I began using his manuscript for both academic and clinical purposes. I had my students read it for credit in my courses at Wright State University. I also had my clients read it for therapeutic benefit in my clinical practice. For example, below is an excerpt from my syllabus at Wright State University describing how I used his story as a learning experience:

Man's Search for Redemption: The Lavender Scare, the Development of a Gay Identity, and the Beginning of Sex Offender Treatment in Ohio. Read a private manuscript by an individual who served time in prison for his sex crimes. This is an opportunity to understand the psychology of both a sex offender as well as the psychology of incarceration. Report your responses to reading it, including what you learned and your emotional responses to his story. Submit a summary for 50 points.

Mr. Myers knows a great deal about struggling with personal demons and a subsequent search for redemption. *Man's Search for Redemption* refutes the widely held notions that sex offenders voluntarily choose to be attracted to minors, that they make no effort to change their attractions, that they are typically violent, and that the criminal justice system is fair to harshly punish them (even keeping them incarcerated beyond their court-ordered sentence, a process known as civil commitment).

Man's Search for Redemption refutes these notions by telling a surprising tale of a young boy's confusion regarding his own personal experiences of being sexually abused, hungering for a father to protect and guide him, becoming sexually fixated on teenage boys, and having a lifelong engagement with the justice system. He tries everything to feel better, from spending years as a street fighter to years of intensive psychotherapy. In a general sense, Mr. Myers' story is also one about the 21st century American male being fitted for his own personal strait jacket of cultural and emotional restraints affecting his masculinity, sexual expression, and his struggle for humanity.

Beyond the academic and therapeutic value of *Man's Search for Redemption,* my hope is for older baby boomers to relate to approaching their later stages of life and seeking redemption from whatever transgression they regret. This is a common experience as people age into their later years: To search for a path to redemption. Some do it through service to others, some through charitable giving, and some through writing a book like Mr. Myers. This is what Mr. Myers has accomplished and he knows that he can die confident that his life has greater meaning by leaving *Man's Search for Redemption* as his legacy.

Before ending this introduction to his book, it occurs to me that some may question the validity of the narrative you are about to read. Understandably so. After all, there is precedent for very articulate "con men" to weave a tale that puts themselves in a positive light. As one reads his story, there will be numerous occasions where it becomes apparent that he shares details regarding himself – unflattering and/or incriminating details that he could have excluded with the reader never knowing. These details may be hard for some to understand but they also make clearer the internal struggle Mr. Myers confronted every day.

It may be of value to know that steps were taken to examine the historical veracity of Mr. Myers' historical account. This was done through several means, including public records that were simple to verify (imprisonment records and sex offender registry). Of more importance is documentation relative to the details surrounding letters of correspondence and lawsuits. For example, he was able to supply a copy of the "Right to Treatment" lawsuit against the Governor of the State of Ohio (for the lack of specific sex offender treatment in Ohio prisons). This lawsuit was filed for him by two professors at the College of Law of The Ohio State University. In addition, I verified many details of Mr. Myers' story from information shared with me by his former therapists. Primary verification came from Mr. Theodore "Ted" Smith, retired from the Ohio Department of Corrections in 1996. Mr. Smith served as a psychologist in the prison and was 74 years old when I interviewed him. He remembered Mr. Myers very well and provided valuable historical context to where Mr. Myers spent so much of his adult life: Lima State Hospital for the Criminally Insane (he stated that the prison was a "snake pit," telling stories which would make one's skin crawl).

As many thousands of men find each day (across Ohio and the nation), the double stigma of being a felon as well as a sex offender made it exceedingly difficult for Mr. Myers to find employment as well as acceptance socially. His epilogue addressed this dilemma after his most recent release from incarceration in 2017. In this account, the members of a Columbus church exercised their right to be as fearful, bigoted, and discriminatory towards a 77-year-old man in poor health and in clear need of support.

It may also be of interest to readers to know that I have never met Mr. Myers and I never will. I only talked to him by phone. Our last conversation was during the start of the COVID-19 pandemic when he was experiencing a pulmonary emergency and was waiting for the paramedics to arrive. He is likely one of the 1 million+ Americans lost to the pandemic, although I have not been able to verify his cause of death. Like many Americans (including myself), some people stop making contact and are never heard from again.

I did not know him personally, professionally, nor was he a relative of mine or of anyone I know. I only knew him through the manuscript that found its way to me. I do know that I have been so moved by what I've read that I decided to do what I can to help have Mr. Myers' story be told. Those interested in his full manuscript can contact me to have it sent to them. It has been my privilege to have written this introduction to give some context to his story and include the following abbreviated version of his story within this text. It is my hope that you will see the humanity within and be moved as well.

Docpete, June 2022
Yellow Springs, Ohio
Kansas City, Missouri

Chapter One: My Father

My early life offered a hint of what was to come. Because my father had abandoned the family well before my birth in 1940, this left me with my mother and three older sisters in Old North Dayton for the first 7 years of my life. Deprived of my father's income, my mother had to apply for child welfare. That, plus my mother's reclusiveness, tended to set us off from our neighbors a bit.

All in all, life wasn't bad, though I was disturbed by my father's absence. Because I frequently compared my situation with that of other children in the area, I came to feel ashamed of being fatherless and told my first-grade classmates and teacher that my father was a war hero who had been killed blowing up a tank.

The adults in my family were too uncomfortable with sex to talk about it, and their discomfort with it conveyed the message that it was dirty or bad, something that shouldn't be thought about. My experience was like that of other American children, in that I was loaded with shame and guilt about my sexual impulses when I was very young, and thus forced underground, where I was left to grope at other children guiltily in the dark.

My life took an unexpected turn at age 7½ when my father showed up "out of the blue." Although I initially basked in the glory of finally having a father, I soon learned that I had three younger stepbrothers and a stepsister to compete with for my father's love. I was 9 when my mother decided to leave my father and take my sister Doris and me back to Dayton. Although I didn't know it until I was considerably older, my father shattered the three families he started over a period of many years by sexually abusing some of the young female family members. The whole experience of finally meeting my father at age 7½ and then losing him again at age 9 was traumatic, leaving me in a state of grief. During the first year back in Dayton, my mother, Doris, and I lived in cheap one-room space of a two-room apartment. It was hard times in cramped living quarters, and there was very little money for anything.

Intensifying the loss of my father, my mother went to work cleaning offices on the 4:30 pm - 1 am shift and became more socially withdrawn than ever. It was as if I had lost both parents. Mother also became increasingly verbally abusive of me. She was bitter over her failed marriage, and because I looked enough like my father to remind her of him, she took her bitterness out on me.

Our family situation improved in 1950 when we moved into a duplex. But I continued to feel inferior to most of the other children in Old North Dayton because, in addition to the verbal abuse I got from my mother, our family seemed to be one of the poorest in the area. This perception on my part came not only from the shabbiness of our house and furniture, but the fact that Mother was very thrifty – and stingy – with money. While my friends always seemed to have a refrigerator packed with Pepsi that could be taken freely, and parents who could give them money to go swimming on summer days, I saw pop only if I bought a bottle with my tiny weekly allowance. When I wanted to go swimming, I had to hustle the neighborhood for empty pop bottles to return for deposit. Perhaps my greatest shame was our small downstairs bathroom, which was unusual in that it had no sink or bathtub, and thus forced us to take turns closing off the kitchen, where we bathed at the sink.

After we moved to the duplex, my schoolwork improved slightly, and I managed to pass my classes, though I had little interest in academics. However, I stood out in speech class. My dramatic attention-seeking speeches never failed to provoke roaring laughter from my classmates and male teacher. I also excelled in all sports. Yet, by the early part of the sixth grade in late 1952, I had been placed at a desk in the rear corner of my classroom for disciplinary reasons, and my "incorrigibility" at school had come to the attention of the Board of Education. I also developed a record at the Juvenile Court for petty thievery type of offenses, including an arrest with another boy for stealing items from the glove compartments of neighborhood cars, and another for taking money from a woman's purse at a nearby church. At the request of my sister Virginia, my brother-in-law Fred attempted to counsel me about the thefts. While I politely listened to him, my private attitude was one of resentment of any man who tried to replace my father.

Chapter Two: A Conspiracy of Silence

While still 12, I had several sexual experiences, mostly with girls. I found them to be less than a big deal. A one-time encounter with a 16-year-old male cousin made a greater impression. When he began thrusting between my buttocks, I experienced some intense emotion even though the thrusting lasted less than a minute and there was no actual penetration. I would describe my feelings as intense pleasure as well as guilt, shame, and concern about what the pleasure meant.

This was 1953, when there were no visible gay role models because virtually all homosexuals were "in the closet." At the same time and somewhat contradictorily, U.S. Senator Joseph McCarthy was conducting his witch hunt, not only for Communist subversives in government, but also homosexuals in the State Department. Not that I had any awareness. In fact, the very word "homosexual" was largely taboo and couldn't be used on radio or television. Rather, the silence about, and invisibility of, other homosexuals effectively isolated me and made homosexuality seem incomprehensible, like it existed only in the secrecy of my depraved mind.

Desperate for information about sex, I began peeping into the bedroom windows of my male and female peers after dark. I also took a younger boy into my garage and performed oral sex on him, which is interesting because I had never seen or experienced oral sex. I also impulsively touched the crotch of a pre-school girl when I entered her yard across the alley from my house to retrieve my basketball. The next day, I was arrested by the police on the charge of "morals" for this latter incident and taken from my seventh-grade class to a juvenile detention home.

The detention home officials seemed to be at a loss for how to deal with me. Apparently fearful of tarnishing my innocence if they acknowledged that something sexual had happened, the juvenile staff opted to bury the matter. There was no counseling nor even any mention of the incident for which I had been arrested. But it was ignorance, not innocence, that they were preserving in me when they released me on probation two weeks later, saying simply, "Stay out of trouble!"

The incident that most revealed what I was experiencing at age 13 occurred one night when I found myself at home alone. In a trance-like state, I put on some of my sister's clothing. I proceeded to walk out of the house into the darkness as if I had a destination or purpose. However, after crossing the street and taking several steps down the sidewalk, it dawned on me that I could be recognized even in the dark. I quickly returned home, put the clothing back in my sister's drawer, and resumed my normal behavior.

During the year I was 14, I had a close friend named Ray who suggested that we steal his next-door neighbor's '47 Plymouth because he knew where the keys were kept. Our adventure turned out to be a fiasco after about 12 hours on the road. I fell asleep while driving and flipped the car over in the middle of the highway! Fortunately, we incurred only rug burns from the wreck, but the Georgia Highway Patrol spotted us trying to get away on the hillside and arrested us for auto theft.

In February 1955, I was sentenced to the Boys' Industrial School (B.I.S.) of Ohio. The school emphasized military discipline as a supposed means of rehabilitation. The key to the military regimen was an inmate monitor system in which the three toughest boys in each cottage were chosen to be monitors. Discipline usually consisted of standing silently at attention in the cottage basement with one's toes on a groove in the cement floor (called "stand-on-line"), and it wasn't unusual to see a monitor sucker-punch a boy for failing to keep an erect posture and to do so with the blessing of the cottage parent who sat at a desk near the line.

Although for most of my stay at B.I.S. I kept a low profile, I surprised myself one morning toward the end of my term when a monitor my size started harassing me in the steam room (restroom) and I impulsively threw a solid blow to his jaw that knocked him flat on his back. I jumped on top of him to continue my attack. Upon hearing the commotion in the steam room, the head monitor rushed to the scene, pulled me off his second-in-command, and ordered me to stand-on-line. I obeyed the order and got online, though not out of fear and with an unmistakable new pride.

It was in the spring of 1956 that I was paroled back to Old North Dayton to live with my mother and sister. As if trying to compensate for my heterosexual shortcomings, I pursued street-fighting with a vengeance, won several battles, and found myself being challenged by older males in Old North Dayton who felt that my growing reputation as a tough guy was overblown. In what turned out to be the climactic incident of the summer, a college athlete 3 years my senior came to the park one afternoon to challenge me. There was a brief flurry of punches but the fight ended quickly when I broke his jaw.

Chapter Three: A Self Divided

I was returned to B.I.S. for assault and battery. I became more aware of my attraction to the slightly built boys in the 12-15 age range. Plagued by doubts about my masculinity, I escaped from the reform school no sooner than I was returned there. They caught me before I got even 10 miles away.

I escaped again and made it back to Old North Dayton this time. My friends kept me hidden from the police, and after a couple of weeks, I went to stay with my sister Barb in Buffalo. When I arrived at Barb's house, she asked me if I'd be interested in trying my hand at boxing. I began training in downtown Buffalo six nights a week.

Before going to Buffalo, I was well aware that my father was living there. He was cool toward my pursuit of a boxing career and felt that I should get a job instead. But he had waited far too long to show an interest in me. His absence from my life over the years had left a deep, painful emptiness in me where love should have been, and I was unable to embrace him.

Partly because of the lack of acceptance and support from my father, I became restless and disillusioned with boxing. I abruptly left Buffalo without explanation. Two days later, I was arrested in Dayton and transported to B.I.S. I escaped from the school a third time and was spared a transfer to the dreaded Mansfield Reformatory only because I turned myself in. This time, I managed to stay at B.I.S. until I earned parole.

I eventually resumed hanging out with my old friends. Even though I enjoyed considerable popularity with my heterosexual peers, I wasn't always able to keep homosexual fantasies repressed. For that reason, I felt alienated underneath my façade. I found myself fantasizing about a pretty, younger, teen boy named Mike to whom I'd been attracted in reform school. I decided to seek him out.

To get the money necessary for a 200-mile trip to Warren, Ohio (where Mike lived), I stole some payroll checks and recruited a couple of neighborhood peers to assist me in passing them. I had no idea how Mike would respond to sexual overtures from me. Nevertheless, I justified the trip to my friends by telling them Mike could help us steal more checks in a city where we were unknown. We learned when we got there Mike was still in reform school. At that point, I had little choice but to follow through with the plan to steal more checks, even though in my mind, stealing checks was secondary to making contact with Mike.

Though we made it back to Dayton, we were arrested soon afterward. I was returned to B.I.S. for a third term as a juvenile but was released in May 1958 because I had reached my 18th birthday. I was now legally an adult, but a very unhappy one for reasons I only dimly understood. Looking back, I would characterize my pain as that of a terrified young gay boy who was trapped inside an emerging macho self who eventually predominated at the expense of younger boys in lopsided relationships. Only the macho streetfighter had access to other people, and I always felt a hollowness.

During the summer of 1959, I had sexual intercourse with a girl for the first time. While the experience was physically pleasurable, the relationship seemed to have no meaning to me other than being a means to prove my manhood. I was still 19 when Frank, a 15-year-old I had kissed once, came home from the boys' reform school. Another of my neighborhood peers, Jim, and I stole some checks, used them to buy a used car, and the three of us – Jim, Frank, and I, drove to California.

We rented an apartment in a suburb of Los Angeles. Even though the three of us shared the same bedroom at our South Pasadena apartment, I continued to pursue sexual relations with Frank at night when I thought Jim had fallen asleep. But Frank refused to take the passive role. He and I never once discussed what was going on between us or how we felt about it, and our relationship had become more a competition over who would conquer whom than the simple, harmonious romance I had envisioned back in Dayton. But given the rigid macho indoctrination that each of us had received in reform school, I'm not sure that anything less competitive could have been expected of us.

Jim returned home to Dayton. Now that Frank and I were alone, I wanted to start a life with him in California. On a Sunday afternoon shortly afterward, Frank and I prepared a meal together at the apartment. We broiled steaks, and I can still see Frank standing at the kitchen table mashing the potatoes I had peeled and cooked. When we had finished eating, Frank decided to take a nap, and I promptly joined him, though I was not able to sleep. Summoning all of my courage, I disregarded gender-role stereotypes for a moment and, with a sense of great urgency, performed oral sex on Frank. I felt tremendous relief at having gratified my desire, but when I returned home from work the next day. Frank was gone.

I had never felt lonelier and more isolated. Choked with shame and self-disgust, I packed my bags and drove east on U.S. Route 66 the following day. I returned to Dayton and the next thing I knew, I was looking up at a judge.

Chapter Four: Hiding the "Woman" Within

"You are hereby sentenced to serve the term prescribed by law, for burglary, in the Ohio State Reformatory at Mansfield," the judge said. "Perhaps you will use this period of time to rehabilitate yourself, Mr. Myers." That hypocritical proposition about rehabilitation was still ringing in my ears when I got my first glimpse of the reformatory. A few brisk steps and I was inside the formidable walls.

On my 2nd day at the adult reformatory, I was one of a company of about 30 newcomers marched to the administration area for orientation classes. Various prison officials lectured us on how to get along in prison. A major theme was that an inmate's ability to follow institutional rules reflected his readiness to live a law-abiding life on the outside and hence his readiness for parole. "If you want to get along here, obey the rules," one official told us. "You'll get out that much sooner."

However, if the goal was to encourage respect for the law, Capt. Dyer, one of the speakers, was the worst possible role model. Capt. Dyer was the most corrupt official at the institution. For the right number of cigarettes or a $5 bill, one could buy the cellmate of his choice. For the same price, one could buy a desirable job assignment. The actual lesson, then, was that rules were not to be taken seriously. At least not if you had cigarettes or cash money to put on the table. Just don't get caught when you break a rule!

Yet it was neither the ghastly physical facilities nor the corruption that had the most brutalizing effect on me. It was the fact that, in an all-male prison population, definitions of masculinity shift to an extreme position. The definitions, imported from the outside culture, shift to the degree of causing victimization. Fights over an inmate's perceived slight to his manhood by another inmate were common, and not long after I was assigned to a job in the tailor shop, a young co-worker buried a pair of scissors in the chest of an older inmate who'd been pressuring him for sex.

I couldn't let anyone know of the gnawing loneliness I felt, but it led me to pay Capt. Dyer's clerk to move a 17-year-old I'd known at B.I.S. into my cell. Ernie was of somewhat small stature with a slender adolescent physique that had me mesmerized, and although I had no reason to believe he was homosexually inclined, I wanted him as my cellmate, nevertheless. I believed that his mere physical presence would make life in a steel cage more bearable, and there was a possibility I might be able to seduce him. But despite his slight build, Ernie was streetwise and tough, and it eventually became clear that he wasn't about to succumb to passivity in any sexual liaison. The only possibility of having an encounter with him was if I were to be passive myself.

But unlike the situation with Frank in California, there were potentially grave consequences for taking a passive sexual role in Mansfield. If caught, the passive partner (but not the active one) was segregated on a special range exclusively for homosexuals who were, in effect, put on display to the general inmate population.

Despite my awareness of the potentially horrific consequences, I became emotionally attached to Ernie and increasingly more willing to risk being sexually passive with him. Indeed, I became unable to resist touching him when I saw him sleeping in undershorts after lights-out, which caused him to move to another cell.

Just as Ernie was moving out of my cell, Frank showed up at the reformatory, and to my surprise, blatantly offered himself to me sexually to become my cellmate. I had him moved in with me, but even though I took the active or penetrator's role with him in bed that night, the experience was emotionally empty and lacking in excitement. This was no doubt because I was still emotionally attached to Ernie, but in addition, Frank simply didn't have the powerful effect on me that he'd had in California nearly 2 years prior. He had lost some of his youthful beauty and become somewhat hardened and cold. Additionally, he seemed to have a reputation for being homosexual among inmates he'd done time with in juvenile institutions, and I feared that being closely associated with him might make the inmates view me as homosexual also. So, when he was put in the hole for some misbehavior at his prison job the very next day, I decided not to have him moved back to my cell. Ironically, he got into the boxing tournament after his release from the hole, and with a killer instinct I seemed to have lost, he won the featherweight championship.

The 2 years and 2 months that I spent in Mansfield were otherwise uneventful. I got into only one fist fight during this period and won it easily. I was certainly not rehabilitated, as that would have required recognizing and treating my gender-identity conflict, emotional detachment, and my obsessive attraction to adolescent males.

Chapter Five: Eliminating the "Woman" Within

In June 1962, I was paroled back to my mother in Old North Dayton and found work as a city truck driver. My social life didn't change much from what it had been before my stretch in Mansfield. I continued to hang around the same Old North Dayton boys with whom I'd grown up. After about 4 months on parole, I met Gaile, an 18-year-old male youth who lived only a few blocks away. It seemed too good to be true – an attractive young man I'd fallen in love with was actually reciprocating my love! While walking down a dark street between bars, I stopped, turned, and kissed Gaile.

We then went straight to his house, upstairs to his bedroom, and into bed. As if following a script from my dreams about how our love should be expressed, Gaile automatically assumed a passive position on his stomach and waited for me. It was a long wait, for I found myself paralyzed by anxiety and sexually dysfunctional. Realizing that I was unable to perform the role of "the man," I felt humiliated. Things were never the same between us after that night. Although we continued to feel a closeness for months and even years, Gaile adopted a new pattern of behavior in which he would entice me, then reject me.

At the same time, I learned that he had two girlfriends who stopped by to have sex with him periodically. One night, Gaile, his hetero friend Bill, and I went to a dance hall in a neighborhood where Gaile used to live. I was drunk, and for some reason Gaile and Bill began bragging to Gaile's former friends about how tough I was. Their local tough guy eventually rose to the bait, and, apparently sober, had no trouble landing a solid blow that knocked me down. Amazingly, I picked myself up off the floor, and fired a straight right to his head that knocked him down. I went on to hit the security cop who was trying to stop the fight and knocked him down! About 5 minutes later, I was arrested by two armed deputies and taken to the local jail for assault and battery on a peace officer.

I was sentenced to 6 months in jail for the assault and battery, and while serving that sentence, I became concerned that this violent incident might result in my parole being revoked and my being returned to the reformatory. Seeing a vague connection between my sexual self-image and my propensity to get into trouble with the law, I decided to write a letter to my parole officer (P.O.) stating that I believed I was homosexual and that my homosexuality was the cause of all my troubles.

In this mid-1963 environment, my P.O. helped me stay out of jail by referring me to the Adult Psychiatric Clinic in Dayton, Ohio. Ultimately, my case was assigned to a psychiatric social worker named Jett. Mr. Jett and I began weekly therapy sessions that would continue for nearly 2 years. I became enchanted with an idea of being transformed into a "normal" heterosexual man.

About this same time, I met Paulette. She managed to initiate a relationship with me. During the early months, I could take her or leave her. Paulette made sure that we got together at least once a week, and almost invariably, we spent the night at a motel having sex. I thought it was kind of neat having a pretty, young girl interested in me. The sexual relations with her made me feel more like a man, since I believed that to be masculine was to have sexual desire only for women.

I gradually developed feelings for Paulette and declared my love for her. It was as close as I'd ever been to feeling like an ordinary person and as if I was on equal footing with my hetero peers. During this period, I helped to raise Paulette's daughter, a toddler who was a delight to interact with. We were a little family, and I believed that this new lifestyle had restored my sexual health.

I had been in therapy at the clinic and in a relationship with Paulette for a year when Frank was released from the reformatory. His release was immediately threatening to me because of the possibility of his revealing my homosexuality. He wanted me to help him get some money to send to his ex-lover in the reformatory, and to appease him, I assisted him in breaking into a local restaurant. We were apprehended by a policeman after exiting the restaurant and then put in jail on the charge of breaking and entering.

In January of 1965, the court sent me to the Lima State Hospital in Lima, Ohio, for 30 days of observation to determine whether or not I had a conscience and was amenable to rehabilitation. Although their finding was that I was amenable to treatment, the court rejected the hospital's recommendation of outpatient therapy and sentenced me to 1-15 years. Therefore, I ended up in London Reformatory, a medium-security prison in London, Ohio. My time at London certainly seemed to pass by slowly and without anything noteworthy happening, other than a visit from Paulette to tell me that our relationship was over. What could I say?

Chapter Six: A Complete Split

After only a year, I was paroled from the London prison just prior to my 26th birthday, and I left that institution determined to be a heterosexual man. I again lived with my mother and grandmother in Old North Dayton. Almost immediately, I got a job as a route salesman for Mechanic's Uniform Rental. I was strongly motivated to stay out of trouble with the law and to fit into society, though questions about human sexuality lingered in my thoughts.

Late one night toward the end of summer in 1966, I was alone at an East Dayton bar that featured go-go dancers. My purpose for being there was to meet a young woman I could pick up and take to a motel for the night. This was what a man was supposed to do. I recall having an unusually clear sense of being "out of my element" in this setting and decided to leave the bar.

When I got into my car in the parking lot, I had only a vague idea of what I was about to do. I simply started fantasizing about boys I'd been attracted to in reform school and began combing the streets of this East Dayton neighborhood for such a boy. I found one and invited him to come with me. He readily accepted my invitation, jumped into my car, and we sped off.

I couldn't stop myself, but as I reached across the car seat toward the boy, my arm stopped in mid-air, visibly shaking as I fought against the urge. Noting my nervousness, the boy said, "I've been out with men before!" as if he were telling me to relax. My hand then dropped down on him, and I felt great relief with a wave of emotion coming over me.

This was the first time as an adult man that I had sexual relations with a minor adolescent male, but certainly not the last. At the time, I believed that this was the way it had to be. I and the Adult Psychiatric Clinic had missed an opportunity to unify me, to help me help myself make my sexuality an integral and wholesome part of my being. That missed opportunity was not without consequence. By continuing to view my homosexual desires as a disease during nearly 2 years of "therapy," I remained split and may have even deepened what I saw as my split between "healthy heterosexuality" and an "unhealthy homosexuality." During the year of 1967 and beyond, I continued to classify myself as heterosexual and to maintain my position in the world of my heterosexual peers. To the extent that I acknowledged the encounters with male hustlers, I saw them as nothing more than a temporary fill-in for the woman I had not yet found.

My occasional secret excursions to East Dayton turned into episodic sexual compulsions that I could not control. At these times, I seemed to suddenly switch from one state of consciousness to another. In early 1968, I impulsively picked up a 15-year-old boy I saw walking down the street. After we drove off, I reached over and touched the boy's crotch, which offended or frightened him enough to make him jump out of the car while it was still moving. He then memorized my license number and reported the incident to the police.

Within about 24 hours, I was arrested. Word of my arrest and the nature of the charge got around to my peers in Old North Dayton. Once I was released on bond, I found some of my closest friends pulling back from me, and it was extremely hurtful.

I was sentenced to Lima State Hospital as a sex offender. I was fortunate to have a man named Jim Seitz as my psychotherapist. One of my earliest encounters with Jim was when he came on the ward one morning and unexpectedly walked into the room where I may have been overly harsh with another patient. I can′t remember what else was said at that point, but he was probably focusing on my macho façade. He walked over to where I was sitting, put his hand on my shoulder and said, "What's the matter? Do you think it's unmanly to have feelings?" I don't think any therapeutic maneuver had ever hit me more squarely between the eyes, and the second I felt Jim's hand on my shoulder and heard his words, tears came pouring down my cheeks. It was an emotional moment, and I was impressed by how quickly and skillfully Jim had gotten through my defenses.

I was returned to the Dayton court for a hearing in January 1970 and was granted probation. It was a great relief to have been spared prison. However, within about 2 weeks of my release, I found myself experiencing a high level of anxiety about the possibility of resuming my sexual behavior with boys. It was pretty scary, and I decided to make a long-distance phone call to Jim in Lima. Jim drove down to Dayton that weekend to meet with me. Although I appreciated his "above and beyond call-of-duty" efforts, I had sex with another teen hustler before the week was out. When Jim heard of this relapse on his next trip to Dayton, he acknowledged the compulsive nature of the problem and remarked, "You're a slave to your past conditioning."

Over the next several weeks, he gave me a series of homework assignments, such as wearing a rubber band around my wrist and snapping it hard against my skin each time I had a fantasy of a boy, thereby interrupting the obsessive fantasies and hopefully my overt sexual behavior as well. Another assignment was to interrupt the inappropriate fantasies by shouting the word "Stop!" aloud. Still another was a masturbatory reconditioning technique in which I was to masturbate to fantasies of adolescent boys but switch to fantasies of adult women at the point of orgasm, using Playboy magazine to stimulate the latter and thus reinforce sexual fantasies of women. However, none of these classical and operant conditioning methods were effective, and I was still unable to go beyond about 2 weeks without having sex with an adolescent male.

I believe that the failure of these behavioral intervention methods only added to my feelings of helplessness and defeat. And the failure baffled Jim, possibly because the way in which my compulsion had developed confounded the reward/punishment laws of learning enshrined in both psychology and common sense. At that point in my life, I was once again socially isolated and lonely. My sense of worth as a human being was nearly nonexistent.

Chapter Seven: A Father Figure

When the various strategies failed to curtail my sexual activity with minor adolescent boys, Jim arranged for me to consult with Dr. Elizabeth Wales, a renowned behavioral psychologist and sex educator at the local medical school. Dr. Wales opened the discussion by saying, "You've got quite a friend here," in reference to Jim, and I replied simply, "I know." I was well aware that Jim was a friend and that I'd be hard put to find another person who'd go to so much trouble to help me. He had become like a father to me. Dr. Wales recommended that I get myself admitted to one of the few behavior modification hospitals in the country. I responded to her suggestion by saying that I didn't want to lose my freedom, and she said, "What freedom?" – obviously concurring with Jim that I was a slave to my past conditioning.

I called the following day, only to find that the hospital treated only psychotics and the mentally retarded, not sex offenders. When I told Jim what the hospital had said, he indicated that I might have to move to Lima if I wanted him to remain my therapist. It was in May 1971, that I was granted permission to move to Lima and live under Jim's supervision. Jim had a halfway house for sex offenders who'd been released from Lima State Hospital and who sincerely wished to live within the law.

My sexual fantasies of adolescent boys were rampant, and the more I made them forbidden, the more compulsive they became. Jim had devised what he called a "shock box" to enable him to carry out a crude form of aversion therapy. During treatment sessions, Jim repeatedly paired my obsessive fantasies of adolescent boys with an unpleasant electric shock with the goal of conditioning me to experience anxiety each time I had such a fantasy. We had at least two therapy sessions per week for a period of 8-10 weeks.

The aversion therapy didn't affect me much, though I kept fantasies of boys suppressed for about 4 weeks after the therapy ended. Then, while walking through a nearby park, I seduced a boy, giving him oral sex behind some bushes. This was an innocent boy, meaning he wasn't a hustler or someone actively seeking sex, and he was only 14 years old. When I told Jim what I'd done, he grounded me and informed the Dayton court of my behavior. While waiting to hear back from the court, he called a house meeting to deal with me, and I was harshly confronted about my sexual behavior. I recall feeling tremendous shame and self-loathing during the confrontation, but I also recall experiencing confusion about what people expected of me.

Both Jim and Dr. Wales had indicated that I was a slave to my past conditioning. If I was a slave, then nothing I did would make a difference. So why do anything at all?

I was allowed to remain at the half-way house, but was still not permitted to leave the premises unless accompanied by another adult. As Christmas of 1971 approached, there was talk among the residents about having a Christmas Eve party at the house. Scant few females showed up. But a rather plain-looking woman in her middle 20s, along with one of her girlfriends, finally arrived and I put some suave heterosexual role-playing into action, talking, drinking, and dancing with the young woman in the living room.

Around 3 a.m., the woman and I left the house for her apartment, where we had sexual relations. However, the experience left me feeling just as unhappy, just as empty, and dissatisfied as I had been before the party. We must've dozed off for a while after the sex, but I remember lying in bed fixated on the nearby photo of the woman's two young sons sometime after daybreak. While driving the woman's car to the store for cigarettes, I began to experience sexual fantasies again. My trip to the store was uneventful, but while returning, I seemed to lapse into a fugue-like state and began combing the streets for an adolescent boy to have sex with. And I found one. After he got in the car, I had no sooner persuaded the boy to let me unbutton his jeans when a carload of his adult male relatives pulled up in front of us, blocking me from driving off. I was arrested by the Lima police within about 30 minutes.

My actions had hurt Jim. He incurred considerable expense throughout that period and risked his reputation as a psychologist by starting a halfway house in his own community to give people like me a chance at life. All those selfless acts on Jim's part taught me more about love than I was ready to incorporate into my behavior and daily living at that point. I could feel it but didn't know how to utilize it. Rather, I single-handedly brought the wrath of the community down on the man who'd been like a father to me by committing a sex crime on Christmas Day. Because of my actions, I would be incarcerated for the next 7½ years, first at Lima State Hospital and then at the state prison at Chillicothe. At Lima, Ted Smith would be my therapist this time around instead of Jim.

Even though I could see Jim's hurt and knew that I had messed up big-time, I had no idea of what to do about it. But I felt that I had to do something. I sought help from the top experts in the world as I was convinced I had to "go big" and show Jim (and myself) that I was committed to change. I decided to ask for help by writing B. F. Skinner (at Harvard) and Hans J. Eysenck (at the University of London in the UK), two of the most distinguished behavioral psychologists in the world. I did not have any sustained correspondence from my efforts, although I spent the next 3 years writing to dozens of behavioral therapists throughout the U.S. in search of one who treated sex offenders. It wasn't until late 1974 that I finally discovered a state-of-the-art treatment program for sex offenders run by Gene G. Abel, a behavioral psychiatrist at the University of Mississippi. After receiving my records from the Lima State Hospital, Dr. Abel accepted me into his program which was being relocated to the University of Tennessee in Memphis.

Chapter Eight: The Fight for Treatment

From the time I received Dr. Abel's initial letter, I felt that his program was one worth fighting for. I wrote letters to many attorneys before receiving a positive response from LeRoy Pernell of The Ohio State University College of Law in Columbus. Mr. Pernell agreed to take my case. He would spend the next 4 years fighting in the courts for my right to treatment.

An influential event was that I met a 19-year-old man in the Lima Unit around 1973 and fell in love with him. Chuck was intelligent, sensitive, and had boyish good looks. Unfortunately, he was heterosexual. Although I had much difficulty pulling back from Chuck emotionally, it eventually dawned on me that if I could have such a young man on the outside, I should be able to stay away from minor boys and live within the law! So it was that realization at age 35 – less than 3 years after Ohio had decriminalized sodomy between males – that I decided I wanted to live a gay lifestyle. At my request, Ted, my therapist, arranged for me to make a long-distance phone call to Dr. Abel in Tennessee and ask him if I could change my treatment goal to developing an attraction to adult men instead of adult women. Dr. Abel replied, "Sure."

It was in late 1975 when the hospital returned me to the Lima court for a hearing. Despite strong testimony from the OSU doctor that my age was a critical factor in this kind of treatment, and that the treatment therefore shouldn't be delayed, the Lima court denied my probation request and sent me to Chillicothe Correctional Institution to be punished for my December 1971 offense (on Christmas with the 14-year-old-boy).

Mr. Pernell filed a civil lawsuit on my behalf, arguing that I had a constitutional right to access to a treatment program. Before the court battle even began, I'd been having serious difficulty adjusting to prison life. There was intense pressure on me in the prison environment to keep my homosexual orientation hidden so as to avoid being labeled a "sissy," a term of scorn that meant "like a woman." Knowing about the special hell that other inmates reserved for those labeled "Baby Rapers," I became a loner at Chillicothe in order to keep the sexual nature of my crime a carefully guarded secret. That was often difficult to do in the crowded institution. I eventually had to see the psychiatrist and get prescriptions for anti-anxiety medications, but none of the meds relieved my pain when there was the slightest noise in my living area.

At one point, I had an unforgettable break with reality. It was touched off when another inmate approached me and wanted to know if he could have sex with me, specifying that he wanted me to take the passive role in anal intercourse. I was shocked. He apparently had found out that I was a "Baby Raper" with a male victim. Trying hard to sound calm and confident, I responded to the inmate with a simple, "I'm not into that kind of thing," realizing that he knew I was lying if he did in fact know about my crime.

While in my room one evening in October 1978, I became extremely tense. I heard what at first sounded like clicking noises in the hallway outside my room. I bolted out of my room more frightened than I can possibly describe. With my chest still heaving and my heart pumping like it was about to explode, I walked the aisles of the library to try to calm down. After about 10 minutes, I left the library because it occurred to me that it wasn't a good place to be. I again broke out running at full speed and did not slow down until I was back inside my room at the dorm.

Even there, I felt trapped or pinned down, like it was totally impossible to get away from this inmate. I tried to cope by sitting down and began writing a long, apparently irrational kite (letter) to the psychiatrist who visited the prison once a week.

The next day was the psychiatrist's day to be at the prison. When I reiterated what I believed was going on, he kept saying "No, no, no." I respected his opinion. He said he wanted to put me in the segregation (isolation) cellblock "to get away from it all for a while," and to give me a prescription for an anti-psychotic medication called Mellaril.

Although the psychotic symptoms would not recur, I would remain sensitive to noise in prison dorms and experience more pain from such noise than I could possibly put into words.

I was suddenly and unexpectedly scheduled for a "special reconsideration" hearing with the Ohio Parole Board in March of 1979. I had less than a week to prepare for it. At that point, I didn't feel that I could take prison life any longer and believed that I should be able to change my sexual preference from adolescent boys to young adult gay men on my own. I therefore told the board that I no longer needed Dr. Abel's treatment program and – presto! – I was released on parole in April 1979.

Chapter Nine: A Bastard Science

I quickly realized that telling the parole board that I no longer needed treatment was a huge mistake. It was one thing to decide that I wanted to live a gay lifestyle with an adult man. It was quite another thing to do it. I was paroled to Columbus, Ohio, where there was no sex offender treatment at all. When I went to Dayton to visit my mother on my first weekend on the outside, I went to a couple of gay bars for the first time in my life. I went to the bars alone, only to find that I was terrified in such settings.

Once again, I began cruising the streets for an adolescent boy I could have sex with soon after my harrowing experience at the bars, and I was arrested for sexual offenses against two young teenaged boys roughly 30 days after my release on parole.

Around November 1979, I was convicted of both sex crimes, and I was returned to the Chillicothe prison with a combined 9-35 year sentence plus a parole violation. It would be 12 years before I'd see freedom again.

In February 1980, the bloodiest, most savage riot in the history of American prisons erupted at the New Mexico Penitentiary at Sante Fe. The image of a child molester being hacked and incinerated with a blowtorch during the riot was forever etched into my memory. I knew that the same thing could happen at Chillicothe or almost any other American prison. Indeed, even without a riot, an attempt was made on my life at Chillicothe around May of 1980. I was struck in the head from behind with a metal pipe while walking up a dark stairway into my cellblock one evening. I managed to stay on my feet, but couldn't see my assailant, who quickly disappeared. Two of my inmate friends told me independently that a contract had been authored against my life by a relative of my crime victims.

It was a great relief when Dr. Pinta had me placed in a special cellblock for inmates who needed quiet and solitude. As far as my overall hopelessness was concerned, my salvation turned out to be Ohio University's decision to establish a college campus inside the Chillicothe prison. I excelled in all of my classes, and in particular developed a reputation as someone knowledgeable about psychology. I spent 4 years as an O.U. student, earning both an associate degree in Human Services Technology and a bachelor's degree in Psychology, graduating with a 3.94 grade point average.

Much to my surprise, the Ohio prison system decided to start a pilot sex offender treatment program at Chillicothe in 1986. It was not a highly sophisticated, behaviorally oriented program like Dr. Abel's in Tennessee, but rather one based upon the victimological paradigm. I knew nothing of victimology at the time and was one of the first to volunteer for the pilot treatment program at Chillicothe. Treatment consisted of group therapy twice a week and relevant classes 5 days a week.

I began trying to answer the question of whether sex between a man and an adolescent boy was actually harmful to the adolescent boy. Many of the victim/offender adults were described as being unable to empathize with their victims, and it was felt that this might reflect a denial process in which the adult denies his own experiences and his own feelings. That "clicked" for me as an area I needed to explore, since I had always regarded the sexual encounter with my cousin as mere childhood experimentation and had not worked through any trauma in previous therapy. I came to accept that cross-generational sex between males was often harmful to the younger participant and that I myself had been harmed at age 12.

I eventually came to understand the victimology perspective and developed a genuine empathy for victims of sexual abuse, including the two adolescent boys I had abused in 1979 (as well as other victims). I then vowed to give up sex with adolescent boys for the rest of my life and began going through a grieving process just by imagining what that was going to be like.

Chapter Ten: Last Chance at Freedom

I was paroled to Dayton in March of 1991. While I was certainly enjoying my freedom in many respects, I was also experiencing anxiety about whether the intensive work I had done on myself in the Polaris program (the sex-offender program at the Chillicothe prison) had been adequate.

I got my own apartment, and within a couple of days of moving in, I unexpectedly crossed paths with a boy walking down the sidewalk. I didn't trust myself as I passed the boy, and to make sure that I kept walking, I silently yelled to myself, "Leave him the f--- alone!" After walking another ten feet or so, I repeated "Leave him the f--- alone!" even more emphatically. It was only at that point that I allowed myself to think back to what I had experienced while passing the boy. I had felt nothing sexual, no urge toward him at all. Reflecting upon what had happened, I said to myself something like, "So okay! This is good! Looks like I may be able to do this!" and my anxiety disappeared for the first time since my release from prison.

My efforts to become acquainted with the Dayton gay community were not, in retrospect, all they could have been or even always appropriate, because I was determined to meet a young man in his early- to mid-20s even though I was now 51. My reasoning was that it would be unrealistic to try to move up the age ladder any higher, at least initially. By the time I'd been on parole about 2½ months, I had successfully removed myself from many unanticipated high-risk situations with adolescent boys. The relapse prevention plan I had devised while in the Polaris program called for never being alone with a minor boy under any circumstances, and I was sticking to that plan.

I'd been out for 3 months when I met Sean, a 23-year-old man with strawberry-blond hair and the physique of an adolescent. I met him at a restaurant in the university area where he worked. As we started to spend time together and become acquainted, we were rapidly drawn into an emotional bond. My need to provide nurturing to a younger male was matched by Sean's need to feel safe with an older male who could provide maturity and paternalism in a relationship.

Sean and I fell into the habit of cooking meals at each other's apartments, going for long walks together, and occasionally spending the night together. In fact, I stopped my efforts to socialize and develop friendships with others so that I could be with Sean all the time. I seemed to believe that I could meet all my needs with just one person! However, our relationship soon became one of constant emotional ups and downs. During the up times, I was happy, and my life had meaning. However during the down times, I felt desperate, as if I couldn't survive without Sean.

By late September when I'd been out of prison for 6 months, everything fell apart. I had been warned that May/December relationships usually don't last very long. Sean and I met for the last time on Friday, October 4, 1991. I had taken a job in advertising sales (telemarketing) and was on my lunch hour. We talked for about 30 minutes. When Sean said he wanted to end our relationship, it was what I'd been expecting to hear. I covered up the panic inside me, like I was calmly accepting his decision. But even as I dropped him off and return to work, I was asking myself how on earth was I going to survive this loss.

I then began pretending that everything was normal, and I promised myself that I would simply go out to the gay disco on Saturday night and find myself another young man. In the meanwhile, I drove through a male prostitution cruising area in North Dayton known as "the levee," a spot where young adult male hustlers could be picked up. I wanted a back-up plan in case I didn't meet anyone at the disco. Sure enough, when I went to the disco Saturday night, all I could think about was when Sean and I had gone dancing there, and I became so depressed that I left the disco around midnight and went home to bed.

On Sunday morning, I was still depressed and drove through the cruising area again on my way to cash in some food stamps. I spotted a young male and picked him up. Even after he said he was 15 years old, I allowed myself to continue driving to my apartment and had sex with him here. I was then arrested at my apartment because the boy's stepfather had seen me pick him up and gave my license number to the police. I pled guilty to Corruption of a Minor. That was 25 years ago, and I have never been released.

Yet subjectively, I have not felt that my sentence was sufficient punishment for what I did. The fact that the boy admitted to the police that the sexual relations with me were consensual means little. He turned out not to be a hustler soliciting for sex, but an innocent 15-year-old. Having stopped caring about myself after the break-up with Sean, I was unable to care about anyone else on the day of the offense. I allowed myself to seduce the boy and thereby put him at risk of serious psychological harm. That was inexcusable.

During the first 5 years of this incarceration, I couldn't stand myself. After 5 years, I began trying to forgive myself, which is something a sex offender must do if he's to engage in a recovery process and to be fit for release. The sex offender with unresolved guilt is more likely to reoffend, and with my history, I want to heed that wisdom. However, I may remain in prison until I die and won't have to worry about unresolved guilt and reoffending.

I'd like to believe I'm not the same person I was in 1991. For when I die, I'd like to be remembered as someone who finally conquered his sex offending and who did what he could to help the public get sex offending into a more accurate perspective.

EPILOGUE

I made my transition into the free world in early 2017 after 25 years of incarceration. I had hoped to join the Unitarian Church of Columbus and had been encouraged to do this by their Senior Pastor. Unfortunately, he retired and I was informed by an assistant pastor that I was not allowed on church property even with a chaperone. In a faltering attempt to justify the decision, the associate pastor said, "It's just something about you."

That rejection led me to leave Columbus and relocate to Dayton, and my experience in Dayton has been rather uneventful because my old friends also opted not to have any contact with me. I have considered trying to join another Unitarian church, but so far have declined to do so because of my experience in Columbus. One can take only so much rejection. My only sources of support have been my niece, my sister, and a professional counselor I see regularly. The counseling has been quite voluntary, as I am not on parole or under any kind of supervision. The counseling is for the purpose of addressing the difficulties of reintegrating back into society after 25 years of incarceration.

In any event, I've had no inclination to reoffend during the 2-3 years I've been out. Have I just grown too old to be interested in sex anymore? Was it that my prostate cancer and the removal of my prostate in 2006 reduced my sex drive? Or is this new freedom due to something I have finally learned at a deep and painful level, something that has given me a new strength that was previously beyond my grasp? I suspect I could probably answer in the affirmative to all of those questions.

My other remaining task before I die is to go up to Lima, Ohio, and visit the grave of Jim Seitz, who had a greater impact on me in the late 1960s than he may have realized. While in Lima, I will visit with Ted Smith. Ted is perhaps the only person who'll understand the closeness I still feel to Jim after all these years and why I'll ask to be alone at his grave.

A Post-Epilogue Note

This is a final note on Mr. Jerry Myers. I know that Mr. Myers (or Jerry as he asked me to call him) visited Lima to visit his old friend and therapist Jim Seitz. He brought flowers and left them on his grave. I know this as both Jerry and Ted Smith told me so. In my interview with Ted Smith, he stated he accompanied Jerry to the cemetery.

Jerry did harm to many adolescent boys over his lifetime. It is impossible to measure the magnitude and longitudinal effects of his behavior on the adolescents he offended. There is no way to deny that he caused this hurt and there is no room for forgiveness – and he asks for none. He eventually took responsibility for that harm and accepted his punishment, even citing it as not being "sufficient."

At the same time and to his credit, he also tried many ways and many times through his life to change in a world that would only condemn him without any effective answers to his requests for assistance. I am glad that he did reach a time when he felt like he had "conquered his demons" (his compulsion to sex offend). He worked hard to get to that place, a place where he felt some satisfaction and redemption.

Life is complex and social determinants of health have come to be understood in medicine as significant influencing factors in the outcomes of an individual life. These are not excuses for an individual's behavior. Yet they are real and potent variables that science bears out. Had he been born 50 years later in 1990, I believe it would be more likely than not, that the trajectory of his life would have been very different. That's what I believe and I could be wrong. However, I chose not to add judgment to him beyond the lifetime of judgment he has already received.

When I came to know Jerry, he was plagued by many medical illnesses, including chronic obstructive pulmonary disorder. He had a distinct voice on the phone and expressed a great deal of humor and appreciation for the good things that happened in his life, such as being cared for by some who knew his worse obsessions and still treated him with dignity. His final conversation with me was in a height of the COVID-19 epidemic and he had just called EMS to take him to the hospital. That is the last I heard from Mr. Jerry Myers. However, I leave you with his final words of gratitude and dedication.

Dedication

This is book is dedicated to the memory of my beloved mother, Isabelle Myers, who stood by me; to the memory of my sisters Doris Rauscher, Virginia Ritter, and to my sister Barbara Lombardo, who all suffered; and to the memory of psychologist James W. Seitz, who was like a father to me, an inspiring mentor, and the greatest man I ever knew.

This book is also for those who attempted to give me legal access to effective treatment, namely the late Judge Carl Kessler and attorneys LeRoy Pernell and Lou Jacobs; and for numerous helping professionals and supportive friends, including Ted Smith III, Sam Craddock, Joan Heidtmann, Earl Stump, Emil Pinta, Gene Siesky, Richard Aucoin, David George, Dave Rickard, Curt Hileman, Jean Scott, Bob Fulmer, Kurt Brickner, Joyce Segreto, Bill Wellmeier, Karen G. Thimmes, Rev. Mark Belletini, Ed Neisz, and the late Robin "Doc" Herman. Most recently, I've been having discussions with Dr. Frederick Peterson, who studied under the famous sex researcher William Masters and, because of Docpete's aid, my chances of having the work published are looking up.

This book is also for paraphilic sex offenders who are struggling to put lust and love back together, and for everyday citizens who wish to understand us.

Finally, this book is for the adolescent boys against whom I offended.

Section VI

Therapist Guides and Patient Handouts

31

American Association of Sexuality Educators, Counselors and Therapists Code of Conduct

Most mental/physical health disciplines have a national society, such as the American Psychological Association or the American Medical Association, that establishes their own codes of ethical conduct. Likewise, most mental/physical health disciplines have governing boards which are mandated by the various states to guide and control the practice of each discipline within that state. In recent years, organizations that certify practitioners to practice in a specialized area of treatment have also set up guidelines for ethical/professional conduct that must be followed within the subspecialty.

These subspecialty codes of ethical conduct are very specific guidelines. The Board of the American Association of Sexuality Educators, Counselors and Therapists (AASECT) has been especially cognizant of the need to guide and control the practice of sex therapy. This subspecialty, more than any other, requires that the therapist be held accountable to practice at the highest possible standards of care and professionalism. Sexuality educators, counselors, and therapists not only have the burden of helping their clients and patients experience a healthy sexual life, they must also do everything in their power to overcome many sex negative attitudes and many misrepresentations of how sexuality educators, counselors, and therapists perform their work as seen in the popular media.

AASECT has kindly granted permission to reprint their Code of Conduct here for the benefit of our readers. The Code of Conduct can also be seen on the AASECT website at www.aasect.org.

Code of Conduct for
AASECT Certified Members*

Article I: Preamble

Recognizing its responsibilities to society and given its own national and international objectives, the American Association of Sexuality Educators, Counselors and Therapists (AASECT) has adopted the following Code of Conduct (Code). The Code applies to all Certified AASECT members and encompasses any activity that directly or indirectly relates to professional identity or training. The Code does not replace or modify the requirements for or purposes of certification as a sex educator, counselor, therapist or Supervisor.

As a professional association, AASECT has a duty to advocate and enforce both high quality services from and proper conduct/professionalism by its members in order to ensure both. Through setting forth standards of ethical conduct for practice-related conditions, qualities, skills and services, the Code is intended to assist AASECT Certified members with judgments made in the course of their professional services.

Certified members of AASECT, in the conduct of all aspects of their life that relates to their professional work and identity, are expected to honor the Code, and AASECT certification is predicated upon adherence thereto.

Article II: Conditions of Certification

AASECT Certification may be terminated for sufficient cause as outlined in the Bylaws and the formal Application for Certification.

Those applying for AASECT Certification must submit the following as part of the application process:

1. Notification in writing to the AASECT Office of:
   a. denial of an application for or disciplinary action taken against any professional license or certification by a state or federal entity, or by a private certification entity;
   b. conviction, guilty plea, or no contest plea of a felony;
   c. conviction, guilty plea, or no contest plea of a misdemeanor directly related to public health or the provision of safe and competent sexual health counseling or therapy;
2. a. Current AASECT Certified members are required to notify the AASECT Board of Directors (Board) in writing within thirty (30) days should an action listed in paragraphs (a) – (c) of the above Section 1 occur.
   b. In the event any professional licensing board or certification entity initiates charges against a current AASECT Certified member, that member shall provide the Board with written notification of the charges, along with any related documentation. Such notifica-

tion must be made within thirty (30) days of the Certified member's knowledge of the charges and any request from AASECT for information or documentation related to such charges must be satisfied within thirty (30) days of such request.

c. Decisions on all applications for AASECT certification or recertification may be suspended until the adjudicatory outcome of charges has been determined. Denial of applications shall be by two-thirds vote of the entire Board in accordance with the policies and procedures established by the Bylaws and the Formal Application for Certification.

Article III: Grounds for Corrective Action

Actions that may constitute grounds for discipline involving a Certified member include, but are not limited to:

1. violation of AASECT Practice Guidelines, Code of Conduct and/or other policies developed and implemented from time to time by the Board (collectively, AASECT Standards);
2. violation of guidelines and ethical standards established by the sexual health community;
3. denial of an application for or disciplinary action taken against any professional license or certification by a state or federal entity, or by a private certification entity;
4. conviction, guilty plea, or no contest plea of a felony;
5. conviction, guilty plea, or no contest plea of a misdemeanor directly related to public health or the provision of safe and competent sexual health education, counseling or therapy;
6. failure to promote the safety and welfare of the public, whether through negligent acts or omission, or through misrepresentation;
7. misuse or reproduction of AASECT certification materials, logos, abbreviations, or emblems that are the exclusive property of AASECT without the express written permission of AASECT;
8. failure to relinquish and/or refrain from using AASECT Certificates, the AASECT logo and/or emblems, the AASECT name, and/or AASECT abbreviations, when so directed by AASECT;
9. misrepresentation or falsification of material information in connection with an application, credentials, assessment documentation, continuing education reports, or other materials or information submitted to AASECT;
10. engaging in inappropriate conduct in connection with the certification or certification renewal processes, including, but not limited to:

    1. noncompliance with assessment procedures or instructions;
    2. violation of confidentiality agreements signed in accordance with the candidate application and/or assessment administration; or
    3. publishing, reproducing, or distributing assessment materials or information.

11. termination from an employment position involving the use of AASECT certification and where the conduct leading to such termination involved:

    1. child or elder abuse;
    2. sexual abuse;
    3. substance abuse; or
    4. job-related crimes.

12. filing a complaint with AASECT deemed to be false, frivolous or intended to harm a member, certified member or applicant and not intended to protect the public;
13. discipline by or expulsion from a grievance board of a university, college, governmental agency, or professional organization to which the Certified member belongs;
14. failure to comply with a duly entered order of the Board;
15. failure to cooperate with an investigation conducted by the Board;
16. failure to report known or suspected violations of AASECT Standards within thirty (30) days of such knowledge or suspicion;
17. unprofessional conduct as determined by the Board.

The information available to, as well as the deliberations of the Board, shall be deemed confidential. The outcomes, negative determinations and sanctions may be published on the AASECT website. Any action taken regarding continued or terminated membership, with concomitant conditions made by the Board is final and cannot be appealed. The Certified member will be notified in a timely fashion by the Board in writing of any decision regarding membership or certification status.

Article IV: Administrative Sanctions

Sanctions imposed by AASECT may include, but are not limited to:

1. Temporary or permanent loss of eligibility for certification or membership.
2. Suspension of Certificate or membership.
3. Probation of Certificate or membership.
4. Revocation of Certificate or membership.
5. Assessment of monetary sanctions to recover costs associated with the investigation and administrative prosecution by AASECT.

Article V: Additional AASECT Authority and Disclosure

In the interest of protecting the public and the integrity of the profession, AASECT shall have the authority to:

1. Disclose an individual's certification and/or membership status on its website.
2. Disclose a member and/or certified member's AASECT disciplinary history on its website.
3. Provide AASECT disciplinary history and/or complaints filed regarding a Certified member to the agency(s) responsible for state licensure, employers, and/or other professional certification or credentialing organizations.

Please see Disciplinary Procedures for concerns related to enquiries or complaints.

Article VI: Code Of Conduct

Principle One: Competence and Integrity

Competence

AASECT Certified members shall be committed to maintaining high standards of scholarship and practice and shall be accountable as an individual to the AASECT Standards. Additionally, Certified members shall perform any professional service in accord with the prevailing standards of performance in professional activities when measured against generally prevailing peer performance.

The Certified member shall have training in sexuality education, counseling, therapy, and/or supervision that is in accord with AASECT Standards and the laws relevant to the jurisdiction in which the Certified member practices.

The Certified member shall recognize the necessity and benefit of professional growth by participating in continuing education as determined by the Practice Guidelines and by the Certification standards.

Informed Consent

The Certified member shall recognize his/her limits of competence and shall communicate them at the earliest possible time and at any time thereafter to the consumer. When the Certified member's level of competence does not afford optimal benefits to the consumer, the Certified member shall, in a timely and efficient manner, recommend referral to better-qualified sources.

The Certified member shall not knowingly permit any consumer to misunderstand the Certified member's competency and shall clarify credentials, training, affiliations, experiences and skills in an honest and accurate manner.

Aiding/Abetting Unqualified Practice

The Certified member shall not enter into association for professional practice with or assist, aid, or promote in any manner the practice of an unqualified or incompetent person which shall include any person whom the Certified member knows or has reason to believe, does not adhere to the Code or is in violation of any law. This shall include, but is not limited to, making a referral to an unqualified or incompetent person.

The Certified member shall not provide any remuneration, regardless of form, to any source for receiving the referral of a consumer for professional services unless the source of the referral maintains continued involvement in the care of the consumer. Conversely, the Certified member shall not receive any remuneration regardless of form from any source for providing the referral of a consumer for professional services unless the Certified member maintains continued involvement in the care of the consumer. Any such financial arrangement must be disclosed to and approved and acknowledged in writing by the consumer.

The Certified member who becomes emotionally, physically or otherwise impaired or disabled to a degree that it impacts on the best interest of the consumer shall, in a timely and efficient manner, make a referral of the consumer to a qualified and appropriate professional source so as to avoid any undue abandonment of the consumer.

Principle Two: Moral, Ethical, and Legal Standards

The Certified member shall accept that the quality of his/her professional services (are) is dependent upon both personal morality and professional ethics and on the ability to maintain legal standards.

The Certified member shall be aware of and monitor the fact that his/her personal needs may influence judgments and actions in the therapeutic relationship and shall, regardless of experience or training, have a qualified review source such as a supervisor available to assist in safeguarding against unwise or inappropriate judgments and acts.

The Certified member shall not enter into any dual relationship regardless of nature that jeopardizes the well-being of the consumer.

The Certified member shall avoid any action that might violate or diminish the legal and civil rights of the consumer.

The Certified member shall not engage in or condone practices by any source that are inhumane or that result in illegal or unjustifiable action relevant to race, handicap, age, gender, sexual orientation, religion or national origin.

The Certified member shall make only factual, honest, and clearly stated (not misleading) public announcements, statements or communications such as (but not limited to) for advertising or promotional purposes.

The Certified member shall not set forth identification with AASECT such as (but not limited to) membership or certification status in an announcement statement, or communication, whatever the form, that also includes a college or university degree, unless that degree is based on academic merit and is from an appropriately accredited higher education institution.

The Certified member shall act in accord with AASECT ethics, standards and guidelines related to education, counseling, therapy, supervision and research.

The Certified member shall act in accord with the standards and guidelines for the protection of consumers promulgated by other professional associations with which the Certified member is affiliated and the laws of the jurisdiction(s) in which the Certified member provides professional services.

The Certified member shall report any ethical, regulatory, or legal complaint or judgment relevant to their practice filed against the member with this report being submitted in writing within thirty (30) days of knowledge to the Chair of the AASECT Disciplinary Committee.

Principle Three: Welfare of the Consumer

Given that consumers are in unique and vulnerable positions with respect to the sensitive nature of services related to sexuality education, counseling, therapy, research and supervision, Certified members shall constantly be mindful of the responsibility for protection of the consumer's welfare, rights and best interests and for the rigorous maintenance of the trust implicit in the consumer relationship.

1. The member shall, from the onset of professional contact with a consumer or a potential consumer, clarify:

    a. Professional training, experiences and competencies;
        i. AASECT's mission includes responsibility for providing education and certification for sexual health professionals. One of AASECT's objectives is consumer protection and to ensure that the public is not misled by inaccurate claims of those AASECT members.
        ii. If a Certified member lists certification among his/her credentials, that member must specify the area of certification (i.e., as a sexuality educator, sexuality counselor, sex therapist or supervisor) in any manner, media or forum. For example, a certified sexuality counselor may not advertise him or herself as a certified sexuality educator. Only AASECT Certified Supervisors may advertise themselves as offering AASECT supervision.
        iii. AASECT members who are candidates for degrees, certification or supervisor may not state their candidacy as part of their identification in any manner, media or forum. For example, a candidate for a degree program such as a doctorate or for AASECT sex therapy certification may not advertise that status. Consumers can be misled by titles such as "PhD Candidate" or "Sex Therapy Certification Candidate."
    b. The nature of the professional services available to the consumer (with an explanation of mutual roles and duties);
    c. The limits of intervention effectiveness;
    d. Personal values or professional preferences that reflect biases rather than being responsive to the needs and well-being of the consumer;
    e. Any exceptions to confidentiality and privileged communications (e.g. duty to warn, mandatory reporting, etc.); and
    f. Any financial issues, especially the payment obligations of the consumer.

2. The Certified member shall treat all information received about a consumer as confidential including, but not limited to, the mere existence of an educational counseling or therapeutic relationship with the consumer. Where required by law, the Certified member will develop a policy consistent with reporting requirements under HIPAA/PIPPA and follow all legal requirements protecting consumer privacy.
3. The Certified member shall advocate the consumer's privileged communication as granted by the laws of the jurisdiction applicable to the consumer and/or the Certified member. In the event that there is uncertainty about the effectiveness or validity of the consumer's consent to release information that is potentially confidential and/or privileged, the Certified member shall obtain appropriate legal determination.
4. The Certified member shall divulge information received from a consumer or prospective consumer to the extent required only in the following circumstances:

    a. When the consumer provides written and informed consent, which indicates:

        i. The type and nature of information to be released;
        ii. Knowledge of the purpose for which the information will be used;
        iii. Designation of the source that will receive the information;
        iv. That the consent is given voluntarily and with competency; and
        v. The consumer's name and the date on which the consent is given.

b. When there is clear and imminent danger of bodily harm or to the life or safety of the consumer or another person; such disclosure shall be made in accord with the laws of the jurisdiction in which the member practices.
c. When applicable law declares that such information may be released.

5. The Certified member may only use identifiable information about the consumer for purposes of education, training, research or publication, but may not do so without the consumer's written informed consent.
6. The Certified member may reveal information about a consumer's treatment and treatment plan only to the extent that such is revealed in consultation with another professional, such as a supervisor or coworker, for treatment purposes. Such information may not include any confidential or identifying information about the consumer, unless the consumer provides written consent.
7. The Certified member shall keep meaningful records relevant to the professional services provided to and contacts (of any nature) with the consumer and shall have a secure system for the preservation of records with the minimal contents and duration of retention being in accord with the laws that are applicable to the jurisdiction in which the Certified member practices, but no less than the following:

   a. A full record shall be retained intact for no less than 7 years after completion of the last date of professional services or contact or more as required by applicable provincial, state or federal/national law. In the case of minor clients, a full record shall be retained intact for no less than 7 years after the client reaches the age of majority and after completion of the last date of professional services or contact or more as required by applicable provincial, state or federal law;

8. The Certified member shall have a formal (written) arrangement for the preservation of consumer records upon his/her ceasing of practice, death or incapacity. This arrangement must be in accord with the laws of the jurisdiction in which the Certified member practices.
9. The Certified member shall, when providing professional services in a group context or to a couple or family, make a reasonable effort to promote safeguarding of confidentiality on the part of each consumer in the group, couple or family.
10. The Certified member shall orient the minor consumer to the limits of confidentiality pertaining to a parent's right to know as defined by the laws of the jurisdiction in which the member practices.
11. The Certified member shall, regardless of the reasons for which the consumer sought professional services and regardless of the theory or technique being used by the Certified member, predicate every sex counseling or therapy intervention with an assessment and a meaningful discussion with the consumer(s) as to planning for counseling or therapy. Such plan shall be consistently documented in writing, justified academically, evaluated for effectiveness, monitored for strengths and weaknesses and periodically modified accordingly.
12. The Certified member shall not engage in any dual relationship, regardless of nature or circumstances, with a consumer or with persons who have a primary relationship with a consumer served by the Certified member if such dual relationship could potentially be detrimental to or jeopardize the well-being of a consumer. A dual relationship occurs when a Certified member is in a professional role with a person and (1) is simultaneously in another role with the same person, and/or (2) is simultaneously in a relationship with a person closely associated with or related to the person with whom the Certified member has the professional

relationship, and/or (3) promises to enter into another relationship in the future with the person or a person closely associated with or related to the consumer.

13. The Certified member practicing education, counseling or therapy shall not engage, attempt to engage or offer to engage a potential, current, or former consumer in sexual behavior whether the consumer consents to such behavior or not. Sexual behavior includes, but is not limited to, kissing; sexual intercourse and/or the touching by either the Certified member or the consumer of the other's breasts or genitals; sexual solicitation, physical advances, or verbal or nonverbal conduct that is sexual in nature, that occurs in connection with the Certified member's activities or roles as an educator, counselor or therapist, and that either (1) is unwelcome, is offensive, or creates a hostile workplace or educational environment, and the Certified member knows or is told this or (2) is sufficiently severe or intense to be abusive to a reasonable person in the context.
14. The Certified member shall terminate professional services to the consumer when it is reasonably evident or should be evident that the consumer is not obtaining benefits sufficient to justify continued services by such Certified member. Upon termination, the Certified member shall make referral to another professional source and/or offer reasonable follow-up to further the best interests of the consumer.

Principle Four: Welfare of Students, Trainees and Others

The Certified member shall respect the rights and dignity of students, trainees and others (such as employees), maintain high standards of scholarship and preserve academic freedom and responsibility.

1. The Certified member shall, from the onset of professional contact with students, trainees and others over whom the Certified member has administrative, educational or supervisory authority clarify: the Certified member's professional qualifications and competencies; the objectives, responsibilities and duties of all concerned and any financial issues, especially any payment obligations.
2. The Certified member shall maintain in confidence personal information regarding a student, trainee, or others obtained in his/her professional role; the provision of confidentiality does not, however, preclude fulfilling a professional responsibility or duty to consumers, educational or training institutions or programs, professional associations or governmental/regulatory or legal sources.
3. The Certified member shall maintain high standards of scholarship and present information that is accurate and timely in all administrative, educational and supervisory activities.
4. The Certified member shall keep meaningful and systematic records of all administrative, educational and supervisory activities.
5. The Certified member shall not coerce or require a student, trainee or other to serve as a subject for a research project.
6. The Certified member shall not provide diagnosis, therapeutic counseling or therapy or any other clinical service to students or trainees or those over whom the Certified member has administrative, educational or supervisory authority.
7. The Certified member shall not harass in any manner a student, trainee or other person over whom the Certified member has administrative, educational or supervisory authority. Certified members do not engage in sexual relationships with students or supervisees who are in their department, agency, or training center, or over whom Certified members have, or are likely to have, evaluative authority.

8. The Certified member shall not, during the administrative, educational or supervisory period enter into any dual relationship, regardless of nature, that jeopardizes the well-being of the student, trainee or other.
9. The Certified member shall not, during the administrative, educational or supervisory period, engage, attempt to engage or offer to engage the student, trainee or other in sexual behavior.
10. The Certified member shall be cognizant that a dual relationship subsequent to the administrative, educational or supervisory period may potentially jeopardize the well being of the student, trainee or other.

Principle Five: Welfare of Research Subjects

Certified members shall conduct their investigations with respect for the dignity, rights and welfare of the subjects. Research must be ethical and legal at its inception and throughout the course of the investigation, with Certified members being mindful of not justifying investigative techniques that are solely considered by the intended or achieved outcome.

1. The Certified member shall be involved only with sex research that is carried out by persons qualified to perform such investigations or under the direct supervision of persons so qualified.
2. The Certified member shall be involved only with sex research that designates and identifies (in writing) to the potential subjects the names and professional qualifications of the person(s) or persons with ethical scientific and legal responsibility for the conduct of the investigation.
3. The Certified member shall be involved only with sex research that provides adequate protection(s) to human subjects at risk. Any research project must:

   a. Include the voluntary and informed consent of each subject; and
   b. Be in accord with applicable legal authority of the jurisdiction within which such research is being conducted.

4. The Certified member shall only be involved with sex research that protects the confidentiality of research data including the identity of participants or others revealed during the investigation.
5. The Certified member shall only be involved with sex research that requires all investigators to be honest and accurate in their dealings with research subjects and all persons receiving information about the research.
6. The Certified member shall only be involved with sex research that offers to provide an explanation of the purpose of the investigation and of the individual and collective results to each person who serves as a research subject.
7. The Certified member shall only be involved with sex research that has been prefaced by the submission of a research proposal for peer review with special reference to ethical and legal safeguards for the potential research subjects. This peer review may occur in different forms, such as an institutional review board for evaluation for ethical propriety, and must be in accord with all relevant laws.
8. The Certified member shall not engage in any type of sexual relationship or sexual behavior with research subjects as defined above in Principle Three (3), paragraph thirteen (13).

32

Sexual Health Assessment Questionnaire

R. Brian Denton and Ashley N. Grinonneau-Denton

Since William Masters and Virginia Johnson introduced their revolutionary ideas about how to help people with sexual problems, sex therapists and counselors have been trained about the importance of taking a thorough history of the presenting complaint. Later, sex therapists such as Helen Singer Kaplan introduced the importance of understanding the presenting sexual complaint within the context of the developmental history of the person and/or the couple.

The "Sexual Health Assessment Questionnaire" that follows is a comprehensive questionnaire that asks clients to respond to questions related to their psychosexual development starting with questions about their parent's relationship to each other and to the client, sibling relationships, dating history, abuse history (if any), important relationships prior to the current one, and then the history of the current relationship, as well as some questions concerning their medical history. There are important questions related to sexual development, such as when the client first masturbated and the emotional reaction to the experience, how the client learned about sex, and whether the information was accurate. Although the questionnaire is rather lengthy, most clients feel that it is well worth their time and effort to fill it out because it causes them to think about certain aspects of their development and sexuality that they may not have thought about or considered to be important or relevant to their presenting problem.

Sexual Health
Assessment Questionnaire

INSTRUCTIONS

This questionnaire is provided so that we can address sexuality as part of normative human functioning as quickly as possible. Even if you are not coming in with an acute sexual issue, opening the door to conversation on sexuality early helps to create a positive and open space to include it in treatment when relevant.

Please take your time in answering the following questions. There are no "right" or "wrong" answers to these questions; please answer them in a way that is accurate for you. The information gathered here is important for our assessment of the difficulties you are experiencing and for development of our course of treatment. If you need additional space for an answer, feel free to use additional paper to do so. We will review your answers together in our session and ongoing as needed.

- If you are not in a partnered monogamous or non-monogamous relationship, feel free to skip the partnered sections or answer in past tense when you were in a relationship.
- If meeting for partnered therapy, keep in mind that responses may be used/shared in the therapy context to facilitate conversation. We encourage you to be as honest and open as possible, and try not to skip any. However, if there are things that you do not want shared then do not put them here.
- If something is not applicable, just answer "NA"
- If you have concerns, please let me know so that I can answer any questions.

Client/patient name: ________________________________ Today's date ____/____/____

Age _______ Gender ___________________ Sex assigned at birth _________________

Relationship status (check one)

- ☐ Single
- ☐ Partnered
- ☐ Separated
- ☐ Divorced
- ☐ Remarried
- ☐ Widowed

Name(s) and age(s) of current partner(s) (If applicable) _________________________
____
____

Gender of current partner(s) (if applicable) _____________________________________
____

Sexual orientation ______________________________

Religious/spiritual background(s) ______________________________

Did you grow up living with your birth parents? ☐ Yes ☐ No If no, please explain.

____

____

Describe briefly how your parents (stepparents, guardians, adoptive parents, etc.) got along with and interacted with each other.

____

____

____

Please describe what sexual education you received growing up. Who did you get the information from, what were you told, and how did you respond? This may include both helpful and unhelpful messages about sexuality from the media, family, friends, educational institutions/schools, internet, religious organizations, etc.

____

____

____

____

What were your attitudes about genitalia (i.e., "dirty," etc.)? Or your body and its impact on later attitudes about your body (i.e., oral sex, body image, etc.)? What words were used in your family for body parts or functions? What words do you use today?

____

____

____

____

Was nudity acceptable in the family? How was privacy handled regarding toileting, bathing, etc.? What were the differences between genders?

____

____

____

____

How was affection shown in your family growing up? Were there differences between parents; between different gender children? Was it present at some ages and not others?

____

____

____

____

What was the attitude about masturbation in your childhood household? Shameful, accepted, harmful, healthy, normal, abnormal?

____

____

____

What were you told about sex after marriage? Having children? How was "intercourse" referred to in your family?

____

____

____

What were the expressed attitudes about gay men, lesbian women, bisexuality, other sexual orientations, and transgender individuals in your childhood household?

____

____

____

Were your caregivers open and accessible to questions about sexuality? ☐ Yes ☐ No
If there were not, did you wish they were? ☐ Yes ☐ No
If they were, what was that experience like for you?

____

____

____

What ideas did you have about sexual matters before you knew "the truth" about where babies came from and how they got here? What was your reaction when you learned "the truth?"

____

____

____

Who was the first person you ever thought of as sexually attractive? Why did you find them attractive? How does this now inform you about your "love map" formation (how you conceptualize true affection now)?

____

____

____

Did you ever experience any abuse as a child (physical, sexual, emotional, neglect, etc.)?
☐ Yes ☐ No If yes, please explain.

____

____

____

Please describe your first erotic/sexual experiences and what that experience was like for you. This may include positive and negative consequences, as well as emotional, physical, and psychological aspects of that experience.

____

____

____

Have you ever felt shamed by another for something sexual (e.g., masturbation, fantasies, history, etc.)? ☐ Yes ☐ No If yes, please explain.

____

____

____

Did you ever see anyone engaging in intercourse or other sex acts? ☐ Yes ☐ No
If yes, please explain how you felt about the event then and how you feel about it now.

____

____

____

Have you had any sexual experiences involving person(s) of same sex/gender either as a child or adult? ☐ Yes ☐ No
If yes, please explain how you felt about the event then and how you feel about it now.

____

____

____

Has anyone in your family ever involved you in any sexual activity as a child or as an adult?
☐ Yes ☐ No
If yes, please explain how you felt about the event then and how you feel about it now.

____

____

____

Have you ever engaged in sexual activities with an animal? ☐ Yes ☐ No
If yes, please explain how you felt about the event then and how you feel about it now.

____

____

____

____

Have you or someone you know ever experienced sexual assault and/or rape?
☐ Yes ☐ No
If yes, please explain how you felt about the event then and how you feel about it now.

____

____

____

What do you believe the perfect relationship consists of?

____

____

____

How would you describe your sexual style?

____

____

____

____

Do you feel you most often "give your best" when having sex with your partner(s)?
☐ Yes ☐ No If yes, please explain briefly.

____

____

____

Do you have a comfortable way of declining sexual contact with your partner?
☐ Yes ☐ No If yes, please explain briefly.

____

____

____

Do you have a comfortable way of initiating sex with your partner?
☐ Yes ☐ No If yes, please explain briefly.

____

____

____

How do you talk about sex with your partner?

____

____

____

Are you proud of the way you express your feelings toward your partner at this time?
☐ Yes ☐ No If yes, please explain briefly.

____

____

____

Are you happy with the way things are or would you like things to change? Please describe if there is/are sexual difficulty(difficulties) that you are experiencing currently or have experienced in the past.

____

____

____

Do you WANT your partner during sex or just "want sex?" Do you WANT to be aroused and involved sexually?

____

____

____

How do you know if your partner wants sex?

____

____

____

How do you communicate your desire to have sex with your partner(s)?

____

____

____

What are the "consequences" if you or your partner refuses to accept sexual advances?

____

____

____

What is the approximate frequency of sexual activity (not limited to intercourse)? Is this ideal for you?

____

____

____

Have you been open about your sexual history with your spouse/partner?

____

____

____

Do you have any of the following physical health difficulties? Please check all that apply.

- ☐ Diabetes
- ☐ Cardiovascular disease
- ☐ Take blood thinning medication
- ☐ Smoke cigarettes
- ☐ Alcoholic
- ☐ Binge drinking
- ☐ Substance abuse
- ☐ Sedentary lifestyle (no exercise)
- ☐ Poor diet
- ☐ Risky sexual behavior
- ☐ I never or rarely conduct breast self-exams
- ☐ I never or rarely conduct testicular self-exams
- ☐ I never or rarely conduct vulva self-exams
- ☐ I am on Hormone Replacement Therapy
- ☐ I take anti-depressant medication
- ☐ I have had labor/delivery complications
- ☐ I have a history of groin or straddle injury
- ☐ Testicular, cervical, or ovarian cancer
- ☐ Genital circumcision
- ☐ I take supplements for sexual performance and/or difficulties

Are there any physical difficulties that interfere with your sexual enjoyment or functioning?
☐ Yes ☐ No If yes, please explain.

____
____
____

Do you have any history of sexually transmitted infections/disease, pelvic inflammatory disease, or difficulties with infertility?
☐ Yes ☐ No If yes, please explain.

____
____
____

At what age did you experience pubertal changes (pubic hair, breast development, voice change, rapid growth, menses, etc.)? ____________________

Who provided you information about puberty? ____________________

When and how did you receive this information? What was the tone of the message? Did this information happen too soon or too late?

____
____
____
____

Did you develop earlier or later than peers? What effect did this have upon your body image? Any carryovers in that body image today?

____
____
____
____

At what age did you first begin menstruation? ____________________

How did you learn about menstruation? ____________________

____
____

Do you have any difficulties related to menstruation? ☐ Yes ☐ No
If yes, please explain.

____
____
____

What are your feelings about sexual activity during menstruation?

____
____
____

When and how did you first learn about nocturnal emissions (wet dreams)?

____

____

____

During foreplay, intercourse, or partnered sexual stimulation, do you experience any of the following? Please check all that apply.

- ☐ Lack of arousal
- ☐ Lack of genital sensation (no tingling/warmth/excitement)
- ☐ Difficulty reaching climax
- ☐ Loss of climax intensity (short in duration or strength)
- ☐ Vaginal dryness
- ☐ Erectile difficulties
- ☐ Decreased sense of connection with your partner
- ☐ Lack of focus on sexual feelings/sensations
- ☐ Genital pain
- ☐ Difficulty with sexual response (quick, slow, intermittent)

Do you have the same sexual difficulties when engaged in masturbation that you do with your partner? ☐ Yes ☐ No

Do you feel a lack of sexual interest when your partner initiates sexual activity?
☐ Yes ☐ No

Do you initiate sexual activity with your partner? ☐ Yes ☐ No

Please describe your current interest in sexual activity and how you view your sex drive/ libido.

____

____

____

____

Do you feel any of the following (please check all that apply)?

- ☐ Your partner knows how to sexually satisfy you
- ☐ You know how to sexually satisfy yourself
- ☐ You are comfortable giving direction to your partner to get your sexual needs met, and/ or in order to stimulate you to climax
- ☐ You and your partner are emotionally connected before and after sexual activity
- ☐ You and your partner have good sexual communication
- ☐ You and your partner have a close nonsexual relationship

If you are currently dissatisfied with your sex life, please describe if you have ever been happy about your sex life, and what about it you are currently dissatisfied with.

If you are currently having sexual difficulties, how long have they been present? Do you have any ideas about what may be happening to cause these difficulties?

Please describe your current satisfaction level with your relationship(s) status and functioning.

Do you or your partner(s) have any children? ☐ Yes ☐ No
If yes, who and what are the ages?

Were there changes in your sexual desire or activity following having children?
☐ Yes ☐ No If yes, please describe briefly.

Do you find your partner(s) attractive sexually? Romantically?

Does your partner tell you (verbally/nonverbally) he/she finds you attractive? Can/do you believe him/her?

Would you find someone like YOU sexually attractive? Romantically attractive? If not, how does this impact your own sexual expression?

Describe your thoughts and feelings about the following:

Pregnancy

Being a parent

Being single

Being in a relationship

Masturbation

Mutual masturbation

Oral sex

Anal sex

Sexual fetishes

___

___

___

Orgasm

___

___

___

Sexual bondage/discipline play

___

___

___

Dominance and submission

___

___

___

Semen and/or vaginal lubrication

___

___

___

Viewing genitals (self and/or others)

___

___

___

Toys and accessories

___

___

___

Polyamory/open relationships/swinging

___

___

___

Do you have any sexual fantasies (past or present) that you feel are unfulfilled?

___

___

___

___

If you are currently in a relationship:
Does your partner know you feel the way that you do in regard to the topics and/or difficulties that have been identified in this questionnaire?

☐ Yes ☐ No

If yes, how were they discussed? If no, please discuss the barriers to sharing this information with your partner.

____
____
____
____

Is there anything else that you would like to explain, elaborate on, or identify to assist me further in understanding the information included in this questionnaire?

☐ Yes ☐ No If yes, please describe.

____
____
____
____
____
____
____
____
____
____
____
____
____
____
____
____
____
____
____
____
____
____
____
____
____
____
____
____

Thank you for taking the time to complete this extensive review, and for taking the opportunity to include your sexual health and satisfaction in your life and relationships to our work together!

33

International Index of Erectile Function (IIEF)*

National Library of Medicine

The International Index of Erectile Function is a reliable, brief, self-administered assessment tool for clinicians and clients to assess problems with erectile function with men. The 15-item questionnaire contains five domains: (a) Erectile Function (6 items), (b) Orgasmic Function (2 items), (c) Sexual Desire (2 items), (d) Intercourse Satisfaction (3 items), and (e) Overall Sexual Satisfaction (2 items). Each domain captures a unique dimension of responses relating to male sexual or erectile function. The questions ask about the man's sex life over the last 4 weeks, with ratings on a five-point (1 to 5) Likert scale with lower values indicating relatively more erectile dysfunction or sexual dysfunction, depending on the item. The instrument was validated for use in 10 languages in 12 countries.

SCORING

Items load on the five scales as follows:

Erectile Function:	Items 1, 2, 3, 4, 5, and 15
Orgasmic Function:	Items 9 and 10
Sexual Desire:	Items 11 and 12
Intercourse Satisfaction:	Items 6, 7, and 8
Overall Sexual Satisfaction:	Items 13 and 14

A particular domain score is computed by summing the responses of its individual items, with lower values suggesting more dysfunction. No firm cut-off scores are used; however, some research has suggested using a cut-off score of 25 for the Erectile Function scale. That is, men who scored 25 or less would be likely classified as having erectile dysfunction, while men who score above 25 would be likely classified as not having erectile dysfunction. Other research has suggested that a cut-off score of 21 is preferred.

INTERNATIONAL INDEX OF ERECTILE FUNCTION (IIEF)

HOSPITAL NUMBER (IF KNOWN) ________________

NAME ________________

DATE OF BIRTH ________________ AGE __________

ADDRESS ________________
____
____

Patient Questionnaire

TELEPHONE ________________

These questions ask about the effects that your erection problems have had on your sex life over the last four weeks. Please try to answer the questions as honestly and as clearly as you are able. Your answers will help your doctor to choose the most effective treatment suited to your condition. In answering the questions, the following definitions apply:

- **sexual activity** includes intercourse, caressing, foreplay, & masturbation
- **sexual intercourse** is defined as sexual penetration of your partner
- **sexual stimulation** includes situation such as foreplay, erotic pictures, etc.
- **ejaculation** is the ejection of semen from the penis (or the feeling of this)
- **orgasm** is the fulfilment or climax following sexual stimulation or intercourse

Over the past 4 weeks:

*Please check **one** box only*

☐ Q1 How often were you able to get an erection during sexual activity?

0 No sexual activity
1 Almost never or never
2 A few times (less than half the time)
3 Sometimes (about half the time)
4 Most times (more than half the time)
5 Almost always or always

☐ Q2 When you had erections with sexual stimulation, how often were your erections hard enough for penetration?

0 No sexual activity
1 Almost never or never
2 A few times (less than half the time)
3 Sometimes (about half the time)
4 Most times (more than half the time)
5 Almost always or always

☐ Q3 When you attempted intercourse, how often were you able to penetrate (enter) your partner?

0 Did not attempt intercourse
1 Almost never or never
2 A few times (less than half the time)
3 Sometimes (about half the time)
4 Most times (more than half the time)
5 Almost always or always

☐ Q4 During sexual intercourse, how often were you able to maintain your erection after you had penetrated (entered) your partner?

0 Did not attempt intercourse
1 Almost never or never
2 A few times (less than half the time)
3 Sometimes (about half the time)
4 Most times (more than half the time)
5 Almost always or always

☐ Q5 During sexual intercourse, how difficult was it to maintain your erection to completion of intercourse?

0 Did not attempt intercourse
1 Extremely difficult
2 Very difficult
3 Difficult
4 Slightly difficult
5 Not difficult

☐	Q6	How many times have you attempted sexual intercourse?	0 No attempts 1 One to two attempts 2 Three to four attempts 3 Five to six attempts 4 Seven to ten attempts 5 Eleven or more attempts
☐	Q7	When you attempted sexual intercourse, how often was it satisfactory for you?	0 Did not attempt intercourse 1 Almost never or never 2 A few times (less than half the time) 3 Sometimes (about half the time) 4 Most times (more than half the time) 5 Almost always or always
☐	Q8	How much have you enjoyed sexual intercourse?	0 No intercourse 1 No enjoyment at all 2 Not very enjoyable 3 Fairly enjoyable 4 Highly enjoyable 5 Very highly enjoyable
☐	Q9	When you had sexual stimulation or intercourse, how often did you ejaculate?	0 No sexual stimulation or intercourse 1 Almost never or never 2 A few times (less than half the time) 3 Sometimes (about half the time) 4 Most times (more than half the time) 5 Almost always or always
☐	Q10	When you had sexual stimulation or intercourse, how often did you have the feeling of orgasm or climax?	1 Almost never or never 2 A few times (less than half the time) 3 Sometimes (about half the time) 4 Most times (more than half the time) 5 Almost always or always
☐	Q11	How often have you felt sexual desire?	1 Almost never or never 2 A few times (less than half the time) 3 Sometimes (about half the time) 4 Most times (more than half the time) 5 Almost always or always
☐	Q12	How would you rate your level of sexual desire?	1 Very low or none at all 2 Low 3 Moderate 4 High 5 Very high
☐	Q13	How satisfied have you been with your overall sex life?	1 Very dissatisfied 2 Moderately dissatisfied 3 Equally satisfied & dissatisfied 4 Moderately satisfied 5 Very satisfied
☐	Q14	How satisfied have you been with your sexual relationship with your partner?	1 Very dissatisfied 2 Moderately dissatisfied 3 Equally satisfied & dissatisfied 4 Moderately satisfied 5 Very satisfied
☐	Q15	How do you rate your confidence that you could get and keep an erection?	1 Very low 2 Low 3 Moderate 4 High 5 Very high

Additional Resources

Cappelleri, J. C., Rosen, R. C., Smith, M. D., Quirk, F., Maytom, M. C., Mishra, A., & Osterloh, I. H. (1999). Some developments on the International Index of Erectile Function (IIEF). *Drug Information Journal, 33,* 179-190.

Rosen, R. C., Riley, A., Wagner, G., Osterloh, I. H., Kirkpatrick, J., & Mishra, A. (1997). The International Index of Erectile Function (IIEF): A multidimensional scale for assessment of erectile dysfunction. *Urology, 49*(6), 822-830

34

Female Sexual Function Index (FSFI)

Ray Rosen and Associates

The Female Sexual Function Index (FSFI) is a reliable, self-administered assessment tool for clinicians and clients to assess sexual functioning in women. The 19-item questionnaire assesses functioning in six domains: (a) desire, (b) arousal, (c) lubrication, (d) orgasm, (e) satisfaction, and (f) pain. Each domain captures a unique dimension of responses related to female sexual functioning. The questions ask about the woman's sex life over the last 4 weeks, and the instrument is appropriate to use with women of all adult ages.

INSTRUCTIONS

Participants are asked to check one answer for each question that describes their sexual feelings and responses during the past 4 weeks. It will be helpful to define for participants that "sexual activity" includes caressing, foreplay, masturbation, and vaginal intercourse. "Intercourse" is defined as penile penetration (entry) of the vagina. "Sexual stimulation" includes foreplay with a partner, masturbation, and sexual fantasy. "Sexual desire or interest" refers to feelings of wanting to have a sexual experience, thinking or fantasizing about having sex, and feeling receptive to a partner initiating sex.

SCORING

Each item is scored on just one scale as listed below. In addition, because the number of items on scales varies, a domain factor multiplier is applied as noted.

Domain	Questions	Domain Multiplier	Minimum Score	Maximum Score
Desire	1, 2	0.6	1.2	6.0
Arousal	3, 4, 5, 6	0.3	0	6.0
Lubrication	7, 8, 9, 10	0.3	0	6.0
Orgasm	11, 12, 13	0.4	0	6.0
Satisfaction	14, 15, 16	0.4	0.8	6.0
Pain	17, 18, 19	0.4	0	6.0
		Full Scale Score Range	2.0	36.0

Individual domain scores are obtained by adding the scores of the individual items that comprise the domain and multiplying the sum by the domain multiplier (see preceding page). The full scale score is obtained by adding the six domain scores. Note that within individual domains, a score of zero indicates that no sexual activity was reported during the past 4 weeks. When zero activity is reported in a domain, the full scale score is also lowered. Lower scores indicate increased problems of sexual function. A score of 26 or lower is used as a cut-off for distinguishing members of the normal and clinical samples.

Female Sexual Function Index (FSFI)*

Question	Response Options
1. Over the past 4 weeks, how **often** did you feel sexual desire or interest?	5 = Almost always or always 4 = Most times (more than half the time) 3 = Sometimes (about half the time) 2 = A few times (less than half the time) 1 = Almost never or never
2. Over the past 4 weeks, how would you rate your **level** (degree) of sexual desire or interest?	5 = Very high 4 = High 3 = Moderate 2 = Low 1 = Very low or none at all
3. Over the past 4 weeks, how **often** did you feel sexually aroused ("turned on") during sexual activity or intercourse?	0 = No sexual activity 5 = Almost always or always 4 = Most times (more than half the time) 3 = Sometimes (about half the time) 2 = A few times (less than half the time) 1 = Almost never or never
4. Over the past 4 weeks, how would you rate your **level** of sexual arousal ("turn on") during sexual activity or intercourse?	0 = No sexual activity 5 = Very high 4 = High 3 = Moderate 2 = Low 1 = Very low or none at all
5. Over the past 4 weeks, how **confident** were you about becoming sexually aroused during sexual activity or intercourse?	0 = No sexual activity 5 = Very high confidence 4 = High confidence 3 = Moderate confidence 2 = Low confidence 1 = Very low or no confidence
6. Over the past 4 weeks, how **often** have you been satisfied with your arousal (excitement) during sexual activity or intercourse?	0 = No sexual activity 5 = Almost always or always 4 = Most times (more than half the time) 3 = Sometimes (about half the time) 2 = A few times (less than half the time) 1 = Almost never or never

Question	Response Options
7. Over the past 4 weeks, how **often** did you become lubricated ("wet") during sexual activity or intercourse?	0 = No sexual activity 5 = Almost always or always 4 = Most times (more than half the time) 3 = Sometimes (about half the time) 2 = A few times (less than half the time) 1 = Almost never or never
8. Over the past 4 weeks, how **difficult** was it to become lubricated ("wet") during sexual activity or intercourse?	0 = No sexual activity 1 = Extremely difficult or impossible 2 = Very difficult 3 = Difficult 4 = Slightly difficult 5 = Not difficult
9. Over the past 4 weeks, how often did you **maintain** your lubrication ("wetness") until completion of sexual activity or intercourse?	0 = No sexual activity 5 = Almost always or always 4 = Most times (more than half the time) 3 = Sometimes (about half the time) 2 = A few times (less than half the time) 1 = Almost never or never
10. Over the past 4 weeks, how **difficult** was it to maintain your lubrication ("wetness") until completion of sexual activity or intercourse?	0 = No sexual activity 1 = Extremely difficult or impossible 2 = Very difficult 3 = Difficult 4 = Slightly difficult 5 = Not difficult
11. Over the past 4 weeks, when you had sexual stimulation or intercourse, how **often** did you reach orgasm (climax)?	0 = No sexual activity 5 = Almost always or always 4 = Most times (more than half the time) 3 = Sometimes (about half the time) 2 = A few times (less than half the time) 1 = Almost never or never
12. Over the past 4 weeks, when you had sexual stimulation or intercourse, how **difficult** was it for you to reach orgasm (climax)?	0 = No sexual activity 1 = Extremely difficult or impossible 2 = Very difficult 3 = Difficult 4 = Slightly difficult 5 = Not difficult
13. Over the past 4 weeks, how **satisfied** were you with your ability to reach orgasm (climax) during sexual activity or intercourse?	0 = No sexual activity 5 = Very satisfied 4 = Moderately satisfied 3 = About equally satisfied and dissatisfied 2 = Moderately dissatisfied 1 = Very dissatisfied

Question	Response Options
14. Over the past 4 weeks, how **satisfied** have you been with the amount of emotional closeness during sexual activity between you and your partner?	0 = No sexual activity 5 = Very satisfied 4 = Moderately satisfied 3 = About equally satisfied and dissatisfied 2 = Moderately dissatisfied 1 = Very dissatisfied
15. Over the past 4 weeks, how **satisfied** have you been with your sexual relationship with your partner?	5 = Very satisfied 4 = Moderately satisfied 3 = About equally satisfied and dissatisfied 2 = Moderately dissatisfied 1 = Very dissatisfied
16. Over the past 4 weeks, how **satisfied** have you been with your overall sexual life?	5 = Very satisfied 4 = Moderately satisfied 3 = About equally satisfied and dissatisfied 2 = Moderately dissatisfied 1 = Very dissatisfied
17. Over the past 4 weeks, how **often** did you experience discomfort or pain during vaginal penetration?	0 = Did not attempt intercourse 1 = Almost always or always 2 = Most times (more than half the time) 3 = Sometimes (about half the time) 4 = A few times (less than half the time) 5 = Almost never or never
18. Over the past 4 weeks, how **often** did you experience discomfort or pain following vaginal penetration?	0 = Did not attempt intercourse 1 = Almost always or always 2 = Most times (more than half the time) 3 = Sometimes (about half the time) 4 = A few times (less than half the time) 5 = Almost never or never
19. Over the past 4 weeks, how would you rate your **level** (degree) of discomfort or pain during or following vaginal penetration?	0 = Did not attempt intercourse 1 = Very high 2 = High 3 = Moderate 4 = Low 5 = Very low or none at all

Additional Resources

Rosen, R., Brown, C., Heiman, J., Leiblum, S., Meston, C., Shabsigh, R., Ferguson, D., & D'Agostino, R., Jr. (2000). The Female Sexual Function Index (FSFI): A multidimensional self-report instrument for the assessment of female sexual function. *Journal of Sex and Marital Therapy, 26,* 191-208.

Wiegel, M., Meston, C., & Rosen, R. (2005). The Female Sexual Function Index (FSFI): Cross-validation and development of clinical cutoff scores. *Journal of Sex and Marital Therapy, 31,* 1-20.

35

Sexual Health Self-Assessment Battery

Frederick L. Peterson, Jr.

I. SELF-ASSESSMENT OF FAMILY SUPPORT FOR HEALTHY SEXUAL DEVELOPMENT

This patient questionnaire is a measure of satisfaction regarding 25 dimensions of childhood and adolescent developmental sexuality. It can be self-administered or used as a structured interview. The measure includes key questions concerning satisfaction related to important sexual experiences such as prepubescent sexuality, puberty activation, pregnancy, abortion, and abuse. The range of scoring is zero to 300 and an interpretive guide is included.

II. SELF-ASSESSMENT OF SEXUAL HEALTH AND WELL-BEING SATISFACTION

The second questionnaire is a measure of satisfaction regarding 25 dimensions of childhood and adolescent developmental sexuality. It can also be self-administered or used as a structured interview. The measure includes key questions regarding satisfaction with one's own sexuality, partnered sexual relations, medical aspects of sexuality, and sexual identity. Again, the range of scoring is zero to 300 and an interpretive guide is included.

III. SELF-ASSESSMENT OF YOUR BIG WHEEL OF HEALTH AND WELL-BEING

The third questionnaire is a measure of satisfaction regarding 25 dimensions of one's general health and well-being – all of which can be influential in terms of sexual health. Like the others, it can also be self-administered or used as a structured interview. The measure includes key questions regarding medical, nutritional, environmental, emotional, spiritual, financial and other aspects of health and well-being. This questionnaire is important as sexual health cannot be accurately assessed without consideration of the broader context of overall health. Again, the range of scoring is zero to 300 and an interpretive guide is included..

I. Self-Assessment of Family Support for Healthy Sexual Development

Name: ______________________ Current Age: _______ Date: ______________

Instructions: Select item which best describes your experience and place score in the blank to the right. All questions refer to experiences during childhood/adolescence.

Did your parents allow you to discuss sex in your home? ______

Full discussion was allowed with at least one parent	12 points
Some attempts were made at discussion (some embarrassment)	9 points
Equal amount of encouragement/discouragement for discussion	6 points
Discussion discouraged (with much embarrassment)	3 points
Forget about it! - No discussion allowed at all!	0 points

Did you see your parents share public displays of affection (hugs & kisses)? ______

Yea, they would smooch it up and grab a handful	12 points
Occasional pecks on the cheek and hugs when arriving/leaving	9 points
PDA was equally encouraged/discouraged	6 points
Rarely saw any PDA – generally absent from daily life	3 points
No way on earth (I still don't know how I was conceived)	0 points

Did you feel comfortable giving or getting hugs and kisses as a child? ______

Yes, I enjoyed the affection!	12 points
Yes, I mostly felt comfortable but occasionally did not	9 points
I felt equally comfortable and uncomfortable, depending on situation	6 points
No, I was mostly uncomfortable giving and getting affection	3 points
No, never liked being touched and I am still that way	0 points

Did your family allow you to be partially clothed (or naked) before puberty? ______

Yes, we ran around naked or shared baths – we never thought about it	12 points
Yes, to a limited degree (I was a small child for God's sakes!)	9 points
Nudity as a child was equally encouraged/discouraged	6 points
Not really, when it happened it has definitely frowned upon	3 points
No, that would never have happened in my family!	0 points

Were you comforted by your family when others bullied you or you felt bad? ______

I strongly felt comforted and protected by my family if I was picked on	12 points
Yes, I was usually comforted and protected if I was picked on	9 points
Sometimes I did and other times I did not (or I never got picked on)	6 points
No, I was usually not protected and suffered for it	3 points
I never felt comforted or protected by my family (and suffered a lot for it)	0 points

What messages did you get from school and/or church regarding sex? ______

Overall positive messages	12 points
Mostly positive messages	9 points
Equally positive and negative messages (or did not attend school/church)	6 points
Mostly negative messages	3 points
Overwhelming negative messages	0 points

What was discussed if you actually received the "birds & bees" talk? ______

Talked about anything I wanted to and given information (like a book)!	12 points
Limited discussion of "basics" and was given information (like a book)	9 points
Very limited discussion AND very limited information provided	6 points
Very limited discussion OR very limited information was provided	3 points
No talk at all AND no information (even when dog was humping my leg)	0 points

My family used anatomically correct names of the genitals (or their parts)? ______

Yes, with little embarrassment (even if they also used pet names)	12 points
Sometimes, but mostly used pet names if they talked about it at all	9 points
Equally used anatomically correct names and pet names	6 points
Mostly used pet names when they felt they had to say something	3 points
No, they just did not go there AT ALL (no use of any names of any sort)	0 points

Were you prepared for changes that happened to you in puberty? ______

I was well informed and not surprised by all the changes	12 points
I was a little prepared from a class in school or from "the talk"	9 points
I was about equally prepared as I was unprepared	6 points
I heard some about puberty but was not really prepared	3 points
I was ambushed – Have no idea how I got through	0 points

Was your first period or wet dream a positive experience? ______

Yes, it was acknowledged as positive and even celebrated!	12 points
Yes, it was acknowledged as positive but not really celebrated	9 points
About as positive as it was negative for me	6 points
Not really, it was overall a negative experience	3 points
You have got to be kidding you pagan!	0 points

Where did you learn about masturbation? ______

Got the real story from reliable sources (such as family, books, class)	12 points
Got some information from somewhat reliable sources	9 points
Street corner, locker room, or other unreliable sources	6 points
I learned about masturbation by myself	3 points
I was so scared about masturbation that I never tried it	0 points

How did you <u>feel after masturbation</u>? ______

Felt positive (without shame or embarrassment)	12 points
Felt good but had concern, guilt, or embarrassment about it	9 points
Felt equally positive and negative about it	6 points
Felt mostly negative about it	3 points
Felt guilt, shame, or as if I sinned (or I never masturbated)	0 points

As a teenager, did you <u>feel positive about your body</u>? ______

Yes, I felt very positive overall about my body	12 points
I had mostly positive feelings about my body despite some concerns	9 points
I felt equally positive and negative about my body	6 points
No, I did not like my body much while growing up	3 points
No, I could not stand my body's appearance while growing up	0 points

Based only on teenage sexual experimentation, did you <u>learn to orgasm?</u> ______

Pretty much most times (probably at least 90% of the time)	12 points
Most of the time (probably about 70% of the time)	9 points
Hit and miss (inconsistent frequency but on a 50% basis)	6 points
Had a lot of trouble with orgasm (probably 30% or less of the time)	3 points
I never masturbated or never had orgasm when I did	0 points

When you <u>dated as a teenager</u>, did you discuss your dates with a parent? ______

Yes, I felt free to share whatever I wanted with at least one parent	12 points
Yes, for the most part (with some censoring)	9 points
Not really, I censored a lot of what I said but we did talk	6 points
No way! - I would have been kicked out of the house!	3 points
I was never allowed to date and/or never chose to date	0 points

How do you describe the first <u>messages learned about homosexuality</u>? ______

Mostly very positive messages	12 points
Fairly positive messages	9 points
Equally positive and negative messages	6 points
Fairly negatively messages	3 points
Overwhelming negative messages	0 points

Did you ever have <u>questions about your own sexual orientation</u>? ______

No, I have always been 100% confident of my orientation	12 points
No, not for the most part (at least 80% confidence)	9 points
I have had some question (50% confidence) and turmoil about it	6 points
Yes, but I figured it out with a lot of turmoil at times (30% confidence)	3 points
Yes and I still don't have it figured out (10% confidence with much turmoil)	0 points

Have you questioned whether you were <u>masculine/feminine enough</u>? ______

No, I never thought I wasn't masculine/feminine enough	12 points
Not really, I've been fairly confident that I'm masculine/feminine enough	9 points
Yes, but I decided I was okay (masculine/feminine enough)	6 points
Yes, I occasionally think I am not masculine/feminine enough	3 points
Yes, frequently I question whether I am masculine/feminine enough	0 points

Have you ever questioned yourself about being "<u>good enough</u>" as a lover? ______

No, I never thought I wasn't good enough as a lover	12 points
Not really, I've been fairly confident that I'm good enough as a lover	9 points
Yes, but I decided I was okay (good enough as a lover)	6 points
Yes, I occasionally think I am not good enough as a lover	3 points
I frequently question whether I'm good enough (or I never had sex)	0 points

Were you ever <u>physically abused</u> when you were a child? ______

No, I was never physically abused when I was young	12 points
No, I was never physically abused but I saw/knew of others being abused	9 points
Yes, I was abused but I was given help to heal as a child	6 points
Yes, I was abused and I had to find my own way to heal as a child	3 points
Yes, I was abused and I never did heal as a child	0 points

Were you ever <u>sexually abused</u> when you were a child? ______

No, I was never sexually abused when I was young	12 points
No, I was never sexually abused but I saw/knew of others being abused	9 points
Yes, I was sexually abused but I was given help to heal as a child	6 points
Yes, I was sexually abused but found my own way to heal as a child	3 points
Yes, I was sexually abused and I never did heal as a child	0 points

Were you involved in an <u>unplanned pregnancy or abortion</u> (as male or female)? ______

I was never personally involved in an unplanned pregnancy/abortion	12 points
Never involved but there was unplanned pregnancy/abortion in family	9 points
Had unplanned pregnancy/abortion but got through it okay (mild effects)	6 points
Had unplanned pregnancy/abortion and I had moderate negative effects	3 points
Had unplanned pregnancy/abortion and I had severe/traumatic effects	0 points

How do you describe your overall <u>feelings and thoughts about sex</u> growing up? ______

As very positive	12 points
As mostly positive	9 points
As neutral (equally positive/negative)	6 points
As mostly negative	3 points
As very negative	0 points

How do you rate your <u>level of acceptance</u> about sexuality growing up? ______

As very accepting	12 points
As mostly accepting	9 points
As neutral (equally accepting/non-accepting)	6 points
As mostly non-accepting	3 points
As very non-accepting	0 points

Overall, how do you feel your sexual experiences (or lack of the same) while you were growing up have had an <u>effect on you today</u>? ______

They have had a very positive effect	12 points
They have had a mostly positive effect	9 points
They had a neutral effect (equally positive/negative OR I am not sure)	6 points
They have had a mostly negative effect	3 points
They have had a very negative effect	0 points

Self-Assessment of Family Support for Healthy Sexual Development during childhood/adolescence total overall score: ______

Making Sense of Your Score for the Self-Assessment of Family Support

The range of scores is 0 to 300. The scoring is accumulative (so just add up your total score). Generally speaking, the higher the score, the greater the degree of family support you likely experienced for healthy maturation and sexual development as a child and adolescent.

The scoring key is divided into approximate quasi-thirds. A score in the lower half of range (<150) indicates low support from family for healthy sexual development. A score in the moderate elevation above the mid-point (150) indicates a moderate level of support. Finally, the highest level of family support is reflected by scores greater than 225.

This scaling of scores is based completely upon the clients in my specialized sex therapy practice. Hence, the statements below should not necessarily be considered generalizable to people who do not go to therapy. Therefore, caution is to be exercised while applying the following descriptive interpretations. In other words, take this measure as a general indication of how you did or did not feel supported as a kid learning about sexuality. A low score does not necessarily suggest an indictment of your family or that your chances of gaining sexual health are a long shot.

<u>Score of 225 and above</u>: Suggests overall sex-positive development as a child/teenager with a minimal amount of adverse effects from family influences and sex-induced anxiety during your maturation.

<u>Score between 150 and 225</u>: Suggests overall sex-neutral or sex-ambivalent development as a child/teenager with a moderate amount of adverse effects from family influences and sex-induced anxiety during your maturation.

<u>Score below 150</u>: Suggests overall sex-negative development as a child/teenager with a high amount of adverse effects from family influences and sex-induced anxiety during your maturation.

II. Self-Assessment of Sexual Health and Well-being Satisfaction (SHAWS)

Name: ______________________________ Current Age: ______ Date: ____________

Instructions: Select the item which best describes your experience and place the score in the blank to the right. Then total your individual scores for your total overall score.

Read the definition provided to you for each dimension of sexual health. It is provided to help you understand the aspect of your sexuality which you will be rating. Try your best to answer each question regarding your level of satisfaction. For example, even though you may not know something like your hormone level, please rate your satisfaction based upon what you do know ("Well, I've never had a problem in that area") or your general feeling. Use the following rating scale to answer each question:

12 = very high satisfaction
9 = high level of satisfaction
6 = moderate level of satisfaction
3 = low level of satisfaction
0 = very low level of satisfaction

DNK means you **D**o **N**ot **K**now your level of satisfaction (try not to use this option). Use DNK if you feel the question does not apply to you, like when you are asked to rate your satisfaction with a primary relationship. Well, what if you don't have one? You can either rate the question on your last relationship with a primary partner or just use DNK if you prefer (but adjust your score accordingly).

Self Sexual Satisfaction (This section is just about you)

1. **Sexual health literacy** (knowledge) – Accurate information regarding sexuality that is not biased by prejudices and politics.

   ___ *How satisfied are you with your level of knowledge about human sexuality?*

2. **Sexual self-image** – How you see your own physical appearance, including attractiveness (based on how you see yourself).

   ___ *How satisfied are you with the sexual attractiveness your body?*

3. **Sense of self-love** – A tender feeling of kindness, self-care, and acceptance toward yourself, associated with self-respect and positive feeling.

   ___ *How satisfied are you with your ability to love yourself?* (This does not mean masturbation; that is the next question.)

4. **Sexual self-pleasuring** (sexual function of desire, arousal, and climax through masturbation) – Positive feelings resulting from any physical stimulation which makes you sexual interested and aroused (including but not requiring orgasm and not involving another person).

   a. ___ *How satisfied are you with your ability to experience sexual desire associated with self-pleasure (masturbation)?*

b. ___ *How satisfied are you with your ability to experience sexual arousal (erections for men and vaginal lubrication for women) associated with self-pleasure (masturbation)?*

c. ___ *How satisfied are you with your ability to experience sexual climax (orgasm) associated with self-pleasure (masturbation)?*

5. **Sexual fantasy** – thinking about sexy things which create or increase sexual feelings (whether or not a person masturbates).

   ___ *How satisfied are you with your ability to enjoy sexual fantasy?*

6. **Sexual health service access** – Being able to access sexual health services (such as seeing a doctor, getting reproductive services, getting sex counseling) based upon your location and financial status.

   ___ *How satisfied are you in your ability to access sexual health services?*

Relational Sexual Satisfaction (This section is about you and your partner).

7. **Overall *relationship* satisfaction** – Your total satisfaction resulting from all aspects of your relationship with another person (including, but not limited to, emotional, affectionate, sexual, intellectual, financial, spiritual, and safety aspects of your overall relationship).

   ___ *How satisfied are you with the overall relationship with your primary partner?*

   (If you are not in what you consider a "primary relationship" at present, you may respond to this item based on thinking of a particular partner, your last primary relationship, or use NA if you do not think it applies.)

8. **Overall *sexual* satisfaction** – Your total satisfaction resulting from all SEXUAL aspects of your relationship with another person (including, but not limited to, frequency, duration, climax-consistency, and emotional aspects of your overall sexual relationship).

   ___ *How satisfied are you with the overall SEXUAL relationship with your primary partner?*

   (If you are not in what you consider a "primary relationship" at present, you may respond to this item based on thinking of a particular partner, your last primary relationship, or use NA if you do not think it applies.)

9. **Sense of love for another** – A feeling of affection, tenderness, and connection towards a person, often associated with a feeling of passion and a longing for intimacy with that person.

   ___ *How satisfied are you with your ability to experience love toward another person?*

10. **Sexual pleasuring with a partner** (sexual function of desire, arousal, and climax with another person) – Your ability to experience sexual desire, sexual arousal, and orgasm with a sexual partner.

   a. ___ *How satisfied are you with your ability to experience sexual desire associated with sexual relations with another person?*

   b. ___ *How satisfied are you with your ability to experience sexual arousal (erections for men and vaginal lubrication for women) associated with sexual relations with another person?*

c. ___ *How satisfied are you with your ability to experience sexual climax (orgasm) associated with sexual relations with another person?*

11. **Social acceptance of sexuality** – The average amount of acceptance you feel you receive from people in your social networks regarding your sexuality (including an average of support from family, peers, organizational memberships, or community as a whole).

    ___ *How satisfied are you with how your sexuality is accepted within your social network (such as family, peers, and community-at-large).*

12. **Sexual-Spiritual Relationship** – The degree of alignment between one's spiritual/religious beliefs and one's sexual practices (whether the sexual behaviors are practiced alone or with another person).

    ___ *How satisfied are you with the relationship between your sexuality and your spiritual/religious beliefs?*

    (You can use DNK if you do not think this item applies.)

Medical Sexual Satisfaction

Special note – the previous items are based on the general premise that the more you have – like self-acceptance or ability to orgasm – the higher your satisfaction. With the exception of the question about fertility, the items in this section are the opposite – the less you have, usually means (but not always) the higher your satisfaction.

13. **Sexual pain status** – Pain primarily experienced by women (although men can be affected as well) during or immediately after sexual activity (especially sexual intercourse).

    ___ *How satisfied are you with regards to your degree of comfort (absence of pain) during or after intercourse?*

14. **Sexual injury status** – Sexual trauma or abuse that has been forced upon you by one or more perpetrators against your consent.

    ___ *How satisfied are you with regards to whether all your sexual relations have been with your consent?*

15. **Sexual transmitted infections status** (sometime referred to sexually transmitted diseases) – Illnesses caused by a virus, bacteria, or parasite that have high probability of transmission between people by means of sexual contact.

    ___ *How satisfied are you with regards to your ability to prevent yourself from getting a sexually transmitted infection?* (Please answer regardless of whether or not you actually know if you have a sexually transmitted infection.)

16. **Sexual hormone status** – Natural substances produced by the body (primarily testosterone and estrogen) which make a person more interested in sex as well as increase one's fertility, sense of vitality, and overall health and well-being.

    ___ *How satisfied are you in regard to your status of sexual hormones?* (Please answer regardless of whether or not you have actually had your hormone levels measured).

17. **Sex addiction (compulsivity) status** – When individuals report being unable to control their sexual behavior despite increasingly adverse consequences as a result of their "out-of-control" sexual behavior (such as ruining their health, relationships, and careers).

    ___ *How satisfied are you in regard to your ability to prevent yourself from engaging in sexually compulsive behaviors (also referred to as sex addiction behaviors)?*

18. **Sexual reproductive status** – The natural capacity to conceive and have children as well as the ability to prevent pregnancy (regardless of one's sexual orientation).

    ___ *How satisfied are you with you fertility (your ability to have children and/or keep from having offspring)?*

<u>Sexual Identity Satisfaction</u>

19. **Sex orientation** – Traits of people which make them see themselves as male, female, or transgendered (transgendered defined as a combination of both male and female traits).

    ___ *How satisfied are you with your identified sex (being a man, woman, or transgendered)?*

20. **Sexual orientation** – An enduring pattern of emotional, romantic, and/or sexual attraction you have to men, women, both sexes, or neither sex.

    ___ *How satisfied are you with your sexual orientation (being heterosexual, homosexual, bisexual, or asexual)?*

21. **Sex role orientation** – A person's self-description as being traditionally masculine, traditionally feminine, or androgynous (having high amounts of both masculine and feminine traits).

    ___ *How satisfied are you with your gender role orientation (being masculine, feminine, or androgynous)?*

Domain and Overall Sexual Health
Scoring and Summary

Instructions: This page allows you to summarize your ratings and draw conclusions regarding your sexual health satisfaction.

List how you see your sexual identity:

List your sex orientation
(male, female, or transgender): ________________

List your sexual orientation
(heterosexual, homosexual, bisexual, or asexual): ________________

List your sex role orientation
(traditionally feminine, traditionally masculine, or androgynous): ________________

List your **areas of high satisfaction** (your highest scores). These are the strengths of your sexual health.

____

____

____

____

____

____

____

____

List your **areas of low satisfaction** (your lowest scores). These are the areas of your greatest concern and focus of your self-improvement.

____

____

____

____

____

____

____

____

Sexual Self Satisfaction Total Score _____

Relational Sexual Satisfaction Total Score _____

Medical Sexual Satisfaction Total Score _____

Sexual Identity Satisfaction Total Score _____

Overall Sexual Health Indicator _____
(Total the four domain scores together)

Making Sense of Your SHAWS Baseline Scores

The preceding summary page is designed to help you have a better understanding of your areas of satisfaction and, as noted, draw conclusions what your ratings mean. There is wide variation to the guidelines that follow for understanding your ratings, so remember that exceptions exist for some of the following generalizations.

Scoring is designed to approximate a continuum of 0 to 300, with 100 representing complete (or nearly complete) satisfaction in all areas of sexual health. A score of 300 is meant to represent an ideal model of sexual health. For most people, it is unrealistic to assume they should be anywhere close to a score of 300. People who have been diligently working towards enhancing their sexual health are more likely to be within the 240 to 270 range. This simple 0 to 300 "continuum design" is based upon the following several factors:

- There are twenty-five (25) dimensions of sexual health you have rated 0 to 12 for satisfaction (equaling a possible range of scores from 0 to 300).
- Two items are subdivided into separate sections (questions 4 and 10) and they are to be scored as three equal dimensions of sexual function.
- You are to try your best to give an answer for every area of sexual health. If you cannot, then your total score will be artificially lowered and any missing answer must be taken into account during interpretation.
- If you responded to item 7 or 8 (in the **Relational Sexual Satisfaction** Domain) with "NA" (not applicable) because you are not in a primary relationship or a sexual relationship, then adjust your score accordingly. For example, if you used NA for item 7, your total responses (to a highest possible score) is a total of "288," not 300. Hence, you are not penalized numerically for not being in a primary relationship.
- The following interpretation of scores is similar to what you used in the first questionnaire (Self-Assessment of Family Support). However, it is about your level of satisfaction and again based on my experience with clients:

290 - 300.................. Come on, stop fooling yourself!

250 - 289.................. Very high satisfaction

200 - 249.................. High satisfaction

150 - 199.................. Moderate satisfaction

075 - 149.................. Low satisfaction

000 - 075.................. Stop being so hard on yourself!

The listing of your areas of highest and lowest levels of satisfaction have specific purposes. Your areas of highest satisfaction are represented by your highest rating (typically a rating of 12). These are the strengths of your sexual health and are important in not only "counter-balancing" your areas of low satisfaction, but possibly assisting you in strategies to enhance your sexual health satisfaction.

Your areas of lowest satisfaction are represented by your lowest ratings (typically a rating of 0 to 3). These are the areas of your greatest concern and should guide you in focusing your efforts on your self-improvement journey, recovery program, and/or therapy strategies. Pay particular attention to these areas to focus on for increasing your satisfaction in the areas of your lowest ratings.

III. Self-Assessment of Your Big Wheel of Health and Well-being

Name: ______________________________ Current Age: ______ Date: ____________

Instructions: Please read the definitions provided for each of these dimensions of general health (listed below). They are provided to help you understand the aspects of your general health which you will be rating. Try your best to answer each question regarding your level of satisfaction. For example, even though you may not know your blood pressure or cholesterol level, please rate your satisfaction based upon what you do know (last available information or a lack of noticeable symptoms).

Having multiple heath risk factors, for heart disease and stroke for example, does not mean your life is over or that you have to be resigned to live without a high quality of life. That's the funny thing about personal satisfaction, it is individually defined. Individuals with a terrible sexual abuse history, sexual dysfunction, and/or living with AIDS can report a high level of satisfaction with their sexual health or their life in general. A person without these challenges in their history, who has good general health and living a life of privilege, can be completely miserable. The best approach to health is considered being as informed as you can in order to be better prepared to make health choices. Therefore, if you do not know your blood pressure, go buy a home-version blood pressure monitor. If you do not know your blood sugar or cholesterol level, work with your doctor and get the facts. In the meanwhile, complete the following self-assessment as well as you can and use the questions you don't know as a prompt for getting a healthcare provider to develop a personal health plan.

Use the following rating scale to answer each question:

12 = complete or very high satisfaction
9 = moderate satisfaction
6 = equal amount of satisfaction/dissatisfaction
3 = moderate dissatisfaction
0 = complete or very high dissatisfaction

<u>Overall Health and Well-Being Satisfaction Ratings</u>

- **Nutrition and Health Literacy.** Nutrition is the specific knowledge related to what, how, and when to eat in order to provide our bodies a balanced diet of all required nutrients and to aid us in maintaining positive health (including a body weight something close to ideal). Health literacy is knowing what is important to do to maintain our general health across all areas of the Big Wheel.

___ *How satisfied are you with how often you eat a daily well-balanced diet that includes several servings of fruits and vegetables (half your plate), whole grain cereals, and low fat, low cholesterol proteins and dairy?*

___ *How satisfied are you with your body mass index (BMI) in terms of what is recommend for your height and weight?*

___ *How satisfied are you with your level of knowledge about all that is needed to maintain your overall health and well-being?*

- **Medical Health.** Physical health is measured on a continuum from optimal body function and absence of disease, to disease, and to death that is comprised of cardiovascular, neurological, endocrinological, gastroenterological, respiratory, reproductive, and other aspects of your physical self.

___ *How satisfied are you with your blood pressure?*
___ *How satisfied are you with your cholesterol level?*
___ *How satisfied are you with being able to avoid a chronic illness such as diabetes, cardiovascular disease, respiratory disease, etc.? (If you already have been diagnosed with a chronic illness, how satisfied are you in how well you self-manage the illness?)*

- **Lifestyle Health Factors.** This is a domain of health involving choices people make that significantly affect their risk for developing chronic disease and is related to tobacco and alcohol consumption, drug abuse (prescribed or non-prescribed), and regular health maintenance through exercise, health screenings, and vaccinations.

___ *How satisfied are you that you are not exposed to the health risks of using tobacco products (cigarettes, cigars, or smokeless tobacco) by your own use or the second-hand smoke of others?*
___ *How satisfied are you that you regularly engage in aerobic exercises (at least of 30 minutes duration) and exercises that increase your strength and flexibility 3-4 times per week?*
___ *How satisfied are you that you either do not consume alcohol or do so within recommended limits (no more than one drink per day for women and no more than two drinks per day for men ("drink" being considered a 12 oz. beer, 5 oz. of wine or 1.5 oz. of distilled spirits)?*
___ *How satisfied are you that you regularly engage in health maintenance through recommended health screenings, exams, and vaccinations (including annual dental and vision exams)?*

- **Environmental Health.** This involves having reliable shelter with a supply of clean water and food (free of toxins and contagious diseases), and the living surroundings free of environmental hazards (such as pollutants, second-hand smoke, radiation, etc.), as well as an environment free of violence and cohesion (including domestic violence, gang violence, and war).

___ *How satisfied are you that you have reliable shelter (with little to no risk of being homeless) that has clean water and food supply (free of toxins and contagious diseases)?*
___ *How satisfied are you that you have living surroundings free of environmental hazards and pollutants, such as asbestos, lead, mercury, radon, radiation, and smog?*
___ *How satisfied are you that you have a home environment free of violence and cohesion (including domestic violence, gang violence, and war)?*

- **Mental Health.** This involves the cognitive, emotional, and behavioral factors contributing to personal health, including how an individual feels about changes experienced as he or she goes through life stages and whether he or she has a basic positive or negative sense about his- or herself.

___ *How satisfied are you with your ability to have a positive mood and not be overly bothered by depressed thoughts and feelings?*
___ *How satisfied are you with your ability to relax and not be overly bothered by worries or anxiety?*
___ *How satisfied are you with your level of self-esteem?*

- **Relational Health.** This area includes achieving significant emotional connections with others, including primary relationships with one or more partners; having healthy relations with family members (your biological family or family by choice); maintaining a healthy social network (your friends and coworkers); and defining yourself in relation to the universe (whether that includes what is commonly referred to as GOD).

  ___ *How satisfied are you with your ability to establish and maintain a significant emotional connection in your primary relationship(s) so you feel like part of a "couple?"*
  ___ *How satisfied are you with your sense of connection to, and degree of support from, your friends and family?*
  ___ *How satisfied are you with your sense of spiritual connection to the world and/or sense of meaning in your life (whether that is through a spiritual belief in a God, higher self, or another entity)?*

- **Work and Financial Health.** This domain includes how you are able to provide for yourself (and possibly a family), how you define "work," and how you achieve a sense of productivity or contribution.

  ___ *How satisfied are you with what you do for work or how you support yourself financially?*
  ___ *How satisfied are you with your sense of productivity or the contribution you make to your work, volunteering, or hobbies?*
  ___ *How satisfied are you with your financial status including your ability to reliably support yourself (and family?), your savings and investments for retirement, and your credit rating?*

- **Sexual Health.** Includes the reciprocal relationships between the previous seven domains and all the dimensions of how you are a sexual being (across all the SHAWS domains of self, relational, and medical aspects of sexuality).

  ___ *How satisfied are you with your core sexual identity (the combination of sex orientation, sexual orientation, and sex role orientation)?*
  ___ *How satisfied are you with your overall sexual function (the combination of sexual desire, arousal, and orgasm)?*
  ___ *How satisfied are you with your overall sexual health (the combination of the self, relational, and medical aspects of your sexuality)?*

Making Sense of Your Measure of Overall Health and Well-being Satisfaction

Like the other two questionnaires, just add up your scores and compare them to the range of scores from 0 to 300. Based on your score, different sets of recommendations are offered for your consideration.

How satisfied are you? Remember, it is still important to get actual measures of the health indices you were asked about; such a blood pressure, cholesterol, etc.

<u>Scores above 225</u>: Congratulations! Your general satisfaction is high (average score of at least 9), which is likely an indication of better-than-average health (assuming you were honest with yourself). Enjoy your good overall health and do all you can to preserve it. You are most likely able to achieve optimal health through your own determination and self-help strategies. However, you still may want the aid of a health coach, personal trainer, or have your healthcare provider address specific areas of concern regarding your health (such as any individual rating of 0-3). It's always better to have a "team" in your corner.

Scores between 150 - 224: Good work! You reported an average rating in the moderate range of satisfaction with your overall health (average response at least 6), which indicates you have some areas of strength and that you feel good about many areas of your health. The need for professional help is greater and it is definitely recommended that you work with a team in your corner. You are recommended to use self-help strategies but you really need to work with professionals to help get you where you want to go. Strongly consider consulting the professionals of your choice that are specialists in the area(s) of your lowest satisfaction (such as a financial counselor, minister, health coach, personal trainer, or your healthcare provider). There are many ways to access these services either free or at little cost.

Scores below 150: Okay – there was just a question on this survey about being overly bothered by worry or anxiety. If you scored this low, then you seriously need to be worried! You have reported having pervasive and significant dissatisfaction about many areas of your health, which means there is a good chance you likely have general dissatisfaction with many areas of your life. Your score indicates you may be experiencing difficult challenges regarding your health, and there is no question that you need professional assistance to help you find your way back to the days when you actually felt good about yourself, your health, and your life. You may also be suffering from depression which saps your energy and motivation to make efforts toward positive change. While you are scheduling an appointment with your primary care physician, remember to ask to be screened for anxiety and depression as well.

Again, remember your score can be deceiving in two ways. First, this is a rating of your satisfaction only and you can have high satisfaction partly because you may not be aware of symptoms or a disease process. As mentioned before, one of the purposes of these questionnaires is to prompt you to get the facts on specific health measures in concert with your healthcare providers, including hormone and cholesterol levels as well as having regular screenings and exams.

Secondly, and although unlikely, you could have scored above 225 and had low scores (0-3) on many of the questions for the medical and lifestyle health factors. Hence, take a close look at your lowest scores, build a personal health plan with your team of healthcare providers and advisors, and get started in earnest preserving the health you have. Remember, in the domain of sexuality, the general guideline is "use it or lose it." The same can be said of many of the general areas of your overall health that need to be attended to and maintained such as nutrition, exercise, and relationships.

36

Sharing the Treatment Plan For Sex Therapy

Frederick L. Peterson, Jr.

This chapter focuses on the details of a treatment agreement and an example of what is shared at a results-sharing conference (RSC) for an in-depth client evaluation. The RSC is usually the third (sometimes fourth) meeting in a multiple-session assessment protocol. During the RSC, three basic sets of information are shared with the client (and the partner):

1. a brief summary of the key information learned about the client from all sources (data from interviews, psychological testing, other providers, etc.),
2. what the therapist concludes about the information, including diagnosis, and
3. the therapist's recommendations concerning what to do about the presenting problems.

The RSC document includes the summary of data, diagnosis, desired outcomes, treatment goals, recommendations, evaluation criteria by which to determine if the recommendations are making positive change, and standard language regarding consent and client responsibilities. To avoid overwhelming the clients, they should first be told that the RSC document is a draft to allow client input and modification; that they are in charge of what recommendations to accept; what the time frame will be to implement any recommendations they do accept; and that they are not expected to make an immediate decision regarding the entire plan at the RSC, but that they are asked to take the document with them for their review and decision.

Draft Treatment Agreement

Developed Between Marcia* and Robert and
Dr. Frederick L. Peterson, Jr.

I. DIAGNOSIS, TREATMENT OUTCOMES, AND GOALS

Robert is a 72-year-old Anglo-American male and Marcia is a 61-year-old Anglo-American female who have been married about 2 years. Whereas Marcia and Robert demonstrate strength in their love for each other in their marriage, each has expressed concerns related to communicating with the other and improving the satisfaction with their sexual relationship. They have experienced a history of health concerns, including Robert's vascular disease, bypass surgeries, congestive heart failure, and a history of erectile dysfunction secondary to heart disease and medication effects. Marcia has a history of ovarian cancer and hysterectomy after which she used hormonal treatment for several years but stopped because she was not sexually active. She has to use vaginal dilators to permit containment during penile-vaginal intercourse because both Marcia and Robert report that her vagina is "small sized." She is not orgasmic during sexual intercourse with Robert but able to have multiple orgasms during masturbation.

Both Marcia and Robert were previously married and both of their spouses are deceased. The couple have known each other for decades and culminated their friendship in a romance after each was widowed. Each has advanced graduate education; Robert is a retired leader of a religious community and Marcia is retired from a job in human services. They are currently seeking treatment to enhance their relationship and sexual satisfaction.

On the Beck Depression Inventory, Robert reported he has less energy and gets fatigued more than he used to but was within the normal range of symptoms for depression. Marcia was within the moderate range of depressive symptoms, reporting less energy than she used to have, thinking of herself as a failure, and not seeing herself as attractive. On the Sexual Health Inventory for men, Robert reported a severe level of symptoms for erectile function but also reported a high level of satisfaction with sexual relations with Marcia. On the Female Sexual Function Index, Marcia reported sexual health symptoms with sexual desire, sexual arousal, orgasm, and sexual satisfaction.

Diagnosis: (R) Erectile Dysfunction
(M) Depressive Disorder, moderate
(M) Female Sexual Interest/Desire Disorder
(M) Female Sexual Arousal Disorder

Robert and Marcia are consulting with Dr. Peterson for a comprehensive mental health and sexual health assessment. As such, they are conjointly developing the components of this Draft Treatment Agreement. Hence, the following are *desired treatment outcomes* for ensuring the mental and sexual health as defined by:

1. enhancing the couple's satisfaction with their overall relationship.
2. specifically enhancing their satisfaction with their sexual relationship.

This outcome will be accomplished through *specific treatment goals*, which include:

1. increasing satisfaction with, and frequency of, nondemand, nongenital touch, employing sensate focus therapy techniques.
2. increasing satisfaction with, and frequency of, sensual and erotic touching, with and without intercourse.

---

* Names and characteristics have been changed to protect confidentiality.

3. increasing satisfaction with, and communication about, their sexual and overall marital relationship, specifically addressing feelings of security, emotional intimacy, and physical intimacy.

These treatment outcomes and goals, as well as the following recommendations, may be accomplished at whatever pace and amount of time Robert and Marcia wish to proceed, acknowledging that these difficulties took considerable time to develop and will not be resolved "overnight." Please take this draft with you, review and discuss it, then decide to start treatment.

II. TREATMENT STRATEGIES

Treatment strategies employed to achieve these outcomes and treatment goals will be:

1. Couples sex therapy, as provided by a therapist of Robert and Marcia's choosing. Should this be Dr. Peterson, multiple techniques will be employed, including but not limited to sex education and therapy (including video-based education), cognitive-behavioral prescriptions/contracting, and existentially focused psychotherapy. Treatment sessions will be on a biweekly basis until such a time as both parties agree to move to a monthly schedule or end treatment.
2. Behavioral prescriptions will be employed, including but not limited to:

    a. Robert effectively overcoming the challenges of erectile dysfunction (ED) through use of a vacuum-constriction device (VCD) or one of the first-line treatment options for the clinical practice guidelines on primary care management of ED.
    b. Sexual self-image affirmations being assigned and completed toward a goal of enhanced self-esteem.
    c. Relaxation exercises enhancing willful control over the level of tension in the body, including optional Kegel exercise or biofeedback training of vaginal tension.
    d. Sensate focus exercises concentrating on the exploration and sharing of each other's sensuality.

3. Marcia employing an at-home female orgasmic training program with support from the couple's sex therapy and involving Robert as indicated by program guidelines.
4. Bibliographic strategies (journaling, reading assignments) focused upon expanding sexual literacy and improving marital communication.
5. A women's therapy group or individual counseling for Marcia to increase emotional support and decrease anxious symptoms. Group treatment can either be on a concurrent or consecutive basis with individual therapy.
6. A men's support group for Robert to increase level of support and buffer the effects of stress related to age-related losses as well as to diminish his cardiovascular risk.
7. Diagramming, monitoring, and engineering the couple's social support system to serve as a mediating buffer to stress and to provide structuring of time for leisure together.
8. Participation in a regular exercise program together, such as walking for a minimal period of 20 to 30 minutes of increased heart rate, several times a week.
9. Testosterone evaluation of Robert to ensure he is within normal limits and, if he is not, consideration of a supplemental hormone treatment.
10. Specific recommendations for sexual adjustment secondary to health changes related to client's medical conditions:

    a. Increased sensual play to change the pattern of sexual relations as "work."
    b. Bathing each other/mutual showers for sensual play and relaxation as well as reduction of spasticity and muscular pain.
    c. Emphasis on morning sensual/sexual activity rather than evening to reduce the impact of the fatigue factor.

d. Maintenance of an air conditioned environment and avoidance of lengthy exposure to heat which can "sap" energy and strength.
e. Employment of different positions when having sexual intercourse, which can add variety and reduce continued pressure of body parts that cause discomfort.
f. Consideration of the use of mild stimulants if fatigue continues to be an obstacle to sexual activity as well as activities of daily living (e.g., caffeine).
g. Use of lubricants to supplement Marcia's vaginal lubricating response.
h. Use of vibration stimulation for increased intensity and reduction of fatigue.

11. Establishment of a personal and family mission for the integration of physical, emotional, and spiritual goals for this stage of the couple's life development, including end-of-life decision planning.
12. Consideration of a second trial of hormonal supplement treatment employing estrogen transdermal patch if behavioral treatment of hypoactive sexual desire disorder does not increase sexual desire to the level of patient satisfaction.
13. If improvements are not witnessed within 3 months of treatment, consideration of psychiatric consultation for evaluation of medication management related to history of depressive episodes.

III. EVALUATION

Evaluation of treatment progress will be conducted on a regular basis using a combination of subjective satisfaction ratings and completion of behavioral contracts. Subjective ratings will be on a 1 to 10 scale (1-10) with 10 representing the highest level of satisfaction. Frequencies are recorded in episodes per time unit (3x/week) or percent of time (10%). Criteria are specific to the client's presenting complaints. This treatment agreement will be for a 3-month period, with review and modification or termination every 3 months thereafter.

Criteria	1 Year Ago	TX Start	Mid-TX	TX End	6 Month F/U
Her Sexual Self-Esteem					
His Sexual Self-Esteem					
Satisfaction With Nondemand Touch					
Frequency of Sexual Desire					
Intensity of Sexual Desire					
Frequency of Female Orgasm With Manual Pleasuring					
Frequency of Female Orgasm With Oral Pleasuring					
Frequency of Female Orgasm With Vibration					
Frequency of Female Orgasm During Intercourse (With Clitoral Stimulation)					

Criteria	1 Year Ago	TX Start	Mid-TX	TX End	6 Month F/U
Frequency of Exercise					
Utilization of Support System					
Frequency of Sexual Relations					
Her Satisfaction With Sexual Relationship					
His Satisfaction With Sexual Relationship					
Her Satisfaction With Overall Relationship					
His Satisfaction With Overall Relationship					

IV. CLIENT RESPONSIBILITIES

1. Maintain personal responsibility for one's own health and satisfaction, using professionals only as consultants and resources for treatment/healing process.
2. Maintain personal safety by removing any weapons from the home and never bringing weapons to the treatment center. Abstain from any acts of physical aggression unless one's own safety is threatened.
3. Keep the therapist informed of any contemplation of suicide, harm to others, or separation and divorce.
4. Participate in treatment plan as conjointly developed and agreed upon at the start of treatment, including, but not limited to, consistently attending sessions, being on time to sessions, completing assignments, and paying fees for services.

V. CONSENT FOR TREATMENT

The contents of this agreement have been developed as a draft for my review and input. The draft agreement has been explained to my satisfaction and I understand I may withdraw from this treatment at any time. I understand the rules of confidentiality and that any disclosure of imminent harm to self or others (intent of suicide or homicide) or abuse to minors or elders will be reported to appropriate authorities, by obligation of law and professional ethics. The signatures below represent an agreement to this statement of treatment outcomes, goals, strategies, and evaluation methods.

______________________	______________________
Marcia	Date
______________________	______________________
Robert	Date
______________________	______________________
Dr. Frederick L. Peterson, Jr. Clinical Psychology and Sex Health	Date

37

Sexual Health Word Cue Paradigm

Teja Fuller and Gabriele Mamone

The Sexual Health Word Cue Paradigm is a Galton-Crovitz styled word-cue measure that uses a combination of words in a timed recall method. Its purpose is to determine if a respondent has either positive, negative, or neutral correlations associated with certain sexual themes.

INSTRUCTIONS

When using this word-cue paradigm, the therapist will clearly pronounce a word from the list in the order listed. After stating the word, the participant will be given 90 seconds to recall any thoughts, words, or memories they feel are associated with the word. In the space next to the word, the therapist will write down the responses of the participant.

SCORING

To score the section, each response block has a Likert scale next to it for scoring each response. The scale ranges from 0-10, with 10 being the highest. The ranges for the score are arranged as so:

0-3 (negative associations)
4-6 (neutral associations)
7-10 (Positive associations)

If the majority of the response is observed to be negative, then numbers 0-3 should be selected, with 0 being on the lower end of negative associations and 3 being on the higher end. If the majority of the response observed is thought to be neutral, then numbers 4-6 should be selected, with 4 being on the lower end of neutral associations and 6 being on the higher end. If the majority of the responses observed are thought to be positive, then numbers 7-10 should be selected, with 7 being on the lower end of positive associations and 10 being on the higher end. Please note any behaviors or situations that are observed during the cues.

Thought Perception Scoring Scale										
Negative Association				Neutral Association			Positive Association			
0	1	2	3	4	5	6	7	8	9	10

Words	Response	Score
1. Love		
2. Eggplant		
3. Impulse		
4. Intimate		
5. Vagina		
6. Hug		
7. Violence		

Words	Response	Score
8. Sex		
9. Kiss		
10. Restraint		
11. Woman		
12. Social		
13. Penis		
14. Impulse		
15. Hurt		
16. Man		

Words	Response	Score
17. Fetish		
18. Father		
19. Pleasure		
20. Mother		

Observational notes:

Sensual Pleasuring Through Sensate Focus Exercises*

Building Your Sensual and Emotional Connection

The exercises described below will help you to feel comfortable freely sharing your body with your partner and freely exploring your partner's body. These exercises have been used by sexuality therapists since they were developed and published by Masters and Johnson in their landmark book *Human Sexual Response* (1966). They were originally designed to help couples overcome sexual dysfunctions related to erection, lubrication, and orgasm problems. Therapists have learned over the years that these exercises can also help couples learn to feel more comfort in giving and receiving pleasure.

They are named "sensate focus" because the exercises help the couple learn to focus on the pleasurable sensations one experiences when touched in a sensual manner. They help to greatly reduce and eventually eliminate anxiety that has built up over time as couples struggled to fix their sexual problems or discomforts.

These exercises are here for four purposes:

1. To help people who are having certain problems regain their previous level of functioning;
2. To give couples who cannot have sexual intercourse (permanently or temporarily) ideas about how they can continue to have a loving sexual relationship without intercourse (through loving touch referred to as "outercourse");
3. To encourage couples to take a break from focusing on intercourse and orgasm as the most important aspect of their sexual relationship and learn how to enjoy one another in a less-genitally focused way; and
4. To reconnect as a couple by building an emotionally significant and meaningful connection.

The fourth point deserves some special emphasis because when a couple builds an emotionally significant and meaningful connection, they are building the intimacy bond that is crucial for promoting and sustaining the kind of long-term commitment that most couples hope for. True intimacy requires that two people develop closeness by bonding intellectually, emotionally, spiritually, and sexually in a committed relationship. These exercises provide an excellent tool for bonding emotionally, spiritually, and sexually. When a couple has emotional, spiritual, and sexual bonding, the intellectual part and the commitment part are so much more likely to grow and thrive.

Sexual dysfunctions (such as the inability to have orgasm, ejaculating too fast, no lubrication, and erection problems) are most likely to respond well to these exercises. However, the couple must follow the step-by-step instructions from Sensate Focus I through Sensate Focus III. Here are the ground rules that couples should follow if they decide to do the exercises. These ground rules apply to each phase of the exercises. Remember, you need to follow the instructions carefully, step by step, and not be tempted to jump ahead to the next level too soon if you want to get the full benefit of the experience.

---

*This handout was prepared by Jill W. Bley, PhD, and Frederick L. Peterson, Jr., PsyD.

The first and most important rule for using these exercises is that both partners agree that they will neither try to have intercourse until they progress through the steps to Sensate Focus III, nor have an orgasm or pressure their partner for orgasm. In other words, there must be an agreement to put a ban on intercourse and orgasm during the time that you are going through the steps together. If either partner finds it really difficult not to have an orgasm for the period of time that they are doing these exercises, that partner should masturbate alone, making sure that they do not put any pressure on their partner to provide the orgasm for them.

You should decide ahead of time who will initiate the request to do the exercise. The best way to arrange this is to agree that whoever asks first will not initiate again until the other initiates. That way, each of you will have the responsibility to ask for sexual pleasuring about 50% of the time. Most couples are used to leaving that responsibility to one or the other partner most of the time. If you share the initiating, you will both have an opportunity to learn how to ask for sex and how to say "yes" or "no." If your response is "no," then the rule should be that the one who says "no" must offer an alternative time and then be ready to do the exercise at the designated time without being reminded.

Before you get started, it is helpful for couples to talk about what kind of sexual language they have. If you have none (i.e., you don't say anything when you want sex), just start to kiss or touch or give some other non-verbal indication; you may find it very helpful to figure out together whether that is okay with both of you or if you would like to be able to ask for a sexual encounter. You could also discuss how to say "no" without the other's feelings being hurt.

The person whose turn it is to initiate the pleasuring exercise is responsible to make sure the room temperature is comfortable enough to be nude without clothes or blankets. That person should also set the "mood," paying attention to the lighting and perhaps soft music. Have lotions, oils, or creams available that are at room temperature. Find some fabrics in your home that might feel good if used to touch your partner (e.g., a piece of fur, a silk scarf, a piece of soft felt). The initiator is also responsible to make sure that both partners have paid adequate attention to hygiene before the encounter. You may both like to start the pleasuring time by showering together. Make sure your breath is pleasing to your partner so that you both feel free to kiss and/or use your mouth to provide touching.

A question that most couples have when they are beginning these pleasuring experiences is, "How much time should we do this?" The answer is not always an easy one. If either partner finds touch to be unpleasant, the couple must take things slowly and allow "de-sensitization" to touch to happen. Avoiding touch never solves the issues related to fear of touch. However, forcing prolonged discomfort won't help either. So it needs to proceed at a pace that allows the person to become comfortable with touch gradually. If there are no issues around touch, the general answer is to make sure that you touch your partner long enough that you have been able to touch the entire body and have given yourself the chance to touch until you feel "lost" in the joy of touching. You are now ready to begin Sensate Focus I.

Sensate Focus I: Non-Genital Pleasuring

The Initiator begins to touch the partner all over the body, excluding genitals, breasts, and buttocks. The touch should be like a loving massage, making sure that the pressure is comfortable (not too soft or too hard). The Initiator should be focused on touching the partner for the Initiator's own pleasure, allowing themself to be "lost" in the experience of giving pleasure and touching. The Receiver just relaxes and focuses on the pleasure of receiving loving, sensual touch and allows themself to be "lost" in the sensations of the body. No one talks during the pleasuring except to indicate pleasure or ask the Receiver to turn over or to check out whether or not the touch is comfortable.

The Receiver should enjoy pleasurable touch to both the front and back of the body. The Receiver may talk to indicate if something is uncomfortable and may show the Initiator how to touch in a particular area in order to make the touch more comfortable. When the Initiator feels that they are ready to stop touching, then the two change places. The Receiver becomes the one who touches and the Initiator receives the pleasuring touch. Remember that both should focus on "getting lost" in the sensations of touching and being touched. Repeat these exercises and enjoy Sensate Focus I on several occasions (four to six times is a suggested minimum) before progressing to the next level of exercises.

Sensate Focus II:
Non-Genital and Genital Pleasuring

You are ready to move on to this step only if both partners are enjoying the sensations of "getting lost" in the feelings of pleasure produced by the loving touch they were experiencing while doing Sensate Focus I. The rules and suggestions for Sensate Focus II are the same. Except that this time the genitals and breasts and buttocks are included in the pleasuring touch. However, there should be no more emphasis on the breasts, genitals, and buttocks than on the other parts of the body. In other words, the difference between these two exercises is to merely include the breasts and genitals and buttocks in an overall body sensual massage, with the person whose turn it is to initiate the exercise going first and being responsible to set the mood.

If you are doing these exercises to correct a sexual problem, there continues to be a ban on intercourse and orgasms. Do not sabotage your progress by putting pressure on your partner to violate this ban. If you feel you simply must have an orgasm, do it privately by bringing yourself to climax. This privacy keeps your partner from feeling pressure or guilt for not "giving" you the orgasm.

If you are hoping to correct an orgasm problem, this exercise is great for learning to control the timing of orgasm. If the problem is coming too fast, you can learn how to slow down. If the problem is taking too long (or not at all), you can enjoy the teasing and building of sexual tension.

If you are hoping to correct an erection or lubrication problem, pressure to "use" it right away if an erection or lubrication occurs will usually result in success for the moment but will probably not produce the long-term solution you are hoping for. Ridding oneself of "performance anxiety" and/or inhibitions to receiving pleasure will not be overcome if you try to have intercourse as soon as you have an erection or begin to lubricate.

If you are using these exercises as a way to maintain sexual closeness during a period of time when you cannot have intercourse, or to enhance your sexual relationship, there is no ban on orgasm. However, you may want to have an agreement that you will occasionally decide together to have a ban so that you can keep the emphasis and focus on the touch and loving sensations instead of orgasm. If you are using these sensual play exercises to fix a sexual problem, it is really important to return to these exercises at times in order to ensure that "performance anxiety" never intrudes on your sexuality again. If you are using the exercises to enhance your sexual relationship, we suspect you will want to plan to go back to them just to experience the wonderful, loving, sensual feelings you get from them.

Sensate Focus III: Intercourse Pleasuring

You are ready to move on to these exercises only when (a) both partners are enjoying the feelings of "getting lost" in the sensations of being lovingly touched and caressed all over the body (now including the breasts, genitals, and buttocks) and (b) the partner with the identified sexual problem is feeling comfortable and secure about lubrication or erection (i.e., they can depend on it and do not feel inhibited or worried about their performance).

The rules about how to initiate are the same. Begin this exercise by doing Sensate Focus II. Do not take turns touching each other now. Sort of "choreograph" a mutual "dance" of loving touch. Then when both partners feel ready, begin to pleasure one another with intercourse, starting out in one position and then gracefully and rhythmically changing to another position. After a while, change positions again. NOTE: vaginal lubrication is not necessarily a sign that a woman is ready for vaginal containment. Therefore, it is important for the female partner to indicate when she is ready. Some ideas for various positions for intercourse will be discussed later.

If premature orgasm is the problem, be sure that you do not start this exercise until you are confident in your ability to prolong your pleasure by withholding the ejaculation for an agreed-upon time. Achieving this skill is done by using the "Stop-Start" technique for stimulating the penis during masturbation and then using "Stop-Start" during Sensate Focus II pleasuring. The instructions for doing "Stop-Start" can be found in many books that focus on male sexuality. An "oldie but goodie" is *The New Male Sexuality* by Bernie Zilbergeld (2013).

If inhibited orgasm is the problem, Sensate Focus III, with no pressure at all to produce an orgasm, may help an orgasm to happen. If it does not and you cannot have an orgasm even with masturbation, then you need to give yourself an orgasm with masturbation first and then teach your partner how to touch your genitals to replicate your own touch and then "Bridge" these sensations to intercourse. "Bridging" the orgasm from self-stimulation to partner stimulation requires informing the partner when one is approaching orgasm and then directly involving the partner right before orgasm starts. You only move from one step to the next when you have been able to have orgasm during each step.

Intercourse Positions

Many couples who begin Sensate Focus III (Intercourse Pleasuring) realize that they have a very limited repertoire of positions for intercourse. Most are very familiar with the "male superior" position where the male is facing the female (better known as the "missionary" position). Even though this is the most popular position, it often is not the best position for the female partner to receive as much stimulation of the clitoris and/or G-spot as she may need.

Another "male superior" position is for him to enter her vagina from the rear. She is in a "doggy" pose on her forearms (so that her rear end is elevated higher than the front end) and knees on the bed or floor. This is a great position for her to receive stimulation to the G-spot, so while you are pleasuring with intercourse you will have an opportunity to see if you can experience pleasure from the G-spot. This position also allows for the opportunity for him to stroke and caress her buttocks and/or anus.

There are many "female superior" positions. They are similar to the above except, of course, she is on top. In the superior position the female can guide the penis into her vagina. She can decide how fast or how slow she wants to let the penis enter. She can also decide how fast or slow the in and out movements will be.

Being on top also provides an opportunity for her to ask her partner to stroke and caress her clitoris and/or her breast. Women are encouraged to self-stimulate their clitoris especially when "on top" during vaginal containment of a penis or vibrator (but really time during sexual arousal). They are encouraged to be confident, comfortable, and assertive with self-stimulation while being with a partner. If the partner is uncomfortable with the woman touching her own clitoris during sex, simply say, "It's my clitoris and I'll touch it when I wish."

She can also turn and be in the superior position with her back to him and her legs and feet toward his head. In this position she provides the opportunity to have her partner stroke and caress her buttocks and/or her anus.

The side-by-side position is a face-to-face position with neither partner "superior." Couples may have to practice a bit and play with positioning in order to make this a comfortable and pleasurable position for both of them. Most couples find that if she opens her legs so that he can put one leg between hers, he can enter her vagina more easily. So, it is really a side-by-side entwined position.

There are many variations on the "male superior" and the "female superior" which can be accomplished by sitting, squatting, standing, or kneeling. When experimenting with any position, good support and balance is required. Be sure to check how sturdy the furniture is, if the chandelier will hold your weight, and if you are able to support one another's weight. It can be rather painful to fall with an erect penis inside the vagina.

Remember, the point of Sensate Focus III is to be playful, enjoy, and experiment with intercourse together with no pressure for orgasm. Of course, the standard illustrated reference guides are recommended to make the many positions of lovemaking clear in your mind. The ancient classic of the *Kama Sutra* (the book, not the movie) is the ultimate sex guide from antiquity. More recently, *The Joy of Sex: The Ultimate Revised Edition* is the American classic illustrated guide to sex (Comfort, 2009). Of course, let's not forget the highly recommended and favorite reference guides of the first author, *Sex for Dummies* (Westheimer, 2007) and *The Complete Idiot's Guide to Amazing Sex* (Locker, 2005).

Kegel Exercises (Pelvic Floor Exercises)*

The exercises that your therapist has asked you to do are very important because they are a key element to the success of your treatment. These exercises, if done as directed, will strengthen the muscles of your "pelvic floor." The pelvic floor is a large group of muscles that stretch from side to side across the floor (bottom) of your pelvic area. The muscles are attached to the pubic bone which is in front of your body, and to the lowest part of your spine (the coccyx), which is in the back of your body. All of the openings in the lower part of your body pass through these muscles, that is, the urethra, anus, and vagina. These muscles support your pelvic organs and control the flow of urine and feces. The primary muscle group in the pelvic floor is the pubococcygeal muscle (PC muscle).

How to Do Pelvic Floor Exercises

The first thing to do is to clearly identify the muscles that you need to control. Other muscles near the pelvic floor muscles can easily get involved. Therefore, you should spend some time making sure that you are working only with those muscles in the pelvic floor by making sure that you are not pulling in your stomach, not tightening your buttocks, not tightening your thighs, and not holding your breath. To make sure that you are not using muscles that should not be included, place your hand on your abdomen while you do the exercises. Your abdomen should not move.

Now try to isolate your PC muscle. To accomplish this, sit on the toilet. Spread your legs. Begin to urinate. Squeeze the muscles that will stop the flow of urine. Pay attention to the muscles that you are contracting in order to stop the flow. Finish urinating and then insert your finger into your vagina or just rest your finger on the opening of the vagina and see if you can feel the muscle contract. If you can insert your finger, you will feel the muscle contract around your finger. These are the muscles that you will be exercising. Here are the exercises:

- Tighten the PC muscles quickly by contracting them powerfully. Then relax the muscle completely after each contraction. Do 10 repetitions.
- Tighten the PC muscles and hold them for 3 to 5 seconds and then relax them for 3 to 5 seconds.

The quick contractions build muscle strength. The slow contractions build stamina. Do these exercises 3 times per day. Every week increase the number of repetitions by 5 until you reach 30. The contractions that you hold for 3 to 5 seconds should be increased from 3 to 10 seconds.

You need to remember to do these exercises every day. One way to remember to do the exercises is to link them with a predictable daily activity. For example, if you drive to and from work you can decide to do your exercises every time you have to stop your car for a red traffic light. If you are a stay-at-home person, you could decide to do your exercises every time you need to urinate during the day, or every time you have to walk up or down the stairs.

---

*This handout was prepared by Jill W. Bley, PhD.

Personalized Health Maintenance and Relapse Prevention Plan*

Prescription for Health

Having a specific written plan to be healthy is always more effective if it is organized (on paper) and shared with others for accountability rather than just having some ideas rolling around in your head (even good ideas) regarding how to avoid and deal with triggers which lead you to behave in a self-destructive manner. This plan can be used to avoid a relapse of many types of self-harm behavior, including use of alcohol and drugs, sexual acting out, or suicidal thoughts and behaviors. It also goes beyond relapse protection to assist individuals walk a path of intention and healthy daily living. It is recommended that drafting a personalized health maintenance and relapse prevention plan contain the following ten components:

1. A personal mission statement clarifying one's sense of purpose.
2. Identifying what your "bottom lines" are that you do not want to cross/be part of your healthy life.
3. Identification of triggers for acting out, both emotional and situational triggers.
4. Inventory of healthy coping behaviors, both "Tried and True" as well as "Expanding the Toolbox."
5. Creating a Personal Mission Support Team from your social network.
6. Creating a "Prediction Relapse Scenario" identifying an "early warning" thought, feeling, and behavior to help you avoid "going off the tracks."
7. Developing a Model of Positive Sexuality.
8. Time Management schedule for structuring preferred health maintenance practices.
9. Creating a reinforcement schedule by which you reward yourself in a healthy and positive way for effective execution of your plan and practices.
10. Rating your level of satisfaction with the BIG WHEEL OF HEALTH satisfaction questionnaire at the beginning of your efforts (as a baseline measure) and after 3, 6, and 12 months of health practices. For those seeking to enhance their sexual health as well, you can rate your levels of satisfaction in the same way using the SHAWS Scale (Sexual Health and Well-being Satisfaction scale).

*This handout was prepared by Frederick L. Peterson, Jr., PsyD - Clinical Psychologist at the 88th Medical Readiness Operations Squadron, Wright-Patterson Air Force Base Medical Center

1. **Reflect upon and write out a <u>personal mission statement</u> regarding your sense of purpose:**

   Reflect on your values and what is most important to you in life. How would you describe your purpose or how you would prefer to be remembered as a person?

2. **<u>Identify your "bottom lines</u>" that you do not want to cross/be part of your healthy life.**

   Bottom Line #1:

   Bottom Line #2:

   Bottom Line #3:

3. **<u>Identify your triggers</u> for acting out, both emotional and situational triggers.**

   Emotional:

   Situational:

4. **List your <u>Inventory of Healthy Coping Behaviors</u>, both "Tried and True" as well as "Expanding the Toolbox."**

   Tried and True (healthy things that always make you feel better):

   Expanding the Toolbox (things you want to learn in order to help you live a healthy life):

5. Map your social support network and creating a <u>Personal Mission Support Team</u> from this social network.

Measure your social support system to evaluate how robust your network is:

Who do you have for a Personal Mission Support Team?

6. Create a <u>Prediction Relapse Scenario</u> identifying warning thoughts, feelings, and behaviors.

If you were to relapse today or this weekend, describe how it would most likely happen:

Identify any warning thoughts:

Identify warning feelings:

Identify warning behaviors:

7. Develop a <u>Model of Positive Sexuality</u> – How many of the following factors characterize your present life?

___ Having a sense of self-worth as a person.
___ Self-security with an internal loci of control so you do not feel you have to prove your personhood to self or others.
___ Acceptance and appreciation of a positive sexual self-image.
___ Commitment to the principles and practices of consensual sex.
___ Have the ability to avoid or recover from cyclic patterns of problematic sexual behavior (sex addiction/compulsivity).
___ Openness to learning how to be a good sexual partner devoted to your lover's erotic interests/arousal/satisfaction.
___ Positive practice of accepting and exercising self-pleasuring (including sexual self-interest, arousal, and climax).

___ Enhancing communication skills with your partner (and others) regarding sex.
___ Understanding the value for life-long learning regarding the unique aspects of positive sexuality for every stage of life.
___ Developing a personal perspective that views sex as another form of communication serving the overall goal of having a significant and emotionally meaningful connection with another person.

8. **Create a <u>Time Management Schedule</u> for structuring a preferred "recovery practice routine."**

   What health practices will you integrate into your daily and weekly schedule? Create the schedule on a separate page (you may likely need to eliminate some activities to create more time for health practices).

9. **Create a <u>Reinforcement Schedule</u> by which you reward yourself in a healthy and positive way for effective execution of your plan and practices.**

   Make your rewards meaningful and frequent (at least weekly reinforcement).

10. **<u>Rate your level of satisfaction</u> with the BIG WHEEL OF HEALTH satisfaction questionnaire (attached) at the beginning of your efforts (as a baseline measure) and after 1, 3, and 6 months of health practices.** For those seeking to enhance their sexual health as well, you can rate your levels of satisfaction in the same way using the SHAWS Scale (Sexual Health and Well-being Satisfaction Scale).

Use of Mobile Applications To Augment Psychotherapy*

Why Bring Mobile Apps Into the Therapy Session?

- Can help to make treatment more engaging for the patient
- Offers scientifically proven benefit to improvement
- Gains legitimacy in mainstream treatment practices
- Can increase homework compliance
- Covers down on limited treatment availability
- Allows for overcoming barriers to care
  - Stigma of conventional treatment
  - Web-based and mobile apps are anonymous
  - 24/7 access to care, 365 days a year

So how do I Introduce an App to my Patient?

- Assess the patient's use of smartphone technologies
- Describe the purpose of the app
- Have them download it in session and orientate them to the layout
- State expectations for frequency of use (as per treatment plan)
- Emphasize that use of an app is voluntary

Below are several apps and their descriptions.

Psych Drugs

Provides information on all psychotropic medications currently available (including indications, dosages, side effects).

Moodtrack Social Diary

Allows for periodic tracking of mood fluctuations. Can graph results and creates reports to send to providers.

CBT-i Coach

For patients with insomnia or general sleep difficulties. Offers guided imagery, breathing exercises, self-assessment, sleep diary, psychoeducation.

---

*This handout was prepared by Lorenzo E. Aranda, PsyD.

PTSD Coach

Assists those who are experiencing symptoms of PTSD by offering audio-guided meditations, muscle relaxations, breathing exercises, self-assessment of symptoms and graphing of assessment results, CBT exercises, psychoeducation.

Mindfulness Coach

For patients with no familiarity with the practice of mindfulness. Offers psychoeducation, audio mindfulness, meditations/body scans, logging of mindfulness sessions.

Breath2Relax

For patients with anxiety and PTSD. Offers step-by-step audio-guided diaphragmatic breathing exercises.

COVID Coach

Designed to help patients build resilience, manage stress, and increase well-being during the pandemic. Features mood tracker, audio meditations, and resource connection.

To download any of the above apps, visit:

https://www.ptsd.va.gov/appvid/mobile/

or the Apple Apps/Google Play stores

The Nitty-Gritty of Positivity! Sexual Self-Image Exercises*

The reason some individuals do not want to have sex is because of very negative feelings and beliefs about their bodies. Because much of our economy is based on consumerism, we are routinely exposed to advertised messages that reinforce the belief, "I am not good enough." Of course, the rest of the message is that by buying their product or service (such as cosmetic surgery – the list is virtually endless), we can be happy and more attractive to others. Within this type of environment, it is not surprising that so many people have a negative self-image, including poor sexual self-image.

The purpose of the sexual self-image exercise is to feel better, be more accepting, and more confident about your physical body. No matter what shape or level of fitness a person is in, everybody can make themselves feel better or worse emotionally based on what we tell ourselves about our physicality. Many people have a history of criticizing their body in regard to media-based images and standards of beauty. The negative practice of an internalized body-critic is not only unnecessary and unfortunate "BS" but damaging to a person's sense of well-being.

The following exercises are effective strategies you can employ to counter the effects of media-influenced self-criticism and highlight the positive aspects of your body; that is something to appreciate, including the beauty, strength, functionality, softness, and sensitivity of parts of your body often ignored. This is also an opportunity to appreciate the positive aspects of the parts of your body that you may have always cringed about and wished were different. In other words, it's all about how you see yourself and the messages you tell yourself.

There is only one way to do these exercises wrong, and that is to continue to criticize yourself. ***NO CRITICISM ALLOWED*** for the few minutes you are engaged in any of these activities. Even if it is something you always wished was different about you, find something nice to say! Your mission is to identify at least one positive attribute of every part of your body. Not only are you to identify the positive attribute, but you are asked to write down your descriptions for a full list of your body parts, head to toe. If you absolutely can no-way-no-how generate a positive quality or attribute to the body part, leave it blank and go on to the next part. ***NO CRITICISM***.

The list of positive attributes is simply a baseline for your self-image at the time you do it. Your list can then be used to measure your growth over time in self-appreciation and being kind to yourself. If you need to view yourself fully clothed or in your undies, then that's where you are and that's where you start. Be accepting of yourself for where you are. That does not mean that you can't want to lose weight or shape up. Just do it with kindness and appreciation of yourself!

Instructions

Self-Affirmation Sexual Self-Image Exercises

a. Use a room that is warm, well lit, and provides privacy.
b. Commit to no use of criticism for the duration of this exercise.
c. If you can, get naked in front of a large mirror that shows all or most of your body (when starting out, various degrees of undress are acceptable as well).

*This handout was prepared by Frederick L. Peterson, Jr., PsyD

d. Have a pen and paper next to you for recording your responses.
e. Go from the tip of your crown to the tip of your toes finding positive attributes about every part of your body that is visible to you.
f. Commenting on internal features of our anatomy (like your heart) is acceptable, but the emphasis is on your external features.
g. Record in detail your body features on a list and record to the right the positive attributes. To what level of detail, you wonder? Let's use your head as an example:

- Hair color
- Hair texture
- Hair style
- Hair line
- Hair on the face
- Eye color
- Eye shape
- Eyelashes
- Eyebrows
- Eyes' ability to see
- Nose size
- Nose shape
- Nose's ability to smell
- Ear shape
- Ear size
- Ear color
- Ears' ability to hear
- Teeth shape
- Teeth smile
- Teeth ability to eat
- Lips color
- Lips shape
- Lips smile
- Skin complexion
- Cheekbones
- Dimples?
- Chin

h. Go down the rest of your body with the same level of detail while recording what you can appreciate and using positive attributes only. If you have the fortitude, share your list with someone you can trust to affirm you for the positivity of your self-image. This could be a trusted spouse, lover, or therapist. Security tip – make sure you have your list password protected or in a place no one else will discover. Repeating this exercise at a later date (such as several months or several years) gives you the opportunity to compare your new list of attributes with your first list and measure the growth of your positivity regarding self-acceptance, sexual self-image, and your ability to find self-validation (all very important skills for health and well-being).

Self-Sharing
Sexual Self-Image Exercises

Ready to bump up the affirmation? If you have a trusted lover or spouse, repeat this exercise as a couple, and again – only positive comments are allowed! Create two lists – you finding the positive aspects of their body and your partner doing the same with you. ***AFFIRMATIONS ONLY!***

Get naked in front of that person and have them go from the tip of your crown to the tip of your toes identifying only positive aspects of your body. Doing this exercise as a shared exercise not only challenges you to higher levels of positive self-image but also builds trust and greater understanding of what your partner appreciates about your body. Again, it may be the part of you that you dislike the most, but now you may be surprised as to what positive qualities your partner comes up with about that very same thing.

Really want to get crazy with the sexual self-image affirmation? If you think the shared self-image experience is challenging with a person you know and trust – what about a room full of strangers? It happens all the time at self-image workshops around the planet. The objective is you being able to stand naked in front of the world and say, "Hello everybody, this is what a human being looks like and I'm pretty darn happy with me." Talk about positive self-image!

This last "global" version of the sexual self-image experience may not be your cup of tea, and that is perfectly all right. That's why there are so many varieties of tea! You are encouraged to complete the single-person version of enhancing your self-image at the very least to take another step forward in your sexual health. What do you have to lose (besides some self-negativity)?

The idea of this exercise is to give you a new path to more positive self-image. It is also designed to prompt you to apply what you have learned about sexual health and enhance your sexual comfort and confidence. This exercise gets you down to the nitty-gritty of positivity! Keep moving forward – it is all about progress, not perfection!

A Healthcare Professional's Guide to Contemporary Sexual Myths*

Sexual health is defined as the integration of the physical, emotional, intellectual, and social aspects of being sexual in ways that are positively enriching and that enhance personality, communication, and love (World Health Organization, 2000). Hence, sexual misinformation and myths interfere with the intellectual understanding of sexuality, which in turn can affect perceptions of self and others (emotional and social aspects) as well as risk for transmission of disease (physical aspects). In short, the perpetuation of sexual myths serves as a significant obstacle to achieving sexual health. The sexual myths are listed below as "red flags" for misconceptions that complicate sexual lives. This is not by any means a comprehensive list but rather a representative list of some of the most common myths. Review the list and evaluate if you have been (or currently are) influenced by any of them during your own sexual development. Ask yourself, "What impact have these sexual myths had upon my view of sexuality, physical attractiveness, sexual function, self-esteem, relationships, and how I communicate (or do not communicate) about sexual matters?"

Sexual Myths Regarding COVID-19

- You can't get COVID-19 from sex if you use a condom.
- You should not get the COVID-19 vaccine if you are trying to get pregnant.
- COVID-19 may impair people's sexual performance.
- COVID-19 cannot be sexually transmitted.
- The COVID-19 vaccine will threaten sperm or erectile function.
- COVID-19 will lead to infertility in both men and women.

Sexual Myths Regarding Age (Children and Seniors)

- The most potent myth of childhood sexuality is the idea of childhood nonsexuality: The myth that children do not have any interest in sex, or if they do, it is to be discouraged.
- The idea that kids are not sexual also leads to the common myth about sex education of children – talking to children about sex will "pollute" them by putting ideas in their heads.
- Children always tell the truth about sex.
- People have to be young and beautiful to be attractive to others and sexually happy.
- Aging itself will bring an end to sexual function (e.g., old age causes impotence).

Sexual Myths Regarding Cybersex, Virtual Sex, and Sexting

- Cybersex and/or virtual sex is only for the younger generations.
- The use of cybersex is only for heterosexual cisgender males.
- Cybersex will lead to an addiction to it or frequent masturbation.
- Virtual and online sexuality is for porn addicts and "creeps."
- Online sexual acts are always prone to "catfishing" (i.e., someone online is acting like someone who they are not).

---

*This handout was prepared by Eva Hernandez-Cuevas and Kayla Gallagher.

- Cybersex is only for long-distance relationships.
- Virtual sex is a last resort for dysfunctional relationships and to satisfy needs that are not met.
- Online sexual encounters cannot be romantic and are purely sexual.

Sexual Myths Regarding Polyamorous Relationships

- Polyamory is a mental illness or a personality disorder.
- Polyamory will lead to more sexually transmitted infections.
- Participating in polyamory is negative for children's development.
- Monogamous relationships are healthier than those that are polyamorous, and vice versa.
- Polyamory is just an excuse for couples to cheat on each other.
- Couples decide to be polyamorous or "open" just to have more sex.
- Polyamorous couples are just afraid of commitment.
- Polyamory will never work because human nature is jealous and competitive.
- Polyamorous couples are just interested in having orgies.
- Polyamorous individuals are never attached or emotionally committed to others.
- Polyamorous couples have lower relationship and sexual satisfaction.

Sexual Myths Regarding Sex Workers

- There is never a good or valid reason to choose to be a sex worker.
- All sex workers have childhood and/or sexual trauma to be able to choose their job.
- Sex work is easy money.
- Sex workers are uneducated and lack experience for other job opportunities.
- All sex workers are forced, coerced, and manipulated into their jobs.
- All sex workers are overly sexual (and are sexual fiends).
- Allowing and decriminalizing the sex working industry will lead to more human trafficking and manipulation towards the sex industry.
- Sex workers are dangerous to the general population and propagate the spread of STIs.
- Having sexual intercourse with a sex worker means that one is filthy or a sexual fiend.
- One cannot have a stable relationship with a sex worker.
- Sex workers do not have sexual needs outside their field.
- Sex workers have to be beautiful able-bodied cisgender heterosexual women.
- All sex workers are in shame and degraded because of their work.
- Sex workers give women a bad reputation.

Sexual Myths Regarding Asexuality

- Asexuals have no sexuality.
- Asexuality is a choice and is simply abstinence.
- Asexuality is a mental illness.
- Asexual individuals are anti-sex and all find sexuality repulsive.
- Asexual people simply have not found the right partner yet and have not been properly satisfied.
- Asexual individuals should not belong to the LGBTQ+ community.
- People who are asexual do not practice sexual acts, relationships, or intercourse.

Sexual Myths Regarding Anatomy and Physiology

- The size of sexual organs is related to a person's sexual satisfaction.
- The absence of the hymen (maidenhead) proves that a girl is not a virgin.
- Menopause or hysterectomy ends a women's sex drive and sex life.
- Each person has a designated number of sexual experiences (orgasms, ejaculations) and then they are used up; the person is no longer sexual.
- Only men have "wet dreams" and they are a sign of a sexual disorder.
- Masturbation results in physical and mental disorders.

Sexual Myths Regarding Sexual Performance

- Optimal health (as well as athletic performance) is achieved through sexual abstinence.
- Real men are to be the active lovemakers, "doing it" to passive women who tolerate it being "done to them." It is the man's role to initiate.
- If a good girl has to do it, then she should have the decency not to enjoy it.
- Men are "sexual experts" who impart their sex knowledge to pure and virginal brides.
- Honeymoons are times of great sexual satisfaction and release after long "waiting."
- Real men are supposed to have erections at the drop of a bra.
- Good women, God bless them, better fake it well – just smile and moan but never yell.
- To be true to your marriage in love and bliss, you are never to find another attractive enough to kiss.
- Marital sex is a delightful routine of the missionary position only after 9:00 p.m. in the master bedroom with the lights out resulting in mutual and simultaneous orgasms.
- Erections for men and climax for women are necessary for sexual satisfaction.

Sexual Myths Regarding Pregnancy and the Postpartum Period

- Women cannot conceive during their menstruation period.
- Women cannot get pregnant if the man withdraws before climax, or if the woman is on top.
- During pregnancy, the baby can get hurt from the probing penis or it may "break the bag" of amniotic fluid protecting the baby.
- Sex during pregnancy is unnatural and repulsive.
- Pregnancy changes the woman's body in ways that will make her unattractive.
- Natural childbirth doesn't hurt and anyone can do it.
- Breastfeeding is a "woman's thing" and there is no role the father plays.
- Breastfeeding is not as healthy as bottle feeding a baby.
- Breastfeeding mothers don't mind if their husbands "belly up to the bar."
- Resuming your sex life postpartum will be simple and anxiety free.
- Good parents never have thoughts about abusing their children.

Sexual Myths Regarding Sexually Transmitted Infections (STI)

- You can tell a person has an STI by their appearance.
- Just by chance, there is a low probability of getting an STI.
- An STI is a punishment for bad behavior more than a result of an infection.
- If a person does not have any symptoms of anything wrong, they don't have to worry.
- With all the medicines today, I can get treated and cured if I get an STI.
- Rubbers (condoms) don't really make a difference in protecting a person from STIs.
- People cannot get an STI if they don't have sex.

- There are no sexual activities that protect you from AIDS that are still satisfying.
- In general, men have more severe consequences of STIs than women do.
- By law, physicians have to report all cases of an STI to the public health authorities.

Sexual Myths Regarding Sex Offending (Rape, Child Molestation)

- Women want to be raped and "ask for it."
- Women are primarily raped by strangers.
- Women can always avoid being raped if they want to.
- Women "cry rape" for revenge.
- Rapists are always crazy (psychotic) or low-life sociopaths.
- Child sexual abuse is rare and only happens in poor families with uneducated parents.
- When child sexual abuse occurs, it usually gets reported and the child gets help.
- Child sexual abusers are usually strangers to the child.
- Child sexual abuse usually involves force and physical coercion.
- Child sexual abuse really doesn't hurt the child as there are no long-term effects.

Sexual Myths Regarding Same-Sex Attraction

- You either are or are not gay.
- Homosexuality (or heterosexuality for that matter) is a lifestyle choice.
- Feminine men HAVE to be gay and highly masculine men HAVE to be straight.
- Masculine women HAVE to be lesbians and highly feminine women HAVE to be straight.
- Gay people are out to recruit or turn heterosexuals gay.
- The LGBTQ+ community is more promiscuous and sexual than heterosexuals.
- The LGBTQ+ community is more prone to and are infected with STIs than heterosexuals.
- Homosexuality is only towards/for cisgender people and not transgender or nonbinary individuals.
- Homosexuality (and sexuality as a whole) is for the able-bodied, White, and cisgender community.
- Queer people are pedophiles that want to have sex with children.
- Transgender and nonbinary individuals will solely be with same-gendered people or attempt to be heterosexual.
- Same-sex activity is doing something unnatural and immediately means one is homosexual.
- A child conceived through rear-entry coitus will be homosexual.
- A child raised under same-sex parenting will be homosexual and/or queer.

Sexual Myths Regarding People with Varied Abilities

- People with disabilities are asexual, innocent, and childlike, or predatory.
- People with disabilities should only be sexual with other disabled individuals or they will have disabled offspring.
- Sexual problems experienced by people with disabilities are caused by their disability.
- If an able-bodied person has a sexual relationship with a person with a disability, it is because the nondisabled person cannot attract anyone else or is predatory.

Sexual Myths About Sex Therapy and Sexual Medicines

- Sex medicines give all men instant, sustained erections that do not subside after climax.
- Using a pill to resolve concerns about erections will make your sex life satisfying.
- It is safe to "try out" sex pills by borrowing some from a friend.

- Sex therapy involves being observed while having sex or having sex with a therapist.
- My physician, psychologist, or therapist received training in sex therapy while completing academic requirements and is comfortable discussing sex.

Sexual Myths About Masturbation

- Masturbation is abnormal and unhealthy.
- Masturbation is unnatural and it is not observed in animal behavior.
- Masturbation leads to illness or disability, such as blindness or insanity.
- Men have limited sperm, so don't waste them through masturbation.
- Men with available sex partners shouldn't want or need to masturbate.
- Masturbating is immature and should never be discussed with a partner.
- Young children do not masturbate and if they do, it is a sign of sex abuse.
- Elderly people do not masturbate because they lose interest in sex.
- The Bible condemns masturbation as the "sin of Onan."
- There is no room for masturbation in a "Christian marriage."
- Parents should be punitive towards children caught masturbating.
- Masturbating more than a couple times per week, and especially more than once per day, is always a sure sign of "sex addiction."

References

Abbas, A. M., Fathy, S. K., Khamees, A. A., Salem, A. S., & Ahmed, L. (2020). A focused review on the genital and sexual affection of COVID-19 patients. *Journal of Gynecology, Obstetrics and Human Reproduction, 49*(8), 101848. https://doi.org/10.1016/j.jogoh.2020.101848

Alpalhão, M., & Filipe, P. (2020). The impacts of isolation measures against SARS-CoV-2 infection on sexual health. *AIDS and behavior, 24*(8), 2258-2259. https://doi.org/10.1007/s10461-020-02853-x

Banerjee, D., & Rao, T. S. S. (2021). "#Intimacy" at Times of COVID-19: The renewed impetus behind cybersex. *Journal of Psychosexual Health, 3*(1), 13-17. https://doi.org/10.1177/26318318211004397

Conley, T. D., Moors, A. C., Ziegler, A., & Karathanasis, C. (2012). Unfaithful individuals are less likely to practice safer sex than openly nonmonogamous individuals. *The Journal of Sexual Medicine, 9*(6), 1559-1565.

Conley, T. D., Ziegler, A., Moors, A. C., Matsick, J. L., & Valentine, B. (2013). A critical examination of popular assumptions about the benefits and outcomes of monogamous relationships. *Personality and Social Psychology Review, 17*(2), 124-141.

Coy, M., Smiley, C., & Tyler, M. (2019). Challenging the "prostitution problem": Dissenting voices, sex buyers, and the myth of neutrality in prostitution research. *Archives of Sexual Behavior, 48*, 1931-1935. https://doi.org/10.1007/s10508-018-1381-6

Döring, N. (2020). How is the COVID-19 pandemic affecting our sexualities? An overview of the current media narratives and research hypotheses. *Archives of Sexual Behavior, 49*, 2765-2778. https://doi.org/10.1007/s10508-020-01790-z

Li, G., Tang, D., Song, B., Wang, C., Qunshan, S., Xu, C., . . . Cao, Y. (2020). Impact of the COVID-19 pandemic on partner relationships and sexual and reproductive health: Cross-sectional, online survey study. *Journal of Medical Internet Research, 22*(8), e20961. https://doi.org/10.2196/20961

Mumm, J., Vilsmaier, T., Schuetz, J. M., Rodler, S., Zehni, A. Z., Bauer, R. M., . . . Falk Batz, F. (2021). How the COVID-19 pandemic affects sexual behavior of hetero-, homo-, and bisexual males in Germany. *Sexual Medicine, 9*(4). https://doi.org/10.1016/j.esxm.2021.100380

Oliva-Farrell, D. (2018). Asexuality: To include or not to include a slice of cake in the LGBTQ+ community. *Tredway Library Prize for First-Year Research.* https://digitalcommons.augustana.edu/libraryprize/8

Purvis, A., Symons, E., Bruckert, C., & Chabot, F. (n.d.). Myths and facts. *Sex Work is Real Work.* https://www.sexworkisrealwork.com/myths-facts

Ross, M. W. (2005). Typing, doing, and being: Sexuality and the internet. *The Journal of Sex Research, 42*(4), 342-352. http://www.jstor.org/stable/3813787

Rubel, A. N., & Bogaert, A. F. (2015). Consensual nonmonogamy: Psychological well-being and relationship quality correlates. *The Journal of Sex Research, 52*(9), 961-982.

Sahoo, S., Padhy, S. K., Ipsita, J., Mehra, A., & Grover, S. (2020). Demystifying the myths about COVID-19 infection and its societal importance. *Asian journal of psychiatry, 54*, 102244.

Sheff, E. (2013). *The polyamorists next door: Inside multiple-partner relationships and families.* Rowman & Littlefield.

Studer, J., Marmet, S., Wicki, M., & Gmel, G. (2019). Cybersex use and problematic cybersex use among young Swiss men: Associations with sociodemographic, sexual, and psychological factors. *Journal of behavioral addictions, 8*(4), 794-803. https://doi.org/10.1556/2006.8.2019.69

Urban Justice Center/ Working Group on Sex Work and Human Rights. (n.d.). Sex worker myths vs reality. *Sex Workers Project.* https://sexworkersproject.org/media-toolkit/downloads/08-Myths.pdf

Weinstein, A. M., Zolek, R., Babkin, A., Cohen, K., & Lejoyeux, M. (2015). Factors predicting cybersex use and difficulties in forming intimate relationships among male and female users of cybersex. *Frontiers in Psychiatry, 6*(54). https://doi.org/10.3389/fpsyt.2015.00054
Willingham, E. (2021, August 24). Covid vaccines show no signs of harming fertility or sexual function. *Scientific American.* https://www.scientificamerican.com/article/covid-vaccines-show-no-signs-of-harming-fertility-or-sexual-function/
World Health Organization. (2000, May 19-22). *Promotion of sexual health: Recommendations for action.* Proceedings from a regional consultation convened by Pan American Health Organization and the World Health Organization in collaboration with the World Association for Sexology, Antigua, Guatemala. https://www.paho.org/hq/dmdocuments/2008/PromotionSexualHealth.pdf

Subject Index